Ruptured Abdominal Aortic Aneurysm

Benjamin W. Starnes • Manish Mehta
Frank J. Veith
Editors

Ruptured Abdominal Aortic Aneurysm

The Definitive Manual

Springer

Editors
Benjamin W. Starnes
Harborview Medical Center
University of Washington
Seattle, WA
USA

Frank J. Veith
Bronx, NY
USA

Manish Mehta
Albany Medical Center
Albany, NY
USA

ISBN 978-3-319-23843-2 ISBN 978-3-319-23844-9 (eBook)
DOI 10.1007/978-3-319-23844-9

Library of Congress Control Number: 2016963217

Printed on acid-free paper

This Springer imprint is published by Springer Nature
The registered company is Springer International Publishing AG
The registered company address is Gewerbestrasse 11, 6330 Cham, Switzerland

Foreword

The editors—Benjamin Starnes, Manish Mehta, and Frank Veith—are to be congratulated on their contemporary manual on the management of ruptured abdominal aortic aneurysms. This brand-new textbook is the first of its kind to address rupture exclusively, and the result is a truly exceptional educational reference for aortic surgeons.

Rupture remains a life-threatening complication of aortic disease. Aortic rupture may occur in a previously unrepaired section from a de novo aneurysm or as a late complication of prior repair in patients who are known to have aortic disease and are participating in a surveillance protocol to monitor aortic dimensions. In patients with undiagnosed aortic disease, aortic rupture is an unexpected complication—delay related to the inability to establish diagnosis or for other reasons further increases the risk of death. In consideration of the challenge that repair poses in patients who present with aortic rupture, the editors of this manual have presented a thorough review of operative strategies for the treatment of rupture, including the entire range of open and endovascular approaches and the use of protective techniques such as hypotensive hemostasis. Additionally, the editors have tackled the equally critical aspects of clinical presentation and diagnostics, which are necessary for reducing the misdiagnosis of ruptured abdominal aortic aneurysms.

I began my surgical career under the tutelage of the late E.S. Crawford at a time in which rupture of an aortic aneurysm portended devastating consequences. Today, despite the advent of itemized improvements in operative techniques and the use of surgical adjuncts, mortality rates associated with acute rupture of the abdominal aorta remain high. Collaborative efforts such as this text are critical if we wish to reduce these rates, and the editors' and authors' devotion to this goal is made evident by their inclusion of several chapters dedicated to tackling postoperative complications after rupture, postoperative ICU management, and improved quality of life. The manual's focus on rupture is additionally beneficial because bringing more attention to this life-threatening condition may improve patient adherence to surveillance imaging protocols, thereby reducing the risk of rupture in future patient populations.

In conclusion, this manual provides a comprehensive overview of the clinical presentation and management of rupture, providing aortic surgeons a convenient resource to consult. Drs. Starnes, Mehta, and Veith are to be applauded for their efforts in compiling this exhaustive body of work. This guide represents a substantial step forward in our collective understanding of ruptured abdominal aortic aneurysms.

Joseph S. Coselli, MD
Cullen Foundation Endowed Chair
Chief, Division of Cardiothoracic Surgery
Michael E. DeBakey Department of Surgery
Baylor College of Medicine
Chief, Adult Cardiac Surgery
Texas Heart Institute

Contents

List of Contributors

Shahram Aarabi, MD Fellow Division of Vascular Surgery, Department of Surgery, University of Washington, Seattle, WA, USA

Zachary M. Arthurs, MD, RPVI, FACS Department of Vascular Surgery, San Antonio Military Medical Center, San Antonio, TX, USA

S. Bahia St. Georges University Hospitals NHS Trust, St. Georges University of London, London, UK

R. A. Benson Department of Vascular Surgery, University Hospitals Coventry and Warwickshire NHS Trust, Coventry, UK

Todd L. Berland, MD Division of Vascular Surgery, New York University Langone Medical Center, New York, NY, USA

Sanjeev Bhalla, MD Mallinckrodt Institute of Radiology, Washington University School of Medicine, St. Louis, MO, USA

Martin Björck Department of Surgical Sciences, Section of Vascular Surgery, Uppsala University, Uppsala, Sweden

James Budge St George's Vascular Institute, St George's Hospital, London, UK

Marlin Wayne Causey, MD University of California-San Francisco, San Francisco, CA, USA

Neal Cayne, MD Division of Vascular Surgery, New York University Langone Medical Center, New York, NY, USA

Joseph Cuschieri Department of Surgery, University of Washington, Seattle, WA, USA

Ron Dalman, MD Stanford Vascular Surgery, Stanford, CA, USA

Sira M. Duson, MD MedStar Health Vascular Surgery, MedStar Vascular Program, Department of Vascular Surgery, Georgetown University, Washington, DC, USA,

Matthew J. Eagleton, MD Department of Vascular Surgery, H32, Cleveland Clinic Lerner College of Medicine-CWRU, Cleveland, OH, USA

Jay P. Heiken, MD Mallinckrodt Institute of Radiology, Washington University School of Medicine, St. Louis, MO, USA

R. J. Hinchliffe Bristol Centre for Surgical Research, University of Bristol, Bristol, UK

Kim J. Hodgson, MD Division of Vascular Surgery, Southern Illinois University School of Medicine, Springfield, IL, USA

Andrew Holden, MBChB Department of Interventional Radiology, Auckland Hospital, Auckland, New Zealand

Benjamin M. Jackson, MD University Of Pennsylvania, Philadelphia, PA, USA

Kaj H. Johansen, MD, PhD, FACS Vascular Surgery, Swedish Medical Center, University of Washington School of Medicine, Seattle, WA, USA

Kevin Kniery, MD Department of Surgery, Division of Colorectal Surgery, Madigan Army Medical Center, Tacoma/Fort Lewis, WA, USA

Bernard Krüger Vascular Surgery Unit, University of Palermo, University Hospital 'P. Giaccone', Palermo, Italy

John Kuckelman, DO Department of Surgery, Madigan Army Medical Center, Tacoma, WA, USA

Mario Lachat, MD Division of Cardiovascular Surgery, University Hospital of Zurich, Zurich, Switzerland

I. M. Loftus St Georges University Hospitals NHS Trust, St Georges University of London, London, UK

Sean P. Lyden, MD Department of Vascular Surgery, The Cleveland Clinic Foundation, Cleveland, OH, USA

Samuel P. Mandell, MD, MPH Department of Surgery, University of Washington, Harborview Medical Center, Seattle, WA, USA

Matthew J. Martin, MD, FACS Department of Surgery, Madigan Army Medical Center, Tacoma, WA, USA

Surbhi Mathur, MD Department of Surgery, University of Washington, Seattle, WA, USA

Dieter Mayer, MD The Division of Vascular Surgery, University Hospital of Zurich, Zurich, Switzerland

Manish Mehta, MD, MPH Division of Vascular Surgery, Albany Medical College, Albany, NY, USA

Vascular Health Partners, CCP, Gloversville, NY, USA

Matthew Mell, MD, MS Division of Vascular Surgery, Stanford University School of Medicine, Stanford, CA, USA

Vincent M. Mellnick, MD Mallinckrodt Institute of Radiology, Washington University School of Medicine, St. Louis, MO, USA

Khanjan H. Nagarsheth, MD, MBA Division of Vascular Surgery, Rutgers – Robert Wood Johnson Medical School, New Brunswick, NJ, USA

Koichiro Nandate Department of Anesthesiology and Pain Medicine, University of Washington, Seattle, WA, USA

Derek P. Nathan, MD University of Washington, Seattle, WA, USA

Deepika Nehra, MD Department of Surgery, Harborview Medical Center, Seattle, WA, USA

Alexander Niven, MD Department of Internal Medicine, Madigan Army Medical Center, Tacoma, WA, USA

Hernando Olivar Department of Anesthesiology and Pain Medicine, University of Washington, Seattle, WA, USA

James Pan, MD Division of Vascular Surgery, Southern Illinois University School of Medicine, Springfield, IL, USA

Benjamin Patterson St George's Vascular Institute, St George's Hospital, London, UK

Philip S. K. Paty, MD Surgery, Albany Medical College, Albany, NY, USA

Felice Pecoraro Clinic for Cardiovascular Surgery, University Hospital, Zurich, Switzerland

Institute for Cardiovascular Anesthesia, University Hospital, Zurich, Switzerland

Elina Quiroga, MD, FACS Division of Vascular Surgery, Department of Surgery, University of Washington, Seattle, WA, USA

Saum A. Rahimi, MD, FACS Division of Vascular Surgery, Rutgers – Robert Wood Johnson Medical School, New Brunswick, NJ, USA

Zoran Rancic Clinic for Cardiovascular Surgery, University Hospital, Zurich, Switzerland

Constantine A. Raptis, MD Mallinckrodt Institute of Radiology, Washington University School of Medicine, St. Louis, MO, USA

William P. Robinson, MD Division of Vascular and Endovascular Surgery, University of Virginia School of Medicine, Charlottesville, VA, USA

Anthony M. Roche Department of Anesthesiology and Pain Medicine, University of Washington, Seattle, WA, USA

Caron B. Rockman, MD Divisions of Vascular Surgery, New York University Medical Center, New York, NY, USA

Divisions of Vascular Surgery, The Cleveland Clinic, Cleveland, OH, USA

Sean P. Roddy, MD Albany Medical College/Albany Medical Center Hospital, Albany, NY, USA

April Rodriguez, MD Division of Vascular Surgery, Department of Surgery, University of Washington, Seattle, WA, USA

Jarrad Rowse, MD Department of Vascular Surgery, H32, Cleveland Clinic Lerner College of Medicine-CWRU, Cleveland, OH, USA

Andres Schanzer, MD University of Massachusetts Medical School, Worcester, MA, USA

Marc L. Schermerhorn, MD, FACS Department of Surgery, Division of Vascular Surgery, Beth Israel Deaconess Medical Center, Boston, MA, USA

Jessica P. Simons, MD, MPH University of Massachusetts Medical School, Worcester, MA, USA

Niten Singh, MD University of Washington, Seattle, WA, USA

Peter A. Soden, MD Department of Surgery, Division of Vascular Surgery, Beth Israel Deaconess Medical Center, Boston, MA, USA

Benjamin W. Starnes, MD Division of Vascular Surgery, Department of Surgery, Regional Vascular Center at Harborview Medical Center, University of Washington, Seattle, WA, USA

Scott R. Steele, MD Department of Surgery, Division of Colorectal Surgery, Madigan Army Medical Center, Tacoma/Fort Lewis, WA, USA

Johnny Steuer Clinic for Cardiovascular Surgery, University Hospital, Zurich, Switzerland

Department of Surgery, Section for Vascular Surgery, South Hospital, Stockholm, Sweden

Matt Thompson St George's Vascular Institute, St George's Hospital, London, UK

Nam T. Tran, MD University of Washington, Seattle, WA, USA

Frank J. Veith Clinic for Cardiovascular Surgery, University Hospital, Zurich, Switzerland

Divisions of Vascular Surgery, New York University Langone Medical Center, New York, NY, USA

Divisions of Vascular Surgery, The Cleveland Clinic, Cleveland, OH, USA

Anders Wanhainen Department of Surgical Sciences, Section of Vascular Surgery, Uppsala University, Uppsala, Sweden

Edward Y. Woo, MD MedStar Health Vascular Surgery, MedStar Vascular Program, Department of Vascular Surgery, Georgetown University, Washington, DC, USA

Chapter 1
Historical Perspective on the Treatment of Ruptured Abdominal Aortic Aneurysms

Frank J. Veith

When an abdominal aortic aneurysm (AAA) ruptures and is not repaired or excluded from the circulation, the patient almost always dies – although the time course of his or her demise may vary considerably. Because of the lethal nature of ruptured AAAs, surgeons have attempted to repair them as soon as the diagnosis of rupture is made or even suspected. The first successful open surgical repairs of a ruptured RAAA were reported in 1954 using transperitoneal approaches [1–3]. These early reports by pioneering giants in the field make for fascinating reading.

Thereafter open surgical repair was widely accepted as the treatment of choice for this lethal condition [4]. However, intraoperative and postoperative mortality remained high, in the 55–41 % range, even in the hands of experienced vascular surgeons [5]. The reasons for this were many. Patients with ruptured AAAs were often profoundly hypotensive by the time the diagnosis of rupture was made. Often this delay was exacerbated by the tendency of ruptured abdominal aneurysms to masquerade as other diagnoses, particularly a ureteral stone, diverticulitis, myocardial infarction, or other conditions causing acute abdominal or back pain [6, 7]. In addition, patients with ruptured aneurysms are usually elderly with many comorbidities that can complicate a major intra- or retroperitoneal procedure in an already hypovolemic patient. The possibility of major organ or other vascular injuries, especially of large adjacent veins, during a hasty open repair in a surgical field obscured by hemorrhage further adds to the excessive risk of morbidity and mortality from open repair of ruptured AAAs. These risks are further enhanced by the chances that these emergent procedures must often be undertaken by surgeons less experienced in major vascular procedures and by the frequent development of hypothermia in this setting. For all these reasons, the mortality of open repair of ruptured AAAs has

F.J. Veith, MD
New York University – Langone Medical Center, New York, NY, USA

Cleveland Clinic, Cleveland, OH, USA
e-mail: fjvmd@msn.com

B.W. Starnes et al. (eds.), *Ruptured Abdominal Aortic Aneurysm*,
DOI 10.1007/978-3-319-23844-9_1

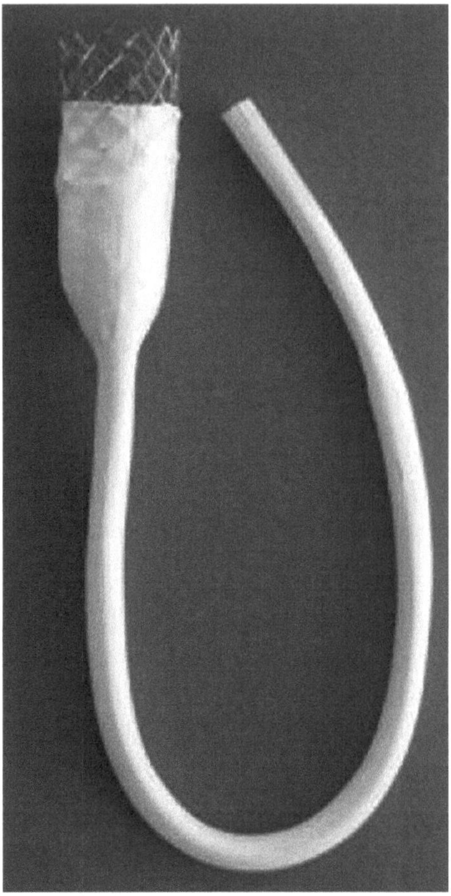

Fig. 1.1 A surgeon-made aortic stent graft consisting of a large Palmaz stent which was sutured to a tulip-shaped PTFE graft. The superior proximal half of the stent was bare and the inferior distal half was covered with the graft. Grafts like this aorto-uni-femoral (AUF) graft were used to treat many ruptured AAAs in our early experience

remained high despite strategic and technical attempts to improve outcomes with earlier operation, supraceliac aortic clamping, minimizing dissection by working within the opened AAA sac as soon as proximal aortic control was obtained [4–8].

The introduction of endovascular aneurysm repair or EVAR in 1991 [9] presented an opportunity to overcome many of these problems by using an intraluminal approach to excluding the ruptured AAA by introducing an endograft from a remote site in the femoral artery and guiding it into position fluoroscopically using local or much lighter anesthesia than that required by an intra-abdominal procedure. However, the feasibility of using EVAR to treat ruptured AAAs was limited by the emergent nature of these procedures and the fact that time would be required to make the measurements and obtain the grafts that would be required.

Our group was fortunate to have an available surgeon-made endovascular graft consisting of a large proximal balloon expandable Palmaz stent sutured to a tulip-shaped PTFE graft which could be prepared, sterilized, and stocked in the operating room (Fig. 1.1) [10]. This aorto-uni-femoral (AUF) graft could be used to treat

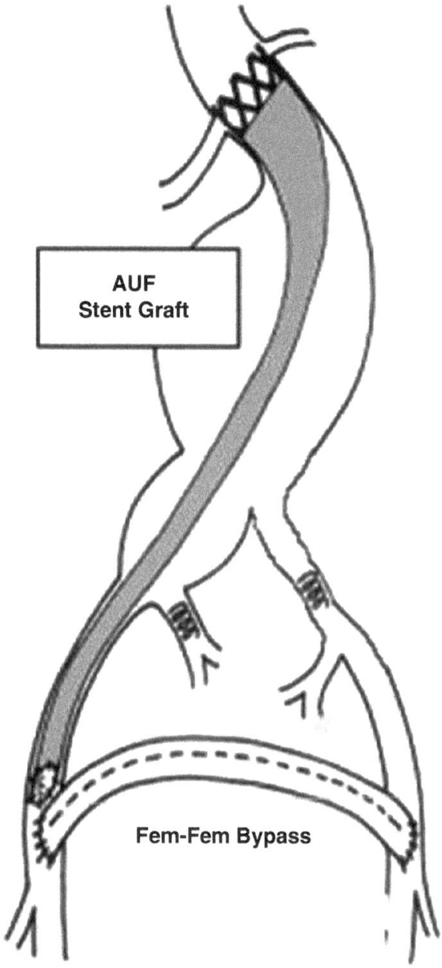

Fig. 1.2 This shows diagrammatically how this stent graft was positioned just below the renal arteries and extending to the ipsilateral (*right*) common femoral artery where an endovascular anastomosis was performed. The procedure was completed by placing an occluder in the contralateral (*left*) common iliac artery and performing a femoro-femoral (fem-fem) bypass. If an ipsilateral common iliac aneurysm was present, the hypogastric artery was occluded by placement of coils

AAAs with proximal necks from 20 to 27 mm because the balloon on which the graft was mounted was partly distensible. Moreover the graft's excessive length could be trimmed to just end within the femoral artery at the device's insertion site so an endovascular graft-to-host artery anastomosis could be performed. The AAA exclusion was then completed by insertion of an occluder in the contralateral common iliac artery and performance of a femoro-femoral crossover graft (Fig. 1.2). Subsequently as modular aortic stent grafts became available for use in EVAR and stocks of components could be kept in the operating room for use in emergency situations like ruptured AAAs, these grafts were used preferentially by our and other groups.

Because wc had this graft available for emergent use, we were able to perform the first EVAR for a ruptured AAA on April 21, 1994, on a patient who was hypotensive and categorically unsuitable for an open repair for anatomical and systemic reasons [10]. The rupture was sealed and the patient survived for more than 3 years after which he died from his medical comorbidities. Another ruptured AAA patient, successfully treated by EVAR at a later date than our patient, was reported in 1994 by Yusuf, Hopkinson, and their colleagues [11].

Thereafter in 1994 and 1995, we performed EVAR treatment on 11 other ruptured AAA patients who were prohibitive risks for an open repair. The leaking AAA was excluded in all 12 patients, and ten survived over 2 months despite serious comorbidities. This prompted us to hypothesize that EVAR would be the preferential treatment for all ruptured AAA patients with suitable anatomy [12, 13]. This hypothesis was also supported by the intuitive superiority of EVAR over open repair. EVAR would minimize dissection and the need for deep anesthesia; it would also reduce blood loss and avoid hypothermia, coagulopathy, and large vein injury. On the other hand, EVAR would require special equipment and skills and had the potential to delay aortic control and repair of the AAA. However, it turned out that this latter potential problem could be offset in most (~75 %) cases by strictly restricting fluid resuscitation and inducing the patient's arterial blood pressure to fall (hypotensive hemostasis) until endograft exclusion of the rupture site was obtained [7, 12–15]. Adequate circulation for short periods was deemed acceptable if the patient was moving and talking even if he or she was profoundly hypotensive. In addition, when hypotensive hemostasis failed and circulatory collapse occurred (arterial pressure <50 mm Hg), supraceliac aortic control could be achieved with appropriate rapid placement, over a previously placed guidewire, of a large hemostatic sheath and a large compliant balloon. The technique of balloon placement and use is complex, but is well described in a recent article [16] and in other chapters in this text.

Between 1994 and 2009, our group treated 57 consecutive patients with ruptured AAAs using EVAR whenever the anatomy was suitable even if the patient was in profound shock [14]. The determination of anatomic suitability was often made on the basis of an intraoperative catheter arteriogram if the patient was unstable or severely hypotensive, but was sometimes made on the basis of a contrast computerized tomographic scan if one could be obtained rapidly. EVAR was performed on 45 of the 57 patients, while open repair was required in 12 patients. Only seven of these 57 patients died within 30 days of their procedure, giving a surprisingly low periprocedural mortality of 12 %. Only 13 or 23 % of these 57 patients required balloon aortic control for circulatory collapse, and several required open abdomen treatment for abdominal compartment syndrome [14, 15].

We concluded from this and other similar collected experience from 12 other centers which also performed EVAR to treat ruptured AAAs, whenever it was feasible, that EVAR was a better way to treat these patients than open repair. This conclusion was based on superior 30-day mortality rates from these 13 preferential EVAR centers of 19.7 % after EVAR and 36.3 % after open repair. This conclusion was reinforced by the ~12 % of ruptured AAA patients who were prohibitive risks for open repair but who could be treated successfully by EVAR [14].

However, there were several groups who disagreed with this conclusion mostly on the basis of single-center or registry controlled trials showing no mortality benefit from EVAR compared to open repair for ruptured AAA treatment. These groups believed that the good results reported for EVAR were based on case selection rather than EVAR superiority, while we believed that the good EVAR results were based on the strategies, techniques, and adjuncts for performing EVAR [14, 15].

Nevertheless it is fair to say that EVAR remains controversial in this setting, and randomized controlled trials (RCTs) have been demanded by many. Three such RCTs have recently been completed and their results published [17–19]. All three of these RCTs concluded that there was no mortality benefit from EVAR when compared to open repair for ruptured AAAs. As discussed in Chapter XX and a recent article [20], it is our belief that all three of these trials were flawed in various ways and that these RCTs were either inconclusive or reached a conclusion that was misleading.

Two other recent studies support the superiority of EVAR for ruptured AAA treatment. In one study from two institutions, one in Zurich Switzerland and one in Orebro Sweden, of 70 ruptured AAAs seen in a 2-year period, only three patients were turned down for reparative treatment, and all the rest were treated by EVAR – although 24 % required a chimney graft or other adjunct. The 30-day mortality for these 70 patients was only 24 % [21]. In the other study, surgeon-modified fenestrated grafts were used to treat RAAAs on an emergent basis with excellent results [22].

It therefore appears likely that EVAR will gain increasing acceptance for the treatment of ruptured AAAs. In addition, as skills, equipment and technology improve. It is also likely that an increasing proportion of ruptured AAAs will be amenable to endovascular treatment. Improved patient outcomes will be the likely result.

References

1. Cooley DA, DeBakey ME. Ruptured aneurysms of abdominal aorta: excision and homograft replacement. Postgrad Med. 1954;16:334–42.
2. Gerbode F. Ruptured aortic aneurysm: a surgical emergency. Surg Gynec Obst. 1954;98: 759–64.
3. Javid H, Dye WS, Grove WJ, Julien OC. Resection of ruptured aneurysms of the abdominal aorta. Ann Surg. 1995;142:613–21.
4. Lawrie GM, Crawford ES, Morris GC, Howell JF. Progress in the treatment of ruptured abdominal aortic aneurysms. World J Surg. 1980;4:653–60.
5. Bown MJ, Sutton AJ, Bell PRF, Sayers RD. A meta-analysis of 50 years of ruptured abdominal aortic repair. Brit J Surg. 2002;89:714–30.
6. Veith FJ. Emergency abdominal aortic aneurysm surgery. Compr Ther. 1992;18:25–9.
7. Veith FJ, Cayne NS, Berland TL, Mayer D, Lachat M. Open surgical and endovascular management of ruptured abdominal aortic aneurysms. Chapter 41. In: Moore WS, editor. Vascular and endovascular surgery: a comprehensive review. 8th ed. Philadelphia: Elsevier/Saunders; 2013. p. 685–90.
8. Veith FJ, Gupta S, Daly V. Technique of occluding the supraceliac aorta through the abdomen. Surg Gynec Obstet. 1980;151:648–50.

9. Parodi JC, Palmaz JC, Barone HD. Transfemoral intraluminal graft implantation for abdominal aortic aneurysms. Ann Vasc Surg. 1991;5:491–9.
10. Marin ML, Veith FJ, Cynamon J, et al. Initial experience with transluminally placed endovascular grafts for the treatment of complex vascular lesions. Ann Surg. 1995;222:449–65.
11. Yusuf SW, Whitaker SC, Chuter TA, Wenham PW, Hopkinson BR. Emergency endovascular repair of leaking aortic aneurysms. Lancet. 1994;344:1645.
12. Ohki T, Veith FJ, Sanchez LA, et al. Endovascular graft repair of ruptured aorto-iliac aneurysms. J Am Coll Surg. 1999;189:102–23.
13. Veith FJ, Ohki T. Endovascular approaches to ruptured infrarenal aorto-iliac aneurysms. J Cardiovasc Surg. 2002;43:369–78.
14. Veith FJ, Lachat M, Mayer D, Malina M, Holst J, Mehta M, Verhoeven ELG, Larzon T, et al. Collected world and single center experience with endovascular treatment of ruptured abdominal aortic aneurysms. Ann Surg. 2009;250:818–24.
15. Lachat M, Mayer D, Labler L, et al. Abdominal compartment syndrome following ruptured AAA. In: Becquemin JP, Alimi YS, editors. Controversies and updates in vascular surgery. Turin: Minerva Medica; 2006. p. 103–07.
16. Berland TL, Veith FJ, Cayne NS, Mehta M, Mayer D, Lachat M. Technique of supraceliac balloon control of the aorta during endovascular repair of ruptured abdominal aortic aneurysms. J Vasc Surg. 2013;57:272–5.
17. IMPROVE Trial Investigators, Powell JT, Sweeting MJ, Thompson MM, Ashleigh R, Bell R, Gomes M, Greenhalgh RM, et al. Endovascular or open repair strategy for ruptured abdominal aortic aneurysm: 30 day outcomes from IMPROVE randomised trial. BMJ. 2014;348:f7661.
18. Reimerink JJ, Hoornweg LL, Vahl AC, Wisselink W, van den Broek TA, Legemate DA, Reekers JA, Balm R. Endovascular repair versus open repair of ruptured abdominal aortic aneurysms: a multicenter randomized controlled trial. Ann Surg. 2013;258:248–56.
19. Desgranges P, Kobeiter H, Katsahian S, Boufi M, Gouny P, Favre J-P. ECAR (Endovasculaire vs. Chirurgie dans les Anevrysmes Rompus): a French Randomized Controlled Trial of endovascular vs. open surgical repair of ruptured aorto-iliac aneurysms. Eur J Vasc Endovasc Surg. 2015;50:303–10.
20. Veith FJ, Rockman CB. The recent randomized trials of EVAR versus open repair for ruptured abdominal aortic aneurysms are misleading. Vascular. 2015;23:217–9.
21. Mayer D, Aeschbacher S, Pfammatter T, Veith FJ, Norgren L, Magnuson A, Rancic Z, Lachat M, Hörer T, Skoog P, Larzon T. Complete replacement of open repair for ruptured abdominal aortic aneurysms by endovascular aneurysm repair: a two-center 14-year experience. Ann Surg. 2012;256:688–95.
22. Starnes BW. Physician-modified endovascular grafts for the treatment of elective, symptomatic, or ruptured juxtarenal aortic aneurysms. J Vasc Surg. 2012;56:601–7.

Chapter 2
Background Scope of the Problem

Nam T. Tran

Aneurysm of the abdominal aorta is very often diagnosed when not present, and when present, the symptoms may be so obscure that the nature of the trouble is overlooked.

Sir William Osler, 1905

Abdominal aortic aneurysm (AAA) is a commonly found disease affecting approximately 7–9 % of the population over the age of 65 years with higher prevalence in those that are smokers [1]. It is a lethal disease with those presenting with ruptured AAAs having an overall mortality of over 90 %. Annually, ruptured AAA accounts for approximately 15,000 deaths in the United States, and it is the 15th leading cause of death. Unfortunately, the first clinical presentation of an AAA is when it ruptured [2]. The classic triad of abdominal pain, pulsatile abdominal mass, and hypotension is presented in only 25–50 % of patients, and many patients with ruptured AAA are misdiagnosed [3, 4]. In recent years, endovascular therapy has advanced and is now the first-line treatment of ruptured AAA. Endovascular aneurysm repair for ruptured AAA has led to reduce mortality with centers of excellence reporting 30-day mortality as low as 25 % with an endovascular first approach and formalized treatment protocols [5, 6]. As such, the rapid recognition and diagnose of a ruptured AAA is critical so that the patient can be appropriately triaged and offered definitive lifesaving therapy.

Epidemiology

Overall, the incidence of AAA has been increasing in the last two decades, likely secondary to improvement in diagnostic imaging, the aging population, better screening program, and the number of male smokers [7]. The Aneurysm Detection and Management (ADAM) Trial examined a defined demographics classified as

N.T. Tran, MD
University of Washington, Seattle, WA, USA
e-mail: nam@uw.edu

B.W. Starnes et al. (eds.), *Ruptured Abdominal Aortic Aneurysm*,
DOI 10.1007/978-3-319-23844-9_2

"high risk," namely, those adult male patients over the age of 65 years at various VA medical centers across the United States. In this study, the overall prevalence of those with aortic diameter of 3.0 cm or more was 4.6 % with AAAs greater than 4.0 cm detected in 1.4 % of study subject. Furthermore, smoking was most strongly associated with large AAAs with odd ratio of 5.57. In particular, 78 % of those AAAs that are 4.0 cm or larger were associated with smoking. On the other hand, female sex, diabetes, and African Americans were negatively associated with AAA [1].

As stated, ruptured AAA was the 15th leading cause of death accounting for approximately 15,000 deaths annually in the United States [8]. Most recently, advances in surgical management, namely, endovascular ruptured AAA repair, have reduced this mortality to just under 10,000 deaths per year in 2013 [9]. Ruptured AAA patients have the highest chance of survival if prompt treatment is delivered by a specialized team with high caseload of AAA surgery [10–12]. Consequently, if a patient with a ruptured AAA is not diagnosed promptly at the initial clinical encounter, appropriate triage and transfer to centers of excellence can be delayed and can adversely affect clinical outcome thus resulting in higher mortality. Moving forward, surgical mortality of ruptured AAA can be lowered further with centralized care at regional vascular centers where higher volume has been shown to improve overall survival [13].

Clearly, the rapid diagnose of a patient who presents with a ruptured AAA is critical to ensure access to the best possible surgical care. Screening guidelines proposed in 2005 by the US Preventive Services Task Force have not lead to significant reduction in annual incidence of ruptured AAA [14]. Even with advances in medical imaging, the rate of misdiagnosis of a ruptured AAA has been reported as high as 42 %. The classic triad of ruptured AAA of abdominal pain, hypotension, and pulsatile abdominal mass is usually present in only 42–61 % of cases. Rate of misdiagnosis is as equally high. There is no "typical" presenting symptom that the clinician can count on when it comes to the presentation of ruptured AAA. A recent meta-analysis of over 700 patients showed that other commonly presenting symptoms consist of back/flank pain, syncope, and nausea or vomiting [15] (Fig. 2.1).

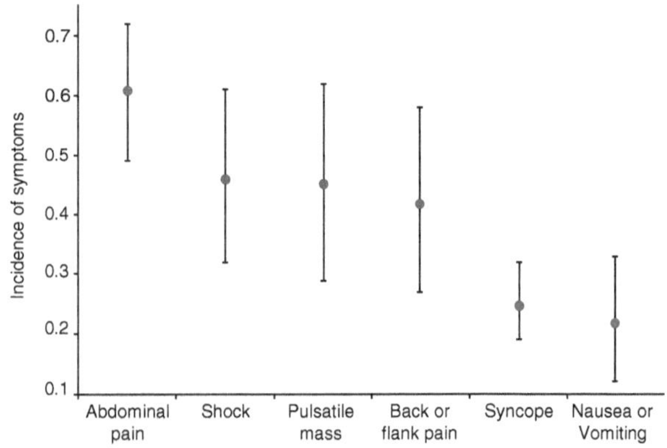

Fig. 2.1 Common presenting clinical symptoms of ruptured AAA (From Azhar et al. [15])

Thus, accurate and timely diagnosis can be elusive and the initial diagnosis of these patients varied greatly. In a pooled series of over 900 patients with ruptured AAA, the initial diagnosis was listed as renal colic in 6 %, myocardial infarction in 6 %, colonic inflammation in 3 %, gastrointestinal pathologies such as perforation/obstruction in 3 %, and unknown diagnosis in 12 % [4].

Clinical Presentations and Sites of Ruptured AAA

In order to better understand and diagnose ruptured AAA, one needs to understand the pathophysiology of ruptured AAA, specifically the sites of ruptured. Commonly, the AAA will rupture and bleed into either the retroperitoneal space posteriorly or into the peritoneal cavity anteriorly. In rare instances, the AAA can erode or rupture into adjacent structures such as abdominal veins (inferior vena cava or left renal) or gastrointestinal track such as the duodenum. These different scenarios offer distinct clinical presentations that a clinician must astutely recognize in order to rapidly arrive at the correct initial diagnosis of a ruptured AAA.

Anterior Intraperitoneal Rupture

It is estimated that an AAA will ruptured freely anteriorly into the intraperitoneal cavity in about 20 % of cases. Usually, this will manifest as sudden severe abdominal or back pain with cardiovascular collapse. Often, the clinical picture is that of a patient found down with hypotension and a distended abdomen. Intraperitoneal rupture will result in rapid exsanguination into the peritoneal cavity as it is a large space without the potential of localized tamponade. In the majority of cases, the patient expired prior to reaching medical care [3]. For those that are fortunate enough to reach medical care, rapid and effective aortic control is the patient's only chance of survival. The use of aortic occlusion balloon has shown great promises as a method of aortic control, even in the emergency department resuscitation bay so that the patient can undergo definitive surgical treatment [16].

Posterior Retroperitoneal Rupture

In the remaining 80 % of cases, the ruptured AAA is directed toward the retroperitoneal space, usually in the lateral posterior direction. In this classic presentation, the patient often experienced transient hypotension due to bleeding into the retroperitoneal space. Subsequent to the initial bleed, the localized effect of the retroperitoneal hematoma will temporarily tamponade and halt the hemorrhage. Typically, back/flank pain, transient hypotension, and syncope are the presenting symptoms.

In the thin patient, the clinician can often palpate a pulsatile abdominal mass. The presence of blood in the retroperitoneal space can also lead to other uncommon clinical presentations such as groin pain, testicular pain, testicular or flank ecchymosis, iliofemoral DVT, or nephrolithiasis [3].

Chronic Contained Rupture AAA

Despite the acute nature of ruptured AAA often leading to death within hours of presentation, a small subset of patients (4 %) can present with a chronic contained ruptured AAA. These patients typically have chronic back pain with radiation to the groin region. Other reporting symptoms can include lower limb weakness/neuropathy, lumbar vertebral erosion, and even obstructive jaundice [17]. In these patients, a high level of vigilance is required to make the correct diagnosis and offer the patient the appropriate surgical therapy.

Aortocaval Fistula

In rare instances, the abdominal aorta can erode/rupture into the inferior vena cava with overall prevalence reported as 3–6 % of all ruptured aneurysms [18]. Clinically, the patient can present with the classic triad of abdominal pain, hypotension, and pulsatile abdominal mass with the addition of an abdominal bruit. These symptoms can be presented from as low as 17 % to as high as 90 % of patients based on the reported clinical series [18–20]. Other presenting symptoms can include high-output heart failure, angina, oliguria, fever, hematuria, and diminished lower limb pulses. Usually, the diagnosis is made at the time of surgery. If suspected, a contrast-enhanced CT scan is the imaging modality of choice. Loss of fat plane, effacement of the IVC, and direct contrast flow into the cava are typical findings. Endovascular repair is preferred over open surgical as open aneurysm repair can result in massive blood loss from the cava upon entering the aneurysm sac [20].

Aorto-left Renal Vein and Aortoduodenal Fistulae

Rare cases of aorta to the left renal vein and aorta to the duodenal erosion/rupture have been reported in the literature [7]. In the case of erosion into the left renal vein, hydronephrosis, hematuria, and previous history of aortic surgery should alert the clinician to the diagnosis. Erosion into the bowel usually occurs in those individuals with prior aortic replacement surgery rather than as the initial presentation of a ruptured AAA. In the case of an aortoduodenal fistula, the patient will often present with a "herald bleed" of either upper or lower GI in nature. The presence of GI bleeding in any individual with a history of prior aortic surgery should prompt the clinician to rapidly workup the patient with an abdominal CT scan looking for obliteration of the fat plane between the aorta and the third portion of the duodenum. Upper GI endoscopy can also be helpful as it is specific but not sensitive. A high index of suspicion and prompt surgical intervention are critical to salvage these patients.

Diagnostic Tests

Traditionally, abdominal palpation during a physical examination was touted as an important diagnostic test to detect AAA. However, many factors can affect the sensitivity, specificity, and overall accuracy of AAA detection by physical exam. In a study where internists were solely tasked with using the physical abdominal exam to detect AAA, overall sensitivity was 68 % and increased, as the diameter of the AAA gets larger with 82 % sensitivity for AAAs of 5.0 cm or larger. Abdominal girth has an important contribution to the accuracy rate of AAA detection with sensitivity of over 90 % in those having abdominal girths of < 100 cm versus sensitivity of just 53 % for those with abdominal girths of > 100 cm [21]. With increasing obesity rate in the United States, the use of abdominal palpation for the detection of AAA should not be relied upon to diagnose the presence or absence of AAA in patients presenting to the emergency department.

As mentioned, a high index of suspicion for ruptured AAA is required especially for those who fit the demographics of an elderly male over the age of 65 years, smokers, and with a history of hypertension. If a patient presents with any of the previously mentioned symptoms, the clinician should be aggressive in ruling out a ruptured AAA before pursuing other less acute differential diagnoses. The most expedient and sensitive diagnostic study that a clinician should order is a contrast-enhanced CT scan of the abdomen. Traditionally, ultrasound was suggested as the initial screening imaging study. While it can detect the present of an AAA, ultrasound likely will not be able to visualize a rupture or the retroperitoneal hematoma [22]. In cases of renal insufficiency, a non-contrast CT is sufficient to make the diagnosis and can be used as preliminary planning for endovascular repair. With the median interval between admission and death of over 10 h, one has ample times to stabilize the patient and obtained a CT scan [23].

Conclusions

A ruptured AAA can be a lethal event and often is the first clinical sign of an abdominal aneurysm in an elderly patient. The classic "triad" of symptoms can be misleading and often not present in a patient with a ruptured AAA. High vigilance, awareness of the risk factors associated with AAA, and rapid recognition of possible clinical signs are critical to ensure that the clinician can make the correct initial diagnosis of ruptured AAA. With timely diagnosis, the patient with this potentially lethal disease can receive the appropriate surgical treatment and likely will survive, especially in the era endovascular first approach to ruptured AAA management.

References

1. Lederle FA. Prevalence and associations of abdominal aortic aneurysm detected through screening. Ann Intern Med. 2009;126(6):1–9.
2. United Kingdom Small Aneurysm Trial Participants. Long-term outcomes of immediate repair compared with surveillance of small abdominal aortic aneurysms. N Engl J Med. 2002;346(19): 1445–52.
3. Assar AN, Zarins CK. Ruptured abdominal aortic aneurysm: a surgical emergency with many clinical presentations. Postgrad Med J. 2009;85(1003):268–73.
4. Eisenhoffer JL, Marston WA, Ahlquist RA, Johnson GA. Misdiagnosis of ruptured abdominal aortic aneurysms. J Vasc Surg. 1992;16(1):0017–22.
5. Starnes BW, Quiroga E, Hutter C, Tran NT, Hatsukami T, Meissner M, et al. Management of ruptured abdominal aortic aneurysm in the endovascular era. J Vasc Surg. 2010;51(1):9–17; discussion 17–8.
6. Mehta M, Byrne J, Darling RC, Paty PSK, Roddy SP, Kreienberg PB, et al. Endovascular repair of ruptured infrarenal abdominal aortic aneurysm is associated with lower 30-day mortality and better 5-year survival rates than open surgical repair. J Vasc Surg. 2013;57(2): 368–75.
7. Sakalihasan N, Limet R, Defawe OD. Abdominal aortic aneurysm. Lancet. 2005;365(9470): 1577–89.
8. Battelle. Deaths: Final Data for 1999. 2001 Sep 24;1–114.
9. National Center for Health Statistics. Deaths: Final Data for 2013. 2014 Dec 29;1–71.
10. Mehta M, Kreienberg PB, Roddy SP, Paty PSK, Taggert JB, Sternbach Y, et al. Ruptured abdominal aortic aneurysm: endovascular program development and results. Semin Vasc Surg. 2010;23(4):206–14.
11. Mayer D, Pfammatter T, Rancic Z, Hechelhammer L, Wilhelm M, Veith FJ, et al. 10 years of emergency endovascular aneurysm repair for ruptured abdominal aortoiliac aneurysms: lessons learned. Ann Surg. 2009;249(3):510–5.
12. Metcalfe D, Holt PJE, Thompson MM. The management of abdominal aortic aneurysms. BMJ Br Med J Pub Group. 2011;342:644–9: d1384–4.
13. Karthikesalingam A, Hinchliffe RJ, Loftus IM, Thompson MM, Holt PJ. Volume-outcome relationships in vascular surgery: the current status. J Endovasc Ther. 2010;17(3):356–65.
14. Harris R, Sheridan S, Kinsinger L. Time to rethink screening for abdominal aortic aneurysm? Arch Intern Med. 2012;172(19):1–2.
15. Azhar B, Patel SR, Holt PJE, Hinchliffe RJ, Thompson MM, Karthikesalingam A. Misdiagnosis of ruptured abdominal aortic aneurysm: systematic review and meta-analysis. J Endovasc Ther. 2014;21(4):568–75.
16. Karkos CD, Papadimitriou CT, Chatzivasileiadis TN, Kapsali NS, Kalogirou TE, Giagtzidis IT, et al. The impact of aortic occlusion balloon on mortality after endovascular repair of ruptured abdominal aortic aneurysms: a meta-analysis and meta-regression analysis. Cardiovasc Intervent Radiol. 2015;38(6):1425–37.
17. Saiki M, Urata Y, Katoh I, Hamasaki T. Chronic contained rupture of an abdominal aortic aneurysm with vertebral erosion: report of a case. Ann Thorac Cardiovasc Surg. 2006;12(4): 300–2.

18. Adili F, Balzer JO, Ritter R-G, Schmandra TC, Tenholt M, Vogl TJ, et al. Ruptured abdominal aortic aneurysm with aorto-caval fistula. J Vasc Surg. 2004;40(3):582–1.
19. Iriz E, Ozdogan ME, Erer D, Uslu M, Koksal P, Kurtipek O. A giant aortocaval fistula due to abdominal aortic aneurysm. Int J Cardiol. 2006;112(3):e78–80.
20. Lin PH, Bush RL, Lumsden AB. Aortocaval fistula. J Vasc Surg. 2004;39(1):266–1.
21. Fink HA, Lederle FA, Roth CS, Bowles CA, Nelson DB, Haas MA. The accuracy of physical examination to detect abdominal aortic aneurysm. Arch Intern Med. 2002;160(6):1–4.
22. Walker A, Brenchley J, Sloan JP, Lalanda M, Venables H. Ultrasound by emergency physicians to detect abdominal aortic aneurysms: a UK case series. Emerg Med J. 2004;21(2):257–9.
23. Lloyd GM, Bown MJ, Norwood MGA, Deb R, Fishwick G, Bell PRF, et al. Feasibility of preoperative computer tomography in patients with ruptured abdominal aortic aneurysm: a time-to-death study in patients without operation. J Vasc Surg. 2004;39(4):788–91.

Chapter 3
The Epidemiology of Ruptured Abdominal Aortic Aneurysm (rAAA)

Peter A. Soden and Marc L. Schermerhorn

Key Points

- There is a decreasing incidence of mortality attributed to rAAA, but it is still a highly lethal condition.
- It is important to report turndown rates for rAAA, which vary by country, in future analyses. As rEVAR utilization increases, there is already evidence that turndown rates are decreasing.
- Use of EVAR for rAAA has lagged behind elective AAA repair, but popularity is growing and perioperative mortality from rAAA is decreasing as a result.
- Broad use of EVAR has increased elective repair in the older population, which correlates with a consistent downward trend in rAAA incidence and mortality.
- Pre-hospital mortality from rAAA is hard to estimate given the low clinical autopsy rates in current times.
- Risk factors for rupture of AAA with strong evidence include female gender, current smoking, aneurysm diameter, rapid aneurysm expansion, high aortic wall stress, symptom status, mycotic aneurysm, and high blood pressure.
- Females have a lower prevalence of AAA but are four times more likely to rupture, and current screening guidelines don't account for this increased risk in females.

P.A. Soden, MD • M.L. Schermerhorn, MD, FACS (✉)
Department of Surgery, Division of Vascular Surgery, Beth Israel Deaconess Medical Center, 110 Francis St 5B, 300 Brookline Ave, Boston, MA 02215, USA
e-mail: mscherm@bidmc.harvard

B.W. Starnes et al. (eds.), *Ruptured Abdominal Aortic Aneurysm*,
DOI 10.1007/978-3-319-23844-9_3

Introduction

Ruptured abdominal aortic aneurysm (rAAA) has a high mortality both in the field and for those who arrive at the hospital [1–3]. It has been difficult to estimate the exact incidence of this highly lethal condition because of problems estimating pre-hospital mortality as a result of low autopsy rates. The studies that address total incidence of rAAA, through high autopsy rates, are outdated and located in isolated geographic areas making it difficult to generalize their results. Furthermore, as will be discussed in this chapter, there have been dramatic changes over time and by geographic region, in the in-hospital incidence and reported mortality for rAAA, further compounding this problem with generalizability [1, 4, 5]. Management of AAA disease has also evolved over this time, with the disruptive technology of endovascular abdominal aortic aneurysm repair (EVAR) also potentially changing the perioperative mortality and number receiving intervention for rAAA [4–8]. Before the introduction of EVAR, open surgery was the only option for operative management of rAAA, with minimal improvement in survival over decades [9–11]. Since wide acceptance of EVAR for both intact and increasing rAAA, there have been significant improvements in mortality from rAAA (Fig. 3.1). There has also been a decline in the incidence of rAAA, as judged from hospital admission statistics [4]. Increased detection of incidental AAAs secondary to imaging; increased

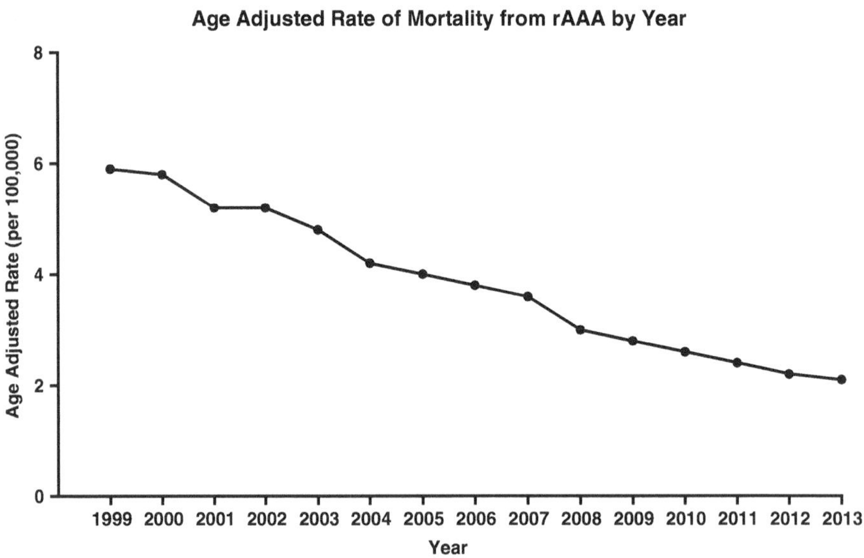

Fig. 3.1 Age-adjusted rate of mortality from rAAA by year in the US population over 44 years old (From Centers for Disease Control and Prevention, National Center for Health Statistics: Compressed Mortality File 1999–2013. CDC WONDER Online Database, compiled from Compressed Mortality File 1999–2013 Series 20 No. 2S, 2014, as compiled from data provided by the 57 vital statistics jurisdictions through the Vital Statistics Cooperative Program. Accessed at http://wonder.cdc.gov/cmf-icd10.html on May 29, 2015 12:44:04 PM)

elective repair, especially in high-rupture risk patients such as the elderly; lower perioperative mortality; and decreasing overall incidence of AAA have all likely led to the reduction in incidence and mortality of rAAA.

History

The first reported operation for ruptured abdominal aneurysm repair was in 1817 by Astley Cooper, who ligated the aortic bifurcation in a 38-year-old man for a ruptured left external iliac artery [12]. However, the first successful aortic ligation for ruptured aneurysm did not occur until 1928, when Rudolph Matas ligated a ruptured syphilitic aortic aneurysm in a 28-year-old [13]. Definitive surgical reconstruction did not come about until 1951, when Charles Dubost performed the first successful homograft reconstruction of the aorta [14]. By 1954 Cooley and DeBakey had treated six patients with a 50 % survival, and soon after open repair was widely accepted as a viable option for AAA [15]. During this same time, Arthur Voorhees developed and used the first synthetic aortic graft, using Vinyon-N cloth, on a rAAA in 1952 and by 1954 had reported on 17 synthetic implants in the abdominal aorta [16].

The first use of EVAR was reported in 1991 by Juan Parodi, in Argentina [17]. The first case of EVAR use for rAAA was reported in Nottingham, England, in 1994, 4 years after Parodi described its use in elective aneurysm repair [18]. However, it was not until 2000 that a code was developed for the procedure in the International Classification of Diseases, 9th Revision, Clinical Modification (ICD-9-CM) after FDA approval in the USA in 1999.

Incidence of rAAA

Many rAAA patients die before reaching the hospital, and since autopsies are no longer commonly performed routinely, the more recent estimates of rAAA incidence are likely underestimating the true incidence. Keeping this in mind, from the 1950s to early 2000s, multiple studies reported an increasing incidence of rAAA. In a Swedish population followed from 1952 to 1988, the incidence of rAAA rose from 0.9 to 6.9 per 100,000 persons [19]. Initially, some did not believe this trend as another study from Malmö, Sweden, reported a steady rate of incidence for rAAA at 5.6 per 100,000 persons [20]. This study had an impressive 85 % autopsy rate; however, it was also over a shorter time period, from 1971 to 1986, which was likely the reason for the lack of change. Later, this same population from Malmö was compared with the data from 2000 to 2004 [21]. Migration to and from the region was accounted for, and this time an increased rate of rAAA incidence was found, of 10.6 per 100,000 (Fig. 3.2). The later period in this study only had a 25 % autopsy rate, and so the more contemporary estimate may even be low. Other

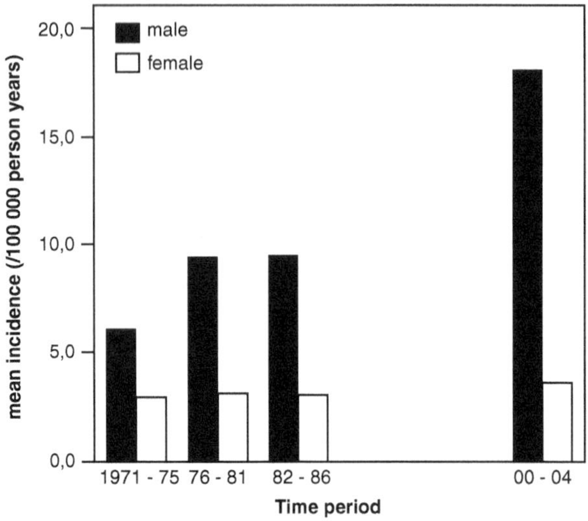

Fig. 3.2 Total population incidence of ruptured abdominal aortic aneurysm in Malmö: evolution between 1971 and 2004 (Acosta et al. [21])

studies have supported such an increase in incidence of rAAA over the same time period [22, 23].

However, this increasing trend has not persisted, and, in fact, there has been a distinct decrease in the incidence of rAAA over the past one to two decades if one uses mortality rates as a surrogate for incidence, see Fig. 3.1, which is reasonable given that mortality from rAAA has been reported to be as high as 80–90 % [1]. In 2013 the mortality rate of rAAA in the US population over 44 years old was 2.5 per 100,000 and in the Medicare-eligible population was 5.2 per 100,000, both down from prior years [24]. Additional studies found similar trends. For example, our group using Medicare data in the USA reported a decrease from 33.4 to 16.8 per 100,000 persons presenting with a diagnosis of rAAA, from 1995 to 2008 (Fig. 3.3) [4]. A second study in the USA, again using Medicare data, supported this same downtrend in hospital admissions for rAAA [25]. Australia had similar trends, as did England, Scotland, and Wales over the same time period (Fig. 3.4) [5, 22]. In England, Scotland, and Wales, the rate of hospital admissions for ruptured AAA over this time period decreased from 18.6 to 13.5 per 100,000; this downward trend was seen across all age groups but was greatest in those under 75 years old.

Incidence of rAAA in the Context of AAA

This decline in rAAA incidence caused much debate and is now thought to be a result of multiple factors. In discussing the trend for rAAA, it is useful to talk about the similar trends seen in AAA disease overall. Historically, there was an increase in AAA incidence similar to that for rAAA [26]. In a countrywide analysis of all admissions in Denmark, from 1977 to 1990, a fourfold increase in diagnosis of

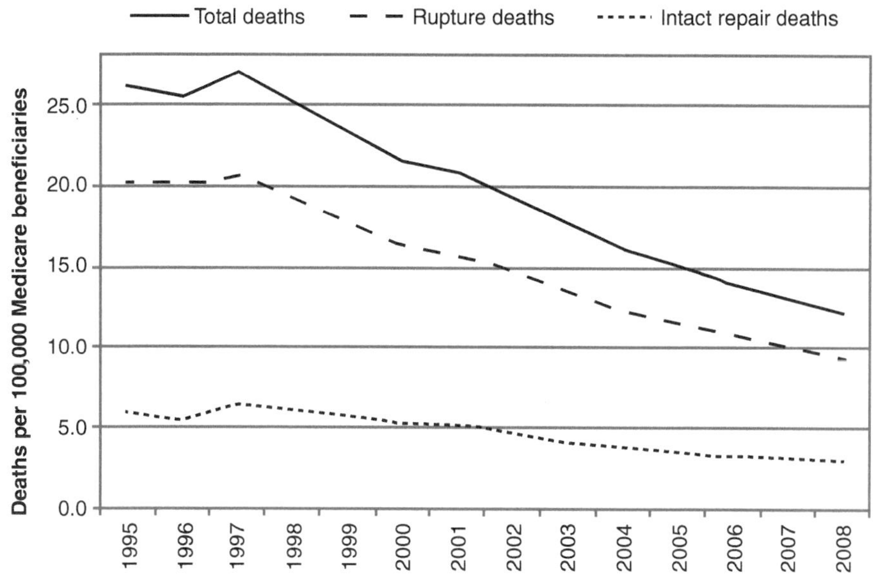

Fig. 3.3 AAA-related deaths in the Medicare population (Schermerhorn et al. [35])

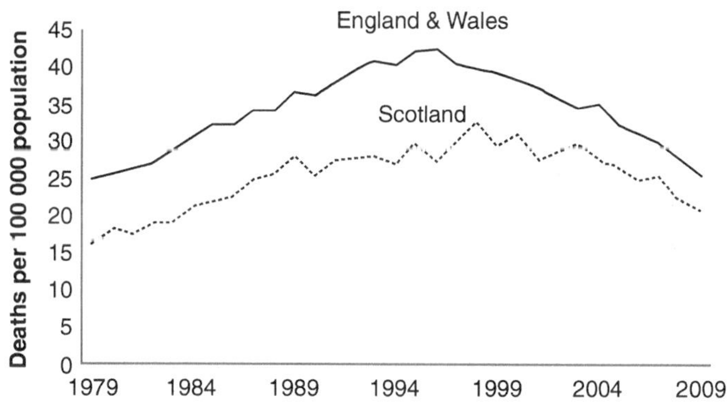

Fig. 3.4 Age-standardized mortality from AAA in England, Wales, and Scotland 1979–2009 (Anjum and Powell [22])

AAA was found [27]. Scotland showed similar results with a large administrative study showing a threefold increase in hospital admission for AAA, both elective and emergent, from 1981 to 2000, with no change in their elective repair rate of approximately 80 % [28]. This same finding was seen in the USA, where from 1951 to 1980, there was a sevenfold increase in AAA diagnosis in a Minnesota population studied [29]. Multiple reasons for this have been cited, including increased incidence, likely related to smoking trends, increased survival of high-risk populations, increased utilization of advanced imaging, and changing diagnostic criteria, but no one reason has been widely accepted. It is logical that the incidence of rAAA should follow that of AAA, unless dramatic changes in screening occurred over the same time interval. Increasing the number of elective operations for AAA as a prophylactic measure against rupture can also be another confounder to such an assumption. AAA and rAAA are now both decreasing in the twenty-first century [30, 31]. Reduction in risk factors, especially smoking, is likely a major reason for both decreases in AAA prevalence and subsequent rAAA incidence, but as important for rAAA is the increasing elective repair of high-risk patients with the wide acceptance of EVAR, to be discussed further below. This downward trend has been seen in much of the developed world. The data are so consistent that most accept the decrease in hospital admissions and mortality reported for rAAA as acceptable measures of a decrease in overall rupture rates of AAA, even without autopsy studies to confirm that the pre-hospital mortality rate is also declining or at least staying the same.

A Note on Pre-hospital Incidence of rAAA

In order to accurately measure pre-hospital rates of rAAA, it is necessary to have autopsy studies, but few areas have the systems set up to study such events retrospectively. There has been a dramatic decline in the rate of clinical autopsy, making replication of more complete historical studies difficult [32]. Population-based studies have attempted to develop surrogates for the clinical autopsy, but these efforts have not been satisfactory in giving an accurate incidence rate of pre-hospital rAAA. This leaves us with only historical data when trying to determine incidence of current pre-hospital rAAA rates. Such a dependence on outdated estimates is problematic, given the changing prevalence of AAA and incidence of rAAA that present to the hospital. Nevertheless, it is still important to understand the findings of these studies. Caution should be used when comparing studies that report on trends of incidence or total mortality for rAAA as the definition for what is included in these measures may differ.

rAAA Repair in the Era of EVAR

After introduction of EVAR, multiple RCTs showed an early morbidity and mortality benefit with EVAR in elective repair, leading to the wide-scale acceptance of EVAR in this setting. This benefit did not persist over the long term, where open repair and EVAR were shown to be more equivalent [33–35]. Nonetheless, EVAR is now performed for a majority of elective AAA cases in the USA [36]. EVAR for rAAA (rEVAR) was slower to gain acceptance, as there were concerns over the ability to expedite repair, the need for imaging, the comfort level with the technology, and the incomplete data on its efficacy in the emergent setting. There was interest, however, and by 2006–2007 a number of large retrospective studies looking at the use of rEVAR emerged. Our study, using the National Inpatient Sample from 1993 to 2005, showed a decrease in the diagnosis of rAAA by 30 % and reported a stable intervention rate for rAAA presenting to the hospital of 65 %, using either open repair or rEVAR, and notably found that by 2005 17 % of rAAA repairs were done by rEVAR [36]. These findings were further supported by our Medicare study from 1995 to 2008, which showed that 31 % of rAAA repairs in this population were by EVAR in 2008 [4]. During this same time period, the incidence of rAAA presenting to the hospital was decreasing as elective repair in the older population was increasing. Increasing use of rEVAR was bolstered by the mortality benefit shown in early prospective feasibility studies that employed protocols to encourage a rEVAR first approach when feasible in the management of rAAA, from both Albany Medical Center and the University of Washington [37, 38].

In Europe there was also acceptance of EVAR for rAAA, with certain centers adopting an EVAR-whenever-possible strategy [39]. However, wide variation persisted across European centers and between countries in the utilization of rEVAR. A comparative study using national administrative datasets from 2005 to 2010 found utilization of rEVAR in the USA to be 21 % compared to only 9 % in England [40].

Variation is also evident in the proportion of rAAA repairs out of total aneurysm repairs across countries, as Mani et al. demonstrated from 2005 to 2009, where the percent of rAAA repairs to total AAA repairs ranged from 9.8 to 30.9 % across Australia and eight European countries [41]. This difference could partially be explained by screening practices and criteria for elective AAA repair but could also be influenced by the difference in populations and presence of risk factors for rupture within these populations. As a comparison, the proportion of rAAA repairs compared to total repairs in the Medicare population in the USA ranged from 8 to 9 % from 2005 to 2008 [4]. Such variation highlights the need for caution when generalizing incidence numbers from a distinct geographic region to other populations.

Retrospective and prospective studies have shown that rEVAR is associated with lower mortality and perioperative morbidity compared to open repair [8, 36, 37, 39, 40, 42, 43]. However, the RCTs have not shown this difference; whether that is from problems with implementing an RCT in this acute population or a selection bias that confounds the nonrandomized studies is not clear at this point [44–46]. In addition, centers within these RCTs likely have a benefit in their open rAAA repairs as well, due to the systems put in place to triage such patients for purposes of the RCT.

The Incidence of Rupture After Prior Repair

A multicenter prospective registry analysis in the USA studied rupture after AAA repair by EVAR and found 20 out of 1736 EVARs (1.2 %) presented after initial EVAR with rupture [47]. Of these 20 ruptures, two had presented as ruptured and four as symptomatic for their initial EVAR. The 30-day and 1-year mortality for those receiving repair for subsequent rupture were 42.9 % and 64.3 %, respectively.

Data from the UK EVAR trials 1 and 2, which studied only initial elective AAA repair, reported no rupture in those treated with open aortic repair but a 3.2 % rupture rate in the EVAR group (total of 27 ruptures) over a mean of 4.8 years follow-up, and a 67 % 30-day mortality rate, for those treated by rEVAR [48]. Five of the 27 ruptures (18.5 %) occurred within 30 days of the index operation, with a 60 % 30-day mortality in this subset. Our group found a subsequent rupture rate of 5.4 % after initial elective EVAR compared to 1.4 % after elective open repair at 8 years of follow-up in the Medicare population [35]. Furthermore, Mehta et al. followed 1768 patients after elective EVAR and emergent EVAR for rupture from 2002 to 2009 and found a higher incidence of rupture after rEVAR compared to elective EVAR, 2.8 % versus 1.4 %, respectively [49]. Multiple studies have identified technical risk factors for rupture after EVAR, which include endoleaks (most notably Type I), stent-graft migration, sac enlargement, stent-graft tears and fractures, and infection [50, 51]. Whether the rate of such risk factors are higher for rEVAR is unclear at this point, but the urgent nature of the repair could presumably increase the frequency of endograft size mismatch and therefore endoleak. However, many clinicians who favor rEVAR believe that the mortality and morbidity benefits of rEVAR outweigh this risk of subsequent ruptures.

Risk Factors for rAAA

Algorithms for risk of rupture remain imprecise, and improving upon them has been confounded by the decreasing incidence of rAAA and lack of data on the most unstable patients who die before presentation to the hospital. Even if high autopsy rates were possible, certain important anatomic details would likely be inaccurate from autopsy, such as aneurysm diameter, which is underestimated postmortem as the vessel is depressurized, making morphology difficult to assess. Given such limitations to identifying clear risk factors, this section will address what is known and suspected to increase the chance of rupture. Identified below are numerous anatomic, demographic, and other risk factors for AAA rupture.

Aneurysm Diameter

Starting in 1966, Szilagyi et al. showed larger aneurysms (>6 cm) were more likely to rupture than smaller aneurysms (<6 cm) (Fig. 3.5) [52]. This size relationship with risk of rupture was further supported by autopsy studies [53, 54]. The UK Small Aneurysm Trial (UKSAT) gave a comprehensive estimate of AAA rupture risk for small aneurysms, size 4.0–5.5 cm, and found no difference in survival for early operation versus surveillance [55]. Brown et al. used the randomized UKSAT population prior to any surgery and added in the 1167 patients ineligible for randomization in this study, and who were also followed, and did find a difference in

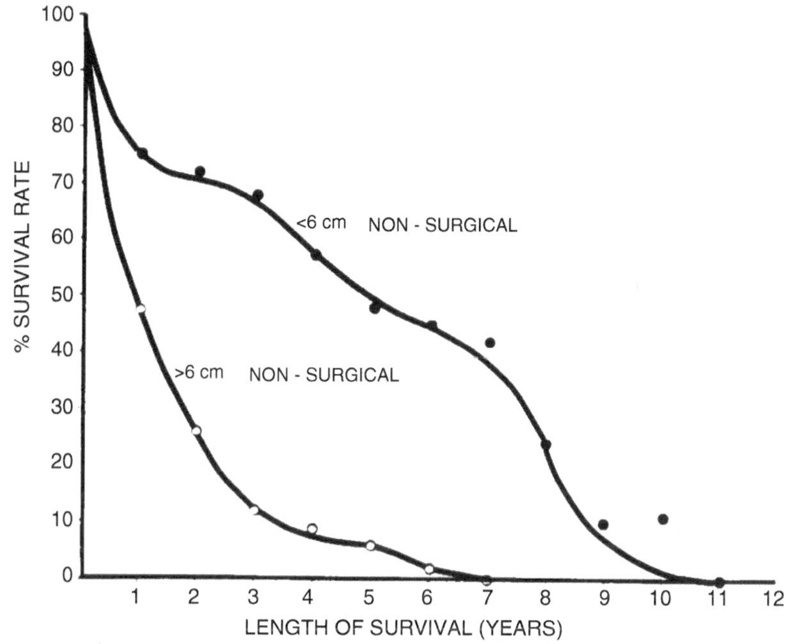

Fig. 3.5 Observed cumulative 13-year-survival experience for small (<6 cm) and large (>6 cm) nonsurgical abdominal aortic aneurysms standardized for age, cardiac status, blood pressure, and renal function (Szilagyi et al. [52])

rupture risk for smaller aneurysms; rupture risks per 100 patient-years were 0.3 % for AAA <4.0 cm, 1.5 % for AAA 4.0–4.9 cm, and 6.5 % for AAAs 5.0–5.9 cm [56]. A population-based study from Minnesota followed 176 patients selected for non-operative management and found an annual rupture risk of 0 % for AAAs <4 cm, 1 % for AAAs 4.0–4.9 cm, and 11 % for AAAs 5.0–5.9 cm [57].

For larger aneurysms, Parkinson et al. performed a meta-analysis of 11 studies, including 1514 patients who were deemed unfit for elective operation but had aneurysms larger than 5.5 cm [58]. Within this study, the rate of rupture was found to be 3.5 % per year (95 % CI 1.6–8.7 %) for aneurysm size 5.5–6.0 cm, 4.1 % (0.7–9.0 %) for 6.1–7.0 cm, and 6.3 % (1.8–14.3 %) for aneurysms >7.0 cm. However, although initially deemed unfit, some patients in these series underwent elective repair. Thus these rates likely underestimate the true rupture risk. Another consideration is that this populations' increased risk is not entirely related to diameter as patients deemed unfit for elective repair have additional risk factors for rupture, such as gender, smoking status, additional wall stress factors, and comorbidities (e.g., COPD and hypertension), which will be discussed below. As a result, caution should be used when generalizing these rupture risks to the general population, who presumably have fewer comorbidities than those deemed unfit for repair. All-cause mortality in this unfit for repair group is known to be high, with a 2-year survival rate as low as 35 % [59].

Aneurysm Shape and Wall Stress

Laminar flow is easily disturbed in the blood vessels, especially with aneurysmal degeneration, and over time forces from this disturbance can lead to adverse effects on the vessel wall. Laplace's law states that the wall tension of a symmetric shape is directly proportional to the radius and intraluminal pressure and inversely proportional to wall thickness. Aneurysms are not symmetric shapes, and logic would tell us that eccentric or saccular aneurysms present a greater risk for rupture than more diffuse and fusiform ones. This has been difficult to quantify, but computer modeling, such as that by Vorp et al., has shown that aneurysm shape is almost as important for wall stress, and likely rupture risk, as is diameter [60]. Furthermore, commonly seen intraoperatively and on preoperative CT scans, small blebs on aneurysm sacs are postulated to pose an added risk for rupture and occur in equal frequency on small and large aneurysms. Histologically, these blebs often show an imbalance of matrix degradation and repair, leaving them especially vulnerable to wall stress [61].

Work is underway to improve our assessment of risk for rupture using models that factor in shape and asymmetry, as well as diameter, to determine overall wall stress. Initial studies have suggested using finite element analysis of wall stress, aided by advances in CT imaging, to advise patients on risk of rupture [62, 63]. This finite element model is basically a stress analysis model for AAA and includes the geometry of the AAA, the mechanical behavior of the AAA tissue, and the boundary conditions (e.g., blood pressure) [64]. As this idea gains momentum, the clinical applicability of such a complex algorithm has been called into question, and studies to simplify it by identifying the essential components of this stress analysis are in progress. Fillinger et al. attempted to show important anatomic details for risk of rupture after matching a group of 259 elective and rAAA by age, gender, and diameter [65]. They found that ruptured AAAs tend to be less tortuous but have more diameter asymmetry than their size matched intact counterparts. What is becoming clear is that to use AAA diameter as the only anatomic measure for risk of rupture and indication for elective repair is likely too simplistic. Fillinger et al. showed a model using wall stress to be superior to aneurysm diameter in predicting rupture and that wall stress was predictive in small aneurysms that rupture as well (Fig. 3.6) [62]. Newer models of wall stress are not ready for general use as of yet but are predicted to become part of common practice as methods improve.

Aneurysm Expansion Rate

It makes sense that more rapid expansion would cause a higher risk for rupture, but it has been hard to distinguish this risk from that of increased aneurysm size alone. In 2011 Powell et al. published a meta-analysis evaluating expansion rates and showed that larger aneurysms tend to increase in size at a faster rate; specifically a 10-mm increase in diameter size was associated with a mean of 1.62 (SEM 0.20) mm/year increase in growth rate (Fig. 3.7) [66]. In addition to diameter cutoffs, rapid

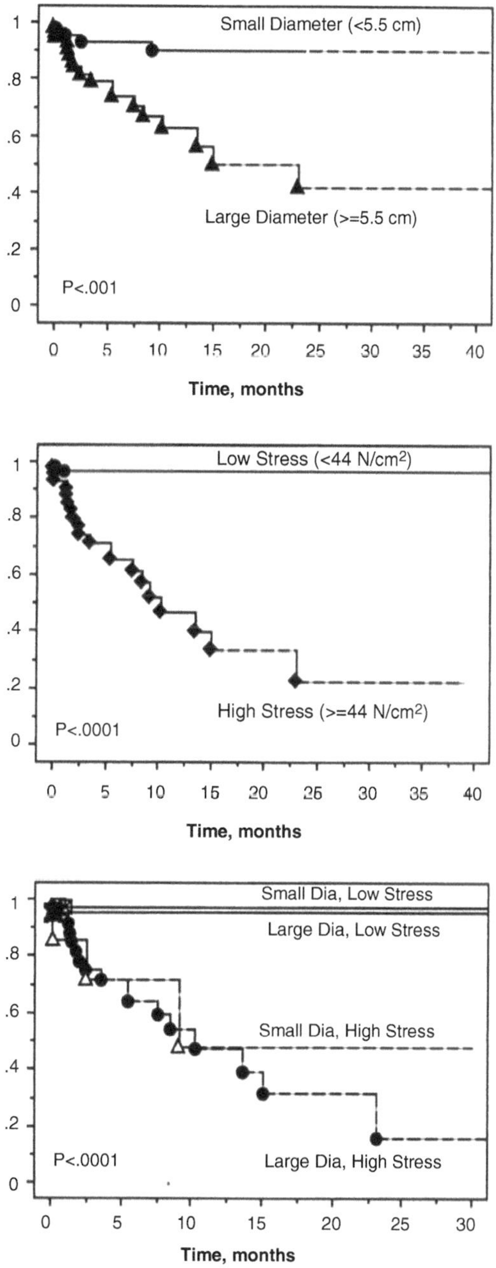

Fig. 3.6 Life tables for Freedom from Rupture or Emergency Surgery because of acute symptoms. *Top* Larger diameter significant predictor for rupture; *Middle* High wall stress significant predictor of rupture; *Bottom* Subgroups were analyzed for combinations of small and large diameter and low and high wall stress, with the same thresholds as used in other life tables. Low-stress aneurysm had a low rupture rate, whether they were small or large, and high-stress aneurysms had a high rupture rate regardless of size (Fillinger et al. [62])

AAA expansion is often used as an indication for elective repair, with expansion rate of >1 cm/year being the most commonly used rate for repair. In addition to diameter, another factor that increases the growth rate of aneurysms is presence of thrombus [67]. Thrombus is thought to induce hypoxia-driven inflammation that weakens the

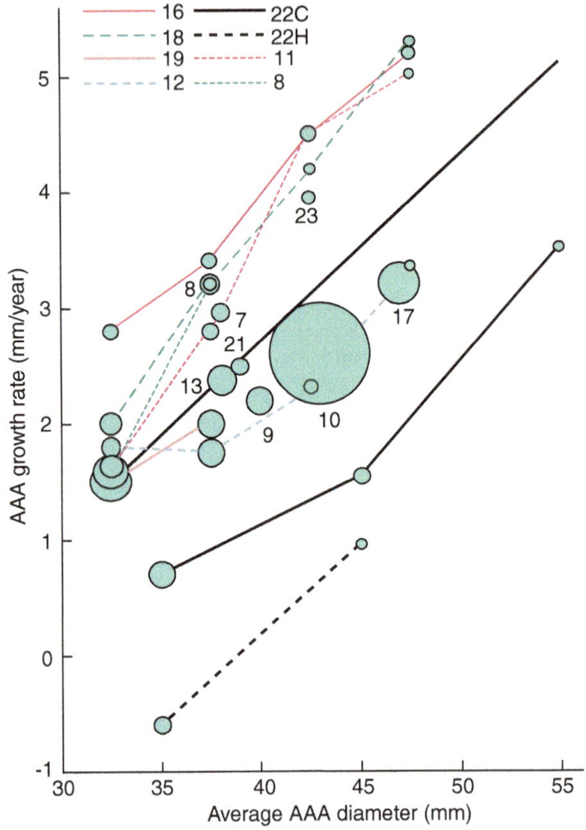

Fig. 3.7 Meta-regression of abdominal aortic aneurysm (AAA) growth rates by AAA diameter. The overall regression line is shown by the solid bold line (Powell et al. [66])

wall of the aneurysm [68]. Please see Chaps. 4 and 5 for more specific details on the role of the thrombus. Rate of expansion is a marker of aneurysm instability and should continue to be used in the identification of high-risk patients who warrant repair.

Current Smoking

One of the most modifiable risk factors that could continue to have a large impact on reduction of ruptures from AAA is smoking cessation. Many credit smoking to part of the decline already seen in the incidence of rAAA. Early studies established a clear link between cigarette smoking and aneurysm development, dating back to 1958 [69]. This link with aneurysm development and mortality from AAA has been supported by multiple subsequent studies from both Europe and the USA [5, 30, 31]. A large screening study of US veterans attributed >70 % of all AAAs in the veteran population to smoking [70]. Sweeting et al. performed a meta-analysis using individual patient data from 18 studies analyzing factors that affected growth and rupture of small AAAs [71]. After adjusting for aneurysm diameter, there was a strong association between smoking and both growth rate and rupture, growth mean

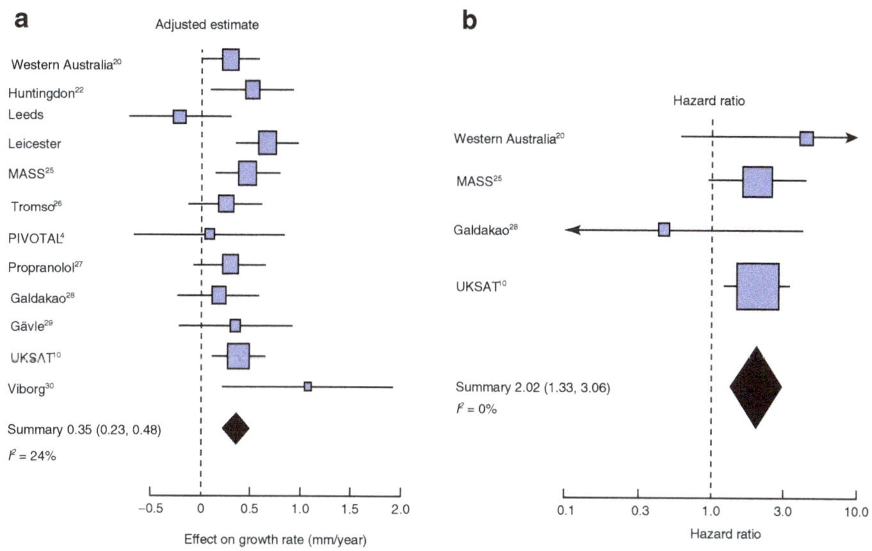

Fig. 3.8 Individual studies and meta-analysis of smoking on (**a**) the effect on growth rate and (**b**) on aneurysm rupture rates using hazard ratios, with 95 % confidence intervals, adjusted for aneurysm diameter. *MASS* Multicentre Aneurysm Screening Study, *UKSAT* UK Small Aneurysm Screening Trial (Sweeting et al. [71])

was 0.33 mm/year (SEM .07) faster, and risk of rupture was twofold higher in current smokers compared to ex- and never smokers (Fig. 3.8). Despite limitations relevant to any meta-analysis, such as heterogeneity of definitions and self-reporting reliability, these results are convincing.

Anjum et al. analyzed health statistics for England and Wales from 1979 to 2009 and estimated that the decrease in prevalence of smoking in England and Wales led to an avoidance of 8–11 deaths from rAAA per 100,000 persons [23]. This study also suggested treatment of hyperlipidemia, and coronary artery disease played a role in the decline rAAA deaths (Fig. 3.9). There are multiple reasons that seem plausible for the reduction in rAAA mortality, but it seems likely that smoking cessation has contributed greatly.

Age

It has been clearly established that the incidence of AAA increases with age [26, 72].

The UKSAT did not find age to be associated with rupture after adjusting for known risk factors, including diameter; however multiple other studies found age strongly predictive [56, 71, 73, 74]. A possible explanation for the lack of predictive ability found in the UKSAT data is the collinear (overlapping) effects of covariates included in the model, such as aneurysm diameter and declining FEV1, which are closely related to increasing age.

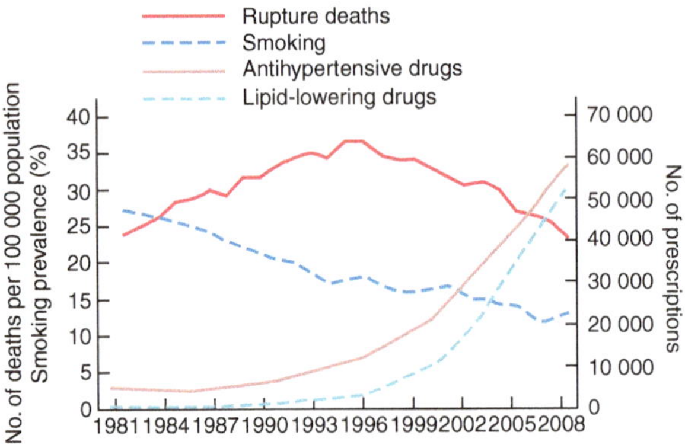

Fig. 3.9 Changes in deaths from rAAA, prevalence of smoking for total population over 65 years, and prescription of blood pressure and lipid-lowering medications in England and Wales from 1981 to 2008 (Anjum et al. [23])

Studies are now showing that the decline in the incidence of rAAA is also being felt across most age groups, although at variable rates. In England and Wales, from 1997 to 2009, there was a decrease in aneurysm rupture across all age ranges, significant in all except the >85-year-old group [23]. This oldest group was also found to have the highest incidence of hospitalization for rAAA at 94.7 per 100,000 people.

In general, older patients with rAAA have a higher in-hospital mortality rate, but a large part of this may be explained by disproportionate intervention rates favoring younger patients [23]. These in-hospital-mortality and rAAA-intervention-rate differences by age are consistent across countries, as highlighted by Karthikesalingam et al. . who compared mortality from rAAA between England and the USA from 2005 to 2010 (Fig. 3.10) [40]. However, this difference between age groups may be closing thanks to the incorporation of rEVAR and presumably a lower turndown rate for those older patients getting rEVAR who would have been less likely to get open repair compared to their younger counterparts. Using National Inpatient Sample data from 2000 to 2005, our group showed the mortality benefit of rEVAR compared to open repair in those over 70 years old: in-hospital mortality rate of 36.3 % after rEVAR compared to 47 % after open repair ($p<.001$) for this age group [73]. Using Medicare data from 1995 to 2008, our group also showed that all ages had a decline in short-term AAA-related death, but this was most evident in the >80-year-old age group, and most of this mortality benefit was related to a steep decline in rupture deaths (Fig. 3.11) [4]. This age group had the largest increase in elective AAA repairs over the same time period suggesting that more aggressive management of intact AAAs in this high-risk group was preventing subsequent ruptures and related deaths.

Symptom Status

Symptoms of abdominal, back, groin, or buttock pain related to an AAA have long been considered an indicator of impending rupture. Tenderness to palpation is a particularly ominous sign when associated with symptoms, and many clinicians have anecdotally used tenderness to palpation in the absence of pain symptoms as an indication for semi-urgent repair given the suspected rupture risk [56]. In the pre-EVAR

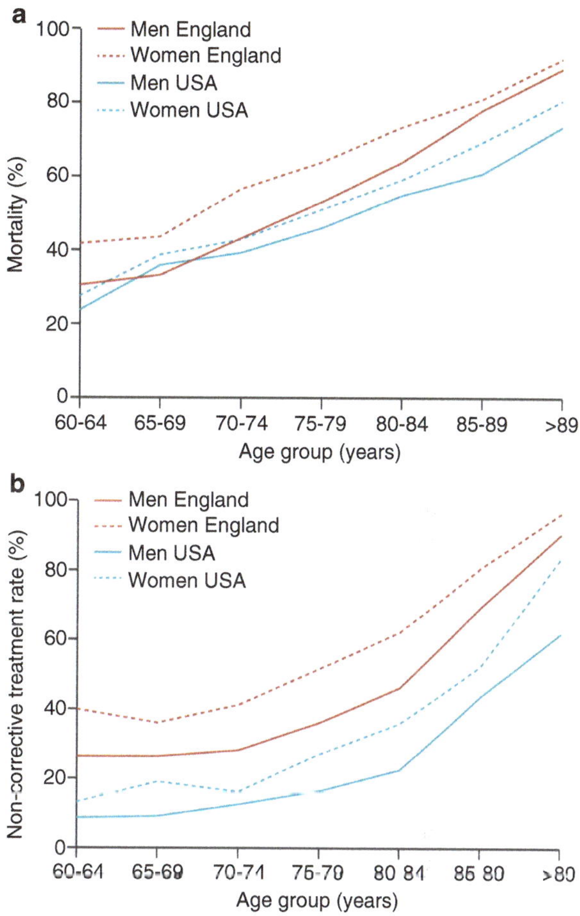

Fig. 3.10 (**a**) In-hospital mortality from rAAA and (**b**) non-corrective (nonoperative) treatment of rAAA, stratified by age and sex, across both England and the USA (Karthikesalingam et al. [40])

era, multiple studies consistently showed worse 30-day and in-hospital mortality rates for repair of the symptomatic but non-ruptured AAA, from 5 to 26 %, compared to elective repair [75–77]. While there is general agreement on the need for urgent repair in this population, Cambria et al. helped clarify the value in a delay of surgery to medically optimize and have a full operating team available for repair of symptomatic patients who can wait [75]. More recent data have suggested that the gap between mortality in the elective versus symptomatic patients may be closing, perhaps due to increasing EVAR use and optimization of comorbid conditions (Table 3.1) [78].

Gender

Multiple clinical trials and epidemiologic studies have identified a lower prevalence of AAA in females, with the male to female ratio of 5–1 [79–81]. Despite having a lower prevalence of AAA disease, women with AAA had a fourfold increased risk

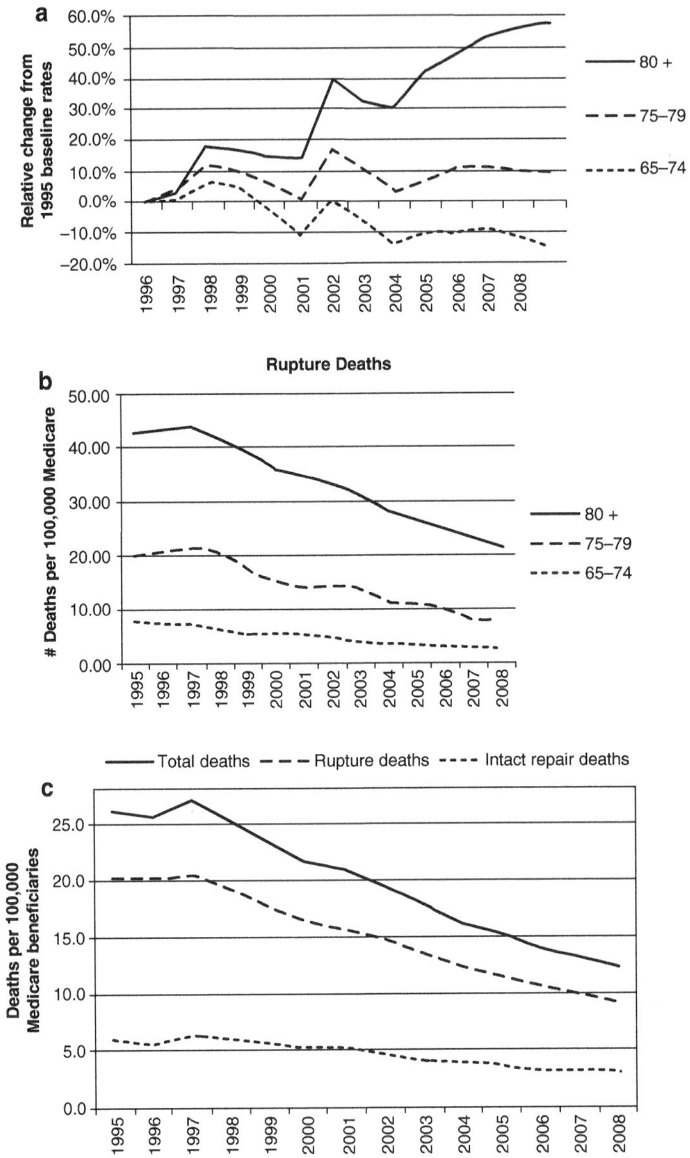

Fig. 3.11 (**a**) Changes in intact AAA repair rates subsequent to 1995 by age and year (sex adjusted). All short-term AAA-related deaths in Medicare population stratified by (**b**) age and (**c**) indication for AAA repair (age and sex adjusted) per 100,000 US Medicare beneficiaries (Schermerhorn et al. [4])

Table 3.1 Mortality and method of repair for prior series reporting symptomatic abdominal aortic aneurysms

First author	Year	Sx-AAA No.	Reported open %	Reported EVAR %	Mortality %
Johnson	1980	84	100	0	16
McCabe	1981	56	100	0	14.3
Sullivan	1990	19	100	0	26
Olsen	1991	151	100	0	17.2
Cambria	1994	36	100	0	11.1
Aune	1995	52	100	0	17
Darling	1996	103	100	0	12.6
Sayers	1997	80	100	0	16
Kantonen	1997	156	100	0	13.5
Bradbury	1998	156	100	0	14.1
Leo	2005	42	100	0	9.5
Antonello	2006	42	100	0	11.9
Franks	2006	20	45	55	5
Oranen	2006	22	0	100	5
Nevala	2008	14	0	100	0
Current	2009	156	62	38	1.3

De Martino et al. [78]

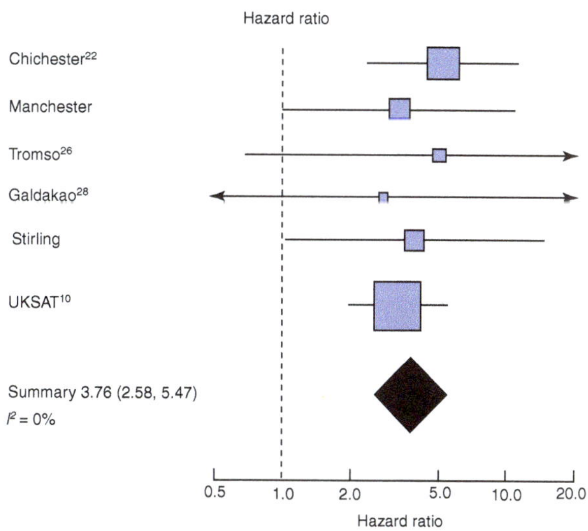

Fig. 3.12 Effect of female sex on AAA rupture states in individual studies and meta-analysis. Hazard ratios, adjusted for aneurysm diameter, are shown with 95 % confidence intervals. *MASS* Multicentre Aneurysm Screening Study, *UKSAT* UK Small Aneurysm Screening Trial (Sweeting et al. [71])

for rupture in the UKSAT trial, after adjustment for age, AAA diameter, smoking status, and mean blood pressure compared to men [56]. In this study the mean diameter at time of rupture was 5 cm for women and 6 cm for men. Further meta-analysis has supported an increased rupture risk in females (Fig. 3.12) [71]. A possible explanation is that female aortas are smaller and more compliant than males;

therefore a smaller aneurysm is of greater risk in the female population [82]. Another possible reason for worse outcomes in females is that they undergo elective repair at relatively larger aneurysm sizes compared to males. By indexing aortic size to body surface area, the Aortic Size Index (ASI), our group showed that women in New England are undergoing repair at larger ASI measurements compared to males for elective AAA repair [83]. ASI has already been shown to be more reliable than aneurysm diameter in predicting rupture, death, and dissection in patients with thoracic aortic aneurysms and has been incorporated into a nomogram used for prediction of rupture risk by both the Society for Thoracic Surgeons and the American College of Cardiology [85].

Currently the US Preventive Services Task Force recommends AAA screening for men aged 65–75 years with a history of smoking but recommends against screening for women who have never smoked and also states there is insufficient evidence to support screening for women who have smoked [86]. A recent Markov model, which considered the higher rupture rate in women, higher prevalence in the over-75-year-old female population, and increased lifespan of females versus males, found screening for AAA in females older than 75 years old to be cost effective [87]. Furthermore, a Medicare analysis from 1994 to 2003 found that 30–34 % of ruptured AAAs that result in death in the USA occur in women, while only 26 % of elective AAA repairs are performed in women [81]. The in-hospital mortality associated with rupture in this same analysis was 52.8 % for women and 44.2 % for men ($p<.001$). Given these disproportionate age-adjusted mortality figures, a reevaluation of current screening guidelines and incorporation of an adjustment for female patients, such as ASI, should be considered.

For those women who receive intervention for rAAA, further administrative studies have shown that rEVAR is less likely to be offered to females, accounting for 28–32.4 % of all repairs for females versus 44.3–46.7 % for men [81, 88]. The aortic anatomy of women that adds difficulty to performing EVAR, such as shorter aortic neck and smaller iliac vessels, may contribute to this difference [89]. As a result of these sex differences, female sex has been found to be an independent predictor of mortality during repair of both elective AAA and rAAA repair when not adjusting for ASI [81, 84]. This highlights the challenge that lies ahead in ensuring equal access and benefit from the gains that have been made with regard to the treatment of AAA disease and subsequent rupture rates.

Blood Pressure

In 1985 Cronenwett et al. was first to note the impact of blood pressure on increased rupture risk [90]. Later, the UKSAT identified higher mean blood pressure as a risk factor for rupture with a HR (95 % CI) of 1.04 (1.02–1.07) for each 1 mmHg increase in mean blood pressure [56]. Now it is accepted that the higher the pressure in the aorta the higher the wall stress and thus increased risk of rupture. The shape of the aorta also plays an important role in determining the vector of force from blood flow on the aortic wall and the surface area this energy is spread over. Interestingly, in a large meta-analysis, mean arterial pressure was found to have no effect on rate of aneurysm growth but did increase the risk of rupture for small aneurysms, HR (95 % CI) for each 10 mmHg increase was 1.32 (1.11–1.56), suggesting the mechanism is not through growth [71]. The association between a decrease in rAAA mortality and blood pressure control has been supported in population studies as well (see Fig. 3.9) [23].

Family History

A family history of AAA disease increases the chance of a first-degree relative having an AAA. In a study evaluating the family pedigree of 542 consecutive patients with AAA, 86 individuals were found to have a first-degree relative with AAA, and 40.7 % of the 86 had a history of aneurysm rupture in their family [91]. This was higher than the general population rupture rate at the time. This study also showed that the frequency of rupture increased with the number of first-degree relatives one had with AAA: 15 % with two first-degree relatives, 29 % with three, and 36 % with four or more. Another pedigree study published 6 years later found rupture rates again higher in the familial AAAs compared to sporadic, 32 % vs. 9 %, respectively, and that these ruptures tend to happen 10 years earlier in the familial group [92]. A population-based cross-sectional study from Denmark in 2008 to 2011 found similar results with a higher prevalence of AAA in individuals with a family history of AAA (6.7 % vs. 3.0 %) [93]. In addition, this study found a larger mean maximum aortic diameter in those with positive family history versus those with no family history, 20.50–19.07 mm ($p < .0001$). This diameter difference brings up a noteworthy limitation regarding possible confounding not adjusted for in pedigree analysis, such as diameter. That said, it is likely that family history plays an important role, but further research is needed to elucidate the reason, whether it be genetic (e.g., collagen maintenance or alpha 1-antitrypsin), lifestyle, or environment related. The reader should continue to take a thorough family history and pay attention to mention of sudden death or aneurysmal disease for any patient being evaluated for vascular disease.

Other Risk Factors

Large meta-analysis and population studies have assessed other potential risk factors for both aneurysm growth and risk of rupture, including statins, antiplatelet agents, individual blood pressure medications, COPD, and FEV1 levels. A brief discussion of notable risk factors follows: in the UK Small Aneurysm Trial, FEV1 levels were stratified into tertiles, and an inverse relationship was found between FEV1 and rate of rupture [56]. The study reported that increasing FEV1 was protective against rupture with a HR (95 % CI) of 0.62 (0.45–0.86) per liter increase, after adjusting for age, sex, and initial AAA diameter. The collinear effect of FEV1 and smoking confounds the results of this analysis given that smokers are more likely to have a low FEV1 and vice versa. Nevertheless, pulmonary reserve and COPD status have been found to be possible risk factors for rupture and remain a point of investigation [90].

The effect of lipid control on the development of AAA has been conflicting. From two prospective studies, one found a 2.3-fold relative risk increase for those in the fourth quartile of serum cholesterol (>240 mg/dl) compared to those in the first (<193 mg/dl) and no association with triglyceride levels, while the other found no association between the level of cholesterol and risk of death from abdominal aneurysm [94, 95]. The ADAM trial found a significant association in both cohorts between high cholesterol level and presence of AAA, combined OR (95 % CI) 1.44 (1.27–1.63) [70]. UKSAT, however, did not show an association between serum cholesterol and risk of rupture from AAA [56]. Improved medical management of hypercholesterolemia is at least temporally related to the reduction in rupture-related mortality (see Fig. 3.9), and so it seems plausible that lipid control may have a small effect that is intermittently noted [23].

Connective tissue disorders, such as Ehlers-Danlos and Marfan syndromes, lead to a number of medical conditions including aneurysmal disease that includes the abdominal aorta. These pathologies offer insight into what is important for the integrity of the aortic wall. The underlying pathophysiology in collagen disorders is a genetic alteration in sequences that affect the synthesis and processing of different forms of collagen. Ehlers-Danlos has a vascular form with a prevalence of 1 in 100,000 and that makes up 4 % of all Ehlers-Danlos cases. Arterial rupture occurs in iliac, splenic, renal vessels, or the aorta, and is usually not preceded by detection of an aneurysm given that most are psuedoaneurysms [96]. Eighty percent of patients experience a vascular event or rupture by age 40. In Marfan the aortic root is the major problem that develops aneurysmal dilatation, aortic regurgitation, and dissection.

Finally, mycotic AAAs, which in a single institution study were found to make up as much as 1 % of all AAAs treated, increase risk of rupture [97]. Mycotic aneurysm refers to any infected aneurysm, whether from bacteremia, septic emboli, or colonization through the vasa vasorum. The overall mortality in this group has been reported to be as high as 30 % and the risk of rupture to be 50–80 %, with a rupture mortality rate of 70 % [26, 97, 98]. Common organisms found in this condition include *Staphylococcus spp.*, *Salmonella spp.*, and *Streptococcus spp.* Additionally, *Campylobacter spp.* has been reported [99].

Protective Effect of Diabetes

Diabetes mellitus is thought to be protective against the development of AAA, aneurysm growth, and rAAA. Historical screening studies have shown a low prevalence of diabetes among persons with abdominal aneurysms [100–102]. In every one of

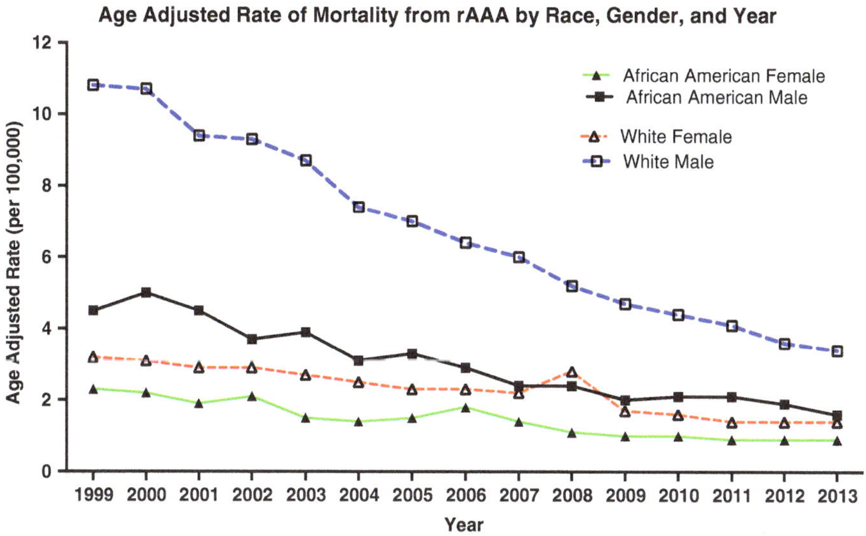

Fig. 3.13 Age-adjusted mortality rate from rAAA by race, gender, and year from 1999 to 2013 in the over-44-year-old population (From Centers for Disease Control and Prevention, National Center for Health Statistics: Compressed Mortality File 1999–2013. CDC WONDER Online Database, compiled from Compressed Mortality File 1999–2013 Series 20 No. 2S, 2014, as compiled from data provided by the 57 vital statistics jurisdictions through the Vital Statistics Cooperative Program. Accessed at http://wonder.cdc.gov/cmf-icd10.html on May 29, 2015 12:44:04 PM)

the 18 studies used in the meta-analysis by Sweeting et al., which included 15,475 people, an overall reduced growth rate was seen in diabetics with aneurysms [71]. Unfortunately, no distinction between Type I and Type II diabetes could be made from the included studies. This consistent trend in diabetics suggests there is change to the aortic wall, possibly through glycosylation or calcification, which stiffens the aorta and protects it against expansion and subsequent rupture.

Race and rAAA

Multiple population-based studies have shown a reduced prevalence of AAA in African Americans [102–104]. Kent et al. performed a screening study in over 3 million individuals and found nonwhite race to be protective for diagnosis of an AAA on multivariable analysis: African American (OR 0.72, 95 % CI 0.66–0.78) and Asian (OR 0.72, 95 % CI 0.59–0.75) [104]. In 1990 the age-adjusted AAA death rate for African American males was 1.6 per 100,000 compared to whites, 3.6 per 100,000, for the >44-year-old population in the USA [103]. Data from the CDC support these findings reporting a decreased mortality from rAAA in African Americans compared to whites over the last 15 years (Fig. 3.13).

Mortality of rAAA

To get a full picture of mortality from rAAA, in addition to in-hospital and perioperative mortality, one must also analyze pre-hospital mortality and the turndown rate (no-intervention rate).

Pre-hospital Mortality

Reimerink et al. attempted to give a complete picture of mortality in a meta-analysis of 24 retrospective studies from 1977 to 2012 [1]. To be included, studies needed to report both mortality of patients admitted to the hospital with rAAA and also report the community/pre-hospital mortality rate from rAAA. This study showed a pooled total mortality of 81 % from rAAA (95 % CI 78–83 %) and a reduction in total mortality over time (Fig. 3.14). Pre-hospital mortality for rAAA was relatively stable throughout the study period: 37 % (95 % CI 28–47 %) before 1990 and 32 % (17–49 %) after 1990, although the autopsy rate over all the studies was poorly and inconsistently defined, so this percentage is likely underestimating the true proportion who die outside of the hospital.

Historically studies from the 1970s and 1980s have a pre-hospital rAAA mortality rate, as percentage of total mortality, of approximately 40–57 % with autopsy rates of 61–85 % [20, 105]. Bengtsson et al. found that of the 215 persons with ruptured AAA in Malmö, Sweden, from 1971 to 1986, 124 were alive on arrival to the hospital, 61 of which were considered operative candidates, and 26 of those operated on survived. It is possible that over time the pre-hospital mortality for rAAA has decreased similar to the in-hospital and total rupture death rates, but the current clinical autopsy rates make this difficult to prove with a robust epidemiologic study [32, 106]. We can say that it is unlikely to have increased given current awareness and improvement in emergency medical services for out of hospital care.

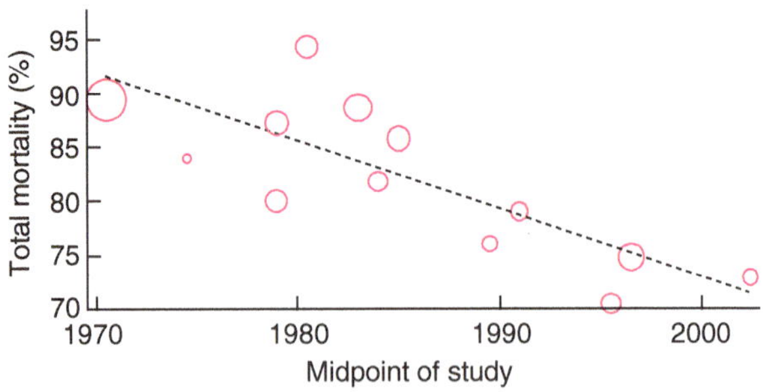

Fig. 3.14 Meta-regression analysis of total rAAA mortality in high-quality studies. Each study is represented by a circle, with size according to number of included patients. Plotted regression line (Reimerink et al. [1])

Table 3.2 Baseline characteristics of patients with an RAAA in the Amsterdam ambulance region undergoing surgical intervention versus patients not undergoing surgical intervention

	No surgical intervention			Surgical intervention (n=467)
Patient characteristics	All patients (n=57)	Subgroup 1 (n=26)	Subgroup 2 (n=24)	
Age in years	83 (75–88)	88 (81–90)	78 (71–82)	76 (69–80)
Male: female	74 %:26 % (42:15)	19 %:81 % (21:5)	25 %:75 % (18:6)	81 %:19 % (378:89)
Previous history of cardiac disease	52 % (25/48)	60 % (15/25)	44 % (7/16)	41 % (193/452)
Previous history of cerebrovascular disease	15 % (7/48)	16 % (4/25)	19 % (3/16)	15 % (69/451)
Previously diagnosed with AAA	16 % (8/49)	19 % (5/26)	13 % (2/16)	NA
Referred from other hospital	11 % (6/57)	19 % (5/26)	0	30 % (140/467)
Systolic blood pressure in the ER in mmHg	90 (50–120)	115 (90–140)	50 (0–64)	106 (80–132)
Cardiopulmonary resuscitation	40 % (23/57)	0	96 % (23/24)	10 % (48/447)
Haemoglobin in the ER in mmol/L	6.9 (5.6–7.6)	7.2 (6.2–7.9)	6.6 (4.9–7.5)	7 (5.9–8.0)
Creatinine in the ER in μmol/L	130 (90–188)	125 (93–187)	131 (95–183)	107 (87–134)
CTA made	49 % (28/57)	77 % (20/26)	13 % (3/24)	82 % (385/467)

van Beek et al. [107]

Continuous data are presented as median (interquartile range) and categorical data as percentage (number). Subgroup 1 included patients not treated because of patient decision, comorbidity, age, or aortic anatomical considerations, and subgroup 2 included patients with cardiopulmonary resuscitation (CPR) and patients with shock as reason for not intervening

CTA computed tomographic Angiography, *NA* not available

Turndown Rate for rAAA

It is also important to know the turndown rate, for those who make it to the hospital with a rAAA but do not get an operation, especially when comparing in-hospital mortality rates between studies. In the Reimerink et al. meta-analysis, the pooled turndown rate for rAAA was 40 % although this reduced over time from 46 % before 1990 to 26 % after 1990 [1]. What cannot be deduced from this study is why someone did not get an intervention. Possible reasons include patient/family choice, some may be considered too hemodynamically or medically compromised on arrival such that operation was thought futile by the surgeon, or inadequate infrastructure/staff on-site to expeditiously triage and treat the rAAA. Van Beek et al. attempted to answer this question by describing characteristics of patients who did not receive intervention, stratified into no intervention by patient choice, age, or comorbidity burden versus too clinically unfit, defined as needing CPR or in shock [107]. Table 3.2 shows these

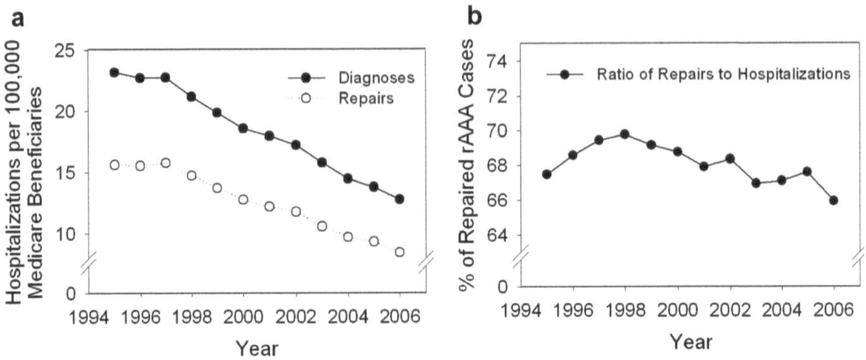

Fig. 3.15 Trends in the (**a**) hospitalizations with diagnosis (*black circles*) and repairs (*white circles*) of rAAA and (**b**) ratio of repairs to hospitalizations with rAAA diagnosis among Medicare beneficiaries from 1995 through 2006 (Mureebe et al. [25])

groups compared to a surgical intervention group; notably only a small percentage of both rupture subgroups actually had known aneurysms. Only half of those turned down were hemodynamically unstable, while the mean age was 88 for those turned down who did not have hemodynamic compromise on admission. A subset of hemodynamically stable patients with a 98 % (95 % CI 89–100 %) 2-h survival were also identified, highlighting the point that not all rAAAs are the same. This is important when evaluating the safety of referral for rAAA patients to tertiary centers and also for the development of systems and protocols for managing rAAA.

The turndown rate in the USA has been relatively stable. Our analysis of Medicare data from 1995 to 2008 demonstrated a relatively steady intervention rate of 68 % for those admitted with rAAA, in the setting of a decreasing incidence of rAAA [4, 25]. This steady turndown rate has been shown in other national datasets in the USA, although none have data beyond 2008, as rEVAR was starting to gain acceptance, and it is our suspicion that this turndown rate may now be lower (Fig. 3.15) [25, 36]. Reasons for this include more centers becoming facile and having around-the-clock facilities to use rEVAR and subsequently becoming more aggressive in their attempts to save the patient with a rAAA. Studies have demonstrated that a more aggressive intervention practice improves mortality from rAAA [39, 108]. Amsterdam, in the setting of an ongoing RCT for intervention on rAAA, has a contemporary turndown rate of 12 % [107]. There is variation in turndown rates across geographic regions. Karthikesalingam reported that the difference in in-hospital mortality from rAAA between the USA and England from 2005 to 2010 was entirely due to a difference in turndown rates [40].

The optimal intervention rate is unknown and is subjective. Such a topic requires cost-effectiveness analysis and input from all stakeholders, which is not the focus of this chapter, but needs to be considered from a policy and hospital standpoint as we move forward. What is important to remember is that the intervention rate will have a big impact on the mortality for a given study, and so care should be taken when comparing results across studies, especially if the turndown rate is not given.

In-Hospital and Perioperative Mortality for rAAA

The Reimerink et al. meta-analysis gives one of the most complete and contemporary insights into overall mortality trends for rAAA [1]. The pooled total mortality was shown to decrease over time in high-quality studies, from 86 % (95 % CI 83–89 %) before 1990 to 74 % (72–77 %) after 1990, with the trend line demonstrated in Fig. 3.14. Pooled perioperative mortality also decreased from 57 % (52–63 %) to 49 % (45–55 %) over this same time period, despite the fact that the intervention rate for rAAA had increased.

The Vascunet report from 2005 to 2009, which included nine countries, eight European and Australia, identified 40,848 primary AAA repairs, 18.3 % of which were performed for rupture (range 9–30.9 % by country) [41]. No overall rAAA mortality rate was quoted, as this study was not set up to do so, but the perioperative mortality for rAAA was 31.6 % (range 27–39 % by country) and decreased over time.

In the USA a similar decline in mortality from rAAA has been seen. Estimates from our analysis of the National Inpatient Sample (NIS), which compared aggregate rates between 1993–1999 and 2000–2005, showed that the diagnosis of rAAA decreased by 30 %, the intervention rate remained constant at 63 %, and the perioperative mortality decreased from 44.3 to 40.8 % [36]. Interestingly, the in-hospital mortality of the no-intervention group was 68 %, which is lower than expected with rAAA and could represent coding inaccuracy or patients being transferred to tertiary care centers or to hospice. NIS is only able to give in-hospital mortality, and so to analyze additional patient variables and 30-day mortality, we performed a follow-up study using the Medicare population from 1995 to 2008 [4]. In this study we found that hospital admissions for rAAA decreased from 33.4 to 16.8 per 100,000 Medicare beneficiaries, 30-day mortality decreased from 20.2 to 9.1 per 100,000, and the 30-day mortality rate fell from 44.1 to 36.3 %. The reduction seen in overall and in-hospital rAAA mortality, further illustrated with data from the CDC, is likely multifactorial (Fig. 3.16). First, our group showed that the greatest reduction in rAAA mortality occurred in the >80-year-old population, which coincided with a similar increase in elective EVAR for the same age group. Despite this temporal relationship, some argue that increasing elective EVAR repair was unlikely to represent a major reason for this reduction as the downtrend in rAAA mortality was noted before EVAR's FDA approval. However, prior to FDA approval, patients unfit for open repair, the majority of whom would be at high risk for rupture, were being enrolled in clinical trials with EVAR and likely were the reason for this pre-FDA approval decrease in mortality. Another important contributing factor to the decrease in incidence of rAAA is the reduction in risk factors, smoking in particular [22]. However, a more gradual rather than sudden change in all short-term AAA and rAAA-related deaths after 1997, as seen in Fig. 3.13, would be expected if smoking were the only major reason.

The decline in perioperative mortality for rAAA points to the added benefit of rEVAR. Contributing to this is the maturation of rEVAR technology and clinician

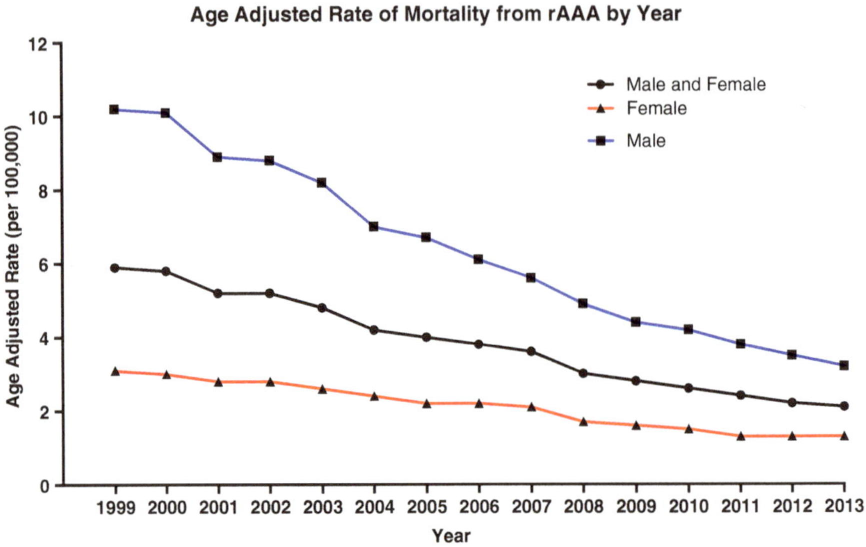

Fig. 3.16 Age-adjusted mortality rates for the over-44-year-old population in the USA from 1999 to 2013 (From Centers for Disease Control and Prevention, National Center for Health Statistics: Compressed Mortality File 1999–2013. CDC WONDER Online Database, compiled from Compressed Mortality File 1999–2013 Series 20 No. 2S, 2014, as compiled from data provided by the 57 vital statistics jurisdictions through the Vital Statistics Cooperative Program. Accessed at http://wonder.cdc.gov/cmf-icd10.html on May 29, 2015 12:44:04 PM)

skills, and more recently systems preparedness programs to expedite care for these patients [24, 38, 109, 110]. Such system improvements can also improve the mortality of open rAAA by expediting multidisciplinary care and resuscitation. Furthermore, perioperative mortality has declined in the setting of at least stable if not higher intervention rates, which is opposite of what one would expect if more aggressive care is being pursued in a highly lethal condition, further endorsing rEVAR use. Our group has shown the clear reduction in mortality from ruptured AAA in the era of EVAR; see Fig. 3.11.

rEVARs Role in rAAA Mortality

The Food and Drug Administration-approved EVAR in 1999 in the USA after pivotal studies from Aneurx and Ancure showed lower mortality than open repair [111, 112]. Multiple randomized controlled trials from Europe confirmed the perioperative benefit followed by our nonrandomized Medicare study, which showed these results were generalizable broadly in the USA, and then the OVER RCT was published from the USA [113–116]. Subsequent to this, long-term results from each of these studies were published showing more equivocal long-term outcomes between EVAR

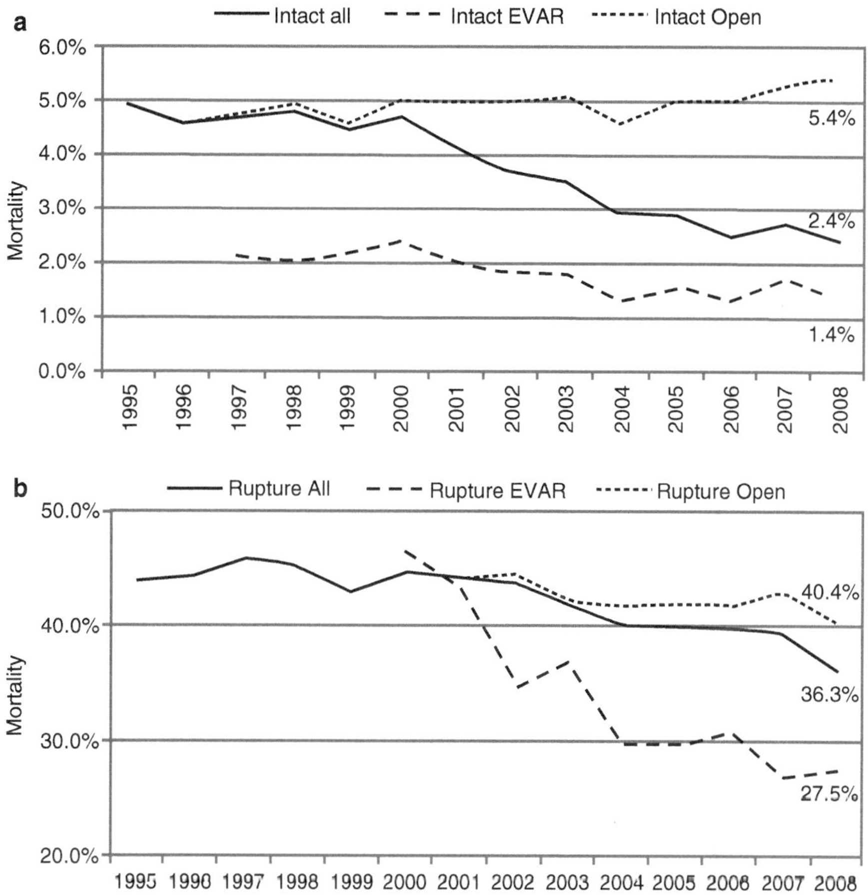

Fig. 3.17 Operative mortality for EVAR, open repair, and total AAA repairs for US Medicare beneficiaries, 1995-2008. (**a**) Intact AAA and (**b**) ruptured AAA (Schermerhorn et al. [4])

and open surgery for elective AAA repair [33–35, 117]. The use of EVAR for rAAA lagged behind elective repair, but by 2008 it was being performed in 31 % of rAAA in the Medicare population [4]. From this Medicare study, we showed that for the first time in decades total operative mortality for rAAA declined as EVAR utilization rose (Fig. 3.17). It is important to note that open operative mortality did not rise during the same time period, thus disputing claims that the more stable and healthy patients were simply being selected for rEVAR. Early retrospective analysis of rEVAR versus open repair further supported this reduction in 30-day mortality [39, 42, 118]. Multiple studies suggested that rEVAR had fewer adverse effects on the cardiac, respiratory, and renal systems and therefore should be better for rAAA than open repair [119–121]. This led to the initiation of RCTs, which have shown less convincing results, but there have also been a number of criticisms of the methods in these studies. Please see Chaps. 4 and 5 for a full discussion of these trials [46, 122].

Long-term outcomes are also important when comparing rEVAR to open repair, as comparison in the elective setting has shown. Our group, using a propensity score-matched cohort of Medicare patients from 2001 to 2008, showed that rEVAR had a survival benefit out to 4 years compared to open repair of rAAA [42]. In addition, a meta-analysis of three RCTs comparing rEVAR to open surgical repair showed a non-significant trend for lower mortality with rEVAR at 1 year and suggested a wider adoption of rEVAR [123]. For many, including the authors, data are strongly suggestive of a benefit to rEVAR, and we will continue to aggressively try to place EVAR for most rAAA. We will also continue to use femoral sheath placement in the awake patient for fluoroscopy-guided balloon control of the aorta, for open repair patients, to avoid hemodynamic instability that often occurs with induction of anesthesia and laparotomy.

Turndown Rates for Elective Repair and Its Effects on rAAA

Patients turned down for elective AAA repair are at higher risk for rupture. It is estimated that in the USA up to 13 % of patients presenting with an AAA will fall into the category of aneurysm >5.5 cm and considered unfit for elective repair [59, 124]. This turndown number is higher in other parts of the world [40]. In the EVAR 2 RCT, which compared EVAR versus nonoperative management for patients unfit for open repair with aneurysms of 5.5 cm or larger, two of the total 172 patients ruptured in the nonoperative group [125]. Even in those randomized to EVAR, 3 of 166 patients had rupture prior to repair (see Chaps. 4 and 5 for detailed discussion). A subsequent meta-analysis further analyzed the fate of patients unfit for elective repair and reported a rupture rate of 5.3 % (95 % CI 3.1–7.5 %) per year [58]. Out of those who did rupture, 32 % received an operation with an overall 58 % perioperative mortality. Rupture rate was likely underestimated as this meta-analysis did not exclude 173 of the 228 patients who crossed over to repair after becoming symptomatic or eligible for repair. It is also lower than reported previously from the 1970s to 1990s, which ranged from 9.4 to 40 % per year for aneurysms >6.0 cm [126, 127]. The definition of medically unfit is not standardized, and so interpretation of these data should be made with caution.

The above meta-analysis stratified risk of rupture by aneurysm size, and so it is possible that a treating clinician could move someone from medically unfit to fit if the benefits of repair begin to outweigh the risks of operation based on aneurysm diameter changes [58]. This size stratification may also help patients and families in their decision-making and goals of care. Careful consideration should be made about what an acceptable elective turndown rate should be, knowing that this population is more likely to return to the hospital with a rAAA.

Conclusion

rAAA is still a highly lethal entity, but over the past one to two decades, we have made significant improvements in rAAA mortality. There has been a decrease in the incidence of rAAA, related to decreases in the prevalence of AAA disease secondary to reduction of risk factors, primarily smoking, as well as an increase in elective treatment of the elderly patients with EVAR who in the past would not have been good candidates for open repair. Along with this, there has been a steady increase in the use of advanced abdominal imaging and more recently the institution of screening programs. As a result, there has been a decline in the overall mortality from rAAA. Our current numbers for total mortality cannot accurately estimate pre-hospital mortality from rAAA, secondary to low autopsy rates, but estimates have been relatively precise from population-based studies, so it is reasonable to extrapolate from hospital admission data the overall mortality rate. Also, alongside the reduction in overall mortality from rAAA, there has been a reduction in perioperative mortality despite steady to possibly decreasing turndown rates. This coincides with heavier adoption of rEVAR and, more recently, systems to expedite the care of those with rAAA, both of which have shown improvements in perioperative mortality.

References

1. Reimerink JJ, et al. Systematic review and meta-analysis of population-based mortality from ruptured abdominal aortic aneurysm. Br J Surg. 2013;100(11):1405–13.
2. Reite A, et al. Epidemiology of ruptured abdominal aortic aneurysms in a well-defined Norwegian population with trends in incidence, intervention rate, and mortality. J Vasc Surg. 2015;61(5):1168–74.
3. Sachs T, Schermerhorn M. Ruptured abdominal aortic aneurysm. Minerva Chir. 2010; 65(3):303–17.
4. Schermerhorn ML, et al. Changes in abdominal aortic aneurysm rupture and short-term mortality, 1995–2008: a retrospective observational study. Ann Surg. 2012;256(4):651–8.
5. Norman PE, Spilsbury K, Semmens JB. Falling rates of hospitalization and mortality from abdominal aortic aneurysms in Australia. J Vasc Surg. 2011;53(2):274–7.
6. Hadjibashi AA, et al. Decreases in diameters of treated abdominal aortic aneurysms and reduction in rupture rate. JAMA Surg. 2013;148(1):72–5.
7. Lee AM, Chaikof EL. Is the abdominal aortic aneurysm rupture rate decreasing? Adv Surg. 2013;47:271–86.
8. Nedeau AE, et al. Endovascular vs open repair for ruptured abdominal aortic aneurysm. J Vasc Surg. 2012;56(1):15–20.
9. Bown MJ, et al. A meta-analysis of 50 years of ruptured abdominal aortic aneurysm repair. Br J Surg. 2002;89(6):714–30.
10. Visser P, Akkersdijk GJ, Blankensteijn JD. In-hospital operative mortality of ruptured abdominal aortic aneurysm: a population-based analysis of 5593 patients in The Netherlands over a 10-year period. Eur J Vasc Endovasc Surg. 2005;30(4):359–64.
11. Heller JA, et al. Two decades of abdominal aortic aneurysm repair: have we made any progress? J Vasc Surg. 2000;32(6):1091–100.
12. Brock RC. The life and work of Sir Astley Cooper. Ann R Coll Surg Engl. 1969;44(1):1–18.
13. Matas R. Ligation of the abdominal aorta: report of the ultimate result, one year, five months and nine days after ligation of the abdominal aorta for aneurism at the bifurcation. Ann Surg. 1925;81(2):457–64.
14. Cervantes J. Reflections on the 50th anniversary of the first abdominal aortic aneurysm resection. World J Surg. 2003;27(2):246–8.
15. Cooley DA, Debakey ME. Ruptured aneurysms of abdominal aorta; excision and homograft replacement. Postgrad Med. 1954;16(4):334–42.

16. Blakemore AH, Voorhees Jr AB. The use of tubes constructed from vinyon N cloth in bridging arterial defects; experimental and clinical. Ann Surg. 1954;140(3):324–34.
17. Parodi JC, Palmaz JC, Barone HD. Transfemoral intraluminal graft implantation for abdominal aortic aneurysms. Ann Vasc Surg. 1991;5(6):491–9.
18. Yusuf SW, et al. Emergency endovascular repair of leaking aortic aneurysm. Lancet. 1994;344(8937):1645.
19. Drott C, et al. Age-standardized incidence of ruptured aortic aneurysm in a defined Swedish population between 1952 and 1988: mortality rate and operative results. Br J Surg. 1992;79(2):175–9.
20. Bengtsson H, Bergqvist D. Ruptured abdominal aortic aneurysm: a population-based study. J Vasc Surg. 1993;18(1):74–80.
21. Acosta S, et al. Increasing incidence of ruptured abdominal aortic aneurysm: a population-based study. J Vasc Surg. 2006;44(2):237–43.
22. Anjum A, Powell JT. Is the incidence of abdominal aortic aneurysm declining in the 21st century? Mortality and hospital admissions for England & Wales and Scotland. Eur J Vasc Endovasc Surg. 2012;43(2):161–6.
23. Anjum A, et al. Explaining the decrease in mortality from abdominal aortic aneurysm rupture. Br J Surg. 2012;99(5):637–45.
24. Prevention CfDCa, National Center for Health Statistics: Compressed Mortality File 1999–2013. CDC WONDER Online Database, compiled from Compressed Mortality File 1999–2013 Series 20 No. 2S, 2014, as compiled from data provided by the 57 vitals statistics jurisdictions through the Vital Statistics Cooperative Program. 2014.
25. Mureebe L, et al. National trends in the repair of ruptured abdominal aortic aneurysms. J Vasc Surg. 2008;48(5):1101–7.
26. Blanchard JF. Epidemiology of abdominal aortic aneurysms. Epidemiol Rev. 1999;21(2):207–21.
27. Eickhoff JH. Incidence of diagnosis, operation and death from abdominal aortic aneurysms in Danish hospitals: results from a nation-wide survey, 1977–1990. Eur J Surg. 1993;159(11–12):619–23.
28. Best VA, Price JF, Fowkes FG. Persistent increase in the incidence of abdominal aortic aneurysm in Scotland, 1981–2000. Br J Surg. 2003;90(12):1510–5.
29. Melton 3rd LJ, et al. Changing incidence of abdominal aortic aneurysms: a population-based study. Am J Epidemiol. 1984;120(3):379–86.
30. Svensjo S, et al. Low prevalence of abdominal aortic aneurysm among 65-year-old Swedish men indicates a change in the epidemiology of the disease. Circulation. 2011;124(10):1118–23.
31. Lederle FA. The rise and fall of abdominal aortic aneurysm. Circulation. 2011;124(10):1097–9.
32. Xiao J, et al. The impact of declining clinical autopsy: need for revised healthcare policy. Am J Med Sci. 2009;337(1):41–6.
33. De Bruin JL, et al. Long-term outcome of open or endovascular repair of abdominal aortic aneurysm. N Engl J Med. 2010;362(20):1881–9.
34. United Kingdom ETI, et al. Endovascular versus open repair of abdominal aortic aneurysm. N Engl J Med. 2010;362(20):1863–71.
35. Schermerhorn ML, et al. Long-term outcomes of abdominal aortic aneurysm in the medicare population. N Engl J Med. 2015;373(4):328–38.
36. Giles KA, et al. Decrease in total aneurysm-related deaths in the era of endovascular aneurysm repair. J Vasc Surg. 2009;49(3):543–50; discussion 550–1.
37. Starnes BW, et al. Management of ruptured abdominal aortic aneurysm in the endovascular era. J Vasc Surg. 2010;51(1):9–17; discussion 17–8.
38. Mehta M, et al. Establishing a protocol for endovascular treatment of ruptured abdominal aortic aneurysms: outcomes of a prospective analysis. J Vasc Surg. 2006;44(1):1–8; discussion 8.
39. Mayer D, et al. Complete replacement of open repair for ruptured abdominal aortic aneurysms by endovascular aneurysm repair: a two-center 14-year experience. Ann Surg. 2012;256(5):688–95; discussion 695–6.

40. Karthikesalingam A, et al. Mortality from ruptured abdominal aortic aneurysms: clinical lessons from a comparison of outcomes in England and the USA. Lancet. 2014;383(9921): 963–9.
41. Mani K, et al. Treatment of abdominal aortic aneurysm in nine countries 2005–2009: a vascunet report. Eur J Vasc Endovasc Surg. 2011;42(5):598–607.
42. Edwards ST, et al. Comparative effectiveness of endovascular versus open repair of ruptured abdominal aortic aneurysm in the Medicare population. J Vasc Surg. 2014;59(3):575–82.
43. Mehta M, et al. Endovascular repair of ruptured infrarenal abdominal aortic aneurysm is associated with lower 30-day mortality and better 5-year survival rates than open surgical repair. J Vasc Surg. 2013;57(2):368–75.
44. Investigators It, et al. Observations from the IMPROVE trial concerning the clinical care of patients with ruptured abdominal aortic aneurysm. Br J Surg. 2014;101(3):216–24; discussion 224.
45. Hinchliffe RJ, et al. A randomised trial of endovascular and open surgery for ruptured abdominal aortic aneurysm - results of a pilot study and lessons learned for future studies. Eur J Vasc Endovasc Surg. 2006;32(5):506–13; discussion 514–5.
46. Ambler GK, et al. Survival following ruptured abdominal aortic aneurysm before and during the IMPROVE Trial: a single-centre series. Eur J Vasc Endovasc Surg. 2014;47(4):388–93.
47. Candell L, et al. Early and delayed rupture after endovascular abdominal aortic aneurysm repair in a 10-year multicenter registry. J Vasc Surg. 2014;60(5):1146–52.
48. Wyss TR, et al. Rate and predictability of graft rupture after endovascular and open abdominal aortic aneurysm repair: data from the EVAR Trials. Ann Surg. 2010;252(5):805–12.
49. Mehta M, et al. Treatment options for delayed AAA rupture following endovascular repair. J Vasc Surg. 2011;53(1):14–20.
50. Brewster DC, et al. Long-term outcomes after endovascular abdominal aortic aneurysm repair: the first decade. Ann Surg. 2006;244(3):426–38.
51. Hinnen JW, et al. Aneurysm sac pressure after EVAR: the role of endoleak. Eur J Vasc Endovasc Surg. 2007;34(4):432–41; discussion 442–3.
52. Szilagyi DE, et al. Contribution of abdominal aortic aneurysmectomy to prolongation of life. Ann Surg. 1966;164(4):678–99.
53. Darling RC, et al. Autopsy study of unoperated abdominal aortic aneurysms. The case for early resection. Circulation. 1977;56(3 Suppl):II161–4.
54. Sterpetti AV, et al. Factors influencing the rupture of abdominal aortic aneurysms. Surg Gynecol Obstet. 1991;173(3):175–8.
55. Mortality results for randomised controlled trial of early elective surgery or ultrasonographic surveillance for small abdominal aortic aneurysms. The UK Small Aneurysm Trial Participants. Lancet. 1998;352(9141):1649–55.
56. Brown LC, Powell JT. Risk factors for aneurysm rupture in patients kept under ultrasound surveillance. UK Small Aneurysm Trial Participants. Ann Surg. 1999;230(3):289–96; discussion 296–7.
57. Reed WW, et al. Learning from the last ultrasound. A population-based study of patients with abdominal aortic aneurysm. Arch Intern Med. 1997;157(18):2064–8.
58. Parkinson F, et al. Rupture rates of untreated large abdominal aortic aneurysms in patients unfit for elective repair. J Vasc Surg. 2015;61(6):1606–12.
59. Karthikesalingam A, et al. The fate of patients referred to a specialist vascular unit with large infra-renal abdominal aortic aneurysms over a two-year period. Eur J Vasc Endovasc Surg. 2011;42(3):295–301.
60. Vorp DA, Raghavan ML, Webster MW. Mechanical wall stress in abdominal aortic aneurysm: influence of diameter and asymmetry. J Vasc Surg. 1998;27(4):632–9.
61. Hunter GC, et al. Incidence and histologic characteristics of blebs in patients with abdominal aortic aneurysms. J Vasc Surg. 1996;24(1):93–101.
62. Fillinger MF, et al. Prediction of rupture risk in abdominal aortic aneurysm during observation: wall stress versus diameter. J Vasc Surg. 2003;37(4):724–32.

63. Venkatasubramaniam AK, et al. A comparative study of aortic wall stress using finite element analysis for ruptured and non-ruptured abdominal aortic aneurysms. Eur J Vasc Endovasc Surg. 2004;28(2):168–76.
64. Fillinger MF, et al. In vivo analysis of mechanical wall stress and abdominal aortic aneurysm rupture risk. J Vasc Surg. 2002;36(3):589–97.
65. Fillinger MF, et al. Anatomic characteristics of ruptured abdominal aortic aneurysm on conventional CT scans: implications for rupture risk. J Vasc Surg. 2004;39(6):1243–52.
66. Powell JT, et al. Systematic review and meta-analysis of growth rates of small abdominal aortic aneurysms. Br J Surg. 2011;98(5):609–18.
67. Speelman L, et al. The mechanical role of thrombus on the growth rate of an abdominal aortic aneurysm. J Vasc Surg. 2010;51(1):19–26.
68. Vorp DA, et al. Association of intraluminal thrombus in abdominal aortic aneurysm with local hypoxia and wall weakening. J Vasc Surg. 2001;34(2):291–9.
69. Hammond EC, Horn D. Smoking and death rates: report on forty-four months of follow-up of 187,783 men. 2. Death rates by cause. J Am Med Assoc. 1958;166(11):1294–308.
70. Lederle FA, et al. The aneurysm detection and management study screening program: validation cohort and final results. Aneurysm Detection and Management Veterans Affairs Cooperative Study Investigators. Arch Intern Med. 2000;160(10):1425–30.
71. Sweeting MJ, et al. Meta-analysis of individual patient data to examine factors affecting growth and rupture of small abdominal aortic aneurysms. Br J Surg. 2012;99(5):655–65.
72. Singh K, et al. Prevalence of and risk factors for abdominal aortic aneurysms in a population-based study: the Tromso Study. Am J Epidemiol. 2001;154(3):236–44.
73. Giles KA, et al. Population-based outcomes following endovascular and open repair of ruptured abdominal aortic aneurysms. J Endovasc Ther. 2009;16(5):554–64.
74. Howard DP, et al. Age-specific incidence, risk factors and outcome of acute abdominal aortic aneurysms in a defined population. Br J Surg. 2015;102(8):907–15.
75. Cambria RA, et al. Symptomatic, nonruptured abdominal aortic aneurysms: are emergent operations necessary? Ann Vasc Surg. 1994;8(2):121–6.
76. Sullivan CA, Rohrer MJ, Cutler BS. Clinical management of the symptomatic but unruptured abdominal aortic aneurysm. J Vasc Surg. 1990;11(6):799–803.
77. Franks S, et al. Endovascular treatment of ruptured and symptomatic abdominal aortic aneurysms. Eur J Vasc Endovasc Surg. 2006;31(4):345–50.
78. De Martino RR, et al. Outcomes of symptomatic abdominal aortic aneurysm repair. J Vasc Surg. 2010;52(1):5–12. e1.
79. Lederle FA, et al. Abdominal aortic aneurysm in women. J Vasc Surg. 2001;34(1):122–6.
80. Johnston KW. Influence of sex on the results of abdominal aortic aneurysm repair. Canadian Society for Vascular Surgery Aneurysm Study Group. J Vasc Surg. 1994;20(6):914–23; discussion 923–6.
81. Dillavou ED, Muluk SC, Makaroun MS. A decade of change in abdominal aortic aneurysm repair in the United States: have we improved outcomes equally between men and women? J Vasc Surg. 2006;43(2):230–8; discussion 238.
82. Sonesson B, et al. Compliance and diameter in the human abdominal aorta–the influence of age and sex. Eur J Vasc Surg. 1993;7(6):690–7.
83. Matyal R, et al. Impact of gender and body surface area on outcome after abdominal aortic aneurysm repair. Am J Surg. 2015;209(2):315–23.
84. Lo RC, et al. Relative importance of aneurysm diameter and body size for predicting abdominal aortic aneurysm rupture in men and women. J Vasc Surg. 2014;59(5):1209–16.
85. Davies RR, et al. Novel measurement of relative aortic size predicts rupture of thoracic aortic aneurysms. Ann Thorac Surg. 2006;81(1):169–77.
86. U.S. Preventive Services Task Force. Screening for abdominal aortic aneurysm: recommendation statement. Ann Intern Med. 2005;142(3):198–202.
87. Wanhainen A, et al. Cost-effectiveness of screening women for abdominal aortic aneurysm. J Vasc Surg. 2006;43(5):908–14; discussion 914.

88. McPhee JT, Hill JS, Eslami MH. The impact of gender on presentation, therapy, and mortality of abdominal aortic aneurysm in the United States, 2001–2004. J Vasc Surg. 2007;45(5):891–9.
89. Lo RC, et al. Gender differences in abdominal aortic aneurysm presentation, repair, and mortality in the Vascular Study Group of New England. J Vasc Surg. 2013;57(5):1261–8. 1268.e1–5.
90. Cronenwett JL, et al. Actuarial analysis of variables associated with rupture of small abdominal aortic aneurysms. Surgery. 1985;98(3):472–83.
91. Darling 3rd RC, et al. Are familial abdominal aortic aneurysms different? J Vasc Surg. 1989;10(1):39–43.
92. Verloes A, et al. Aneurysms of the abdominal aorta: familial and genetic aspects in three hundred thirteen pedigrees. J Vasc Surg. 1995;21(4):646–55.
93. Joergensen TM, et al. Abdominal aortic diameter is increased in males with a family history of abdominal aortic aneurysms: results from the Danish VIVA-trial. Eur J Vasc Endovasc Surg. 2014;48(6):669–75.
94. Reed D, et al. Are aortic aneurysms caused by atherosclerosis? Circulation. 1992;85(1):205–11.
95. Strachan DP. Predictors of death from aortic aneurysm among middle-aged men: the Whitehall study. Br J Surg. 1991;78(4):401–4.
96. Pepin MG, Byers PH. Ehlers-Danlos syndrome type IV. In: GeneReviews(R). Pagon, RA et al., editors. Seattle (WA): University of Washington; 1993.
97. Muller BT, et al. Mycotic aneurysms of the thoracic and abdominal aorta and iliac arteries: experience with anatomic and extra-anatomic repair in 33 cases. J Vasc Surg. 2001;33(1):106–13.
98. Oderich GS, et al. Infected aortic aneurysms: aggressive presentation, complicated early outcome, but durable results. J Vasc Surg. 2001;34(5):900–8.
99. Takano H, et al. Mycotic aneurysm of the infrarenal abdominal aorta infected by Clostridium septicum: a case report of surgical management and review of the literature. J Vasc Surg. 2003;38(4):847–51.
100. Alcorn HG, et al. Risk factors for abdominal aortic aneurysms in older adults enrolled in The Cardiovascular Health Study. Arterioscler Thromb Vasc Biol. 1996;16(8):963–70.
101. Smith FC, et al. Ultrasonographic screening for abdominal aortic aneurysm in an urban community. Br J Surg. 1993;80(11):1406–9.
102. Lederle FA, et al. Prevalence and associations of abdominal aortic aneurysm detected through screening. Aneurysm Detection and Management (ADAM) Veterans Affairs Cooperative Study Group. Ann Intern Med. 1997;126(6):441–9.
103. Gillum RF. Epidemiology of aortic aneurysm in the United States. J Clin Epidemiol. 1995;48(11):1289–98.
104. Kent KC, et al. Analysis of risk factors for abdominal aortic aneurysm in a cohort of more than 3 million individuals. J Vasc Surg. 2010;52(3):539–48.
105. Johansson G, Swedenborg J. Ruptured abdominal aortic aneurysms: a study of incidence and mortality. Br J Surg. 1986;73(2):101–3.
106. Shojania KG, Burton EC. The vanishing nonforensic autopsy. N Engl J Med. 2008;358(9):873–5.
107. van Beek SC, Valh AC, Wisselink W, Balm R, Amsterdam Acute Aneurysm Trial Collaborators. Fate of patients unwilling or unsuitable to undergo surgical intervention for a ruptured abdominal aortic aneurysm. Eur J Vasc Endovasc Surg. 2015;49:163–5.
108. Basnyat PS, et al. Mortality from ruptured abdominal aortic aneurysm in Wales. Br J Surg. 1999;86(6):765–70.
109. Mehta M, et al. Ruptured abdominal aortic aneurysm: endovascular program development and results. Semin Vasc Surg. 2010;23(4):206–14.
110. Mehta M. Endovascular aneurysm repair for ruptured abdominal aortic aneurysm: the Albany Vascular Group approach. J Vasc Surg. 2010;52(6):1706–12.
111. Zarins CK, et al. AneuRx stent graft versus open surgical repair of abdominal aortic aneurysms: multicenter prospective clinical trial. J Vasc Surg. 1999;29(2):292–305; discussion 306–8.

112. Moore WS, Brewster DC, Bernhard VM. Aorto-uni-iliac endograft for complex aortoiliac aneurysms compared with tube/bifurcation endografts: results of the EVT/Guidant trials. J Vasc Surg. 2001;33(2 Suppl):S11–20.
113. Greenhalgh RM, et al. Comparison of endovascular aneurysm repair with open repair in patients with abdominal aortic aneurysm (EVAR trial 1), 30-day operative mortality results: randomised controlled trial. Lancet. 2004;364(9437):843–8.
114. Prinssen M, et al. A randomized trial comparing conventional and endovascular repair of abdominal aortic aneurysms. N Engl J Med. 2004;351(16):1607–18.
115. Schermerhorn ML, et al. Endovascular vs. open repair of abdominal aortic aneurysms in the Medicare population. N Engl J Med. 2008;358(5):464–74.
116. Lederle FA, et al. Outcomes following endovascular vs open repair of abdominal aortic aneurysm: a randomized trial. JAMA. 2009;302(14):1535–42.
117. Lederle FA, et al. Long-term comparison of endovascular and open repair of abdominal aortic aneurysm. N Engl J Med. 2012;367(21):1988–97.
118. Lee WA, et al. Impact of endovascular repair on early outcomes of ruptured abdominal aortic aneurysms. J Vasc Surg. 2004;40(2):211–5.
119. Baxendale BR, et al. Haemodynamic and metabolic response to endovascular repair of infrarenal aortic aneurysms. Br J Anaesth. 1996;77(5):581–5.
120. Boyle JR, et al. Improved respiratory function and analgesia control after endovascular AAA repair. J Endovasc Surg. 1997;4(1):62–5.
121. Hinchliffe RJ, Braithwaite BD, Hopkinson BR. The endovascular management of ruptured abdominal aortic aneurysms. Eur J Vasc Endovasc Surg. 2003;25(3):191–201.
122. Reimerink JJ, et al. Endovascular repair versus open repair of ruptured abdominal aortic aneurysms: a multicenter randomized controlled trial. Ann Surg. 2013;258(2):248–56.
123. Sweeting MJ, et al. Ruptured aneurysm trials: the importance of longer-term outcomes and meta-analysis for 1-year mortality. Eur J Vasc Endovasc Surg. 2015. 50(3):297–302.
124. Tambyraja AL, et al. Non-operative management of high-risk patients with abdominal aortic aneurysm. Eur J Vasc Endovasc Surg. 2003;26(4):401–4.
125. Participants Et. Endovascular aneurysm repair and outcome in patients unfit for open repair of abdominal aortic aneurysm (EVAR trial 2): randomised controlled trial. Lancet. 2005;365(9478):2187–92.
126. Szilagyi DE, Elliott JP, Smith RF. Clinical fate of the patient with asymptomatic abdominal aortic aneurysm and unfit for surgical treatment. Arch Surg. 1972;104(4):600–6.
127. Buth J. Endovascular repair of abdominal aortic aneurysms. Results from the EUROSTAR registry. EUROpean collaborators on Stent-graft Techniques for abdominal aortic Aneurysm Repair. Semin Interv Cardiol. 2000;5(1):29–33.

Chapter 4
Pathogenesis of AAA Rupture

Naoki Fujimura and Ronald L. Dalman

Introduction

Mechanisms of abdominal aortic aneurysm degeneration have been the subject of intense investigation over the last 20 years. As noted in Fig. 4.1, the pathogenesis of abdominal aortic aneurysm disease involves a symphony of interactions between genetic risk, environmental exposures, and interplay between aortic mural inflammation, angiogenesis, smooth muscle cell and elastin depletion, wall strain, and dysfunctional and insufficient regenerative responses of the extracellular matrix [1–10] (Table 4.1).

Epidemiologic studies provide an accurate accounting for demographic and environmental risks. Male gender, age, family history, high cholesterol, hypertension and other cardiovascular diseases, increasing years of smoking and number of cigarettes smoked, and excess weight all carried increased risk for abdominal aortic aneurysm (AAA) disease. The presence of diabetes, smoking cessation, modest levels of regular exercise, consumption of nuts, vegetables, and fruits, as well as African American, Hispanic, or Asians descent are all negatively associated with AAA risk [11].

Much less is known, however, regarding the process(es) that promote aneurysmal progression or rupture in existing "atherosclerotic" aneurysms. As noted in Fig. 4.2, 25-year follow-up data from the Chichester screening study in the UK demonstrates that AAA identified at screening followed a bimodal distribution in terms of aortic diameter enlargement in the years following the baseline imaging study. At both the 5–10-year time intervals, a significant percentage of AAA was noted to either enlarge or remain stable over time. The cellular and molecular mechanisms accounting for these different natural histories, subjects of intense investigation over the last few decades, remain obscure.

N. Fujimura, MD, PhD • R.L. Dalman, MD
Division of Vascular Surgery, Stanford University School of Medicine,
Stanford, CA, USA
e-mail: rld@stanford.edu

B.W. Starnes et al. (eds.), *Ruptured Abdominal Aortic Aneurysm*,
DOI 10.1007/978-3-319-23844-9_4

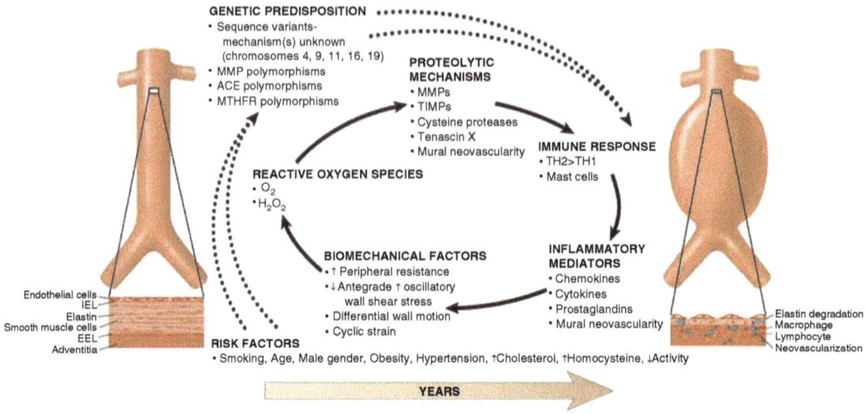

Fig. 4.1 In the setting of specific at-risk haplotypes (such as variability at chromosome 9, p21) and demographic and environmental risks, the interplay of unfavorable hemodynamic influences on expression of reactive oxygen species, proteolytic enzymes, pro-inflammatory immune responses, and mediator production creates conditions for aneurysmal degeneration of the infrarenal aorta, over the course of years to decades (Reproduced from Tedesco and Dalman [91], with permission from Elsevier)

Table 4.1 Results of multivariable regression analysis for predictors of abdominal aortic aneurysm

Variable	Odds ratio	95 % confidence interval	*P* values
Male (vs. female)	5.71	5.57–5.85	<.0001
Age (vs. <55)			
55–59	2.76	2.55–3	<.0001
60–64	5.35	4.97–5.76	<.0001
65–69	9.41	8.76–10.12	<.0001
70–74	14.46	13.45–15.55	<.0001
75–79	20.43	18.99–21.99	<.0001
80–84	28.37	26.31–30.59	<.0001
Race/ethnicity (vs. Caucasian)			
Hispanic	0.69	0.62–0.77	<.0001
African American	0.72	0.66–0.78	<.0001
Asian	0.72	0.59–0.75	<.0001
High blood pressure	1.25	1.21–1.28	<.0001
Coronary artery disease	1.72	1.69–1.76	<.0001
Family history of AAA	3.8	3.66–3.95	<.0001
High cholesterol	1.34	1.31–1.37	<.0001
Diabetes	0.75	0.73–0.77	<.0001
Peripheral arterial disease	1.59	1.54–1.65	<.0001
Carotid disease	1.51	1.46–1.56	<.0001
Cerebrovascular history	1.18	1.14–1.21	<.0001

Table 4.1 (continued)

Variable	Odds ratio	95 % confidence interval	*P* values
Smoking, packs/day			
≤10 years			
<0.5	2.61	2.47–2.74	<.0001
0.5–1	3.19	2.93–3.46	<.0001
>1	3.2	2.88–3.56	<.0001
11–20 years			
<0.5	4.87	4.63–5.12	<.0001
0.5–1	5.79	5.48–6.12	<.0001
>1	6	5.66–6.35	<.0001
21–35 years			
<0.5	7.29	6.97–7.64	<.0001
0.5–1	7.99	7.62–8.38	<.0001
>1	8.41	8.57–9.36	<.0001
>35 years			
<0.5	8.96	8.57–9.36	<.0001
0.5–1	11.19	10.76–11.64	<.0001
>1	12.13	11.66–12.61	<.0001
Quit smoking			
<5 years ago	0.87	0.84–0.912	<.0001
5–10 years ago	0.68	0.65–0.71	<.0001
>10 years ago	0.42	0.41–0.43	<.0001
Fruit and veg. >3 times/week	0.91	0.88–0.92	<.0001
Nuts >3 times/week	0.9	0.89–0.93	<.0001
Exercise ≥1 time/week	0.86	0.85–0.88	<.0001
BMI ≥ 25 kg/m2	1.2	1.17–1.22	<.0001

Reproduced from Kent et al. [11]
BMI body mass index, *CI* confidence interval, *OR* odds ratio, *Veg* vegetable

The term "atherosclerotic" aneurysm is used to distinguish these AAAs from those associated with syndromic (Marfan, Ehlers-Danlos, etc.) or mycotic aortic conditions and recognizes the common risk factors that predispose patients to occlusive or aneurysmal aortic diseases. Despite this shorthand nomenclature, however, the preponderance of available evidence distinguishes aneurysmal and occlusive aortic diseases as distinct entities, each with their own characteristic pathogenic features and natural histories.

Although diameter is the anatomic feature most closely correlated with AAA rupture risk [12], the incidence of rupture varies among series reporting the natural history of large aneurysms not treated due to various circumstances [12–14]. As highlighted by the current Society for Vascular Surgery guidelines regarding AAA disease management, additional circumstances are known or suspected to increase the risk for AAA rupture including saccular vs. fusiform mural contour female gender or rapid

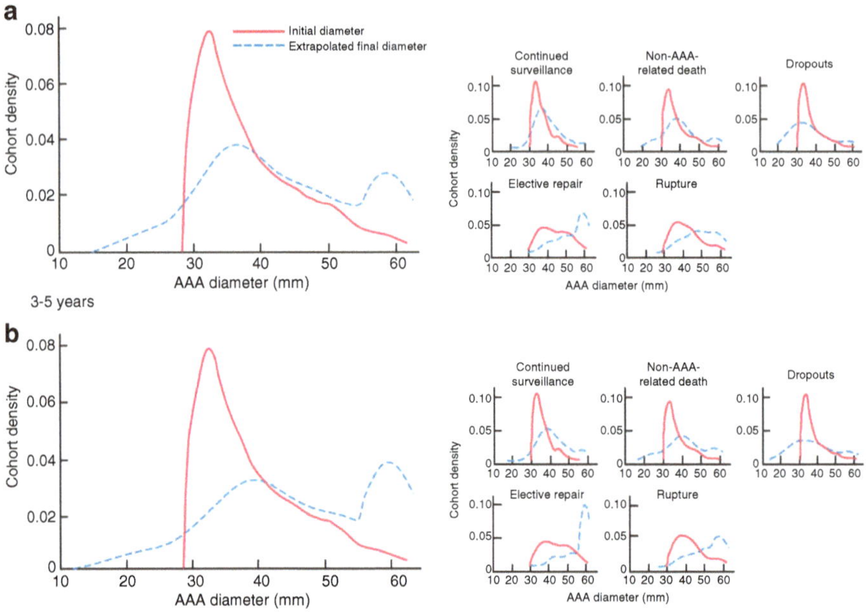

Fig. 4.2 Distribution of initial abdominal aortic aneurysm (AAA) diameters and final diameters at (**a**) 3.5 years and (**b**) 5 years after identification at screening in the Chichester registry. Data shown for the entire cohort and for subjects grouped according to outcome. At both timepoints, only a subset of identified AAAs continue to progress (Reproduced from Thompson et al. [16], with permission from British Journal of Surgery Society)

enlargement at any given diameter, underscoring the reality that additional, still poorly defined, circumstances actually initiate the process of rupture [15]. Female gender, large initial aneurysm diameter, low forced expiratory volume in one second, current smoking history, and elevated mean blood pressure were all identified as specific covariates predicting risk of AAA rupture in the United Kingdom Small Aneurysm trial [16].

The following sections summarize current hypotheses regarding AAA pathogenesis, with particular emphasis on features associated with rupture. Limitations on the latter necessarily stem from the emergent and unpredictable nature of clinical aneurysm progression, limiting access to human AAA tissue immediately preceding the moment of rupture, and the lack of biomarkers or validated animal models to guide mechanistic investigations [17].

Proteolysis and Disease Progression Elastin and collagen type I and III are key structural components of the aortic wall, both extensively investigated in the pathogenesis of AAA disease [6–9, 18–23]. A true pioneer in the field, Phil Dobrin, with colleagues reported that elastin degradation leads to vessel dilation and decreased distensibility, whereas collagen degradation produces greater dilation and ultimate vessel rupture [6, 7]. The accelerated elastin degradation in AAA pathogenesis leads to the phenomenon of collagen loading, where progressively attenuated aortic medial collagen fibers bear a greater share of superimposed hemodynamic strain.

Classification	Trivial Name	Substrates
MMP-1	Collagenase-1	Collagen types I, II, III, VII, VIII, X, gelatin, aggrecan, casein, nidogen, serpins, versican, perlecan, proteoglycan link protein, and tenascin-C
MMP-2	Gelatinase A	Collagen types I, IV, V, VII, X, XI, XIV, gelatin, aggrecan, elastin, fibronectin, laminin, nidogen, proteoglycan link protein, and versican
MMP-3	Stromelysin-1	Collagen types II, IV, IX, X, and gelatin, aggrecan, casein, decorin, elastin, fibronectin, laminin, nidogen, perlecan, proteoglycan, proteoglycan link protein, and versican
MMP-7	Matrillysin-1	Collagen types I, II, III, V, IV, and X, aggrecan, casein, elastin, entactin, laminin, and proteoglycan link protein
MMP-8	Collagenase-2,neutrophil collagenase	Collagen types I, II, III, V, VII, VIII, X, and gelatin, aggrecan, laminin, and nidogen
MMP-9	Gelatinase-B	Collagen types IV, V, VII, X, and XIV, fibronectin, laminin, nidogen, proteoglycan link protein, and versican
MMP-10	Stromelysin-2	Collagen types III, IV, V, and gelatin, fibronectin, laminin, and nidogen
MMP-11	Stromelysin-3	Laminin
MMP-12	Macrophage metalloelastase	Collagen types IV, fibronectin, and elastin; activates pro-MMP-2 and pro-MMP-3
MMP-13	Collagenase-3	Collagen types I, II, III, IV, V, IX, X, XI, and gelatin, aggrecan, fibronectin, laminin, perlecan and tenascin
MMP-14	MT1-MMP	Collagen types I, II, III, and gelatin, aggrecan, dermatan sulphate proteoglycan, fibrin, fibronectin, laminin, nidogen, perlecan, tenascin, and vitronectin; activates pro-MMP-2 and pro-MMP-3
MMP-15	MT2-MMP	Collagen types I, II, III, and gelatin, aggrecan, fibronectin, laminin, nidogen, perlecan, tenascin, and vitronectin; activates pro-MMP-2
MMP-16	MT3-MMP	Collagen types I, III, and gelatin, aggrecan, casein, fibronectin, laminin, perlecan, and vitronectin; activates pro-MMP-2
MMP-17	MT4-MMP	Gelatin, fibrin, fibronectin; activates pro-MMP-2
MMP-24	MT5-MMP	Activates pro-MMP-2
MMP-25	MT6-MMP	Gelatin

Fig. 4.3 Matrix metalloproteinases and their substrates. *MMP* matrix metalloproteinases, *MT* membrane type (Reproduced from Chistiakov et al. [24], with permission from Lippincott Williams & Wilkins)

Degradation of elastin and collagen is primary mediated by proteases expressed by constitutive and infiltrative aortic cells, including matrix metalloproteinases (MMPs), serine proteases, cathepsins, and related enzymes [8, 9]. MMPs are classified according to their substrate specificity [24] (Fig. 4.3). Of the relevant MMPs, many prior studies have suggested a strong relationship between MMP-9 and AAA rupture [18–23]. MMP-9 is primarily expressed from infiltrating macrophages, highlighting the importance of inflammatory rupture pathogenesis [20]. Expression and activity of MMP-2 are also characteristically elevated in both ruptured and non-ruptured AAA tissue [19, 20, 25]; however, MMP-2 may be related more to expansion rather than rupture [21]. Additional MMPs are also elevated in the setting of rupture but with less frequency than MMP-2 and MMP-9 [22, 23].

Tissue inhibitors of metalloproteinases, or TIMPs, are regulatory molecules intimately related to ECM homeostasis and renewal. The role of TIMP activity, or the lack of it, in AAA progression remains uncertain. TIMP-1 binds to MMP-9; this interaction is proposed to be central to the pathological processes of AAA progression [26, 27]. Allaire et al. reported that local overexpression of TIMP-1 prevented AAA rupture in a rat model [18]. Other studies have demonstrated significant endogenous upregulation and expression of TIMP-1 in rat AAA rupture models [28], and no difference was observed in TIMP expression in tissues harvested from ruptured and intact human AAAs [21–23].

Tissue-type plasminogen activator (tPA) and urokinase-type plasminogen activator (uPA) are serine proteases that activate plasminogen and have central roles in blood coagulation and fibrinolysis. In terms of AAA development, Reilly et al. reported that tPA is diffusely present both in the intima and media, and uPA is present only in the infiltrative monocellular cells in the adventitia of the AAA wall [29]. Since plasmin is a potential activator of pro-MMPs [28] and both uPA and tPA can upregulate MMP-2 and MMP-9 [30], uPA and tPA have been reported to contribute to AAA progression [31]. Also, uPA and tPA seem to contribute to the AAA progression through induction of cytokines like IFN-γ, TNF-α, and inflammatory chemokines like monocyte chemoattractant protein-1 (MCP-1) and macrophage inflammatory protein-2 (MIP-2), which lead to monocytes recruitment [30].

There seems to be positive relationship between serine proteases and other related plasminogen activators/inhibitors like plasminogen activator inhibitor-1 (PAI-1) with AAA progression [31], but the effect of serine proteases on AAA rupture has not been investigated thoroughly especially using human AAA tissues [32, 33]. Results from aneurysm models have been mixed [18, 28, 34, 35]. For example, Uchida and associates reported augmented AAA rupture in the angiotensin II infusion in apolipoprotein E-deficient mouse model (Ang II/Apo E -/-) by inhibition of uPA activator in bone-marrow-derived cells [35]. Thus further research is warranted.

Cathepsins are class of lysosomal proteases with high proteolytic activity, also recognized as potential effectors of AAA pathogenesis. Human cathepsins can be classified to B, C, D, F, G, H, K, L, O, S, V, W, and X subtypes, most are either cysteine or aspartic proteases [36]. Expressions of cathepsins in AAA wall and serum are significantly increased compared to control samples [37, 38], and known AAA risk factors such as cigarette smoking, hypertension, and atherosclerosis are all known to induce cathepsin secretion through injury of vascular endothelial cells [36]. Furthermore, pharmacologic cathepsin inhibition inhibits AAA formation in experimental AAA models, reinforcing the potential link to AAA disease [39, 40]. Unfortunately, the role of cathepsins in AAA rupture remains uncertain, however, limited by circumstances similar to those previously discussed.

The concept of progressive aortic mural proteolysis as a modifiable pathogenic mechanism in AAA pathogenesis has been questioned recently on the basis of the Dutch PHAST trial. In this controversial multicenter trial, doxycycline was found to be ineffective in preventing progression of early AAA disease. Rupture, however, was not evaluated as a primary end point [41]. A recent multicenter study (AORTA trial) trialing mast cell inhibitor, which inhibits both MMP-9 and cathepsin G, was also unsuccessful [42]. The work of Shen et al. underscored a potential dual role for MMP-2 in extracellular homeostasis in aneurysm pathogenesis, demonstrating a differential effect of MMP-2 ablation in the progression of thoracic and abdominal disease [43].

Together with the recently reported clinical trial data, these data underscore the complexity of aortic mural homeostasis, and the interplay by which concurrent processes of matrix deposition and degradation occurs. Similar to the concept of autophagy, it is likely that constitutive aortic cells maintain matrix integrity by continuous and concurrent processes of both creation and destruction, and the paucity of medial smooth muscle cell cellularity present in advanced aneurysmal disease leads to progressive deterioration and degeneration of the extracellular matrix (ECM) on the basis of cellular neglect rather than disproportionate proteolysis. Regardless, a larger randomized controlled trial is reexamining the ability of doxycycline, an MMP inhibitor, in limiting progression of early AAA disease (NTA3CT trial, clinicaltrials.gov #NCT01756833). This trial will likely settle the "doxycycline" question once and for all, at least for early (<5 cm in diameter) AAA disease. Remaining to be determined will be the role of proteolysis as a distinct pathogenetic process in AAA disease and whether inhibition with doxycycline can prevent rupture of advanced aneurysms, as the latter are specifically excluded from the study.

Inflammatory Mediators The role of pro-inflammatory chemokines and cytokines expressed by infiltrative inflammatory cells has been extensively investigated in AAA pathogenesis using both human surgical specimens and animal models [1, 2, 4, 44]. For example, the pro-inflammatory cytokine interleukin (IL)-1β is significantly overexpressed in human AAA tissue [45]. Johnston and associates were able to inhibit experimental AAA formation and progression by genetic and pharmacologic inhibition of IL-1β expression [46]. As was the case with MMPs, however, the influence of IL-1β or any specific chemokine/cytokine on AAA rupture remains unknown.

IL-6 is a pro-inflammatory cytokine also known to be overexpressed in explanted human AAA tissue [47]. The importance of IL-6 is underscored by its broad recognition as a systemic marker of increased cardiovascular mortality [48]. Circulating IL-6 levels are increased in ruptured AAA patients compared to patients undergoing elective AAA repair [49, 50]. Similar results have been observed in experimental models of AAA rupture model [28]. Cheuk and associates suggested that since no significant relationship has been recognized between AAA diameter and circulating IL-6 levels, IL-6 may be uniquely related to rupture independent of size [51]. Plasma levels of IL-10, generally recognized as an anti-inflammatory cytokine, have also been demonstrated to be elevated in ruptured AAA patients [50] and are also elevated in animal modeling experiments [28]. Like the MMP-TIMP dyadic, the role of IL- 6 and IL-10 in promoting or preventing aneurysm rupture remains to be defined in higher-fidelity modeling systems yet to be developed.

As to the significance of specific cytokines or chemokines on aneurysm rupture, it remains highly controversial. Wilson and associates reported that tissue (rather than circulating) expression of inflammatory mediators did not differ between intact AAAs and non-ruptured segments of ruptured AAAs, also underscoring the concept that the stimulus for rupture itself, in the advanced but still intact aneurysm, is highly dependent on local (potentially physical) factors. For the record, Wilson et al. also identified lower levels of IL-1β and reduced lymphocyte density at the site of rupture itself vs. intact segments of ruptured AAA. On the basis of their results, these investigators concluded that the biological events leading to AAA rupture may not be dependent on upregulation of the inflammatory process [52]. This observation underscores the growing recognition that processes of aneurysm progression and rupture (as well as initiation) are likely distinct and relatively unique to each respective phase of the disease, and that agents or interventions effective in limiting early or mid-disease progression may not prevent rupture of advanced AAA. A related question remains as to whether the advanced aortic inflammatory response present at the site of rupture precedes the event, or whether inflammation is focally stimulated by the process of rupture itself remains an important area of future investigation.

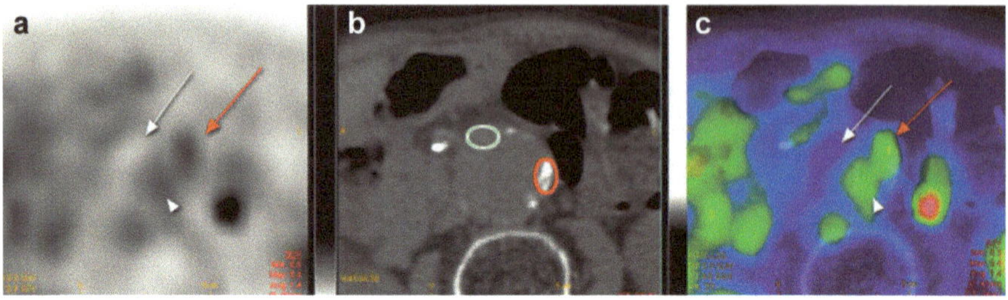

Fig. 4.4 Example of positive ^{18}F-FDG PET/CT representing dense infiltration of leukocytes in the adventitia. (**a**) Transaxial PET (**b**) CT (**c**) fused PET/CT images. *Red arrow*, focus of increased activity; *white arrow*, absence of uptake by thrombus; *arrowhead*, mild uptake by intra-aortic blood pool; *red circle*, intraoperative tissue sampling for positive area; *white circle*, intraoperative tissue sampling for negative area (Reproduced from Courtois et al. [57], with permission from the Society of Nuclear Medicine and Molecular Imaging)

Infiltration of Inflammatory Cells Aortic mural inflammatory cell infiltration, especially the localization of macrophages within the adventitia, is a central pathologic feature of AAA development [2]. Adventitial macrophage density is increased at sites of aortic rupture compared to intact AAA tissue in both clinical [53] and experimental [18, 28] specimens. As previously mentioned, infiltrative inflammatory macrophages (M1 phenotype in the classical characterization) are the predominant source for aortic MMP-9 [20, 54]. These activated macrophages are believed to be strongly related with the pathogenesis of rupture. On the other hand, M2 phenotype macrophages, thought to limit the inflammatory response and promote tissue repair through transforming growth factor-β2 (TGF-β2), may inhibit AAA disease progression [55, 56]. Sakalihasan and associates have demonstrated that inflammatory macrophage localization (as determined by ^{18}F-FDG uptake during positive emission tomography) is characteristic of symptomatic aneurysms and have suggested that this modality may hold promise in predicting impending rupture [57] (Fig. 4.4). Other investigators have failed to identify differences in CD-68- and CD-15-positive cell densities between the site of the rupture and intact AAA wall, however, questioning the broad applicability of macrophage-based molecular imaging strategies in predicting rupture. The recognition that CD-45 cells were less prevalent at the site of rupture again raised the possibility that inflammation itself may be less related to rupture than it is to the process of gradual aneurysm enlargement prior to rupture [23], as previously noted above.

Even less evidence is available for the role of inflammatory cells other than macrophages in AAA rupture. Granulocytes, or neutrophils, are the first cell type to infiltrate thrombus [58], store and release uPA from granules [59], and express MMP-9 in the experimental models of aortic dissection [60]. Increased mural neutrophil infiltration has been observed in experimental models of AAA rupture as well [28]. In human-ruptured AAA tissue, however, a paucity of neutrophils has been identified, highlighting the challenges previously noted in experimental investigations of aneurysm rupture [23, 61]. In summary, although inflammation is unquestionably related to AAA pathogenesis and progression, aortic mural inflammation may be less relevant to the process of aortic tensile failure and rupture in the setting of end-stage disease. Significantly, accelerated AAA progression and rupture have been previously noted in solid organ transplant recipients on massive anti-inflammatory/antirejection medical regimens [62]. Unquestionably, the specific role that inflammatory cells play in precipitating aortic rupture, if any, remains to be determined.

Intraluminal Thrombus The role of intraluminal thrombus (ILT) in promoting or preventing aneurysm rupture has been extensively debated for years [63–65]. Although ILT may reduce AAA wall strain [63], paradoxically advanced ILT has also been associated with accelerated aneurysm enlargement [66]. Empirically, laminar ILT has been shown to induce relative hypoxia in adjacent aortic segments, in turn promoting inflammation [64], MMP-9 activation [26, 67], and downregulation of mural protein synthesis [68]. Many investigators have attempted to draw correlations between ILT burden and deposition pattern and aneurysm size and clinical outcomes based on cross-sectional imaging datasets [65, 69]. However, despite demonstrating a positive correlation between AAA diameter and ILT volume, this ratio was not useful in distinguishing ruptured from intact AAAs, either in clinical series [70] or experimental modeling [28]. Also, Golledge and colleagues recently reported that ILT volume was similar between ruptured and intact AAA [71], making the role of ILT in rupture process even more obscure.

Prediction of Rupture Site Investigators have long recognized that aneurysm rupture occurs most commonly at the retroperitoneum [17, 72], and as originally noted by Darling and associates, ruptures occur more common on the left side of the aorta [17]. ILT, which may contribute to the enlargement of AAA and subsequent rupture [66, 69], accumulates mainly on the anterior aortic wall in mostly asymmetrical patterns, suggesting further influences on rupture risk [70, 73]. Aneurysm morphology, in addition to size, thus likely plays a role as well. Wall strain, related to local hemodynamic factors, may accelerate degradation or precipitate tensile failure of the weakened but still intact aortic wall and seems to correlate in several series to the subsequent risk for aortic rupture [74–76].

Attempts to predict site and likelihood of rupture based on calculated peak wall stress have shown some promises in their early iterations [75–77] (Fig. 4.5). However, efforts to translate these methodologies into clinical practice have proven difficult, since finite element structural analysis used to calculate wall stress is inherently limited by estimations of biological and biomechanical factors, such as elastic properties of the aorta, hemodynamic factors, and patient-specific morphologic features. Recently, Boyd and associates used computational fluid dynamic approach to correlate hemodynamic stress and resulting wall strain, with the site of rupture, and found that rupture occurred not at the sites of high pressure and wall shear stress but at the locations with low wall shear stress and predominant thrombus disposition [78] (Fig. 4.6). Rupture at the low stress region was also reported by Koncar and associates [79]. These reports underscore the importance of incorporating

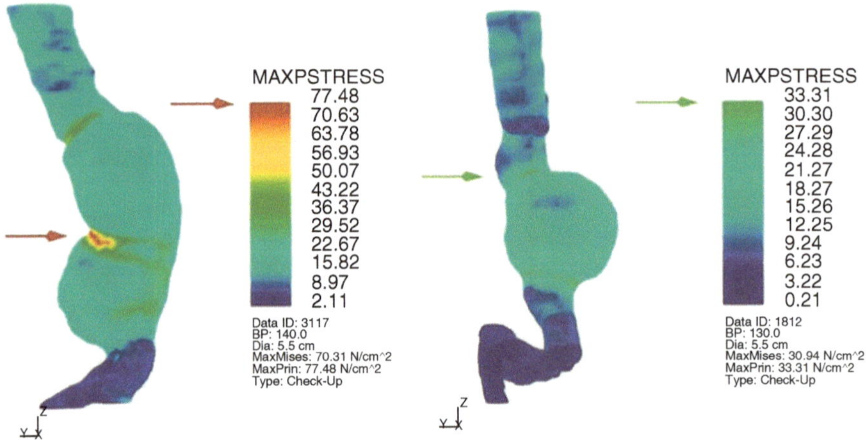

Fig. 4.5 Example of three-dimensional stress distribution mapped by color (*red*, highest; *blue*, lowest) for maximum wall stress at peak systolic blood pressure (Reproduced from Fillinger et al. [75], with permission from the Society for Vascular Surgery)

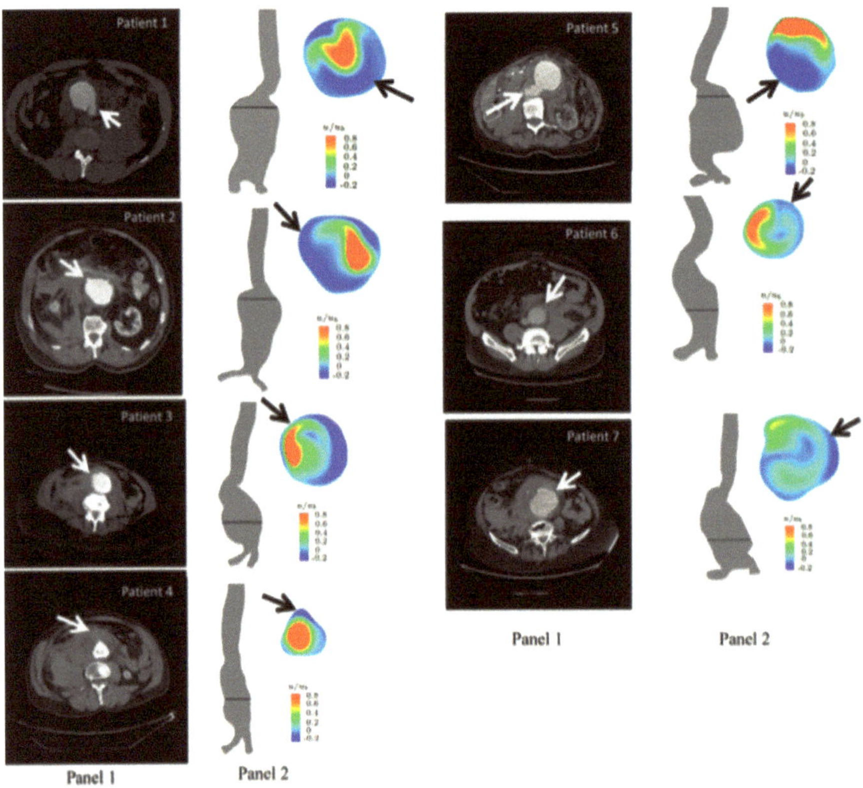

Fig. 4.6 CTA images contrasted with normalized velocity profiles (*high, red*; *low, blue*) showing the nature of flow at the site of rupture (*white* and *black* arrow). Velocity data corresponds with wall shear stress indicating most of the rupture occurring at the site of low wall shear stress (Reproduced from Boyd et al. [78], with permission from Society for Vascular Surgery)

biological and biomechanical factors into consideration for the prediction of rupture risk and localization [80–83].

As the surgical risk for AAA repair has decreased significantly in the endovascular era [84], the clinical utility of predicting rupture, or even elucidating the mechanisms that predispose to rupture, has been substantially reduced. If all or most aneurysms can be safely repaired at earlier stages of the disease, even in patients with substantial comorbidities, what is the relative clinical utility in predicting rupture of advanced disease? As previously emphasized, medical therapies directed at preventing aneurysm progression may not translate to preventing rupture in advanced disease. Given the increasingly prevailing perception that aneurysm rupture may represent the ultimate tensile failure of the atretic and acellular advanced aneurysm, it may be true that no medical intervention short of repopulating medial smooth muscle cells may reduce rupture risk in advanced disease, in essence regenerating the aortic wall. Although rupture-specific clinical trials are underway, regeneration therapy specifically remains an elusive and theoretic possibility [85].

Animal Model of AAA Rupture As we have previously shown throughout this chapter, mechanisms behind pathogenesis of AAA rupture remains poorly understood even compared to the development and progression of AAA. One of the contributing factors to this problem is the lack of established animal model for ruptured AAA. When ease for gene manipulation and handling is considered, rodents, especially mice, are very useful as an experimental animal model. Angiotensin II infusion/Apo E knockout (Ang II) model does acquire rupture in some cases, but they are aneurysms caused by the aortic dissection and also primarily occur at the suprarenal level which is different from the human AAA rupture. The model reported by Allaire et al. had 100 % rate of rupture; however, they used rat as an experimental animal and also a technique of xenograft transplantation coupled with immunization to achieve rupture, which is very different from typical human AAA rupture [18]. On the other hand, English and associates created an AAA rupture in rats by combining the well-established porcine pancreatic elastase (PPE) technique with administration of β-aminopropionitrile (BAPN) [18]. Without question, however, there remains a compelling need for developing high-fidelity animal modeling systems to gain additional insight into the pathogenesis of AAA rupture.

Current Status of AAA Rupture Management Mortality from AAA rupture in the US has been declining for decades [86], most likely related to progressive and continuing reductions in the prevalence of adult cigarette consumption [87, 88] (Fig. 4.7). Worldwide, aneurysm-related mortality has been more variable, with some regions still experiencing relatively high death rates [89, 90] (Fig. 4.8). Thus prevention of aneurysm rupture remains a key priority for public health policy worldwide. Despite ongoing medical therapy trials for early disease management (NTACT, clinicaltrials.gov #NCT01756833) (AARDVARK, clinicaltrials.gov #NCT01118520), (TEDY, clinicaltrials.gov #NCT01683084), little success has been achieved in predicting or limiting rupture risk outside of surgical exclusion. As personalized therapies evolve in the era of precision medicine, additional genetic, biomarker, and biomechanical modeling technologies will almost certainly provide more clarity to the task of predicting and preventing AAA-related mortality.

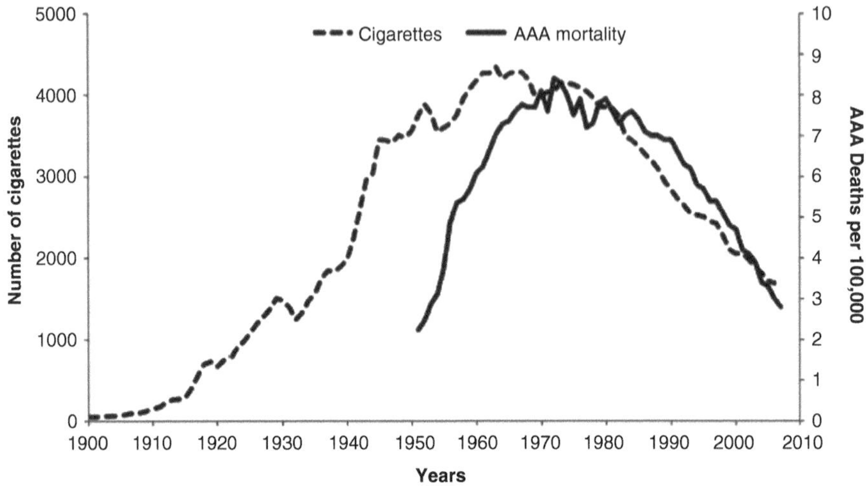

Fig. 4.7 Relationship between US annual adult per capita cigarette consumption and US age-adjusted AAA mortality per 100,000 population by year. A close correlation is clearly present between cigarette consumption and AAA-related mortality in the second half of the twentieth century (Reproduced from Lederle [87], with permission from American Heart Association)

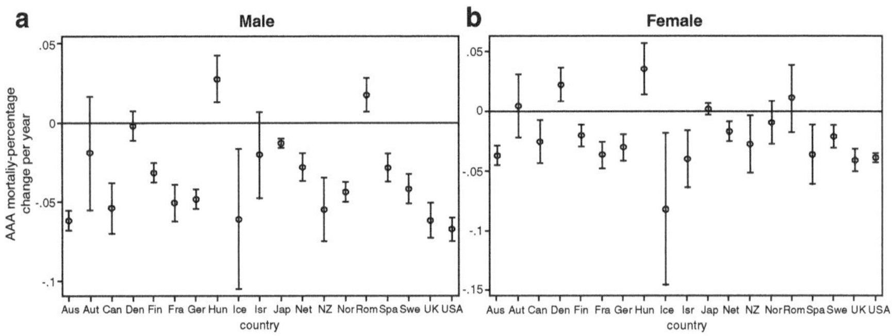

Fig. 4.8 Trends in age-standardized AAA mortality classified by gender showing regional differences around the globe with some regions experiencing higher mortality. (**a**) Male (**b**) Female. *Aus* indicates Australia, *Aut* Austria, *Can* Canada, *Den* Denmark, *Fin* Finland, *Fra* France, *Ger* Germany, *Hun* Hungary, *Ice* Iceland, *Isr* Israel, *Jap* Japan, *Net* the Netherlands, *NZ* New Zealand, *Nor* Norway, *Rom* Romania, *Spa* Spain, and *Swe* Sweden (Reproduced from Sidloff et al. [89], with permission from American Heart Association)

References

1. Nordon IM, Hinchliffe RJ, Loftus IM, Thompson MM. Pathophysiology and epidemiology of abdominal aortic aneurysms. Nat Rev Cardiol. 2011;8(2):92–102.
2. Daugherty A, Cassis LA. Mechanisms of abdominal aortic aneurysm formation. Curr Atheroscler Rep. 2002;4(3):222–7.
3. Daugherty A, Cassis LA. Mouse models of abdominal aortic aneurysms. Arterioscler Thromb Vasc Biol. 2004;24(3):429–34.

4. Thompson RW, Curci JA, Ennis TL, Mao D, Pagano MB, Pham CT. Pathophysiology of abdominal aortic aneurysms: insights from the elastase-induced model in mice with different genetic backgrounds. Ann N Y Acad Sci. 2006;1085:59–73.
5. Trollope A, Moxon JV, Moran CS, Golledge J. Animal models of abdominal aortic aneurysm and their role in furthering management of human disease. Cardiovasc Pathol: Off Jo Soc Cardiovasc Pathol. 2011;20(2):114–23.
6. Dobrin PB, Baker WH, Gley WC. Elastolytic and collagenolytic studies of arteries. Implications for the mechanical properties of aneurysms. Arch Surg. 1984;119(4):405–9.
7. Dobrin PB, Mrkvicka R. Failure of elastin or collagen as possible critical connective tissue alterations underlying aneurysmal dilatation. Cardiovasc Surg. 1994;2(4):484–8.
8. Sakalihasan N, Heyeres A, Nusgens BV, Limet R, Lapiere CM. Modifications of the extracellular matrix of aneurysmal abdominal aortas as a function of their size. Eur J Vasc Surg. 1993;7(6):633–7.
9. Rizzo RJ, McCarthy WJ, Dixit SN, Lilly MP, Shively VP, Flinn WR, et al. Collagen types and matrix protein content in human abdominal aortic aneurysms. J Vasc Surg. 1989;10(4):365–73.
10. Thompson RW, Liao S, Curci JA. Vascular smooth muscle cell apoptosis in abdominal aortic aneurysms. Coron Artery Dis. 1997;8(10):623–31.
11. Kent KC, Zwolak RM, Egorova NN, Riles TS, Manganaro A, Moskowitz AJ, et al. Analysis of risk factors for abdominal aortic aneurysm in a cohort of more than 3 million individuals. J Vasc Surg. 2010;52(3):539–48.
12. Lederle FA, Johnson GR, Wilson SE, Ballard DJ, Jordan Jr WD, Blebea J, et al. Rupture rate of large abdominal aortic aneurysms in patients refusing or unfit for elective repair. JAMA. 2002;287(22):2968–72.
13. Participants ET. Endovascular aneurysm repair and outcome in patients unfit for open repair of abdominal aortic aneurysm (EVAR trial 2): randomised controlled trial. Lancet. 2005; 365(9478):2187–92.
14. Parkinson F, Ferguson S, Lewis P, Williams IM, Twine CP, South East Wales Vascular N. Rupture rates of untreated large abdominal aortic aneurysms in patients unfit for elective repair. J Vasc Surg. 2015;61(6):1606–12.
15. Chaikof EL, Brewster DC, Dalman RL, Makaroun MS, Illig KA, Sicard GA, et al. The care of patients with an abdominal aortic aneurysm: the Society for Vascular Surgery practice guidelines. J Vasc Surg. 2009;50(4 Suppl):S2–49.
16. Thompson AR, Cooper JA, Ashton HA, Hafez H. Growth rates of small abdominal aortic aneurysms correlate with clinical events. Br J Surg. 2010;97(1):37–44.
17. Darling RC. Ruptured arteriosclerotic abdominal aortic aneurysms. A pathologic and clinical study. Am J Surg. 1970;119(4):397–401.
18. Allaire E, Forough R, Clowes M, Starcher B, Clowes AW. Local overexpression of TIMP-1 prevents aortic aneurysm degeneration and rupture in a rat model. J Clin Invest. 1998;102(7):1413–20.
19. Hurks R, Pasterkamp G, Vink A, Hoefer IE, Bots ML, van de Pavoordt HD, et al. Circumferential heterogeneity in the abdominal aortic aneurysm wall composition suggests lateral sides to be more rupture prone. J Vasc Surg. 2012;55(1):203–9.
20. Longo GM, Xiong W, Greiner TC, Zhao Y, Fiotti N, Baxter BT. Matrix metalloproteinases 2 and 9 work in concert to produce aortic aneurysms. J Clin Invest. 2002;110(5):625–32.
21. Petersen E, Wagberg F, Angquist KA. Proteolysis of the abdominal aortic aneurysm wall and the association with rupture. Eur J Vasc Endovasc Surg. 2002;23(2):153–7.
22. Wilson WR, Anderton M, Choke EC, Dawson J, Loftus IM, Thompson MM. Elevated plasma MMP1 and MMP9 are associated with abdominal aortic aneurysm rupture. Eur J Vasc Endovasc Surg. 2008;35(5):580–4.
23. Wilson WR, Anderton M, Schwalbe EC, Jones JL, Furness PN, Bell PR, et al. Matrix metalloproteinase-8 and -9 are increased at the site of abdominal aortic aneurysm rupture. Circulation. 2006;113(3):438–45.
24. Chistiakov DA, Sobenin IA, Orekhov AN. Vascular extracellular matrix in atherosclerosis. Cardiol Rev. 2013;21(6):270–88.

25. Sakalihasan N, Delvenne P, Nusgens BV, Limet R, Lapiere CM. Activated forms of MMP2 and MMP9 in abdominal aortic aneurysms. J Vasc Surg. 1996;24(1):127–33.
26. Khan JA, Abdul Rahman MN, Mazari FA, Shahin Y, Smith G, Madden L, et al. Intraluminal thrombus has a selective influence on matrix metalloproteinases and their inhibitors (tissue inhibitors of matrix metalloproteinases) in the wall of abdominal aortic aneurysms. Ann Vasc Surg. 2012;26(3):322–9.
27. Roderfeld M, Graf J, Giese B, Salguero-Palacios R, Tschuschner A, Muller-Newen G, et al. Latent MMP-9 is bound to TIMP-1 before secretion. Biol Chem. 2007;388(11):1227–34.
28. English SJ, Piert MR, Diaz JA, Gordon D, Ghosh A, D'Alecy LG, et al. Increased 18F-FDG uptake is predictive of rupture in a novel rat abdominal aortic aneurysm rupture model. Ann Surg. 2015;261(2):395–404.
29. Reilly JM. Plasminogen activators in abdominal aortic aneurysmal disease. Ann N Y Acad Sci. 1996;800:151–6.
30. Lee SR, Guo SZ, Scannevin RH, Magliaro BC, Rhodes KJ, Wang X, et al. Induction of matrix metalloproteinase, cytokines and chemokines in rat cortical astrocytes exposed to plasminogen activators. Neurosci Lett. 2007;417(1):1–5.
31. Lindholt JS. Activators of plasminogen and the progression of small abdominal aortic aneurysms. Ann N Y Acad Sci. 2006;1085:139–50.
32. Skagius E, Siegbahn A, Bergqvist D, Henriksson AE. Fibrinolysis in patients with an abdominal aortic aneurysm with special emphasis on rupture and shock. J Thromb Haemost. 2008;6(1):147–50.
33. Hobbs SD, Haggart P, Fegan C, Bradbury AW, Adam DJ. The role of tissue factor in patients undergoing open repair of ruptured and nonruptured abdominal aortic aneurysms. J Vasc Surg. 2007;46(4):682–6.
34. Ang LS, Boivin WA, Williams SJ, Zhao H, Abraham T, Carmine-Simmen K, et al. Serpina3n attenuates granzyme B-mediated decorin cleavage and rupture in a murine model of aortic aneurysm. Cell Death Dis. 2011;2:e209.
35. Uchida HA, Poduri A, Subramanian V, Cassis LA, Daugherty A. Urokinase-type plasminogen activator deficiency in bone marrow-derived cells augments rupture of angiotensin II-induced abdominal aortic aneurysms. Arterioscler Thromb Vasc Biol. 2011;31(12):2845–52.
36. Wang Y, Tang C, Qin Y. Cathepsins: a new culprit behind abdominal aortic aneurysm. Regen Med Res. 2013;1(1):5.
37. Lohoefer F, Reeps C, Lipp C, Rudelius M, Haertl F, Matevossian E, et al. Quantitative expression and localization of cysteine and aspartic proteases in human abdominal aortic aneurysms. Exp Mol Med. 2014;46:e95.
38. Lv BJ, Lindholt JS, Wang J, Cheng X, Shi GP. Plasma levels of cathepsins L, K, and V and risks of abdominal aortic aneurysms: a randomized population-based study. Atherosclerosis. 2013;230(1):100–5.
39. Jadhav PK, Schiffler MA, Gavardinas K, Kim EJ, Matthews DP, Staszak MA, et al. Discovery of Cathepsin S Inhibitor LY3000328 for the Treatment of Abdominal Aortic Aneurysm. ACS Med Chem Lett. 2014;5(10):1138–42.
40. Wang J, Sukhova GK, Liu J, Ozaki K, Lesner A, Libby P, et al. Cathepsin G deficiency reduces periaortic calcium chloride injury-induced abdominal aortic aneurysms in mice. J Vasc Surg. 2014;62(6):1615–24.
41. Meijer CA, Stijnen T, Wasser MN, Hamming JF, van Bockel JH, Lindeman JH, et al. Doxycycline for stabilization of abdominal aortic aneurysms: a randomized trial. Ann Intern Med. 2013;159(12):815–23.
42. Sillesen H, Eldrup N, Hultgren R, Lindeman J, Bredahl K, Thompson M, et al. Randomized clinical trial of mast cell inhibition in patients with a medium-sized abdominal aortic aneurysm. Br J Surg. 2015;102(8):894–901.
43. Shen M, Lee J, Basu R, Sakamuri SS, Wang X, Fan D, et al. Divergent roles of matrix metalloproteinase 2 in pathogenesis of thoracic aortic aneurysm. Arterioscler Thromb Vasc Biol. 2015;35(4):888–98.

44. Abdul-Hussien H, Hanemaaijer R, Kleemann R, Verhaaren BF, van Bockel JH, Lindeman JH. The pathophysiology of abdominal aortic aneurysm growth: corresponding and discordant inflammatory and proteolytic processes in abdominal aortic and popliteal artery aneurysms. J Vasc Surg. 2010;51(6):1479–87.
45. Newman KM, Jean-Claude J, Li H, Ramey WG, Tilson MD. Cytokines that activate proteolysis are increased in abdominal aortic aneurysms. Circulation. 1994;90(5 Pt 2):II224–7.
46. Johnston WF, Salmon M, Su G, Lu G, Stone ML, Zhao Y, et al. Genetic and pharmacologic disruption of interleukin-1 beta signaling inhibits experimental aortic aneurysm formation. Arterioscler Thromb Vasc Biol. 2013;33(2):294–304.
47. Dawson J, Cockerill G, Choke E, Loftus I, Thompson MM. Aortic aneurysms as a source of circulating interleukin-6. Ann N Y Acad Sci. 2006;1085:320–3.
48. Jones KG, Brull DJ, Brown LC, Sian M, Greenhalgh RM, Humphries SE, et al. Interleukin-6 (IL-6) and the prognosis of abdominal aortic aneurysms. Circulation. 2001;103(18):2260–5.
49. Roumen RM, Hendriks T, van der Ven-Jongekrijg J, Nieuwenhuijzen GA, Sauerwein RW, van der Meer JW, et al. Cytokine patterns in patients after major vascular surgery, hemorrhagic shock, and severe blunt trauma. Relation with subsequent adult respiratory distress syndrome and multiple organ failure. Ann Surg. 1993;218(6):769–76.
50. Wallinder J, Skagius E, Bergqvist D, Henriksson AE. Early inflammatory response in patients with ruptured abdominal aortic aneurysm. Vasc Endovascular Surg. 2010;44(1):32–5.
51. Cheuk BL, Cheng SW. Can local secretion of prostaglandin E2, thromboxane B2, and interleukin-6 play a role in ruptured abdominal aortic aneurysm? World J Surg. 2008;32(1):55–61.
52. Wilson WR, Wills J, Furness PN, Loftus IM, Thompson MM. Abdominal aortic aneurysm rupture is not associated with an up-regulation of inflammation within the aneurysm wall. Eur J Vasc Endovasc Surg. 2010;40(2):191–5.
53. Cheuk BL, Cheng SW. Differential secretion of prostaglandin E(2), thromboxane A(2) and interleukin-6 in intact and ruptured abdominal aortic aneurysms. Int J Mol Med. 2007;20(3):391–5.
54. Wang YX, Martin-McNulty B, Freay AD, Sukovich DA, Halks-Miller M, Li WW, et al. Angiotensin II increases urokinase-type plasminogen activator expression and induces aneurysm in the abdominal aorta of apolipoprotein E-deficient mice. Am J Pathol. 2001;159(4):1455–64.
55. Cheng J, Koenig SN, Kuivaniemi HS, Garg V, Hans CP. Pharmacological inhibitor of notch signaling stabilizes the progression of small abdominal aortic aneurysm in a mouse model. J Am Heart Assoc. 2014;3(6):e001064.
56. Gong D, Shi W, Yi SJ, Chen H, Groffen J, Heisterkamp N. TGF beta signaling plays a critical role in promoting alternative macrophage activation. BMC Immunol. 2012;13:31.
57. Courtois A, Nusgens BV, Hustinx R, Namur G, Gomez P, Somja J, et al. 18F-FDG uptake assessed by PET/CT in abdominal aortic aneurysms is associated with cellular and molecular alterations prefacing wall deterioration and rupture. J Nucl Med. 2013;54(10):1740–7.
58. Stewart GJ. Neutrophils and deep venous thrombosis. Haemostasis. 1993;23 Suppl 1:127–40.
59. Heiple JM, Ossowski L. Human neutrophil plasminogen activator is localized in specific granules and is translocated to the cell surface by exocytosis. J Exp Med. 1986;164(3):826–40.
60. Kurihara T, Shimizu-Hirota R, Shimoda M, Adachi T, Shimizu H, Weiss SJ, et al. Neutrophil-derived matrix metalloproteinase 9 triggers acute aortic dissection. Circulation. 2012;126(25):3070–80.
61. Cohen JR, Keegan L, Sarfati I, Danna D, Ilardi C, Wise L. Neutrophil chemotaxis and neutrophil elastase in the aortic wall in patients with abdominal aortic aneurysms. J Invest Surg : Off J Acad Surg Res. 1991;4(4):423–30.
62. Cron DC, Coleman DM, Sheetz KH, Englesbe MJ, Waits SA. Aneurysms in abdominal organ transplant recipients. J Vasc Surg. 2014;59(3):594–8.
63. Di Martino E, Mantero S, Inzoli F, Melissano G, Astore D, Chiesa R, et al. Biomechanics of abdominal aortic aneurysm in the presence of endoluminal thrombus: experimental characterisation and structural static computational analysis. Eur J Vasc Endovasc Surg. 1998;15(4):290–9.

64. Vorp DA, Lee PC, Wang DH, Makaroun MS, Nemoto EM, Ogawa S, et al. Association of intraluminal thrombus in abdominal aortic aneurysm with local hypoxia and wall weakening. J Vasc Surg. 2001;34(2):291–9.
65. Stenbaek J, Kalin B, Swedenborg J. Growth of thrombus may be a better predictor of rupture than diameter in patients with abdominal aortic aneurysms. Eur J Vasc Endovasc Surg. 2000;20(5):466–9.
66. Speelman L, Schurink GW, Bosboom EM, Buth J, Breeuwer M, van de Vosse FN, et al. The mechanical role of thrombus on the growth rate of an abdominal aortic aneurysm. J Vasc Surg. 2010;51(1):19–26.
67. Folkesson M, Silveira A, Eriksson P, Swedenborg J. Protease activity in the multi-layered intra-luminal thrombus of abdominal aortic aneurysms. Atherosclerosis. 2011;218(2):294–9.
68. Choke E, Cockerill GW, Dawson J, Chung YL, Griffiths J, Wilson RW, et al. Hypoxia at the site of abdominal aortic aneurysm rupture is not associated with increased lactate. Ann N Y Acad Sci. 2006;1085:306–10.
69. Scott DJ, Prasad P, Philippou H, Rashid ST, Sohrabi S, Whalley D, et al. Clot architecture is altered in abdominal aortic aneurysms and correlates with aneurysm size. Arterioscler Thromb Vasc Biol. 2011;31(12):3004–10.
70. Hans SS, Jareunpoon O, Balasubramaniam M, Zelenock GB. Size and location of thrombus in intact and ruptured abdominal aortic aneurysms. J Vasc Surg. 2005;41(4):584–8.
71. Golledge J, Iyer V, Jenkins J, Bradshaw B, Cronin O, Walker PJ. Thrombus volume is similar in patients with ruptured and intact abdominal aortic aneurysms. J Vasc Surg. 2014;59(2): 315–20.
72. Assar AN, Zarins CK. Ruptured abdominal aortic aneurysm: a surgical emergency with many clinical presentations. Postgrad Med J. 2009;85(1003):268–73.
73. Tong J, Cohnert T, Holzapfel GA. Diameter-related variations of geometrical, mechanical, and mass fraction data in the anterior portion of abdominal aortic aneurysms. Eur J Vasc Endovasc Surg. 2015;49(3):262–70.
74. Vallabhaneni SR, Gilling-Smith GL, How TV, Carter SD, Brennan JA, Harris PL. Heterogeneity of tensile strength and matrix metalloproteinase activity in the wall of abdominal aortic aneurysms. J Endovasc Ther : Off J Int Soc Endovasc Speci. 2004;11(4):494–502.
75. Fillinger MF, Marra SP, Raghavan ML, Kennedy FE. Prediction of rupture risk in abdominal aortic aneurysm during observation: wall stress versus diameter. J Vasc Surg. 2003;37(4): 724–32.
76. Vorp DA, Raghavan ML, Webster MW. Mechanical wall stress in abdominal aortic aneurysm: influence of diameter and asymmetry. J Vasc Surg. 1998;27(4):632–9.
77. Khosla S, Morris DR, Moxon JV, Walker PJ, Gasser TC, Golledge J. Meta-analysis of peak wall stress in ruptured, symptomatic and intact abdominal aortic aneurysms. Br J Surg. 2014;101(11):1350–7; discussion 7.
78. Boyd AJ, Kuhn DC, Lozowy RJ, Kulbisky GP. Low wall shear stress predominates at sites of abdominal aortic aneurysm rupture. J Vasc Surg. 2016;63(6):1613–9.
79. Koncar I, Davidovic L. Rupture of abdominal aortic aneurysm in the low wall stress zone. Eur J Vasc Endovasc Surg. 2015;49(3):254.
80. Wang Y, Joannic D, Delassus P, Lalande A, Juillion P, Fontaine JF. Comparison of the strain field of abdominal aortic aneurysm measured by magnetic resonance imaging and stereovision: a feasibility study for prediction of the risk of rupture of aortic abdominal aneurysm. J Biomech. 2015;48(6):1158–64.
81. Riveros F, Martufi G, Gasser TC, Rodriguez-Matas JF. On the impact of intraluminal thrombus mechanical behavior in AAA passive mechanics. Ann Biomed Eng. 2015;43(9):2253–64.
82. McGloughlin TM, Doyle BJ. New approaches to abdominal aortic aneurysm rupture risk assessment: engineering insights with clinical gain. Arterioscler Thromb Vasc Biol. 2010;30(9): 1687–94.
83. Reeps C, Gee M, Maier A, Gurdan M, Eckstein HH, Wall WA. The impact of model assumptions on results of computational mechanics in abdominal aortic aneurysm. J Vasc Surg. 2010;51(3):679–88.

84. United Kingdom ETI, Greenhalgh RM, Brown LC, Powell JT, Thompson SG, Epstein D, et al. Endovascular versus open repair of abdominal aortic aneurysm. N Engl J Med. 2010;362(20): 1863–71.
85. Yoshimura K, Aoki H, Ikeda Y, Fujii K, Akiyama N, Furutani A, et al. Regression of abdominal aortic aneurysm by inhibition of c-Jun N-terminal kinase. Nat Med. 2005;11(12):1330–8.
86. Stather PW, Sidloff DA, Rhema IA, Choke E, Bown MJ, Sayers RD. A review of current reporting of abdominal aortic aneurysm mortality and prevalence in the literature. Eur J Vasc Endovasc Surg. 2014;47(3):240–2.
87. Lederle FA. The rise and fall of abdominal aortic aneurysm. Circulation. 2011;124(10): 1097–9.
88. Wang S, Zhang C, Zhang M, Liang B, Zhu H, Lee J, et al. Activation of AMP-activated protein kinase alpha2 by nicotine instigates formation of abdominal aortic aneurysms in mice in vivo. Nat Med. 2012;18(6):902–10.
89. Sidloff D, Stather P, Dattani N, Bown M, Thompson J, Sayers R, et al. Aneurysm global epidemiology study: public health measures can further reduce abdominal aortic aneurysm mortality. Circulation. 2014;129(7):747–53.
90. Sampson UK, Norman PE, Fowkes FG, Aboyans V, Song Y, Harrell Jr FE, et al. Estimation of global and regional incidence and prevalence of abdominal aortic aneurysms 1990 to 2010. Glob Heart. 2014;9(1):159–70.
91. Tedesco MM, Dalman RL. Arterial aneurysms, Rutherford's vascular surgery. Saunders Elsevier: London. 7th ed. 2010.

Chapter 5
Wall Stress

Derek P. Nathan and Benjamin M. Jackson

Introduction

The repair of abdominal aortic aneurysms (AAA) in order to prevent aneurysm rupture and patient death represents one of the central tenets of vascular and endovascular surgery. The ability to predict AAA rupture is therefore of paramount importance. While maximum aortic diameter is an empirically proven metric in the prediction of AAA rupture, it is far from ideal.

Biomechanical analysis has been demonstrated to improve the understanding and prediction of AAA rupture. In particular, wall stress has been shown to predict more accurately the rupture and growth of AAA than maximum diameter. Finite element analysis represents the most commonly employed biomechanical technique to analyze AAA rupture risk, although other methods, including computational fluid dynamics and fluid–structure interaction analysis, have emerged as an important and nuanced means of predicting AAA behavior.

The review of the literature herein highlights the limitations of maximum aneurysm diameter as a predictor of AAA rupture; the use of biomechanical analyses, such as wall stress, to predict AAA rupture; and the evidence in support of wall stress in elucidating the natural history of AAA. While maximum aneurysm diameter remains one of the most important tools available to vascular surgeons in the evaluation and management of AAA, aneurysm diameter is not rigorously predictive of aneurysm rupture, and wall stress represents an important complement and adjuvant in understanding and predicting the behavior of abdominal aortic aneurysms.

D.P. Nathan, MD
University of Washington, Seattle, WA, USA

B.M. Jackson, MD (✉)
University of Pennsylvania, Philadelphia, PA, USA
e-mail: benjamin.jackson@uphs.upenn.edu

B.W. Starnes et al. (eds.), *Ruptured Abdominal Aortic Aneurysm*,
DOI 10.1007/978-3-319-23844-9_5

Maximum Diameter Is a Less than Ideal Predictor of AAA Rupture

Several studies have demonstrated that a not insignificant number of AAAs rupture at a size less than the maximum diameter of 5.5 cm at which repair is typically recommended. One large, single-center study reported that 16 of 161 (9.9 %) ruptured AAAs that presented over a 10-year period were 5 cm or smaller in maximum diameter [1]. This finding led the authors to suggest that in appropriately selected patients, a lower size threshold might be used to recommend repair. The UK Small Aneurysm Trial followed a cohort of over 2000 patients prospectively over time. In that trial, 24 patients with AAAs between 4 and 5 cm ruptured. Patients with AAAs between 4 and 5.5 cm had a crude rupture rate of 2.7 per 100 person-years [2]. It is important to note that in both of the above studies, ultrasound was the primary imaging modality for determining maximum aortic diameter, and ultrasound has been shown to underestimate AAA size compared to computed tomography-based measurements by between 1 and 5 mm depending on the method utilized [3]. Nonetheless, it appears that a number of AAAs rupture prior to reaching the maximum diameter threshold at which repair is recommended. One might ask whether some larger aneurysms are stable over long-term follow-up, which might further impugn the predictive value of aneurysm diameter, but the same UK Small Aneurysm Trial found that very few patients with aneurysms greater than 6 cm survived more than 3 years without rupture. That small aneurysms sometimes rupture highlights the fact that current criteria for aneurysm repair that rely exclusively on maximum diameter are far from ideal in predicting AAA behavior.

Computational Biomechanics in the Prediction of AAA Rupture

Biomechanical analysis utilizing wall stress represents an additional manner of predicting AAA rupture. The Law of Laplace states that wall tension is proportional to pressure times radius for thin-walled spheres or cylinders. Wall stress is wall tension divided by wall thickness. This axiom forms much of the basis for the use of maximum diameter to predict AAA rupture, which, as described above, is the default – but less than ideal – method of predicting AAA rupture. The axiom that an AAA ruptures when the stress on the aortic wall exceeds its strength may offer a more sophisticated and reliable means of predicting the natural history of AAAs. Biomechanical analyses that yield calculations of wall stress and wall strength, as a result, may improve the ability to prognosticate the behavior of aortic aneurysms.

Role of Wall Strength

There are several means of assessing the wall strength of aneurysms of the abdominal aorta. One method is noninvasive and predicated on imaging modalities, such as ultrasound, computed tomography, and magnetic resonance, with cardiac cycle tracking to evaluate the compliance of the aortic wall. Wilson and colleagues employed ultrasound with electrocardiogram gating to measure the aortic wall stiffness at the point of maximum aneurysm diameter in 210 patients over a median follow-up of 19 months [4]. It was found that decreased stiffness, or increased distensibility, conferred a significant increase in rupture risk. Patients with decreased stiffness had almost as great an increased risk of rupture as patients with a 10 % increase in maximum aortic diameter (28 % versus 36 %). While illustrative of the biomechanics of the aortic wall, ultrasound with cardiac cycle tracking has several limitations, including a significant learning curve to master the technique, and moderate interobserver and intraobserver variation [5]. Electrocardiogram-gated computed tomography has been used to quantify circumferential and longitudinal cyclical strain in the aorta; however, this technique remains more of a research-oriented than a practical clinical application at this time [6].

Another manner of calculating AAA wall strength is through the ex vivo analysis of the aortic wall tissue excised from an aneurysm during surgical repair. In this manner, Di Martino and colleagues compared the wall strength of the ruptured and non-ruptured AAA [7]. Aortic wall thickness was measured using a laser micrometer, and wall strength was determined in a uniaxial tensile testing system. The thickness of the ruptured AAA was significantly greater than the non-ruptured AAA; of note, the former were not any greater in maximum diameter than the latter. Moreover, consistent with the findings of the previous study from Wilson and colleagues, decreased stiffness was associated with decreased wall strength. Therefore, both ex vivo and in vivo studies are able to assess the biomechanical properties of the aortic wall and thus aid in the description of AAA behavior. Unfortunately, the most reliable way to determine aortic wall strength is by stretching the surgically excised aortic wall tissue until it ruptures or breaks, which may explain why studies of aortic wall strength have lagged behind those of aortic wall stress.

Finally, Vorp and Vande Geest and colleagues at the University of Pittsburgh, developed circa 2006, a statistical model capable of predicting regional aortic wall strength based on the inputs: age, gender, family history of AAA, smoking status, AAA diameter, normalized regional aortic diameter, and regional intraluminal thrombus (ILT) thickness. The statistical model was validated against ex vivo specimens [8]. This has been implemented in a "rupture potential index," or RPI, elucidated by the same group and described below.

Role of Wall Stress

Calculation of AAA wall stress with finite element analysis (FEA) remains the most widely employed method of investigating in vivo aortic biomechanics. Wall stress determinations with FEA represent a noninvasive, computational method of investigating the biomechanics of aortic aneurysms. Although the specific details of the FEA technique may vary across studies, in general, there are several fundamental steps to the process. First, finite element analysis requires the creation of a precise and robust three-dimensional (3D) reconstruction of the abdominal aorta. This 3D reconstruction is most commonly abstracted from computed tomography imaging [9]. In the case of computed tomography-based methodology, the construction of a 3D model suitable for wall stress analysis requires multi-slice spiral computed tomography scanning with collimation and rotation time that is sufficiently narrow and fast, respectively. The 3D model can be reconstructed and segmented by automatic or manual means. A semiautomatic segmentation method with automated reconstruction based on different material density followed by manual review to confirm that the automatic construction is correct is commonly used. Indeed, this technique is favored by the authors of this chapter and other investigators with extensive experience with FEA and the study of aneurysm wall stress [9, 10].

Early studies of FEA of AAA wall stress only included the wall of the abdominal aorta, while the remainder of the abdominal aorta in the 3D reconstruction was assumed to be the flow lumen. However, as CTA imaging has increased in resolution and availability, and image analysis techniques have become more sophisticated; mural thrombus and atherosclerotic calcifications have been included in models as well. Several studies have demonstrated that the inclusion of mural thrombus and calcifications has important ramifications for AAA wall stress calculations [11, 12]. An additional advancement in FEA technique has been the ability to measure the thickness of the aortic wall. Whereas prior 3D AAA reconstructions were assumed to have uniform wall thickness and improvements in computed tomography imaging provided the spatial resolution necessary to enable patient and region-specific aortic wall thickness measurements; these locally resolved aortic wall thickness measurements have been shown to improve the ability of wall stress to predict AAA behavior [10, 11].

From the 3D reconstruction of the CTA, a mesh is generated, which is composed of thousands of individual nodes and elements representing the abdominal aorta, including the aortic wall, mural thrombus, and calcifications. Computerized algorithms "smooth" the mesh in order to yield a precise 3D model that is suitable for FEA. Boundary conditions and material properties of the model are specified. Boundary conditions include the blood pressure applied to the inside of the modeled aorta, while material properties refer to the mechanical characteristics of the components of the model. The aortic wall, mural thrombus, and calcification are generally given unique material properties, and may behave in an isotropic or anisotropic manner. Elastic or hyperelastic material properties are typically specified. While assigning anisotropic and hyperelastic properties to the various materials may be

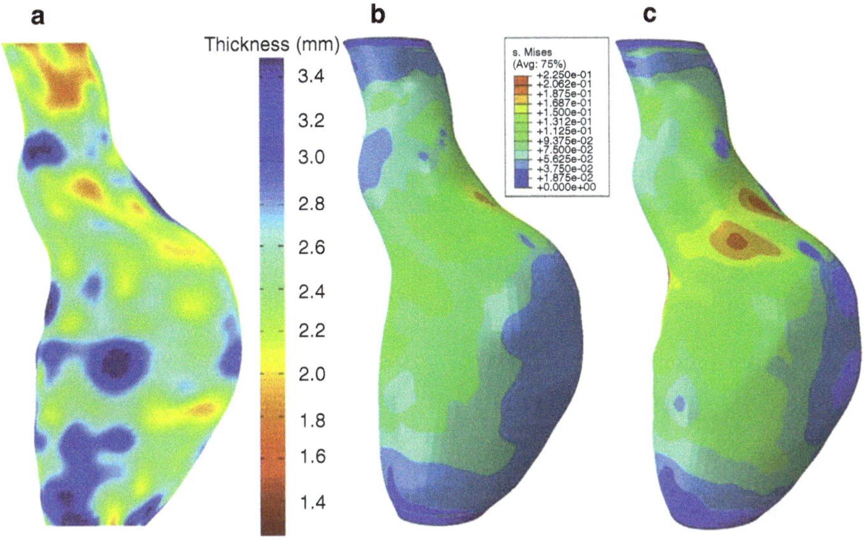

Fig. 5.1 (**a**) Calculated wall thickness map overlaid onto aortic geometry. (**b**) Stress contour map derived from uniform wall thickness aortic geometry. (**c**) Stress contour map derived from variable wall thickness aortic geometry. Note the colocalization of areas with low wall thickness and high peak wall stress, especially in the aneurysm neck (From Shang et al. [10])

more accurate or realistic, these specifications will risk rendering the FEA model computationally unwieldy and time-consuming. In the clinical milieu, time-consuming imaging, image analysis and segmentation, and computational modeling are currently not tenable. Finally, the computational algorithms solve the linked partial differential equations to determine the predicted locally resolved wall stresses. These can easily be depicted visually, as in Fig. 5.1.

Wall Stress as a Predictor of AAA Rupture and Dilatation

In 2002, Fillinger and colleagues at Dartmouth Hitchcock Medical Center employed FEA to assess the association between wall stress and AAA behavior. Patients who underwent elective repair of asymptomatic AAAs, urgent repair of symptomatic AAAs, and emergent repair of ruptured AAAs were included in the study. The peak wall stress of the symptomatic and ruptured AAAs undergoing nonelective repair was significantly greater than that of the asymptomatic AAAs undergoing elective repair [9]. Moreover, even when accounting for differences in maximum aneurysm diameter, the symptomatic and ruptured AAAs still had a significantly greater peak wall stress than the asymptomatic AAAs. Indeed, the smallest ruptured AAA at 4.8 cm had a peak wall stress equivalent to that of an asymptomatic 6.3 cm abdominal aortic aneurysm. The authors also reported that the location of peak wall stress was not at the point of maximum diameter, but in the posterolateral aspect of the AAA. This location of peak wall stress coincided with the area of rupture in the six patients for whom the location of rupture was known. This seminal study from Fillinger and colleagues highlighted that a noninvasive computational biomechanical analysis of 3D AAA geometry might be superior to maximum diameter alone in predicting an aneurysm rupture risk.

Expanding on their work, Fillinger and colleagues analyzed the ability of maximum diameter versus peak wall stress to predict rupture risk over time in a cohort of patients with AAAs under prospective longitudinal observation [13]. One hundred and three patients with AAAs were assessed in an elective setting: 42 underwent observation without intervention within 1 year of their assessment, 39 underwent elective repair within 1 year, and 22 underwent emergent repair for rupture ($n = 8$) or symptoms ($n = 14$). Both index maximum diameter and peak wall stress differed between the groups; however, the latter appeared to better differentiate the AAAs that required emergent repair by receiver operating characteristic curve analysis. Multivariate analysis confirmed that peak wall stress, and not maximum aneurysm diameter, was an independent predictor of rupture risk over time. In addition to these results, the authors reported that almost one-quarter of the patients with ruptured and symptomatic AAAs who underwent emergent repair had maximum aneurysm diameters of 5 cm or less. Approximately three-quarters of the patients who underwent observation without intervention had peak wall stresses lower than the lowest recorded peak wall stress for AAAs that required emergent repair. The findings of this later study by Fillinger and colleagues confirmed those of the previous investigation, suggesting that differences in wall stress could be identified early in the evaluation and treatment of patients with AAA, and thus that FEA might be useful in clinical decision-making.

Additional evidence in support of the role of wall stress in predicting AAA natural history comes from Li and colleagues [14]. Utilizing the rate of AAA expansion as a metric of the risk of aneurysm rupture, these authors sought to analyze the association between wall stress and aneurysm growth. Patients with AAA were included in a longitudinal study with serial computed tomography imaging. Patients with AAA that expanded rapidly ($\geq$4 mm/year) had higher baseline wall stress than slowly expanding AAA ($\leq$4 mm/year). There was no difference in baseline maximum aortic diameter between the two groups. This investigation suggested that AAA with higher wall stress have a greater rate of expansion and consequently a greater risk of rupture. The authors concluded that while the decision to repair AAA remains multifaceted, wall stress could play a role in the management of AAA with diameters in the range of 4–5.5 cm.

As indicated in the prior section, investigators at the University of Pittsburgh have also examined the computationally predicted aortic wall stress in AAAs. However, they have concentrated their efforts on a locally and regionally resolved RPI, instead of peak wall stress alone. They defined the RPI as the ratio between local wall stress and local wall strength, and found that RPI was higher – though the difference was not statistically different – in ruptured than intact AAA [15]. Interestingly, the wall strength was significantly lower in the ruptured group than the intact group, casting some doubt on the clinical utility of wall stress calculations in isolation. Other groups have implemented analyses bases on the RPI formulation: among these is the Munchën group who did find statistically significant increased RPI in symptomatic and ruptured AAA [16].

Our laboratory at the University of Pennsylvania has recently demonstrated the ability to detect the regional aortic wall thickness of the abdominal aorta, including in areas with mural thrombus present [17]. Furthermore, Shang and colleagues in the same lab have shown that the inclusion of locally resolved aortic wall thickness significantly impacts FEA estimates of peak wall stress and that variable wall thickness computational models are more correlated with expansion of AAAs (a putative marker of rupture risk) than are models assuming a uniform aortic wall thickness [10].

Role of Wall Stress in Other Pathologies

Thoracic Aortic Rupture Risk Prediction

While indications for repair of infrarenal AAA are well established, and patients with 6 cm AAA have a high 3-year mortality, similar straightforward and rational indications for the treatment of thoracic aortic pathologies are not uniformly accepted. Historically, an elective repair of descending thoracic aortic aneurysms (DTAA) and thoracoabdominal aortic aneurysms was not universally recommended until maximal diameter exceeded 6.5 cm [18]. But elective repair of even 6.5 cm DTAA is much less compelling than the repair of 5 cm AAA's: only 30 % of 6.5 cm DTAA are expected to be ruptured in 5 years [19]. Surgeons cannot simply ignore relatively small thoracic aneurysms either: the annual risk of rupture, dissection, or death at a diameter of 6.0 cm is 16 % [12]. Therefore, computational stress modeling or other biomechanical indices might play in guiding therapeutic decisions in patients with thoracic aortic aneurysms.

Our laboratory has investigated this possibility and demonstrated that computational peak wall stress was strongly correlated with aneurysm expansion rate, a proxy for rupture risk (Fig. 5.2) [20]. In addition, Shang and colleagues showed that more sophisticated FEA models (Fig. 5.3), incorporating variable aortic wall thickness, intraluminal thrombus, and aortic calcification, predicted very different peak wall stresses, highlighting the importance of choosing an appropriately refined and validated computational model for aneurysm rupture risk prediction [21].

Summary

While computational wall stress modeling of AAAs can better predict rupture than diameter-based risk assessment alone, FEA, RPI, and similar computationally based models have not been implemented clinically to any significant degree. Nevertheless, the clinical insights derived from biomechanical analyses currently can influence our understanding of AAA rupture risk, and future work formally incorporating computational stress modeling into clinical decision-making should be emphasized. Meanwhile, our management of other pathologies, including thoracic aortic aneurysms, should be influenced by predictive biomechanical analyses.

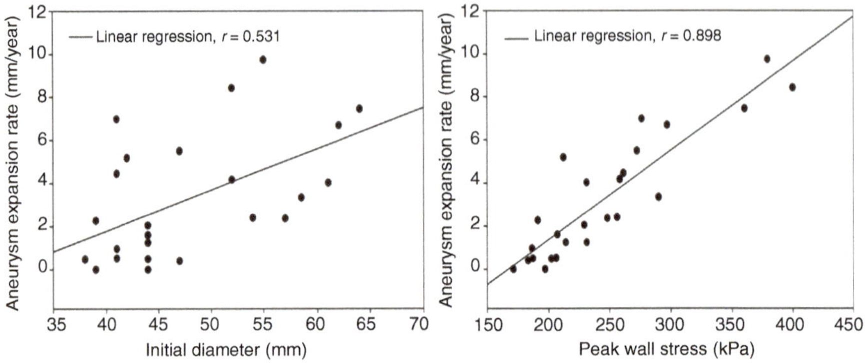

Fig. 5.2 Correlations between thoracic aortic expansion rate and initial diameter (*left*) and between thoracic aortic expansion rate and peak wall stress (*right*), demonstrating that peak wall stress is a better predictor of aneurysm expansion rate (From Shang et al. [13])

Fig. 5.3 Von Mises wall stress distribution in the descending thoracic aorta of a patient with an aneurysm. (**a**) with locally resolved wall thickness. (**b**) with uniform wall thickness (From Shang et al. [14])

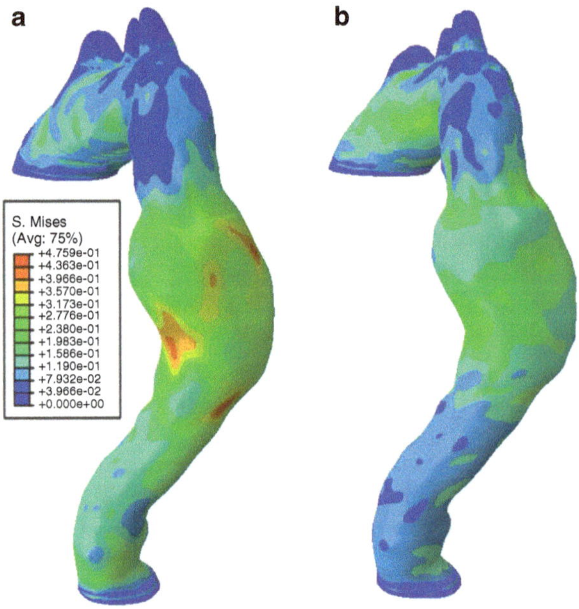

References

1. Nicholls SC, Gardner JB, Meissner MH, Johansen HK. Rupture in small abdominal aortic aneurysms. J Vasc Surg. 1998;28:884–8.
2. Brown LC, Powell JT. Risk factors for aneurysm rupture in patients kept under ultrasound surveillance. UK Small Aneurysm Trial Participants. Ann Surg. 1999;230:289–96.
3. Chiu KW, Ling L, Tripathi V, Ahmed M, Shrivastava V. Ultrasound measurement for abdominal aortic aneurysm screening: a direct comparison of the three leading methods. Eur J Vasc Endovasc Surg. 2014;47:367–73.

4. Wilson KA, Lee AJ, Lee AJ, Hoskins PR, Fowkes FG, Ruckley CV, Bradbury AW. The relationship between aortic wall distensibility and rupture of infrarenal abdominal aortic aneurysm. J Vasc Surg. 2003;37:112–7.
5. Wilson KA, Hoskins PR, Lee AJ, Fowkes FG, Ruckley CV, Bradbury AW. Ultrasonic measurement of abdominal aortic aneurysm wall compliance: a reproducibility study. J Vasc Surg. 2000;31:507–13.
6. Morrison TM, Choi G, Zarins CK, Taylor CA. Circumferential and longitudinal cyclic strain of the human thoracic aorta: age-related changes. J Vasc Surg. 2009;49:1029–36.
7. Di Martino ES1, Bohra A, Vande Geest JP, Gupta N, Makaroun MS, Vorp DA. Biomechanical properties of ruptured versus electively repaired abdominal aortic aneurysm wall tissue. J Vasc Surg. 2006;43:570–6.
8. Vande Geest JP, Wang DH, Wisniewski SR, Makaroun MS, Vorp DA. Towards a noninvasive method for determination of patient-specific wall strength distribution in abdominal aortic aneurysms. Ann Biomed Eng. 2006;34(7):1098–106.
9. Fillinger MF, Raghavan ML, Marra SP, Cronenwett JL, Kennedy FE. In vivo analysis of mechanical wall stress and abdominal aortic aneurysm rupture risk. J Vasc Surg. 2002;36: 589–97.
10. Shang EK, Nathan DP, Woo EY, Fairman RM, Wang GJ, Gorman RC, Gorman 3rd JH, Jackson BM. Local wall thickness in finite element models improves prediction of abdominal aortic aneurysm growth. J Vasc Surg. 2015;61:217–23.
11. Wang DH, Makaroun MS, Webster MW, Vorp DA. Effect of intraluminal thrombus on wall stress in patient-specific models of abdominal aortic aneurysm. J Vasc Surg. 2002;36: 598–604.
12. Li ZY, U-King-Im J, Tang TY, Soh E, See TC, Gillard JH. Impact of calcification and intraluminal thrombus on the computed wall stresses of abdominal aortic aneurysm. J Vasc Surg. 2008;47:928–35.
13. Fillinger MF, Marra SP, Raghavan ML, Kennedy FE. Prediction of rupture risk in abdominal aortic aneurysm during observation: wall stress versus diameter. J Vasc Surg. 2003;37: 724–32.
14. Li ZY, Sadat U, U-King-Im J, Tang TY, Bowden DJ, Hayes PD, Gillard JH. Association between aneurysm shoulder stress and abdominal aortic aneurysm expansion: a longitudinal follow-up study. Circulation. 2010;122:1815–22.
15. Vande Geest JP, Di Martino ES, Bohra A, Makaroun MS, Vorp DA. A biomechanics-based rupture potential index for abdominal aortic aneurysm risk assessment: demonstrative application. Ann N Y Acad Sci. 2006;1085:11–21.
16. Maier A, Gee MW, Reeps C, Pongratz J, Eckstein HH, Wall WA. A comparison of diameter, wall stress, and rupture potential index for abdominal aortic aneurysm rupture risk prediction. Ann Biomed Eng. 2010;38:3124–34.
17. Shang EK, Lai E, Pouch AM, Hinmon R, Gorman RC, Gorman 3rd JH, Sehgal CM, Ferrari G, Bavaria JE, Jackson BM. Validation of semiautomated and locally resolved aortic wall thickness measurements from computed tomography. J Vasc Surg. 2015;61:1034–40.
18. Coady MA, Ikonomidis JS, Cheung AT, Matsumoto AH, Dake MD, Chaikof EL, Cambria RP, Mora-Mangano CT, Sundt TM, Sellke FW. Surgical management of descending thoracic aortic disease: open and endovascular approaches: a scientific statement from the American Heart Association. Circulation. 2010;121:2780–804.
19. Davies RR, Goldstein LJ, Coady MA, Tittle SL, Rizzo JA, Kopf GS, Elefteriades JA. Yearly rupture or dissection rates for thoracic aortic aneurysms: simple prediction based on size. Ann Thorac Surg. 2002;73:17–28.
20. Shang EK, Nathan DP, Sprinkle SR, Vigmostad SC, Fairman RM, Bavaria JE, Gorman RC, Gorman 3rd JH, Chandran KB, Jackson BM. Peak wall stress predicts expansion rate in descending thoracic aortic aneurysms. Ann Thorac Surg. 2013;95:593–8.
21. Shang EK, Nathan DP, Sprinkle SR, Fairman RM, Bavaria JE, Gorman RC, Gorman 3rd JH, Jackson BM. Impact of wall thickness and saccular geometry on the computational wall stress of descending thoracic aortic aneurysms. Circulation. 2013;128:S157–62.

Chapter 6
Clinical Presentation of RAAA

Dieter Mayer

Despite the widespread belief that a ruptured abdominal aortic aneurysm (RAAA) presents with the classical triad of back pain with or without abdominal pain, hypotension, and a pulsatile abdominal mass [1], this triad is only present in one fourth to half of all RAAA patients [2, 3]. Depending on the site of rupture, the comorbidities of the patient, and conditions of the institution or rescue team, RAAA may be misdiagnosed in up to 30 % of patients [2]: myocardial infarction, ureteral stone, peptic ulcer, perforation of the stomach or duodenum, gallstones, or even diverticulitis are often suspected, and their respective diagnostic pathway may considerably delay the diagnosis and treatment of life-threatening RAAA. In contrast, vascular surgeons must be aware that those diseases may mimic RAAA and that these misdiagnoses can be quite troublesome when RAAA is only detected after emergency laparotomy. In chronic contained rupture (CCR) of abdominal aortic aneurysms (AAA) [4, 5], clinical presentation and signs may be even more subtle and misleading. Patients may present with full-blown abdominal compartment syndrome (ACS) [6], which may be missed when the focus is put on the rupture of the aorta and its rapid sealing.

Acute Presentation of RAAA

Individual persons suffering from RAAA may present in many ways. The most typical manifestation of rupture is abdominal and/or back pain with (transient) hypotension or syncope. However, symptoms may be vague and an abdominal pulsating mass may or may not be present. Depending on the localization of rupture (Fig. 6.1), the diagnosis may be confused with acute coronary syndrome, myocardial infarction, congestive heart failure, gastric perforation, renal or ureteral calculus, diverticulitis,

D. Mayer, MD, FEBVS, FAPWCA
Hospital of Zurich, Zurich, Switzerland
e-mail: mayerdieter@hotmail.com

B.W. Starnes et al. (eds.), *Ruptured Abdominal Aortic Aneurysm*,
DOI 10.1007/978-3-319-23844-9_6

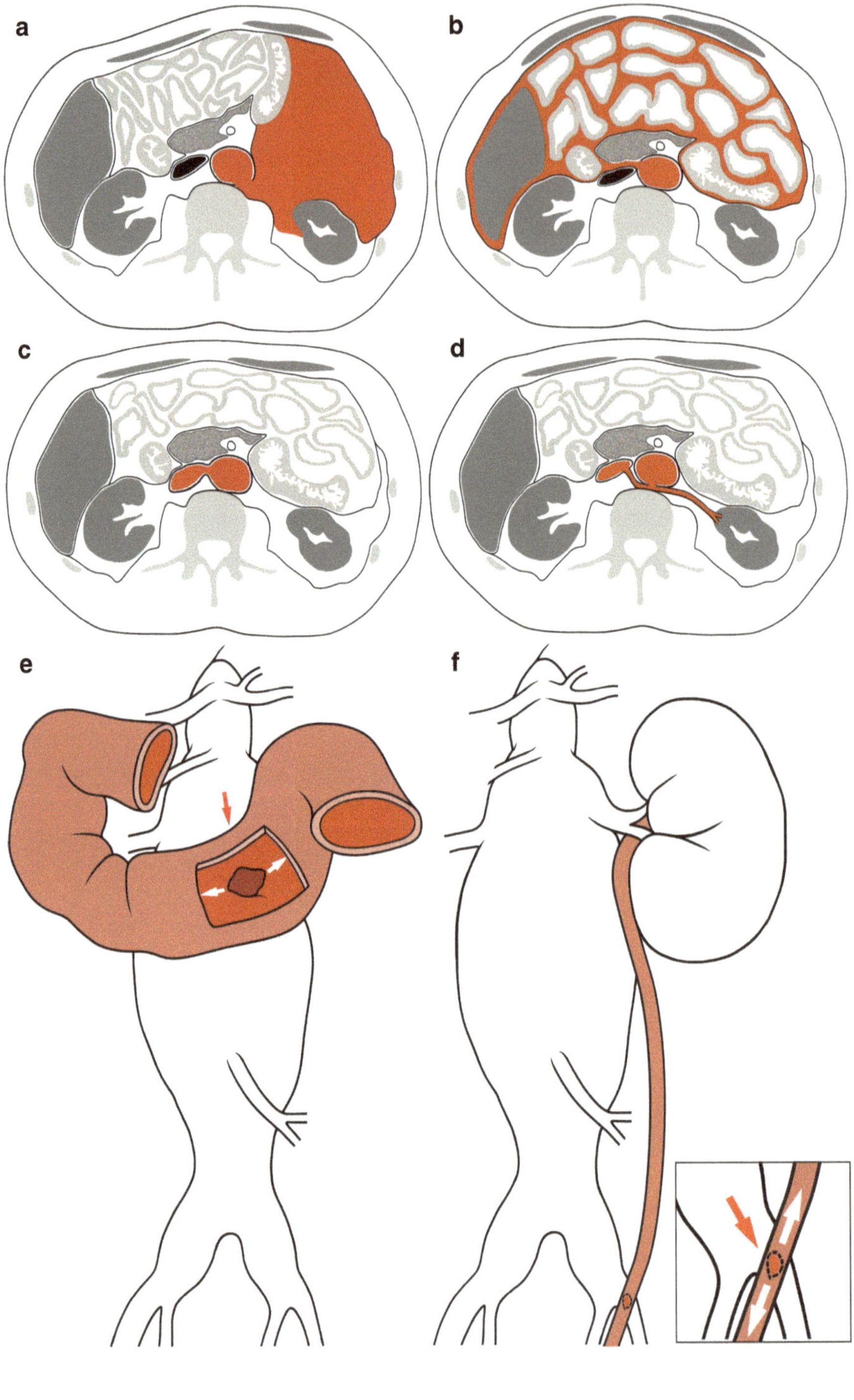
a
b
c
d
e
f

Fig. 6.1 (continued)

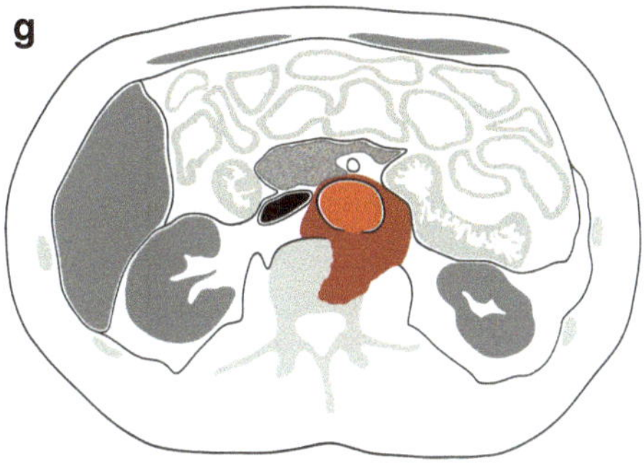

Fig. 6.1 Illustration of various types of ruptures. (**a**) Retroperitoneal rupture. Dorsal or dorsolateral rupture usually leads to a leak into the retroperitoneum, often causing asymmetric displacement and squeezing of the abdominal content. As a consequence, asymmetric bulging of the abdominal wall may be encountered. Due to the restricted retroperitoneal space and the consistency of the retroperitoneal tissues, retroperitoneal leaks often temporarily seal, before definite – sometimes free – rupture. "Contained" rupture is therefore used synonymously to retroperitoneal rupture in the literature. (**b**) Intraperitoneal rupture. More anterior rupture may immediately communicate with the peritoneal cavity, and due to the low resistance in this space and the good compliance of the abdominal wall, massive amounts of blood may flow into this cavity. "Free" rupture is therefore regularly used as a synonym. Bulging of the abdomen usually is symmetric. (**c**) Aortocaval fistula. Right lateral rupture into the vena cava causes a communication of a high-pressure to a low-pressure system. This left to right shunt leads to massive increase in cardiac output and eventually to high-output congestive heart failure. The abdomen is usually unremarkable, although an abdominal thrill may be palpated or auscultated. (**d**) Aorto-left renal vein fistula. Dorsal rupture into a retroaortic left renal vein accounts for 90 % of this type of rupture. In addition to the signs and symptoms of aortocaval fistula, hematuria or varicocele may frequently develop. (**e**) Aortoenteric fistula. Rupture into the bowel creates a communication between usually the third or fourth part of the duodenum and the aorta. However, all parts of the gastrointestinal systems may be involved. Due to the leak into a low-pressure system, blood may immediately ascend to the stomach and pretend an upper GI bleeding. Less frequently, a lower GI bleeding may reveal as an aortoenteric fistula, e.g., the jejunum. (**f**) Arterio-ureteral fistula. Rupture into the ureter most often occurs in the region of the iliac bifurcation either between the native aneurysmatic iliac artery or a previously placed graft for aortoiliac replacement. Hematuria and hydronephrosis are the most common signs of AUF. (**g**) Chronic contained rupture. Retroperitoneal rupture may lead to a slow progressive bleeding that is contained by the resistance of the periaortic tissues and may exert chronic stone mill-like pressure to the adjacent structures such as the vertebral column. Erosion of vertebral bodies has been documented radiologically and surgically. Correspondingly, chronic back pain with or without irradiation to the groin is the most presenting symptom in this type of rupture

incarcerated hernia, or lumbar spine disease, to name only a few. On the other hand, patients with RAAA may present in frank shock, as evidenced by cyanosis, mottling, unconsciousness, tachycardia, and severe hypotension.

Physicians should – independent of their specialties – be aware of the early signs of potential abdominal aortic aneurysm rupture: syncope, transient hypotension, and/or loss of consciousness. Rapid diagnosis due to early suspicion of RAAA may be lifesaving as hemodynamic instability may suddenly ensue due to continuous blood loss, "secondary" rupture, and/or ACS.

Usual Presentation of RAAA

Retroperitoneal Rupture

Rupture of the posterior or lateral aneurysm wall into the retroperitoneal cavity (Fig. 6.1a), generally called retroperitoneal or also "contained" rupture, is the most common site of rupture found in RAAA patients. Due to the posterolateral localization of the tear, the blood will rapidly expand into the retroperitoneal space. However, bleeding will often be temporarily sealed, because of the anatomy and consistency of the retroperitoneal space and tissues that will "contain" bleeding by tamponade due to increased retroperitoneal pressure. Clinically, this manifests as back or flank pain with or without abdominal pain and (temporary) hypotension. The pain is usually severe, constant, and unaffected by position and can radiate to the chest, scrotum, inguinal region, or the thigh. On inspection, patients are pale and sweaty, sometimes restless, and often report feeling cold. Physical examination may show a pulsatile mass in the upper abdomen. The latter is often missing, however, especially in obese patients and/or those with severe hypotension caused by hemorrhagic hypovolemia.

This period of self-tamponade provides the window of opportunity for the treatment of patients with this type of rupture. They remain relatively stable, sometimes even for a few hours, during which patients may rapidly be transferred to an institution familiar with the management of RAAA. Patients are, however, at great risk for "secondary" rupture, especially when reanimation includes aggressive blood pressure and fluid resuscitation as taught for many years. Therefore, these patients should be followed by the principles of hypotensive hemostasis described in the literature: fluid restriction and keeping the systolic blood pressure low [7–9].

If not suspected right away, contained RAAA may develop a variety of misleading symptoms and clinical as well as radiological signs because of the growing intra-abdominal pressure and compression of abdominal organs such as the intestines or the ureters because of the growing hematoma. Even angina-like symptoms may occur, especially when ACS develops leading to low cardiac and coronary filling pressures [6]. Not infrequently, however, true angina pectoris develops due to severe hypotension and hypovolemia caused by the RAAA. The author has experienced situations where patients were kept in the medical emergency department for many hours before RAAA has been detected "incidentally" while performing a (contrast-enhanced) computed tomographic scan for an entire different reason. This kind of diagnostic delay significantly worsens the outcome; the mortality rate increases from 45 to 55 % when diagnosis is delayed for up to 10 h or as high as 100 % when missed even longer [10]. It is strongly suggested, therefore, that in any patient with sudden abdominal and/or back and/or flank pain, RAAA must always be considered in the differential diagnosis. Algorithms and emergency checklists should be updated accordingly. However, retroperitoneal rupture may present in a quite unusual fashion such as painless or painful testicular ecchymosis also called the "blue scrotum sign of Bryant" [11, 12].

Intraperitoneal Rupture

As many as 65 % of patients with ruptured abdominal aortic aneurysms die of sudden cardiovascular collapse before arriving at a hospital. Most of these patients suffer from anterior rupture, also called "free" rupture, with massive bleeding into the peritoneal cavity (Fig. 6.1b). In contrast to the posterior retroperitoneal rupture, there is no resistance that would allow temporary sealing and containment of the rupture. The blood may fill up the intraperitoneal space until the patient's exsanguination. Clinically, sudden severe abdominal and/or back pain is usually followed by collapse because of uncontrolled bleeding. Patients usually remain hemodynamically unstable and do not temporarily recover like the patients suffering from retroperitoneal contained rupture. The abdomen may appear balloon-like due to rapid expansion of the abdominal wall, while in patients with retroperitoneal rupture, an asymmetric bulging may be detected. Some patients may be found dead minutes after free intraperitoneal rupture and therefore mistakenly be diagnosed as cardiac sudden death patients.

Unusual Presentation of RAAA

Rarely, abdominal aortic aneurysms rupture into abdominal veins, small bowel segments, or even the ureter, producing fistulae of the respective hollow structures. The patient's presentation varies depending on the localization of the rupture and the organs involved.

Aortocaval Fistula

Rupture into the inferior vena cava (Fig. 6.1c) will produce an aortocaval fistula (ACF) of varying diameter. Depending on the size of the communication between the aorta and vena cava, variable clinical manifestations may be detected. The classic presentation of patients with ACF is a triad of abdominal and/or back pain, a pulsatile abdominal mass, and a continuous bruit on abdominal auscultation (sometimes accompanied by a palpable thrill) [13–15]. However, the prevalence of this classic triad varies significantly between studies and may be as low as 17 % [14, 15]. High-output congestive heart failure may be the leading manifestation with patients showing dyspnea, pulmonary edema, tachycardia, wide pulse pressure, cyanosis, dilated superficial veins on the abdominal wall or the legs, and lower limb edema [13, 14, 16, 17]. A variety of other symptoms may mislead the clinicians in making the correct diagnosis of RAAA in the form of aortocaval fistula: angina pectoris [13], palpitations [18], fever [19], and rectal bleeding [20] due to rupture of distended veins. Oliguria [15, 19] and renal insufficiency [21–24] caused by decreased renal perfusion and hematuria caused by kidney malperfusion and/or superficial renal or bladder vein rupture [25] may trigger the wrong diagnosis of kidney or bladder disease. Acute hepatorenal failure has been described as a first manifestation at presentation [26]. In fact, probably half of all aortocaval fistulae are missed [19], and ACF is frequently incidentally detected during elective AAA surgery [14]. Hypotension, pulsatile peripheral veins [13], and diminished lower limb pulses [13, 19] may eventually lead to the correct diagnosis when detected. Although rupture of AAA is the main cause of ACF, other causes exist such as trauma and surgery of the lumbar spine [13, 14].

It is important that clinicians and emergency staff be trained in detecting ACF. The outcome of accidentally discovered ACF during surgery is significantly worse because of major blood loss or pulmonary embolism from aortic thrombus caused by the inadequate operative strategy due to ignorance [14]. Preoperative detection of ACF is important and nowadays should be accomplished by contrast-enhanced computed tomographic angiography (CTA) [13, 14, 19, 27].

Aorto-left Renal Vein Fistula

Rupture into the left renal vein (Fig. 6.1d) might be regarded as equivalent to aortocaval fistula with special considerations. Pathophysiologically, this type of arteriovenous fistula behaves similarly to the aortocaval fistula with possible high-output congestive heart failure and all the clinical manifestations as described above. However, due to its site of rupture into the left renal vein, signs and symptoms regarding the kidney and bladder are accentuated. This is best represented by the "abdominal pain, hematuria, silent left kidney" syndrome described in the early 1990s by Mansour et al. [28]. Pain is usually felt in the left flank and radiates to the groin. It is accompanied by hematuria in 85 % of patients [29], and ureteral colic is often suspected rather than an AAA that has ruptured into the left renal vein [30]. Despite the fact that this kind of RAAA is very rare, diagnosis should be promptly made when these symptoms are present [29]. The outcome is similarly worsened because of ignorance of the underlying pathology and the discovery of the condition during surgery. It is important to note that in more than 90 % of the cases, the rupture occurs dorsally into a retroaortic left renal vein, a rare anomaly affecting 1–2.4 % of people [28, 29]. Finally, two patients who presented with a large left-sided varicocele, presumably due to left renal vein hypertension and impaired venous return from the left testicle, have been described [29, 31]. Furthermore, recently, a female patient with a retroaortic left renal vein fistula masquerading as pelvic congestion syndrome has been described by Fassiadis et al. [32]. Of the 32 cases described up to 2013, all but two were male [32–34]. Very recently, Wu et al., in a letter to the editor, describe the case of a 30-year-old man who was brought to the hospital following trauma involving an abdominal stab wound [35]. The postoperative CT scan following emergency abdominal surgery revealed an aorto-left renal vein fistula that was secondarily treated by endovascular repair.

Aortoenteric Fistula

Rupture into the bowel (Fig. 6.1e) creates a communication between a non-sterile compartment, the bowel, and a sterile compartment, the aorta. Anatomically, the third or fourth parts of the duodenum are most commonly involved due to their topographic relationship to the anterior aortic wall and their fixation to the retroperitoneum by the ligament of Treitz [36], but other parts may be involved. Two types of aortoenteric fistulas (AEFs) are recognized: primary and secondary [37]. Primary fistulas occur de novo between the aorta and the bowel, the more common secondary fistulas between an aortic graft and a segment of bowel. Accordingly, clinical presentations vary depending on the size and localization of the communication with the bowel, the dynamic of perforation, and the presence or not of previous open vascular or endovascular interventions. Patients with aortoenteric fistula (AEF) may present with few symptoms beyond abdominal discomfort [38] with or without an elevated CRP and white blood cell count, if perforation is impending or temporarily sealed. In fact, symptoms may be attributed to peptic ulceration, and the proton pump inhibitors prescribed may temporarily relieve the pain [38]. On the other end of the spectrum, AEF patients may present as an emergency, either with massive gastrointestinal (GI) bleeding, with frank sepsis, or both. Patients with significant GI bleeding induced by AEF present with hematemesis, melena, and anemia, sometimes accompanied by syncope or shock [39–41]. Massive hemorrhage is commonly preceded by an episode of small brisk bleeding which stops spontaneously. This so-called herald bleed is characteristic of an AEF [36]. Diagnosis of AEF is often delayed for days or even weeks, and patients sometimes receive multiple blood transfusions before the diagnosis of AEF is established [39]. However, patients may just present with abdominal pain and melena or recurrent rectal bleeding [38]. Melena as the first manifestation of AEF may mislead clinicians to look for peptic ulcer disease, gastritis, esophageal varices, Meckel's diverticulum, or Mallory-Weiss syndrome. Presentation with rectal bleeding and flank pain for 2 weeks before establishing the diagnosis of primary AEF has been described [42]. Unexplained fever may occur in patients with primary [43, 44] or secondary [45] AEF, and missing the diagnosis may end fatally. Some patients present with (recurrent episodes of) sepsis caused by primary [46] or secondary [47] AEF. Diagnosis may be delayed for months, as reported in a 78-year-old female treated for recurrent episodes of *Enterobacter cloacae* sepsis with antibiotics before finally detecting a secondary AEF [47].

In summary, establishing the diagnosis of primary or secondary AEF is very challenging, and a high index of suspicion is required because of the variability of clinical presentation. The classical clinical triad consisting of upper gastrointestinal bleeding, abdominal pain, and a pulsatile abdominal mass is present in only 10 % of patients suffering from primary AEF [48, 49]. Presentation of secondary AEF is even more complex, and the clinical manifestations are often crucial to the diagnosis of AEF, because no single imaging modality is capable of depicting this condition with high sensitivity and specificity. However, if clinically suspected, upper GI endoscopy (to include the entire duodenum), contrast-enhanced computed tomographic angiography, and, sometimes, plain angiography or ultrasound may be required to confirm the diagnosis. Unfortunately, preoperative diagnosis of AEF is reached in only 50 % of the patients [36], exposing half of the patients to a high risk for intraoperative massive bleeding and complications as with aortocaval and aorto-left renal vein fistulas.

Arterio-ureteral Fistula

Rupture into the ureter (Fig. 6.1f) will create a communication between the aorta and the iliac arteries and anastomotic aneurysms or vascular graft material in the aortoiliac position and the ureter [50, 51]. The left and right ureter seems to be involved almost alike, whereas bilateral involvement is only 1 % [51]. Arterio-ureteral fistula (AUF) is an uncommon diagnosis that is often missed due to its misleading presentation. In a recent systematic review of 139 cases from 1899 to 2008 by van den Bergh et al., all patients presented with hematuria [51]. Some patients required acute intervention for massive hematuria, while in most patients hematuria was less intense, and they presented after having experienced multiple intermittent episodes of bleeding. In 74 % of AUF patients, hematuria was the only manifestation, 17 % had accompanying flank or back pain, 7 % showed signs of infection, and 1 % had urinary retention at first presentation. Three quarters of the patients suffered from urologic symptoms for a longer period before initial presentation such as hydronephrosis, ureteral stenosis, a previously damaged ureter, or signs of chronic urinary tract infection. AUF is a life-threatening condition, and the outcome is strongly inversely associated with the length of diagnostic delay [52, 53]. Therefore, all clinicians, especially urologists, and emergency staff should be trained to have a high level of suspicion for the presence of AUF in patients with a background of pelvic oncologic or vascular pathologic features or surgery, abdominal or pelvic radiotherapy, urinary diversion surgery, and ureteral stenting. Further specific diagnostic investigations should be performed immediately, when an AUF is suspected [54]. Often, repeated studies and provocative testing are required to confirm the diagnosis of AUF [55].

Chronic Presentation of RAAA

Chronic Contained Rupture

Retroperitoneal rupture may lead to slow progressive bleeding, eventually forming a large hematoma that is contained by the resistance of the periaortic tissues (Fig. 6.1g) [56, 57]. Clinical presentation is like a colorful bouquet of flowers: most patients suffering from chronic contained rupture (CCR) present with chronic back pain with or without irradiation to the groin [58–61]; other pain-related manifestations reported are lumbar spondylitis-like symptoms [61–63], left lower extremity weakness or neuropathy [64–66], or even crural neuropathy [56]; and vertebral erosion [67–69], left psoas hematoma [60], or even obstructive jaundice [70] are further clinical manifestations. Not surprisingly, RAAA is mostly missed in these patients, and they may be treated, for example, for back pain or neurological symptoms instead. Chronic back pain of unknown origin should raise the clinicians' suspicion for CCR, and further diagnostic investigations (contrast-enhanced CT angiography and/or magnetic resonance imaging) should be performed. Although CCR patients are generally hemodynamically stable, missing the diagnosis, and hence rapid treatment, could lead to fatal free rupture and death [61, 65, 69, 71].

Presentation with Abdominal Compartment Syndrome

The presence of intra-abdominal hypertension (IAH) and abdominal compartment syndrome (ACS) may further confuse the presentation of patients suffering from RAAA. ACS as a consequence of IAH leads to (multiple) organ dysfunction at the early stage, and patients therefore may be investigated for diseases of almost every organ system [6, 72]. If not treated rapidly and appropriately, eventually full-blown multiple organ failure (MOF) will develop. Although ACS usually occurs perioperatively [73], probably as part of the reperfusion injury to the abdominal organs, patients with an RAAA may present with mild to full-blown ACS already on admission. Clinically, renal dysfunction, respiratory insufficiency due to increased airway pressures and decreased pulmonary compliance, cerebral dysfunction due to increased intracranial pressure, decreased cardiac output, signs of right heart failure, angina pectoris-like symptoms, and loss of bowel function due to poor intestinal perfusion may be encountered [72]. Contrary to popular opinion, clinical examination appears to be inaccurate to diagnose IAH/ACS [74–76]. The only reliable diagnostic tool to detect and discriminate ACS is early and repeated measurement of the intra-abdominal pressure (through measurement of the bladder pressure, e.g., using a Foley manometer) [77, 78]. Therefore, regular (1–2 hourly) or continuous IAP monitoring is recommended in RAAA patients [7, 73]. Given the serious consequences of missed ACS and the fact that ACS can imitate many reasons for organ failure, it is strongly recommended that all emergency staff be trained in the recognition of the potentially fatal diagnosis of abdominal compartment syndrome as a consequence of RAAA.

Presentation of Women with RAAA

Despite the ongoing discussion about the gender differences in the outcome of (ruptured) abdominal aneurysm repair and documented worse outcomes of RAAA repair in women [79], little is known about the differences in presentation of women with RAAA compared to men. It seems that women present, at an older age, with smaller aneurysm diameter at rupture and worse vascular anatomy [80, 81]. In a large randomized controlled trial in the UK, comparing an endovascular versus and open repair strategy for RAAA, women were shown to profit from endovascular aneurysm repair [82]. Therefore, RAAAs should be rapidly diagnosed in women so they can be referred to a specialized center with the skills and facilities necessary to perform EVAR, if their anatomy is suitable.

Presentation of Children with RAAA

Abdominal aortic aneurysms in children are distinctly rare and rupture of them even rarer [83, 84]. Acquired AAA in children is associated with various predisposing factors, including infection (e.g., bacteria, tuberculosis, and fungal infection) [85], congenital connective tissue disease (e.g., Marfan's syndrome, Ehlers-Danlos syndrome, and tuberous sclerosis) [86, 87], trauma (e.g., umbilical artery catheterization) [88], and vasculitis (e.g., Takayasu arteritis, polyarteritis nodosa, giant cell arteritis, and Kawasaki's syndrome) [89]. In comparison with acquired abdominal aortic aneurysm, congenital AAA has an unknown etiology [90, 91]. Clinical presentation may vary from a complete lack of symptoms to ruptures [84, 92–94]. Mild abdominal distension is sometimes the only abdominal symptom of rupture in children [93, 94]. A pulsatile abdominal mass may be detected unexpectedly only after laparotomy, and the delay in diagnosis may lead to fatal outcome [93, 94]. Emergency staffs should be aware of the rare and distinct possibility of aortic rupture in children of any age suffering from known or unknown AAA of various etiologies. Immediate further investigation (e.g., contrast-enhanced computed tomographic angiography) is mandatory as soon as signs of major bleeding are present.

Misdiagnosis of RAAA

Hemodynamic stability seems to play a major role when it comes to misdiagnosis of RAAA and as a consequence treatment delay [95]. Among 98 patients undergoing emergency AAA repair, 56 patients were hemodynamically stable at presentation, and misdiagnosis was significantly more common in these patients than in those who were in shock (58.9 % vs 26.2 %, $p=0.002$). Median time delay from presentation to diagnosis was significantly increased (144 min vs 12 min, $p<0.0001$), and median time from diagnosis to arrival in theater was significantly longer (90 min vs 48 min, $p=0.02$) in patients who were hemodynamically stable at presentation. Of the 56 patients who were hemodynamically stable at presentation, 19 underwent hemodynamic decompensation before surgery with a significantly increased mortality compared with those who remained stable (73.7 % vs 37.8 %, $p=0.02$). Of these 19 patients, only five were correctly diagnosed at presentation. Gastrointestinal and renal/urinary tract pathologies were the most frequent misdiagnoses, followed by back, thoracic, or cardiac pathologies [95].

In a recent systematic review and meta-analysis of nine studies comprising 1109 patients eligible for the pooled analysis, a 42 % incidence of misdiagnosis of RAAA was found [96]. In studies reported after 1990, misdiagnosis was seen in 32 %. The most common erroneous differential diagnoses were ureteric colic and myocardial infarction. Abdominal pain, shock, and a pulsatile mass – the classical triad – were presenting features in 61 %, 46 %, and 45 % of RAAA, respectively. A concerning fact is that the rate of misdiagnosis of RAAA has remained consistent over time despite the vast literature and experience available in the medical community. The authors conclude that there is a need for greater awareness of the possibility of an RAAA and an effective clinical decision tool to enable accurate diagnosis and triage when these patients present [96].

References

1. Sakalihasan N, Limet R, Defawe OD. Abdominal aortic aneurysm. Lancet. 2005;365(9470): 1577–89.
2. Marston WA, Ahlquist R, Johnson Jr G, Meyer AA. Misdiagnosis of ruptured abdominal aortic aneurysms. J Vasc Surg. 1992;16(1):17–22.
3. Fielding JW, Black J, Ashton F, Slaney G, Campbell DJ. Diagnosis and management of 528 abdominal aortic aneurysms. Br Med J (Clin Res Ed). 1981;283(6287):355–9.
4. Jones CS, Reilly MK, Dalsing MC, Glover JL. Chronic contained rupture of abdominal aortic aneurysms. Arch Surg. 1986;121(5):542–6.
5. Szilagyi DE, Smith RF, Macksood AJ, Whitcomb JG. Expanding and ruptured abdominal aortic aneurysms. Problems of diagnosis and treatment. Arch Surg. 1961;83:395–408.
6. Mayer D, Rancic Z, Veith FJ, Pecoraro F, Pfammatter T, Lachat M. How to diagnose and treat abdominal compartment syndrome after endovascular and open repair of ruptured abdominal aortic aneurysms. J Cardiovasc Surg (Torino). 2014;55(2):179–92.
7. Mayer D, Pfammatter T, Rancic Z, Hechelhammer L, Wilhelm M, Veith FJ, et al. 10 years of emergency endovascular aneurysm repair for ruptured abdominal aortoiliac aneurysms: lessons learned. Ann Surg. 2009;249(3):510–5.
8. Veith FJ, Ohki T. Endovascular approaches to ruptured infrarenal aorto-iliac aneurysms. J Cardiovasc Surg (Torino). 2002;43(3):369–78.
9. Stern SA. Low-volume fluid resuscitation for presumed hemorrhagic shock: helpful or harmful? Curr Opin Crit Care. 2001;7(6):422–30.
10. Chung WB. The ruptured abdominal aortic aneurysm – a diagnostic problem. Can Med Assoc J. 1971;105(8):811–5.
11. Dargin JM, Lowenstein RA. Ruptured abdominal aortic aneurysm presenting as painless testicular ecchymosis: the scrotal sign of Bryant revisited. J Emerg Med. 2011;40(3):e45–8.

12. Ratzan RM, Donaldson MC, Foster JH, Walzak MP. The blue scrotum sign of Bryant: a diagnostic clue to ruptured abdominal aortic aneurysm. J Emerg Med. 1987;5(4):323–9.
13. Iriz E, Ozdogan ME, Erer D, Uslu M, Koksal P, Kurtipek O. A giant aortocaval fistula due to abdominal aortic aneurysm. Int J Cardiol. 2006;112(3):e78–80.
14. Davis PM, Gloviczki P, Cherry Jr KJ, Toomey BJ, Stanson AW, Bower TC, et al. Aorto-caval and ilio-iliac arteriovenous fistulae. Am J Surg. 1998;176(2):115–8.
15. Quiroga S, Alvarez-Castells A, Hidalgo A, Ruiz-Marcellan C, Castella E, Gifre L. Spontaneous aortocaval fistula: CT findings with pathologic correlation. Abdom Imaging. 1995;20(5): 466–9.
16. Delaney CP, Brady MP. Ruptured aortic aneurysm with aortocaval fistula. J R Soc Med. 1998;91(12):645–6.
17. Bower TC, Cherry KJ, Pairolero PC. Unusual manifestations of abdominal aortic aneurysms. Surg Clin North Am. 1989;69:745–54.
18. Duffy JP, Gardham JR. Spontaneous aortocaval fistula – preoperative diagnosis and management. Postgrad Med J. 1989;65(764):397–9.
19. Tsolakis JA, Papadoulas S, Kakkos SK, Skroubis G, Siablis D, Androulakis JA. Aortocaval fistula in ruptured aneurysms. Eur J Vasc Endovasc Surg. 1999;17(5):390–3.
20. Reckless JP, McColl I, Taylor GW. Aorto-caval fistulae: an uncommon complication of abdominal aortic aneurysms. Br J Surg. 1972;59(6):461–2.
21. Albalate M, Gomez Octavio J, Llobregat R, Fuster JM. Acute renal failure due to aortocaval fistula. Nephrol Dial Transplant. 1998;13(5):1268–70.
22. Brunkwall J, Lanne T, Bergentz SE. Acute renal impairment due to a primary aortocaval fistula is normalised after a successful operation. Eur J Vasc Endovasc Surg. 1999;17(3):191–6.
23. McKeown BJ, Rankin SC. Aortocaval fistulae presenting with renal failure: CT diagnosis. Clin Radiol. 1994;49(8):570–2.
24. Simsek E, Caliskan A, Tutun U, Sahin S. Cause of a rare acute renal insufficiency: rupture aortocaval fistula. Vascular. 2014;22(4):290–2.
25. Takazawa A, Sakahashi H, Toyama A. Surgical repair of a concealed aortocaval fistula associated with an abdominal aortic aneurysm: report of two cases. Surg Today. 2001;31(9):842–4.
26. Kanbay M, Gur G, Boyvat F, Tasdelen A, Boyacioglu S. Spontaneous aortocaval fistula presenting with acute liver and renal failure: a case report. Turk J Gastroenterol. 2004;15(3):169–72.
27. Rosenthal D, Atkins CP, Jerrius HS, Clark MD, Matsuura JH. Diagnosis of aortocaval fistula by computed tomography. Ann Vasc Surg. 1998;12(1):86–7.
28. Mansour MA, Rutherford RB, Metcalf RK, Pearce WH. Spontaneous aorto-left renal vein fistula: the "abdominal pain, hematuria, silent left kidney" syndrome. Surgery. 1991;109(1):101–6.
29. Barrier P, Otal P, Garcia O, Vahdat O, Domenech B, Lannareix V, et al. Aorta-left renal vein fistula complicating an aortic aneurysm: preoperative and postoperative multislice CT findings. Cardiovasc Intervent Radiol. 2007;30(3):485–7.
30. Jabbour N, Radulescu OV, Flogiates T, Stahl W. Hemodynamics of an aorta-left renal vein fistula: a case report and a review of the literature. Crit Care Med. 1993;21(7):1092–5.
31. Meyerson SL, Haider SA, Gupta N, O'Dorsio JE, McKinsey JF, Schwartz LB. Abdominal aortic aneurysm with aorta-left renal vein fistula with left varicocele. J Vasc Surg. 2000;31(4):802–5.
32. Fassiadis N, Macqueen Buchanan E, Wilkins J, Jones K, Edmondson R. Retroaortic left renal vein fistula masquerading as pelvic congestion syndrome: case report. Int J Surg. 2008;6(6): e77–9.
33. Hsu CC, Singh D, Kwan GN, Livsey R. Spontaneous aorto-left renal vein fistula: a rare complication of abdominal aortic aneurysm. ANZ J Surg. 2015;85(6):494–5.
34. Yagdi T, Atay Y, Engin C, Ozbek SS, Buket S. Aorta-left renal vein fistula in a woman. Tex Heart Inst J. 2004;31(4):435–8.
35. Wu Z, He Y, Zhang H. Endovascular aortic repair with the chimney graft technique for abdominal aortic pseudoaneurysms with aorto-left renal vein fistula. J Vasc Interv Radiol. 2015;26(2):290–2.

36. Lemos DW, Raffetto JD, Moore TC, Menzoian JO. Primary aortoduodenal fistula: a case report and review of the literature. J Vasc Surg. 2003;37(3):686–9.
37. Busuttil SJ, Goldstone J. Diagnosis and management of aortoenteric fistulas. Semin Vasc Surg. 2001;14(4):302–11.
38. Pittman M, Sakai L, Craig R, Joehl R, Milner R. Primary aortoenteric fistula following disseminated bacillus Calmette-Guerin infection: a case report. Vascular. 2012;20(4): 221–4.
39. Koshy AK, Simon EG, Keshava SN. Education and Imaging. Gastrointestinal: aortoenteric fistula. J Gastroenterol Hepatol. 2010;25(5):1014.
40. Varetto G, Gibello L, Trevisan A, Castagno C, Garneri P, Rispoli P. Primary aortoenteric fistula of a saccular aneurysm: case study and literature review. Korean Circ J. 2015;45(4):337–9.
41. Batt M, Jean-Baptiste E, O'Connor S, Saint-Lebes B, Feugier P, Patra P, et al. Early and late results of contemporary management of 37 secondary aortoenteric fistulae. Eur J Vasc Endovasc Surg. 2011;41(6):748–57.
42. Vilas-Boas F, Azevedo F, Marques M, Baldaque-Silva F, Cardoso H, Costa-Lima J, et al. Primary aortoenteric fistula. Clin J Gastroenterol. 2013;6(4):299–302.
43. van Olffen TB, Knippenberg LH, van der Vliet JA, Lastdrager WB. Primary aortoenteric fistula: report of six new cases. Cardiovasc Surg. 2002;10(6):551–4.
44. Voorhoeve R, Moll FL, de Letter JA, Bast TJ, Wester JP, Slee PH. Primary aortoenteric fistula: report of eight new cases and review of the literature. Ann Vasc Surg. 1996;10(1):40–8.
45. Arzuaga Torre JA, Tebas Medrano P, Simal Anton A, Estirado de Cabo E, Roman Garcia F, Martinez J, et al. Fever and recurrent bacteremia as presentation form of secondary aortoenteric fistula. An Med Interna. 1993;10(10):495–8.
46. Skourtis G, Papacharalambous G, Makris S, Kasfikis F, Kastrisios G, Goulas S, et al. Primary aortoenteric fistula due to septic aortitis. Ann Vasc Surg. 2010;24(6):825 e7–11.
47. Kibria R, Rao PK, Siva S. Secondary aortoenteric fistula presenting with recurrent episodes of sepsis. South Med J. 2010;103(6):594–5.
48. Lozano FS, Munoz-Bellvis L, San Norberto E, Garcia-Plaza A, Gonzalez-Porras JR. Primary aortoduodenal fistula: new case reports and a review of the literature. J Gastrointest Surg. 2008;12(9):1561–5.
49. Saers SJ, Scheltinga MR. Primary aortoenteric fistula. Br J Surg. 2005;92(2):143–52.
50. Holmes M, Hung N, Hunter M. Hematuria and death secondary to aortoureteric fistula. Urology. 1998;52(4):720–2.
51. van den Bergh RC, Moll FL, de Vries JP, Lock TM. Arterioureteral fistulas: unusual suspects-systematic review of 139 cases. Urology. 2009;74(2):251–5.
52. Bergqvist D, Parsson H, Sherif A. Arterio-ureteral fistula – a systematic review. Eur J Vasc Endovasc Surg. 2001;22(3):191–6.
53. Krambeck AE, DiMarco DS, Gettman MT, Segura JW. Ureteroiliac artery fistula: diagnosis and treatment algorithm. Urology. 2005;66(5):990–4.
54. Darcy M. Uretro-arterial fistulas. Tech Vasc Interv Radiol. 2009;12(3):216–21.
55. Lyon TD, Ferroni MC, McCluskey KM, Maranchie JK. An uncommon cause of gross hematuria: two cases of ureteroarterial fistula. Can J Urol. 2013;20(4):6871–4.
56. Defraigne JO, Sakalihasan N, Lavigne JP, Van Damme H, Limet R. Chronic rupture of abdominal aortic aneurysm manifesting as crural neuropathy. Ann Vasc Surg. 2001;15(3): 405–11.
57. Gandini R, Chiocchi M, Maresca L, Pipitone V, Messina M, Simonetti G. Chronic contained rupture of an abdominal aortic aneurysm: from diagnosis to endovascular resolution. Cardiovasc Intervent Radiol. 2008;31 Suppl 2:S62–6.
58. Akkersdijk GJ, van Bockel JH. Ruptured abdominal aortic aneurysm: initial misdiagnosis and the effect on treatment. Eur J Surg. 1998;164(1):29–34.
59. Al-Koteesh J, Masannat Y, James NV, Sharaf U. Chronic contained rupture of abdominal aortic aneurysm presenting with longstanding back pain. Scott Med J. 2005;50(3):122–3.
60. Cumming MJ, Hall AJ, Burbridge BE. Psoas muscle hematoma secondary to a ruptured abdominal aortic aneurysm: case report. Can Assoc Radiol J. 2000;51(5):279–80.

61. Moran KT, Persson AV, Jewell ER. Chronic rupture of abdominal aortic aneurysms. Am Surg. 1989;55(8):485–7.
62. Amouzougan A, Zenone T, Couret M, Peoc'h M, Barral X, Barral FG, et al. Pseudospondylitis caused by rupture of an aortic aneurysm. J Rheumatol. 2007;34(12):2501–2.
63. Edrees WK, Lee B. A rare case of radiculopathy in an elderly man. Postgrad Med J. 2000;76(899):586, 591–2.
64. Haddad FS, Hatrick NC, Shanahan DJ. An unusual presentation of a ruptured abdominal aortic aneurysm. J Accid Emerg Med. 1995;12(3):220–1.
65. Higgins R, Peitzman AB, Reidy M, Stapczynski S, Steed DL, Webster MW. Chronic contained rupture of an abdominal aortic aneurysm presenting as a lower extremity neuropathy. Ann Emerg Med. 1988;17(3):284–7.
66. Ramasamy PR, Fox D, Narendra G, Carnie L, Watura R. Chronic contained leak of abdominal aortic aneurysm presenting as lumbar neuropathy. J R Coll Surg Edinb. 2001;46(5):307–9.
67. Aydogan M, Karatoprak O, Mirzanli C, Ozturk C, Tezer M, Hamzaoglu A. Severe erosion of lumbar vertebral body because of a chronic ruptured abdominal aortic aneurysm. Spine J. 2008;8(2):394–6.
68. Lai CC, Tan CK, Chu TW, Ding LW. Chronic contained rupture of an abdominal aortic aneurysm with vertebral erosion. Can Med Assoc J. 2008;178(8):995–6.
69. Saiki M, Urata Y, Katoh I, Hamasaki T. Chronic contained rupture of an abdominal aortic aneurysm with vertebral erosion: report of a case. Ann Thorac Cardiovasc Surg. 2006;12(4):300–2.
70. Dorrucci V, Dusi R, Rombola G, Cordiano C. Contained rupture of an abdominal aortic aneurysm presenting as obstructive jaundice: report of a case. Surg Today. 2001;31(4):331–2.
71. Patel SN, Kettner NW. Abdominal aortic aneurysm presenting as back pain to a chiropractic clinic: a case report. J Manipulative Physiol Ther. 2006;29(5):409 e1–7.
72. Mayer D, Veith FJ, Lachat M, Pfammatter T, Hechelhammer L, Rancic Z. Abdominal compartment syndrome. Minerva Chir. 2010;65(3):329–46.
73. Mayer D, Rancic Z, Meier C, Pfammatter T, Veith FJ, Lachat M. Open abdomen treatment following endovascular repair of ruptured abdominal aortic aneurysms. J Vasc Surg. 2009; 50(1):1–7.
74. Malbrain ML, De laet IE, De Waele JJ. IAH/ACS: the rationale for surveillance. World J Surg. 2009;33(6):1110–5.
75. Sugrue M, Bauman A, Jones F, Bishop G, Flabouris A, Parr M, et al. Clinical examination is an inaccurate predictor of intraabdominal pressure. World J Surg. 2002;26(12):1428–31.
76. Kirkpatrick AW, Brenneman FD, McLean RF, Rapanos T, Boulanger BR. Is clinical examination an accurate indicator of raised intra-abdominal pressure in critically injured patients? Can J Surg. 2000;43(3):207–11.
77. Malbrain ML, Cheatham ML, Kirkpatrick A, Sugrue M, Parr M, De Waele J, et al. Results from the international conference of experts on intra-abdominal hypertension and abdominal compartment syndrome. I. Definitions. Intensive Care Med. 2006;32(11):1722–32.
78. Malbrain ML, Chiumello D, Pelosi P, Bihari D, Innes R, Ranieri VM, et al. Incidence and prognosis of intraabdominal hypertension in a mixed population of critically ill patients: a multiple-center epidemiological study. Crit Care Med. 2005;33(2):315–22.
79. Vavra AK, Kibbe MR, Bown MJ, Powell JT. Debate: whether evidence supports reducing the threshold diameter to 5 cm for elective interventions in women with abdominal aortic aneurysms. J Vasc Surg. 2014;60(6):1695–701.
80. Lo RC, Bensley RP, Hamdan AD, Wyers M, Adams JE, Schermerhorn ML, et al. Gender differences in abdominal aortic aneurysm presentation, repair, and mortality in the Vascular Study Group of New England. J Vasc Surg. 2013;57(5):1261–8, 1268 e1–5.
81. Gloviczki P, Huang Y, Oderich GS, Duncan AA, Kalra M, Fleming MD, et al. Clinical presentation, comorbidities, and age but not female gender predict survival after endovascular repair of abdominal aortic aneurysm. J Vasc Surg. 2015;61(4):853–61. e2.
82. Investigators IT, Powell JT, Sweeting MJ, Thompson MM, Ashleigh R, Bell R, et al. Endovascular or open repair strategy for ruptured abdominal aortic aneurysm: 30 day outcomes from IMPROVE randomised trial. BMJ. 2014;348:f7661.

83. Cho YP, Kim SC, Kim SA, Jun H, Kwon TW. An idiopathic congenital abdominal aortic aneurysm with impending rupture in a 23-month-old boy. J Vasc Surg. 2013;57(2):508–10.
84. Wang Y, Tao Y. Diagnosis and treatment of congenital abdominal aortic aneurysm: a systematic review of reported cases. Orphanet J Rare Dis. 2015;10:4.
85. Mechchat A, Idrissi R, El Mahi O, Lekehal B, Sefiani Y, Mesnaoui A, et al. Multiple tuberculous aortic aneurysms in a child. A case report. J Mal Vasc. 2008;33(4–5):218–20.
86. Moon SB, Shin WY, Park YJ, Kim SJ. An abdominal aortic aneurysm in an 8-month-old girl with tuberous sclerosis. Eur J Vasc Endovasc Surg. 2009;37(5):569–71.
87. Yu SC. Marfan's syndrome with spontaneous pneumothorax and abdominal aortic aneurysm. Int Surg. 1976;61(1):30–1.
88. Boumzebra D, Ettaoumi Y, Yaacoubi M, Haddani J, Fehri M, Mehadji BA. Traumatic aneurysm of the bifurcation of the abdominal aorta in an infant. A case report. Eur J Pediatr Surg. 2005;15(3):200–2.
89. Millar AJ, Gilbert RD, Brown RA, Immelman EJ, Burkimsher DA, Cywes S. Abdominal aortic aneurysms in children. J Pediatr Surg. 1996;31(12):1624–8.
90. Belov S. Classification of congenital vascular defects. Int Angiol. 1990;9(3):141–6.
91. Matsushita M, Yano T, Ikezawa T, Sakurai T, Nimura Y, Shionoya S. Fibromuscular dysplasia as a cause of abdominal aortic aneurysm. Cardiovasc Surg. 1994;2(5):615–8.
92. Brekeit KA. Successful repair of a contained rupture of mycotic aortic aneurysm in an 8-year-old child using polytetrafluoroethylene graft. Saudi Med J. 2012;33(7):787–90.
93. Laing AJ, Hussey AJ, Joyce MR, Salmo E, Cassidy M, Flynn J. Ruptured abdominal aortic aneurysm in a 12-month-old boy. J Pediatr Surg. 2002;37(8):1234–5.
94. Mami A, Moront M, Pascasio J, Schlichting C, Finck C. Ruptured abdominal aortic aneurysm in an 11-year-old boy. J Pediatr Surg. 2008;43(4):762–4.
95. Gaughan M, McIntosh D, Brown A, Laws D. Emergency abdominal aortic aneurysm presenting without haemodynamic shock is associated with misdiagnosis and delay in appropriate clinical management. Emerg Med J. 2009;26(5):334–9.
96. Azhar B, Patel SR, Holt PJ, Hinchliffe RJ, Thompson MM, Karthikesalingam A. Misdiagnosis of ruptured abdominal aortic aneurysm: systematic review and meta-analysis. J Endovasc Ther. 2014;21(4):568–75.

Chapter 7
The Ruptured Abdominal Aorta: Diagnostics

Vincent M. Mellnick, Constantine A. Raptis, Jay P. Heiken, and Sanjeev Bhalla

Introduction

Imaging plays an essential role in the diagnosis and treatment planning for ruptured abdominal aortic aneurysms (AAA). The main imaging modality for evaluating the ruptured aorta is computed tomography (CT). CT is widely available, provides rapid image acquisition, and is well suited to image the entire abdomen and pelvis which allows for evaluation of possible alternative diagnoses. Although increasingly used to evaluate the aorta, the applicability of magnetic resonance imaging (MRI) in the clinical setting of a suspected ruptured AAA remains limited. The length of scan time and substantial patient cooperation required confine the role of MRI to evaluate the acute abdominal aorta in stable patients in whom rupture has been excluded by CT. Similarly, although ultrasound is useful in screening for and monitoring abdominal aortic aneurysms, it is generally not used in the setting of suspected ruptured AAA due to limited visibility of the retroperitoneum secondary to bowel gas and an inability to provide complete anatomic depiction of the aorta and its branches. Therefore, this chapter will chiefly focus on CT protocol considerations and imaging features of ruptured AAA. In addition, as both intramural hematoma (IMH) and penetrating atherosclerotic ulcer (PAU) can rarely lead to an unstable and/or ruptured abdominal aorta, the imaging appearance of these conditions will also be discussed.

V.M. Mellnick, MD (✉) • C.A. Raptis, MD • J.P. Heiken, MD • S. Bhalla, MD
Mallinckrodt Institute of Radiology, Washington University School of Medicine,
510 S. Kinghshighway Blvd., St. Louis, MO, USA
e-mail: mellnickv@mir.wustl.edu

B.W. Starnes et al. (eds.), *Ruptured Abdominal Aortic Aneurysm*,
DOI 10.1007/978-3-319-23844-9_7

Imaging Technique and Protocols

CT enables scanning of the entire abdomen and pelvis in 5–10 s with excellent spatial resolution that allows for the generation of high-quality multiplanar reconstructions and 3D images. When a ruptured AAA is suspected clinically, it is appropriate to begin the CT examination with a noncontrast acquisition, which improves the conspicuity of an intramural hematoma or high-attenuating crescent sign. Although abdominal aortic aneurysm rupture or impending rupture may be diagnosed on the noncontrast images alone, postcontrast images usually are required in order to detect the coexistence of a dissection flap and to acquire preoperative aortic measurements for endoluminal stent graft repair. Oral contrast is discouraged when evaluating the aorta, both because of the delay required for the patient to drink and because it may obscure subtle findings, such as an aortoenteric fistula [1]. Oral contrast may also interfere with the generation of 2D and 3D reconstructions that may be needed for endoluminal treatment planning.

A suggested technique (Table 7.1) for evaluating the abdominal aorta in the arterial phase begins with a CT angiogram protocol, injecting 100–125 mL of iodinated contrast (350 mg/mL I) at a rate of 4 mL/s with bolus tracking using a region of interest over the descending thoracic aorta and a 15 s delay. Images are obtained with 2 mm slice thickness and a reconstruction interval of 1 mm with a detector collimation varying from 0.6 to 1.2 mm depending on the scanner used. These settings typically allow for near-isotropic voxels and high-quality coronal and sagittal multiplanar reconstructions as well as 3D-rendered maximum intensity projection (MIP) and volume-rendered images, all of which can aid in diagnosis and in depicting findings for surgeons. While these post-processed images may be helpful, it is important to note that findings on 3D reconstructions should always be verified on the source images. A delayed contrast phase may be acquired to evaluate for periaortic enhancement, to detect an endoleak post endoluminal stent graft repair, or to routinely evaluate the solid organs of the abdomen if another diagnosis is suspected.

When endoluminal repair of an aortic aneurysm is being considered, it is important for the radiologist not only to report the maximum aortic diameter orthogonal to the long axis of the aorta but also to provide measurements of the aorta at the proximal and distal attachment sites, the length and morphology of the aneurysm

Table 7.1 CT protocol for evaluating the acute abdominal aorta

Noncontrast scan first to assess for intramural hematoma
CTA (arterial phase) – 4 mL/s injection rate, bolus tracking at level of descending aorta + 15 s delay
No oral contrast
2 mm slice thickness, 1 mm reconstruction interval
Sagittal and coronal MPRs, 3D post-processing for endoluminal measurements
Delayed images when suspected alternative diagnosis, aortitis, or prior endoluminal graft repair

neck, and the diameter of the iliac and femoral arteries, all of which affect the approach and potential for endovascular repair [2–4].

Many modern scanners automatically aid in selecting an appropriate kVp for the clinical application and patient size. When patient size permits, a lower kVp (100 or 80 when possible) should be considered for CT angiography to maximize the photoelectric effect of iodine and provide high-quality arterial opacification [5]. Dual-energy CT may be a useful adjunct in evaluating the abdomen as it permits the generation of virtual noncontrast images without the added time or radiation dose associated with conventional precontrast scanning [6]. When available, iterative reconstruction techniques can also be employed to reduce dose prospectively. However, radiation dose considerations such as these should not compromise image quality, as acute aortic conditions are potentially life threatening and more commonly seen in older patients for whom radiation dose is not a primary consideration.

Imaging Findings

Ruptured Abdominal Aortic Aneurysm

The primary imaging findings of AAA rupture often are readily apparent and include a retroperitoneal hematoma extending directly from the aneurysm and active extravasation of contrast material (Fig. 7.1) [7]. The vast majority of ruptured AAA patients present with hemorrhage that extends into the retroperitoneum, and

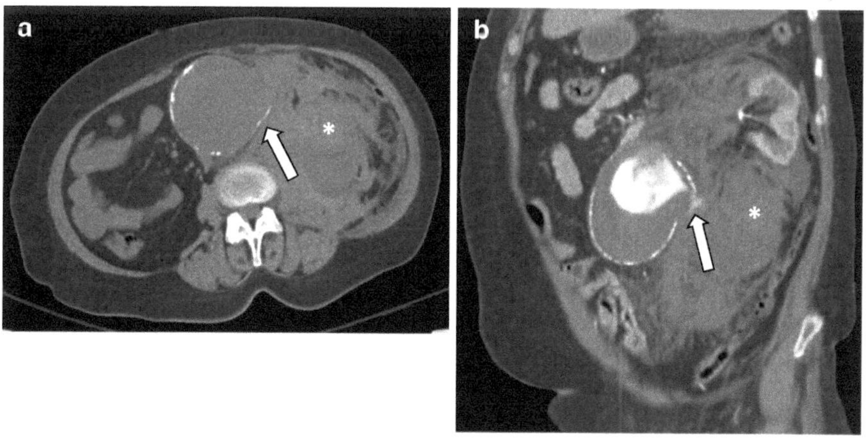

Fig. 7.1 Ruptured abdominal aortic aneurysm. Noncontrast transaxial (**a**) and contrast-enhanced coronal (**b**) CT images demonstrate the "tangential calcium" sign with focal disruption of intimal calcification which points at a tangent from the expected aortic circumference (**a**, *arrow*). Also note the contained active extravasation (**b**, *arrow*) and the large left-sided retroperitoneal hematoma (*)

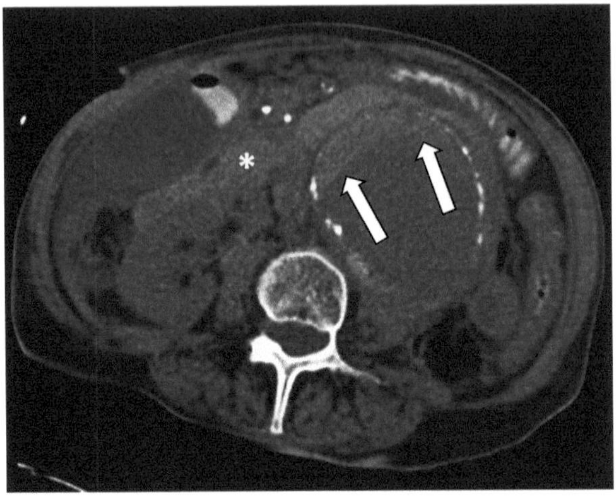

Fig. 7.2 Hyperattenuating crescent sign. Transaxial noncontrast CT image shows an infrarenal aortic aneurysm with a crescent-shaped area of high attenuation in the mural thrombus (*arrows*), representing acute hematoma. There is also rupture, evidenced by surrounding retroperitoneal hematoma (*)

intraperitoneal hemorrhage is far less common. Primary AAA rupture into the inferior vena cava as aortocaval fistula or gastrointestinal tract as aortoenteric fistula is also rare. Although contained AAA rupture can also present with the abovementioned findings, impending rupture may have much more subtle findings, including perianeurysmal soft tissue stranding. Additional CT findings associated with AAA rupture or impending rupture include the hyperattenuating crescent, draped aorta, and tangential calcium signs. Rapidly increasing aneurysm diameter and focal discontinuity of intimal calcification within the wall of the aneurysm also can be indications of aneurysm instability.

A "hyperattenuating crescent" refers to a crescentic area of high attenuation within the wall or mural thrombus of an aneurysm secondary to penetration of blood from the aneurysm lumen into the aortic wall or mural thrombus (Fig. 7.2) [8]. By definition, a "hyperattenuating crescent" has a higher CT attenuation than the luminal blood on unenhanced scans and a higher attenuation than the skeletal muscle on postcontrast scans but is not as high as the attenuation of calcium [9]. Although the reported prevalence of this finding in patients with AAA rupture ranges from 21 to 77 %, the specificity has been reported to be as high as 93% [9, 10].

A "draped aorta" describes the appearance of an AAA wall that bulges posteriorly, either unilaterally or bilaterally, and has lost its fat plane with the adjacent psoas muscle and vertebra (Fig. 7.3). This finding is a sign of aortic wall insufficiency and impending rupture, but also can be seen with a contained aortic leak [11, 12].

Focal discontinuity of intimal calcification within an AAA wall, particularly when shown to be a new finding in comparison with prior studies, has been shown to be a useful sign of acute or impending rupture [9]. The "tangential calcium" sign, defined as calcified atherosclerotic plaque adjacent to an area of focal calcium discontinuity that is divergent from the normal arc of the aorta, is another finding highly associated with AAA rupture (Fig. 7.1) [13].

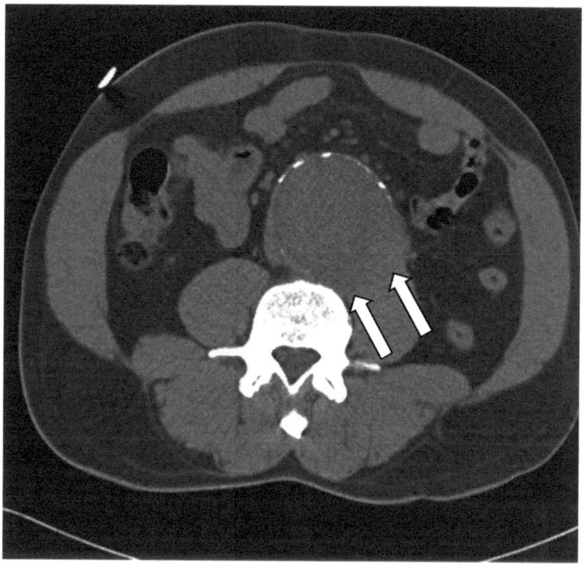

Fig. 7.3 Draped aorta sign. Precontrast transaxial CT shows abnormal contour of the aortic lumen and loss of the fat plane between the aorta and the left psoas muscle (*arrows*), the "draped aorta" sign in an aneurysm with contained rupture

Intramural Hematoma

Aortic intramural hematoma (IMH) represents blood within the aortic wall without persistent flow or an intimomedial flap. Whether this blood arises due to rupture of the vasa vasorum or thrombosis of a dissection is somewhat controversial but probably irrelevant from the perspective of the radiologist as both potential etiologies result in the endpoint of IMH, a condition which is managed similarly to dissection [14, 15]. IMH usually resolves spontaneously, but it may progress to classic dissection, focal aortic ulceration, aortic aneurysm, aortic dissection, and rarely rupture [15, 16]. Factors that predict progression of an IMH to dissection or rupture include the presence of an aortic aneurysm, an ulcer-like projection, persistent symptoms after treatment, and progressive increase in aortic wall thickness and/or aneurysm diameter [17, 18]. IMH most commonly occurs in the descending thoracic aorta, rarely in the abdomen alone.

IMH is seen on imaging as an eccentric, crescent-shaped collection of blood in the aortic wall. On CT, this feature is best seen as hyperattenuation (40–70 HU) on precontrast images, particularly with the use of narrow window settings (Fig. 7.4) [19]. On MRI, precontrast T1-weighted or black blood images may be useful to demonstrate intramural blood products, which can be iso- or hyperintense to the skeletal muscle, depending on the age of the hematoma [20]. Interpretation based on viewing postconstrast images alone may be problematic as the intramural hematoma is less conspicuous when adjacent to the brightly enhancing aortic lumen, thus potentially being confused for mural thrombus. Imaging features that support mural thrombus rather than an IMH include an irregular intraluminal surface (IMH typically is smoothly contoured), isolation to a dilated portion of the aorta (IMH is more common in a normal diameter aorta), and the presence of multiple, interrupted

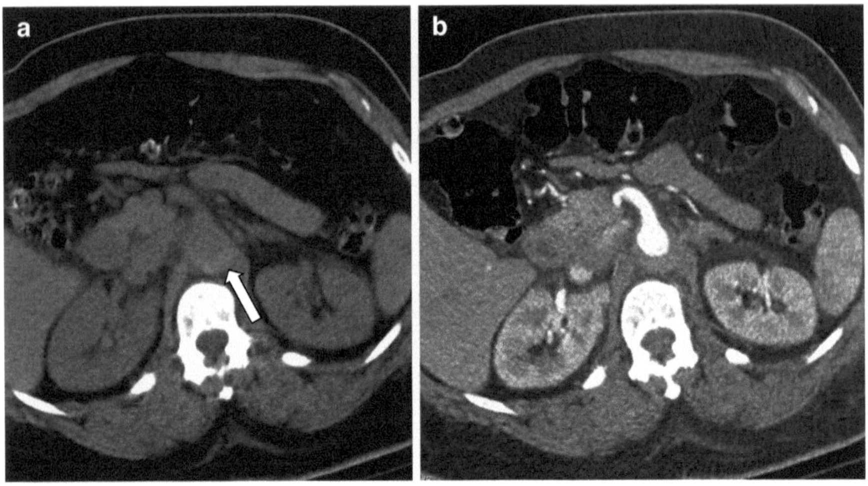

Fig. 7.4 Intramural hematoma. Precontrast (**a**) and contrast-enhanced transaxial CT shows a crescentic area of high signal intensity in the aortic wall (**a**, *arrow*). This area shows no enhancement or ulceration after intravenous contrast administration (**b**)

lesions [15, 20]. Imaging features that help distinguish IMH from aortic dissection include the lack of enhancement of IMH, whereas delayed images generally depict some flow in the false lumen of a classic dissection. Fixed, medial displacement of intimal atherosclerotic calcification rather than a spiraled appearance of displaced intimal calcium also favors an IMH over a classic aortic dissection [21].

Penetrating Atherosclerotic Ulcer

A penetrating atherosclerotic ulcer (PAU) refers to an ulceration of atherosclerotic plaque that allows blood from the aortic lumen to contact the media of the aortic wall. Similar to AAA and IMH, the most lethal complication of PAU is rupture. The reported incidence of rupture from abdominal aortic PAU has ranged from 8 to 37 % [22, 23]. PAU also may resolve spontaneously, but, in addition to rupture, can progress to an enlarging intramural hematoma, dissection, or pseudoaneurysm.

On imaging, PAU presents as a focal outpouching or localized expansion of the aortic lumen with the luminal blood pool communicating with hematoma in the aortic media (Fig. 7.5). Although irregular atherosclerotic plaque without true penetrating ulceration may simulate a PAU and provide a potential pitfall, PAU may be differentiated from irregular plaque by the presence of a saccular outpouching deforming the outer contour of the aortic wall or a circumferentially enlarged aorta. Precontrast CT or T1-weighted MRI also may be useful to show intramural hematoma adjacent to the ulceration, which typically is shorter in length than with classic aortic dissection or a primary intramural hematoma [23].

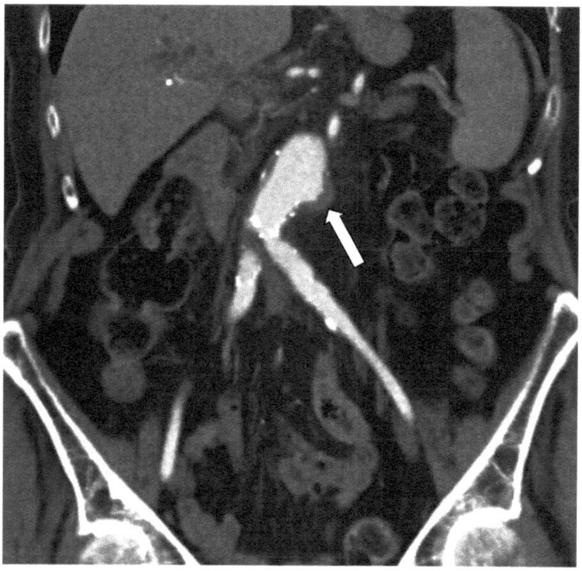

Fig. 7.5 Penetrating atherosclerotic ulcer. Contrast-enhanced coronal CT shows a saccular outpouching from the infrarenal aorta that deforms the external contour of the vessel wall (*arrow*)

Conclusion

CT is the most appropriate imaging modality to diagnose a ruptured AAA and other acute aortic conditions prone to rupture, whereas MRI and US are reserved for assessing stable patients in whom rupture has been excluded. CT protocols for assessing the acute abdominal aorta should include a precontrast phase as well as a high-quality CT angiogram in order to generate multiplanar images for preoperative planning. The CT appearance of AAA rupture and associated conditions often is readily apparent; however, it is critical for radiologists to recognize the more subtle signs of contained or impending rupture. IMH and PAU also may uncommonly lead to aortic rupture, thus requiring familiarity with these entities.

References

1. Puvaneswary M, Cuganesan R. Detection of aortoenteric fistula with helical CT. Australas Radiol. 2003;47(1):67–9.
2. Arko FR, Filis KA, Seidel SA, et al. How many patients with infrarenal aneurysms are candidates for endovascular repair? The Northern California experience. J Endovas Ther. 2004;11(1):33–40.
3. Armerding MD, Rubin GD, Beaulieu CF, et al. Aortic aneurysmal disease: assessment of stent-graft treatment-CT versus conventional angiography. Radiology. 2000;215(1):138–46.
4. Iezzi R, Cotroneo AR. Endovascular repair of abdominal aortic aneurysms: CTA evaluation of contraindications. Abdom Imaging. 2006;31(6):722–31.
5. Siegel MJ, Hildebolt C, Bradley D. Effects of automated kilovoltage selection technology on contrast-enhanced pediatric CT and CT angiography. Radiology. 2013;268(2):538–47.

6. Sommer WH, Graser A, Becker CR, et al. Image quality of virtual noncontrast images derived from dual-energy CT angiography after endovascular aneurysm repair. J Vasc Interv Radiol. 2010;21(3):315–21.
7. Rakita D, Newatia A, Hines JJ, Siegel DN, Friedman B. Spectrum of CT findings in rupture and impending rupture of abdominal aortic aneurysms. Radiographics. 2007;27(2):497–507.
8. Gonsalves CF. The hyperattenuating crescent sign. Radiology. 1999;211(1):37–8.
9. Siegel CL, Cohan RH, Korobkin M, Alpern MB, Courneya DL, Leder RA. Abdominal aortic aneurysm morphology: CT features in patients with ruptured and nonruptured aneurysms. AJR Am J Roentgenol. 1994;163(5):1123–9.
10. Mehard WB, Heiken JP, Sicard GA. High-attenuating crescent in abdominal aortic aneurysm wall at CT: a sign of acute or impending rupture. Radiology. 1994;192(2):359–62.
11. Schwartz SA, Taljanovic MS, Smyth S, O'Brien MJ, Rogers LF. CT findings of rupture, impending rupture, and contained rupture of abdominal aortic aneurysms. AJR Am J Roentgenol. 2007;188(1):W57–62.
12. Halliday KE, al-Kutoubi A. Draped aorta: CT sign of contained leak of aortic aneurysms. Radiology. 1996;199(1):41–3.
13. Wang L, Gratz, B, Peterson, C, Menias, C, Bhalla, S, Heiken, J, Sierra, L, Pilgram, T, Sicard, G, et al. Abdominal aortic aneurysm rupture: diagnostic usefulness of secondary CT signs. Radiological Society of North America 2005 Scientific Assembly and annual meeting, Chicago, 2005.
14. Sawhney NS, DeMaria AN, Blanchard DG. Aortic intramural hematoma: an increasingly recognized and potentially fatal entity. Chest. 2001;120(4):1340–6.
15. Chao CP, Walker TG, Kalva SP. Natural history and CT appearances of aortic intramural hematoma. Radiographics. 2009;29(3):791–804.
16. Sueyoshi E, Matsuoka Y, Sakamoto I, Uetani M, Hayashi K, Narimatsu M. Fate of intramural hematoma of the aorta: CT evaluation. J Comput Assist Tomogr. 1997;21(6):931–8.
17. Nienaber CA, Richartz BM, Rehders T, Ince H, Petzsch M. Aortic intramural haematoma: natural history and predictive factors for complications. Heart. 2004;90(4):372–4.
18. von Kodolitsch Y, Csosz SK, Koschyk DH, et al. Intramural hematoma of the aorta: predictors of progression to dissection and rupture. Circulation. 2003;107(8):1158–63.
19. Holden A. The value of narrow CT window settings in the recognition of subtle acute aortic intramural haematoma. Australas Radiol. 2000;44(1):128–9.
20. Murray JG, Manisali M, Flamm SD, et al. Intramural hematoma of the thoracic aorta: MR image findings and their prognostic implications. Radiology. 1997;204(2):349–55.
21. Rubin GD. Helical CT, angiography of the thoracic aorta. J Thorac Imaging. 1997;12(2): 128–49.
22. Batt M, Haudebourg P, Planchard PF, Ferrari E, Hassen-Khodja R, Bouillanne PJ. Penetrating atherosclerotic ulcers of the infrarenal aorta: life-threatening lesions. Eur J Vasc Endovas Surg. 2005;29(1):35–42.
23. Levy JR, Heiken JP, Gutierrez FR. Imaging of penetrating atherosclerotic ulcers of the aorta. AJR Am J Roentgenol. 1999;173(1):151–4.
24. American Institute of Ultrasound in Medicine, American College of Emergency Physicians. AIUM practice guideline for the performance of the focused assessment with sonography for trauma (FAST) examination. J Ultrasound Med. 2014;33(11):2047–56.

Chapter 8
Predictors of Certain Death

William P. Robinson

Introduction

Ruptured abdominal aortic aneurysm (RAAA) is a common vascular emergency with an overall mortality of 70–90 % [1, 2]. A substantial percentage of patients reach the hospital alive. Without repair, RAAA is uniformly fatal. Any hope of survival depends upon expeditious diagnosis and preoperative care, preparation by the surgical team, and operative repair [3]. However, the operative mortality for patients who undergo repair remains high at 30–50 % in many contemporary reports [4, 5]. The vascular surgeon must make extremely rapid decisions about the patient's chances of survival if repair is to be undertaken. In doing so, the vascular surgeon must balance the opportunity to offer a life-saving procedure against the potential for prolonging the discomfort and emotional stress of both the patient and the patient's family in a scenario where attempts at saving the patient might be futile. Likewise, the patient, if mentating clearly and able to participate in decision making, or the patient's family or healthcare proxies may be forced to make an immediate decision about whether the patient would like to undergo an attempt at repair. The situation is made all the more difficult by its unexpected nature. In only 12–13 % of ruptured aneurysms is the patient aware of the existence of his or her AAA.

In order to allow the vascular surgeon to provide prognostic information to the patient and the family and to aid decision making by the vascular surgeon, attempts have been made to identify factors predictive of in-hospital or 30-day mortality, including "certain death." Presumably identification of factors which are associated with little or no chance of survival could be utilized to exclude the patient from a potentially futile repair of a RAAA. In addition to preventing the patient from

W.P. Robinson, MD
Division of Vascular and Endovascular Surgery, University of Virginia School of Medicine, Charlottesville, VA, USA
e-mail: William.Robinson@umassmemorial.org

B.W. Starnes et al. (eds.), *Ruptured Abdominal Aortic Aneurysm*,
DOI 10.1007/978-3-319-23844-9_8

undergoing an unnecessary and potentially painful procedure, many would also argue for avoiding the considerable cost of a RAAA repair from the standpoint of cost-effective healthcare resource utilization if the repair was thought to have little or no chance of benefit – although some might disagree with this consideration.

Although the stated purpose of these models has been to identify patients with prohibitive operative risk in whom repair might be considered futile, identification of factors predictive of mortality also allows for risk-adjusted comparison of observed and expected outcomes for the purposes of comparative audit. Repair of RAAA has been identified by patients, physicians, and third party payers a key index procedure by which physicians and institutions can be evaluated [6]. As with any outcome measure, accurate risk adjustment is necessary to allow fair and valid comparison between surgeons and institutions and to identify areas of improvement in the care of RAAA. It is worth noting that these prediction models for mortality after RAAA repair have also been used for this purpose.

This chapter will review the literature regarding prediction of short-term mortality following repair of RAAA. It is worth considering these published prediction models individually because in each the ability to predict mortality depended upon a combination of variables according to a specific methodology. It must be remembered that each of factors or combination of factors identified by any particular analysis as predictive of mortality were identified in the context of a unique cohort of patients. These models may or may not be accurate in external cohorts of patients and may not be generalizable to all patients. The goal of this chapter is not to compare the accuracy or validity of each of the proposed models, but rather to cull from these reports those variables which have been consistently identified as the harbingers of an extremely high or certain mortality. For the sake of discussion, these variables have been classified as preoperative, intraoperative, and postoperative.

It must be emphasized that no existing prediction score or combination of variables could be expected to predict death after repair of RAAA with absolute certainty in all patients. Faced with virtually certain death without repair, many patients suffering from a RAAA will desire an attempt at repair even in the face of improbable odds of survival. Vascular surgeons are thus often asked to proceed with repair in the face of unfavorable odds. Many would assert that they have an ethical and professional obligation to do so.

Preoperative Variables

Published mortality prediction models derived from clinical data which utilize variables available before operation include the Glasgow aneurysm score [7], the Hardman index [8], the Vancouver score [9], the Edinburg Ruptured Aneurysm Score [10], the VSGNE RAAA Risk Score [11], and the University of Washington RAAA Score [12] (Table 8.1). Analyses conducted utilizing large "claims" databases were excluded from this review as these databases do not capture the clinical detail necessary to aid the vascular surgeon in a decision at the bedside.

Table 8.1 Risk scoring systems for prediction of in-hospital or 30-day mortality after repair of ruptured abdominal aortic aneurysm

<table>
<tr><th>Risk score</th><th colspan="2">Formula</th></tr>
<tr><td>Glasgow aneurysm score</td><td colspan="2">Age + 17 for shock + 7 for myocardial disease + 10 for cerebrovascular disease + 14 for renal disease</td></tr>
<tr><td>Hardman index</td><td colspan="2">Score from 1 to 5 depending on number of 5 risk factors present
Risk factors: age >76, ECG ischemia, Cr > 0.19 mmol/L, LOC, Hgb <9</td></tr>
<tr><td rowspan="7">Vancouver score</td><td colspan="2">$E^x/(1+E^x)$ where $x=(-3.44)+$[sum of coefficients of significant variables]</td></tr>
<tr><td>Variable</td><td>Coefficient</td></tr>
<tr><td>Age</td><td>0.062 × age</td></tr>
<tr><td>Reduced consciousness: yes</td><td>1.14</td></tr>
<tr><td>Reduced consciousness: no</td><td>−1.14</td></tr>
<tr><td>Cardiac arrest: yes</td><td>.6</td></tr>
<tr><td>Cardiac arrest: no</td><td>−.6</td></tr>
<tr><td>Edinburg ruptured aneurysm score</td><td colspan="2">Score from 0 to 3 summing number of 3 risk factors present
Risk factors: Hob <9, preoperative GCS <15, preop BP <90</td></tr>
<tr><td>Vascular study group of New England RAAA risk score</td><td colspan="2">Score summing integer weights of 4 risk factors:
Age >76: 2
Cardiac arrest: 2
Loss of consciousness: 1
Suprarenal clamp: 1
Total VSGNE RAAA score = 0 – 6</td></tr>
<tr><td>University of Washington RAAA risk score</td><td colspan="2">Score from 0 to 4 summing number of risk factors present
Risk factors: preoperative SBP ever <70, pH < 7.2, age >76, creatinine >2 g/dL</td></tr>
</table>

Glasgow Aneurysm Score (GAS)

The Glasgow score identifies age, "shock," myocardial disease, cerebrovascular disease, and renal disease as the primary predictors of inpatient mortality after open repair of RAAA. The score is additive, with increasing points assigned for the presence of the preceding risk factors (Table 8.1). Application of the GAS resulted in mortality estimates ranging from 0 % for scores below "70 GaAs" to 80 % for scores greater than "95 GaAs" [13].

Hardman Index

The Hardman index identified age >76, electrocardiographic ischemia, creatinine greater than 190 µmoles/liter, loss of consciousness, and hemoglobin less than 9 g/dL as predictive of mortality (Table 8.1). Patients who had three or more factors present had a 100 % 30-day mortality. It must be noted that only eight patients in the data for this study had three or four factors present and no patients had all five factors present [8].

Vancouver Score

The Vancouver score identified age, preoperative unconsciousness, and cardiac arrest as predictive of mortality. The authors created an equation for predicting mortality based upon the coefficients for each independent predictor and derived the variable logistic regression model. Based on application of this equation, 100 % mortality could not be predicted. However, for patients who had sustained cardiac arrest and who were unconscious, the predicted mortality was 88 %, 93 %, 96 %, and 99 % for patients 60, 70, 80, and 90 years of age, respectively [9].

Edinburg Ruptured Aneurysm Score

Developed in 2007, the Edinburg Ruptured Aneurysm Score was developed which predicted mortality based on the presence or absence of three preoperative variables available on admission including hemoglobin less than 9 g/dL, preoperative Glasgow Coma Scale less than 15, and preoperative systolic blood pressure less than 90 mmHg. Tambyraja and colleagues found that there was an 80 % mortality rate in patients who presented with all three factors, although all three factors were only present in five out of 105 patients [10].

VSGNE RAAA Risk Score

This VSGNE RAAA Risk Score, the first derived in a United States cohort, identified age greater than 76, cardiac arrest, loss of consciousness, and the use of a suprarenal clamp as the primary independent predictors of in-hospital mortality on logistic regression analysis. Based on the presence or absence of these variables, an integer score ranging from 0 to 6 can be derived (Table 8.2). This score was demonstrated to accurately predict in-hospital mortality after open repair of RAAA with excellent calibration ($X^2 = 1.96$, $P = .85$) and discrimination (C-statistic = .79) in 242 patients from the Vascular Study Group of New England between 2003 and 2009. A VSGNE RAAA Risk Score of four was associated with an 80 % mortality, while a score ≥5 was associated with an 87 % mortality (Fig. 8.1). No score was associated with 100 % mortality. The VSGNE Risk Score was subsequently validated in the larger cohort of 1165 patients undergoing open and endovascular repair in the Vascular Quality Initiative (VQI) [4].

Table 8.2 Preoperative and intraoperative variables and in-hospital survival

Creatinine	Clamp site	Urine output	Probability survival	95 % range
≤1.3	Infrarenal	≥200	90	76–96
≤1.3	Infrarenal	1–199	76	52–90
>1.3	Infrarenal	≥200	71	53–85
≤1.3	Suprarenal	≥200	65	33–87
≤1.3	Infrarenal	0	52	21–82
>1.3	Infrarenal	1–199	46	32–61
≤1.3	Suprarenal	1–199	39	15–69
>1.3	Suprarenal	≥200	33	9–71
>1.3	Infrarenal	0	23	9–46
≤1.3	Suprarenal	0	18	4–50
>1.3	Suprarenal	1–199	15	4–53
>1.3	Suprarenal	0	6	1–24

From Johnston [14]

For this logistic regression model, constant = 1.834, $b_{\text{creatinine}} = 1.304$, $b_{\text{urine}} = -1.066$, $b_{\text{clamp}} = -1.612$, log likelihood ratio = −61.997, and $p = 0.000$. The codes used were as follows: creatinine (1, ≤ 1.3; 2, > 1.3), aortic clamp site (1 = suprarenal; 2 = infrarenal), and urine output (0, 0; 1, 1–199; 2, ≥ 200)

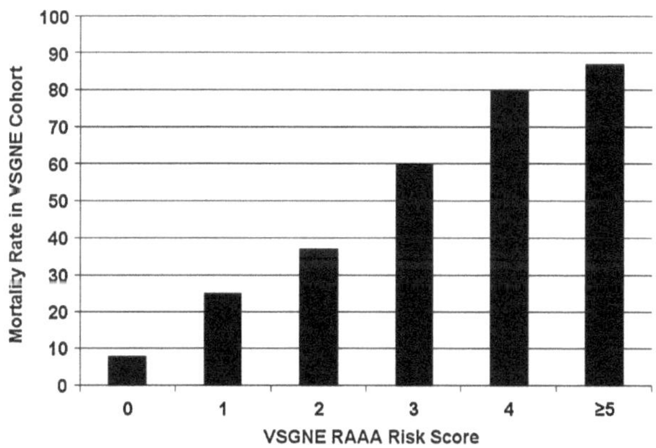

Fig. 8.1 In-hospital mortality rate after open RAAA repair according to VSGNE RAAA Risk Score (From Robinson et al. [11])

The University of Washington RAAA Score

A new score was recently proposed and presented by Garland, Starnes, and colleagues from University of Washington [12]. Age greater than 76 years, pH less than 7.2, systolic blood less than 70 mmHg, and preoperative creatinine >2.0 mg/

dL were found to be most predictive of 30-day mortality. One point each is assigned to the presence of each variable for a total score ranging between 0 and 4. This score is unique in that it predicted 100 % mortality in the cohort from which it was derived. In 303 patients, a score of four was associated with 100 % mortality irrespective of whether the patients underwent open or endovascular repair.

Variables Consistently Associated with High Mortality

Age

It is clear from all the existing prediction models that age is directly related to risk of mortality after repair of ruptured AAA. While this is intuitive, no study has identified a specific age threshold which can predict certain death. In fact, on multivariable analysis controlling for other predictors of mortality, our group found that patients older than 85 had lower mortality than patients aged 80–85 [11]. One must recognize that, the majority of current risk scores utilize a specific age cutoff is a dichotomous variables in their risk prediction models. The Hardman Index, the VSGNE RAAA Risk Score, and the University of Washington RAAA Risk Score all determined age >76 to be significant predictors of death. The VSGNE RAAA authors performed a threshold analysis to determine the optimal age for accurately predicting mortality and determined that age >76 was in fact the optimal threshold for analysis. A variety of other series have identified advanced age as predictive of death. Remarkably, all of these studies identify an age threshold ranging between 70 and 80 years of age [15–17]. It is clear that the physiologic reserve required to survive a ruptured abdominal aortic aneurysm diminishes with age. While it is impossible to identify an absolute age above which repair should not be offered in all instances, it is clear that patients in the eighth or ninth decade of life who have significant premorbid conditions or present in shock have little chance of survival.

Indices of Shock

As expected, all prediction models have identified indices of severe shock including hypotension, cardiac arrest, and loss of consciousness as predictive of mortality. Often the symptoms and signs coexist, making identification of the most accurate predictor of mortality difficult.

Severe Hypotension

In addition to the Edinburg Ruptured Aneurysm Score and the University of Washington RAAA Score, a variety of other studies have identified hypotension as a significant predictor of mortality [18]. In virtually all studies, hypotension was defined as a systolic blood pressure less than 70–90 mmHg. It must be noted that the majority of studies investigating predictors of mortality were conducted before the use of permissive hypotension ("hypotensive hemostasis") was recommended and frequently utilized. This strategy, while not exhaustively investigated, has been increasingly recommended over the last decade [19]. In contrast to a traditional approach to preoperative resuscitation which emphasized aggressive fluid resuscitation to achieve normal attention, permissive hypotension involves maintenance of a systolic blood pressure between 80 and 100 mmHg as long as there is evidence of end-organ perfusion such as maintained consciousness. Until aortic control can be obtained, permissive hypotension is thought to prevent ongoing blood loss secondary to dilution, coagulopathy, and clot disruption that may occur with aggressive fluid resuscitation. Based on the most current evidence, short periods of moderate hypotension (systolic blood pressure less than 80 mmHg) are likely not associated with increased mortality as long as the patient is mentating which is indicative of adequate organ perfusion [20, 21].

Cardiac Arrest

Both the VSGNE RAAA Risk Score and the Vancouver Score identified preoperative cardiac arrest as strong independent predictors of mortality. Similarly, the Hardman Index identifies electrocardiographic ischemia as significant predictor mortality. In addition to these models, multiple additional studies have likewise identified cardiac arrest as predictive of mortality [16, 22, 23].

Loss of Consciousness

The Hardman Index, Vancouver Score, VSGNE RAAA Risk Score, and the Edinburg Ruptured Aneurysm Score all identify diminished consciousness on presentation as predictive of mortality. Other studies have likewise identified loss of consciousness as predictive of mortality [24, 25]. Loss of consciousness represents end-organ malperfusion that will remain an important predictive sign for the clinician, especially when permissive hypotension is employed.

Renal Insufficiency or Increased Creatinine

A number of studies have demonstrated that increased creatinine is associated with mortality, including the Glasgow Aneurysm Score, the Hardman Index, and the University of Washington RAAA Score. Based on these studies and others, a creatinine greater than 180–190 μmol/l (2–2.1 mg/dL) appears to be the threshold associated with increased mortality [15, 26].The detrimental impact of preoperative renal insufficiency is not surprising considering the lethal nature of postoperative renal failure to which these patients are strongly predisposed.

Severe Anemia

Severe blood loss and subsequent disruption of oxygen delivery to vital organs intuitively would predict poor outcome. Accordingly, low hematocrit or hemoglobin (defined in most studies as either as Hgb < 9 g/dL or Hgb < 10 g/dL) has been shown to be another factor predictive of mortality in the Hardman Index, the Edinburg Ruptured Aneurysm Score, and other studies [24, 27]. No studies have investigated whether a hemoglobin less than nine can accurately predict certain death.

Intraoperative Variables

Some studies have analyzed the impact of intraoperative variables on the ability to predict survival [14, 18]. Johnston and colleagues reported that the site of the aorta cross-clamping (suprarenal versus infrarenal), the volume of blood transfusion, and a drop in urine output help predict early survival. For example, a patient who required a suprarenal cross-clamping, was transfused more than 3500 mL of blood, and had no intraoperative urine output was predicted to have a 3 % survival. On multivariable model including preoperative and intraoperative variables, preoperative serum creatinine, cross-clamp site, and intraoperative urine output would predict survival [14] (Table 8.2). A number of other studies, including the VSGNE RAAA Risk Score, also identified the need for a suprarenal clamp as predictive of mortality [11, 28]. In some instances, the need for a suprarenal clamp is not known until operation is undertaken and the abdomen is explored. The need is then based on whether or not patient has hemodynamic collapse and the location of the retroperitoneal hematoma. However, in modern algorithms for RAAA management, 78–93 % of patients who undergo RAAA repair have a preoperative computed tomographic scan [19, 29].The need for a suprarenal clamp can often be readily determined preoperatively. The impact of suprarenal clamp on mortality is an especially important consideration in the current management of RAAA. Increasingly, patients with a suitable infrarenal neck are being offered endovascular repair [4, 5].

Therefore, as time goes on, almost all patients requiring open repair may be unsuitable for endovascular repair and may require a suprarenal clamp. Increased blood loss has also been identified as independently predictive of mortality in an analysis by Panneton et al. and in the derivation of the ruptured AAA POSSUM (RAAA POSSUM) score, which combines both preoperative physiologic and operative variables in predicting mortality [18, 30].

Postoperative Variables

The impact of postoperative complications in instances where the patient survives operation has also been analyzed. Johnston and colleagues reported that the development of myocardial infarction, respiratory failure, coagulopathy, and kidney failure has the greatest impact on in-hospital mortality [14]. Notable was the detrimental impact of a postoperative elevation in creatinine and particularly the need for hemodialysis, even in the absence of other complications. Any patient with two of these variables or the need for dialysis had a chance of survival near zero (Table 8.3).

Table 8.3 Postoperative variables and in-hospital survival

Myocardial infarction	Respiratory failure	Coagulopathy	Kidney damage	Probability survival	95% range
No	No	No	No	96	87–99
No	No	Yes	No	91	27 99
No	Yes	No	No	74	54–87
Yes	No	No	No	66	28–91
No	No	No	Rise in creatinine	66	26–91
No	Yes	Yes	No	58	40–74
Yes	No	Yes	No	49	16–83
No	No	Yes	Rise in creatinine	48	14–84
Yes	Yes	No	No	21	5–57
No	Yes	No	Rise in creatinine	20	4–59
Yes	No	No	Rise in creatinine	15	2–59
No	No	No	Dialysis	15	1–81
Yes	Yes	Yes	No	11	3–37
No	Yes	Yes	Rise in creatinine	11	2–41
Yes	No	Yes	Rise in creatinine	8	1–42

(continued)

Table 8.3 (continued)

Myocardial infarction	Respiratory failure	Coagulopathy	Kidney damage	Probability survival	95 % range
No	No	Yes	Dialysis	8	0–69
Yes	Yes	No	Rise in creatinine	2	0–18
No	Yes	No	Dialysis	2	0–39
Yes	No	No	Dialysis	2	0–33
Yes	Yes	Yes	Rise in creatinine	1	0–10
No	Yes	Yes	Dialysis	1	0–24
Yes	No	Yes	Dialysis	1	0–21
Yes	Yes	No	Dialysis	0	0–8
Yes	Yes	Yes	Dialysis	0	0–4

From Johnston [14]
For this logistic regression model, constant = – 3.058, $b_{\text{infarct}} = 2.389$, $b_{\text{respiratory}} = 2.021$, $b_{\text{renal}} = 0.718$, $b_{\text{coagulopathy}} = 2.413$, log likelihood ratio = – 67.273, and $p = 0.000$. The codes were as follows: myocardial infarction (0 = no, 1 = yes), respiratory failure (0 = no, 1 = yes), coagulopathy (0 = no, 1 = yes), renal damage (0 = no, 1 = increase creatinine > 20 %, 3 = dialysis)

In addition, Panneton and colleagues demonstrated that the development of multisystem organ failure was associated with 100 % mortality. The recommendation of these authors, and others, is to withhold heroic resuscitative measures after repair in these patients [18].

Other Considerations in Predicting Mortality After RAAA Repair

Endovascular Versus Open Repair of RAAA

There has been widespread and rapid adoption of endovascular repair for RAAA over the last 10–15 years. In 2000, only 0.8 % of RAAA in the National Inpatient Sample (NIS) were repaired via EVAR. By 2010, 38.4 % of ruptured abdominal aortic aneurysms in the NIS were repaired via EVAR [5]. In the Vascular Quality Initiative database, which captures clinical data from almost 400 academic and community medical centers across the United States, EVAR for RAAA increased from 0 % of cases in 2003 to 58 % of cases in 2013 [31].

The overwhelming majority of analyses of single and multiple institutional observational studies, large population-based studies utilizing administrative data, and national clinical registries of prospectively collected data indicate that endovascular repair confers a significant survival benefit in comparison to open repair [4, 20, 32, 33]. Furthermore, although the conclusions of the three randomized controlled trials of endovascular versus open repair of RAAA were that endovascular repair did not confer a short-term survival benefit in comparison to open repair, careful scrutiny of these trials has led some to the opposite conclusions [34]. When analyzed in "treatment-received" basis rather than an "intent-to-treat" basis, one sees that patients treated with EVAR had a lower mortality in comparison to those treated with open repair [34]. Interestingly, the majority of sizable series comparing endovascular and open repair of ruptured abdominal aortic aneurysms consistently report in-hospital mortality in the range of 20–25 % for EVAR and 35–40 % for open repair of RAAA.

The preponderance of data on the benefit of EVAR for RAAA has led some authors to recommend an "EVAR-only" approach in which adjunctive endovascular techniques such as snorkels and chimneys are utilized to supplement EVAR in patients whose anatomy is not amenable to standard EVAR. In select centers, this has led to very low "turndown rates" for repair (4 %) and low mortality after EVAR of RAAA (24 %) [35]. Ongoing study will be necessary to confirm the effectiveness and generalizability of an aggressive endovascular approach that utilizes adjunctive techniques in patients whose anatomy will not permit standard infrarenal EVAR. Nevertheless, as endovascular techniques improve and become more widespread, it is likely that endovascular repair will be offered to an increasing percentage of patients who at this time are not offered any repair due to prohibitive risk for open repair and lack of endovascular capabilities. At present, therefore, a proactive approach to endovascular repair of RAAA can be recommended for large number of patients assuming that surgeon ability and institution's endovascular capabilities permit.

It must be noted that the majority of the aforementioned studies which identified predictors of mortality after RAAA where conducted before the adoption of EVAR for RAAA. It is therefore unknown if all the existing risk prediction models are accurate for patients undergoing EVAR or those selected for open repair in the current era. In fact, some authors report that existing prediction models do not predict outcome after endovascular repair with sufficient accuracy [36]. Three prediction models, however, have been validated in a cohort of patients undergoing either open or endovascular repair. Visser and colleagues amended the GAS by adding seven points for open repair and validated this amended model as predictive of mortality after both EVAR and open repair [37]. Likewise, the VSGNE RAAA Risk Score, which was developed in an open cohort of patients between 2003 and 2009, was subsequently shown to have good discrimination (c-statistic = 0.78) and good calibration (Hosmer-Lemeshow test, $P = 0.10$) in a cohort of patients from the VQI undergoing either EVAR ($n = 514$) or open repair ($n = 651$) between 2003 and 2013 [4]. Finally, the University of Washington RAAA Score was shown to be predictive of overall mortality and able to predict 100 % mortality in patients undergoing either open or endovascular repair [12].

Although it is intuitive that EVAR would benefit patients at highest morality risk for open repair, not all evidence suggests that EVAR reduces mortality in patients at the highest risk according to existing risk prediction models. While current risk prediction models accurately capture patient physiology, none of the current risk prediction scores or models adequately account for anatomic variables which almost undoubtedly impact outcome after both endovascular and open repair of RAAA. The major limitation of existing clinical and population-based datasets is that they do not capture all of the anatomic detail relevant to the application of EVAR. The greatest ongoing need to determine the outcomes of EVAR and open repair for RAAA is detailed anatomic data based on careful analysis of preoperative CTA imaging. These imaging data would allow for the determination of the impact of arterial anatomy on short-term and long-term mortality after EVAR and open repair. A robust comparison of EVAR and OR controlling for arterial anatomy as well as physiologic status and comorbidities could then be performed to determine anticipated mortality of each type of repair for specific patients.

Summary

In conclusion, multiple studies have identified patient factors which predict extremely high mortality or "certain death." As we have seen, is very difficult to predict when a patient has zero chance of survival based on preoperative factors alone. Multiple prediction models can identify patients with mortality in excess of 80 %, which some surgeons would consider prohibitive risk. Consistent prediction of 100 % mortality, however, has remained elusive. There has not been external validation of the ability of any proposed prediction model to identify patients with 100 % mortality. Nevertheless, a number of factors have consistently emerged as harbingers of excessive mortality. These variables have typically been markers of extreme patient comorbidity or physiologic insult which renders survival after repair of RAAA highly unlikely. These include age >75–80 years, preexisting renal insufficiency, severe hypotension (SBP<70 mmHg), cardiac arrest, loss of consciousness, and anemia (Hgb<9 g/dL). At the same time, endovascular repair to RAAA has greatly reduced in-hospital mortality after infrarenal RAAA repair, including in some patients in severe shock. Although additional study is needed regarding advanced adjunctive techniques to allow EVAR and the predictors of mortality after EVAR of RAAA, more widespread application of EVAR for RAAA may prove to reduce mortality in patients not currently offered repair because they are thought to be of prohibitive risk for open repair.

When confronted with the patient suffering from RAAA, the vascular surgeon must rapidly assess a patient's opportunity for survival and advise the patient and family accordingly. While the vascular surgeon must always tailor his or her recommendation regarding repair to the individual patient, these variables, which can be rapidly assessed preoperatively, provide valuable prognostic information and guidance. If repair is undertaken and the patient survives operation, additional intraoperative variables and postoperative complications and conditions offer further prognostic information regarding the patient's chances of surviving hospitalization. Knowledge of the determinants of mortality after RAAA repair therefore aids the vascular surgeon in balancing the opportunity to offer a life-saving procedure against the potential for prolonging the suffering and emotional stress of both the patient and the patient's family.

References

1. Bengtsson H, Bergqvist D. Ruptured abdominal aortic aneurysm: a population-based study. J Vasc Surg. 1993;18:74–80.
2. Ernst CB. Abdominal aortic aneurysm. N Engl J Med. 1993;328:1167–72.
3. van Beek SC, Vahl AC, Wisselink W, Balm R. Fate of patients unwilling or unsuitable to undergo surgical intervention for a ruptured abdominal aortic aneurysm. Eur J Vasc Endovasc Surg. 2015;49:163–5.
4. Ali MM, Flahive J, Schanzer A, et al. In patients stratified by preoperative risk, endovascular repair of ruptured abdominal aortic aneurysms has a lower in-hospital mortality and morbidity than open repair. J Vasc Surg. 2015;61(6):1399–407.
5. Dua A, Kuy S, Lee CJ, Upchurch Jr GR, Desai SS. Epidemiology of aortic aneurysm repair in the United States from 2000 to 2010. J Vasc Surg. 2014;59:1512–7.
6. Robinson WP, Huang W, Rosen A, et al. The agency for healthcare research and quality inpatient quality indicator #11 overall mortality rate does not accurately assess mortality risk after abdominal aortic aneurysm repair. J Vasc Surg. 2015;61:44–9.
7. Samy AK, Murray G, MacBain G. Glasgow aneurysm score. Cardiovasc Surg. 1994;2: 41–4.
8. Hardman DT, Fisher CM, Patel MI, et al. Ruptured abdominal aortic aneurysms: who should be offered surgery? J Vasc Surg. 1996;23:123–9.
9. Chen JC, Hildebrand HD, Salvian AJ, et al. Predictors of death in nonruptured and ruptured abdominal aortic aneurysms. J Vasc Surg. 1996;24:614–20; discussion 21–3.
10. Tambyraja A, Murie J, Chalmers R. Predictors of outcome after abdominal aortic aneurysm rupture: Edinburgh ruptured aneurysm score. World J Surg. 2007;31:2243–7.
11. Robinson WP, Schanzer A, Li Y, et al. Derivation and validation of a practical risk score for prediction of mortality after open repair of ruptured abdominal aortic aneurysms in a US regional cohort and comparison to existing scoring systems. J Vasc Surg. 2013;57(2):354–61.
12. Tran NT, Quiroga E, Singh N, Caps MT, Starnes BW, Garland BT, Danaher PJ. Preoperative risk score for the prediction of mortality following repair of ruptured abdominal aortic aneurysms. J Vasc Surg. 2015;61:1.
13. Samy AK, Murray G, MacBain G. Prospective evaluation of the Glasgow aneurysm score. J R Coll Surg Edinb. 1996;41:105–7.
14. Johnston KW. Ruptured abdominal aortic aneurysm: six-year follow-up results of a multicenter prospective study. Canadian Society for Vascular Surgery Aneurysm Study Group. J Vasc Surg. 1994;19:888–900.
15. Calderwood R, Halka T, Haji-Michael P, Welch M. Ruptured abdominal aortic aneurysm. Is it possible to predict outcome? Int Angiol. 2004;23:47–53.
16. Johansen K, Kohler TR, Nicholls SC, Zierler RE, Clowes AW, Kazmers A. Ruptured abdominal aortic aneurysm: the Harborview experience. J Vasc Surg. 1991;13:240–5; discussion 5–7.
17. van Dongen HP, Leusink JA, Moll FL, Brons FM, de Boer A. Ruptured abdominal aortic aneurysms: factors influencing postoperative mortality and long-term survival. Eur J Vasc Endovasc Surg. 1998;15:62–6.
18. Panneton JM, Lassonde J, Laurendeau F. Ruptured abdominal aortic aneurysm: impact of comorbidity and postoperative complications on outcome. Ann Vasc Surg. 1995;9:535–41.
19. Starnes BW, Quiroga E, Hutter C, et al. Management of ruptured abdominal aortic aneurysm in the endovascular era. J Vasc Surg. 2010;51:9–17; discussion –8.
20. Mayer D, Aeschbacher S, Pfammatter T, et al. Complete replacement of open repair for ruptured abdominal aortic aneurysms by endovascular aneurysm repair: a two-center 14-year experience. Ann Surg. 2012;256:688–95; discussion 95–6.
21. Veith FJ, Cayne NS, Berland TL, Mayer D, Lachat M. Current role for endovascular treatment of ruptured abdominal aortic aneurysms. Semin Vasc Surg. 2012;25:174–6.
22. Noel AA, Gloviczki P, Cherry Jr KJ, et al. Ruptured abdominal aortic aneurysms: the excessive mortality rate of conventional repair. J Vasc Surg. 2001;34:41–6.

23. Farooq MM, Freischlag JA, Seabrook GR, Moon MR, Aprahamian C, Towne JB. Effect of the duration of symptoms, transport time, and length of emergency room stay on morbidity and mortality in patients with ruptured abdominal aortic aneurysms. Surgery. 1996;119:9–14.
24. Halpern VJ, Kline RG, D'Angelo AJ, Cohen JR. Factors that affect the survival rate of patients with ruptured abdominal aortic aneurysms. J Vasc Surg. 1997;26:939–45; discussion 45–8.
25. Shackleton CR, Schechter MT, Bianco R, Hildebrand HD. Preoperative predictors of mortality risk in ruptured abdominal aortic aneurysm. J Vasc Surg. 1987;6:583–9.
26. Koskas F, Kieffer E. Surgery for ruptured abdominal aortic aneurysm: early and late results of a prospective study by the AURC in 1989. Ann Vasc Surg. 1997;11:90–9.
27. Kniemeyer HW, Kessler T, Reber PU, Ris HB, Hakki H, Widmer MK. Treatment of ruptured abdominal aortic aneurysm, a permanent challenge or a waste of resources? Prediction of outcome using a multi-organ-dysfunction score. Eur J Vasc Endovasc Surg. 2000;19:190–6.
28. Bauer EP, Redaelli C, von Segesser LK, Turina MI. Ruptured abdominal aortic aneurysms: predictors for early complications and death. Surgery. 1993;114:31–5.
29. Sharif MA, Lee B, Makar RR, Loan W, Soong CV. Role of the Hardman index in predicting mortality for open and endovascular repair of ruptured abdominal aortic aneurysm. J Endovasc Ther. 2007;14:528–35.
30. Prytherch DR, Sutton GL, Boyle JR. Portsmouth POSSUM models for abdominal aortic aneurysm surgery. Br J Surg. 2001;88:958–63.
31. Robinson WP, Schanzer A, Aiello FA, et al. Endovascular repair of ruptured abdominal aortic aneurysms does not reduce later mortality compared with open repair. J Vasc Surg. 2016;63:617–24.
32. Veith FJ, Lachat M, Mayer D, et al. Collected world and single center experience with endovascular treatment of ruptured abdominal aortic aneurysms. Ann Surg. 2009;250:818–24.
33. van Beek SC, Conijn AP, Koelemay MJ, Balm R. Editor's Choice – Endovascular aneurysm repair versus open repair for patients with a ruptured abdominal aortic aneurysm: a systematic review and meta-analysis of short-term survival. Eur J Vasc Endovasc Surg. 2014;47:593–602.
34. Dubois L, Mayer D, Rancic Z, Veith FJ, Lachat M. Debate: whether endovascular repair offers a survival advantage over open repair for ruptured abdominal aortic aneurysms. J Vasc Surg. 2015;61:546–55.
35. Lesperance K, Andersen C, Singh N, Starnes B, Martin MJ. Expanding use of emergency endovascular repair for ruptured abdominal aortic aneurysms: disparities in outcomes from a nationwide perspective. J Vasc Surg. 2008;47:1165–70; discussion 70–1.
36. Bohm N, Wales L, Dunckley M, Morgan R, Loftus I, Thompson M. Objective risk-scoring systems for repair of abdominal aortic aneurysms: applicability in endovascular repair? Eur J Vasc Endovasc Surg. 2008;36:172–7.
37. Visser JJ, Williams M, Kievit J, Bosch JL. Prediction of 30-day mortality after endovascular repair or open surgery in patients with ruptured abdominal aortic aneurysms. J Vasc Surg. 2009;49:1093–9.

Chapter 9
Prehospital Considerations for REVAR

James Pan and Kim J. Hodgson

Ruptured abdominal aortic aneurysms (rAAA) are associated with a high rate of mortality, ranging from 30 to 80 % [1]. These rates most likely underestimate the overall death rate since considerable numbers of these patients die from free rupture prior to presenting to the hospital [2]. As experience with elective endovascular aneurysm repair (EVAR) has grown, it was inevitable that its use would be considered and studied in the ruptured setting, where open abdominal aortic aneurysm repair was the reigning gold standard. Since elective EVAR had been associated with reduced perioperative morbidity and mortality, and results of open repair of ruptured AAAs had not significantly improved over the past several decades, several institutions initiated programs of EVAR for ruptured AAAs (REVAR) to evaluate whether the EVAR advantages extended to the ruptured state. Recent reports of such single institution series have shown that endovascular repair of ruptured abdominal aortic aneurysms led to both lower mortality and morbidity rates, suggesting that it becomes the standard of care for patients with ruptured infrarenal abdominal aortic aneurysms with suitable anatomy [3, 4]. The recently published results of the IMPROVE trial reported no improvement in outcomes, other than discharge to home, for patients randomized to the REVAR strategy group [5]. However, analysis per treatment received rather than by strategy assigned revealed 30-day mortality rates of 26 % for REVAR and 37 % for open repair [6]. Reports such as these, showing REVAR to be at least as effective as open repair, coupled with increasing operator experience with aortic endografting have resulted in more surgeons having attained a level of comfort that allows them to consider adding REVAR to their therapeutic armamentarium. However, optimal outcomes from REVAR come not only from an isolated competent surgeon but also from a system of care that focuses

J. Pan, MD • K.J. Hodgson, MD (✉)
Division of Vascular Surgery, Southern Illinois University School of Medicine, Springfield, IL, USA
e-mail: kimjhodgsonmd@aol.com

B.W. Starnes et al. (eds.), *Ruptured Abdominal Aortic Aneurysm*,
DOI 10.1007/978-3-319-23844-9_9

on rapid diagnosis, permissive hypotension while awaiting treatment or during patient transfer, and therapy customized to the patient's anatomy and coexisting conditions.

This chapter is devoted to preparations that should be undertaken prior to initiating a program of EVAR for ruptured abdominal aortic aneurysms including (1) education of emergency physicians on making a rapid and complete diagnosis, (2) educating those responsible for managing the patient pending or during transfer, (3) outfitting an endovascular operating room with a suitable inventory of devices, and (4) organizing hospital teams. Those interested in improving the outcomes of patients with ruptured AAAs, by whichever means of treatment, through standardization of diagnostic and therapeutic measures may also find the information valuable. Other chapters will review optimal room setups, technical details of REVAR, and potential pitfalls.

Making a Rapid and Informative Diagnosis

The vast majority of patients with ruptured AAAs present to their local emergency room or urgent care center, the sophistication of which can vary widely. While front and center in the minds of vascular surgeons, many emergency medicine physicians will never see a ruptured AAA, so its diagnosis depends on an index of suspicion that comes from education. Given that symptoms may be confused with those of renal colic or a variety of GI conditions, lower-resolution CT scans without IV contrast to evaluate for these conditions are often obtained, with the ruptured AAA being an incidental finding. In this setting, these scans may yield the diagnosis, but their clinical utility to the vascular surgeon is limited by the lack of IV contrast and by their low-resolution acquisition. This leads to the inevitable dilemma about whether or not to take the time to repeat the CT scan with contrast, to be discussed further later. With this common scenario in mind, the focus of education for emergency department physicians and staff should be to explain the value that a contrast-enhanced CT scan brings to the management of patients with a ruptured AAA and to convince emergency room staff that in the overwhelming majority of cases, there is time to obtain such imaging.

For vascular surgeons looking to improve ruptured AAA outcomes, regardless of the ultimate therapeutic modality utilized, education of emergency room personnel in the rapid diagnosis and early management of these patients will yield the best results. In the interest of getting the most possible information, this includes having a low threshold to give IV contrast to patients with suspicious symptoms, acceptable renal function, and no contrast allergies. To reinforce this concept and standardize the diagnostic approach, we developed a ruptured AAA diagnostic algorithm that emphasizes the emergency nature of the suspected condition and guides the provider through the steps of making the diagnosis [7] (Fig. 9.1). An accompanying patient management order set standardizes the management of the patient, particularly emphasizing permissive and even facilitated hypotension, while awaiting transport to your facility or to your site of treatment.

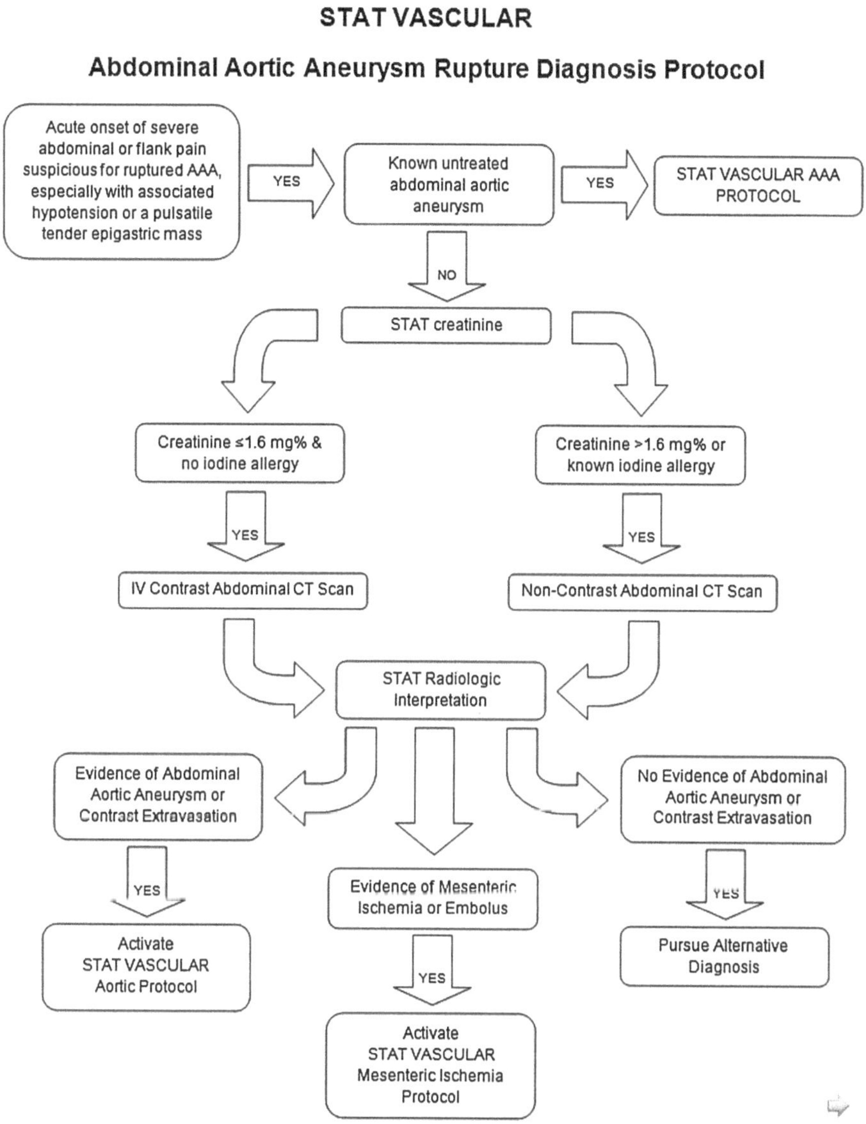

Fig. 9.1 Diagnostic algorithm for patients presenting with symptoms suggestive of a ruptured AAA which emphasizes performance of a CT scan with contrast for maximal diagnostic and therapy-planning information

Unfortunately, the incidentally found ruptured AAA on a non-contrast-enhanced CT scan continues to be an all-too-common scenario. Also common is reluctance on the part of the ED physician to rescan the patient with contrast after the diagnosis is made due to a sense of urgency to get the patient on their way to "somewhere else." Given the rapidity of CT scanning with today's technology, whether that somewhere else is another hospital capable of treating the condition or the OR in the presenting hospital, there should almost always be time for a complete CT scan if time is utilized efficiently. A recent single center series showed that 88 % of patients ultimately diagnosed with a ruptured abdominal aortic aneurysm survived at least two hours after admission, suggesting that there is time for patients to undergo CT scanning to help assist in clinical decision-making [8]. Similarly, in a 2005 Dutch series of 100 ruptured AAA patients, 21 of whom were treated "palliatively," the median time from arrival to death in the palliated group was 435 min (range 15 mins–6 days) [9]. In those undergoing treatment, the median time from presentation to operation was 159 min (range 16–1450 mins) with the mortality in the surgical group not being affected by the length of delay ($p=1.0$) or obtaining CT imaging ($p=0.34$). Since an operating room will rarely be instantly available and interhospital transport, by whatever means, takes time to initiate, there is almost always time to repeat a CT scan with contrast if the surgeon feels it would aid in decision-making.

An alternative strategy for patients with renal insufficiency or other contrast contraindications would be to obtain the non-contrast CT series but leave the patient in the scanner until the imaging is checked for an AAA. If an AAA is present, the scan can be repeated with contrast without having to re-transport the patient in and out of the scanner. This strategy also maintains registration between the pre- and post-contrast scans which can assist in interpretation.

The previous discussion notwithstanding, while contrast-enhanced high-resolution CT imaging is highly desirable, it is not absolutely necessary to successfully perform REVAR. A non-contrast scan coupled with angiographic and/or IVUS evaluations is a common compromise to repeating the CT scan [10, 11]. Furthermore, in the setting of a patient with chronic kidney disease, a CO_2 angiogram can be used to replace iodinated contrast, though visualization may somewhat compromised [12]. In a recently reported series of 40 ruptured AAA patients, ten were hemodynamically unstable and were taken to the endovascular suite without any CT imaging whatsoever, being sized and treated based on angiography and IVUS alone [13].

While compromises may at times be necessary, taking patients for REVAR on the basis of suboptimal imaging will inevitably have a higher failure rate and in the case of a ruptured AAA failure to exclude the aneurysm and staunch the hemorrhage which is not an acceptable outcome. This reinforces the value of an operating endovascular suite, which allows for a relatively seamless transition to open repair if needed. Even more so, it emphasizes the importance of understanding the maneuvers involved in obtaining balloon occlusion of the aorta and subsequently deploying a complete endograft while maintaining balloon occlusion. The exact technique for this will be discussed in another chapter, but it should be recognized that balloon position differs depending on whether the intent is to proceed with REVAR, in which case any balloon deployed needs to be supraceliac, or open repair, in which case the balloon can be a bit lower to allow maintained hepatic and mesenteric perfusion. In either case, the occluding balloon should only be inflated if needed to maintain a reasonable blood pressure and, in the case of open surgery, transitioned to a more distal clamp as soon as possible to minimize the ischemic insult to the visceral organs which can lead to coagulopathy and renal failure [14, 15].

Imaging Is Only Valuable if You Can See It

Under our diagnostic algorithm, since a significant majority of patients will meet the criteria for contrast administration, vascular surgeons can expect high-resolution contrast-enhanced CT scans on most patients they are called about for ruptured AAAs. However, a scan is only as useful as its images are accessible. Fortunately, in today's interconnected world, most regions will have Internet access to CT scans performed in the outlying emergency rooms or at least within their own system. Alternatively, several HIPPA compliant image-sharing Internet-based services are available under contract. More than ever before, vascular surgeons are able to see their future patient's vascular anatomy long before they meet them in the flesh, allowing valuable savings in time by permitting direct patient transfer to the facility best suited to their planned repair. In patients being transferred in from an outside hospital, the ability to scrutinize the CT scans prior to patient arrival can permit the patient to bypass the emergency department entirely, proceeding directly to the therapeutic venue of choice, operating room or endovascular suite, as directed by the CT scan images. Thus, in an ideally functioning program, the ruptured AAA patient's treatment destination will have been determined by a vascular surgeon's review of a contrast-enhanced CT scan shortly after image acquisition, perhaps while the patient is still in an outside hospital's emergency department. The determination of the anticipated mode of repair, REVAR or open, sets in motion a coordinated set of notifications and protocol activations specific to the intended mode of repair, the intent being to minimize the number of additional calls needed to move forward with getting ready to receive and treat the patient.

How Low Can It Go?

Long embraced by surgeons, but only sporadically by emergency personnel, the concept of permissive hypotension is another that needs to be taught to your emergency medical services (EMS) personnel. Admittedly a challenging strategy to get comfortable with initially, allowing a patient to remain hypotensive or even inducing a degree of hypotension (hypotensive hemostasis) is a recognized strategy to maintain hemodynamic stability in a ruptured AAA patient by not stressing the tamponade that had to have happened if the patient is still alive. There are limits, however, to how low a patient's pressure should be allowed to go. Traditionally any pressure in a mentating patient was considered acceptable. A recent analysis of the Immediate Management of Patients with Ruptured aneurysm: Open Versus Endovascular Repair (IMPROVE) trial data, however, suggests that having a blood pressure below 70 mmHg at any time is associated with a 51 % mortality [16]. Others have suggested that blood pressure control is not the only important factor, demonstrating that the total volume of fluids administered before aortic control correlated directly with mortality [17]. A combination approach of fluid limitation to less than 500 ml and systolic blood pressure (SBP) titration to a range of between 50 and100 mmHg, using nitrates as needed to keep it below 100 mmHg, has been reported, although in practice SBP was more often at the upper end of the target range [18].

In our experience, the easiest means to overcome the psychological obstacle to permissive hypotension is to develop specific order sets for emergency physicians and EMS transport personnel to refer to as they manage the patient. In essence, this gives them permission to hold back on resuscitating a hypotensive patient. We have opted to target a SBP range of 70–100 mmHg to avoid potentially detrimental severe hypotension and maintain a level of comfort with EMS personnel. It should not be overlooked that effective pain management is often all that is needed to generate a reduction in SBP to more acceptable levels, with beta blockade further adding to the desired goal. The most critical and not uncommon scenario to avoid is the patient who is hypertensive from pain and, without pain relief, is a significant risk of conversion to uncontained rupture.

Keeping Your Patient's Options Open

The primary advantage of being able to view your patient's imaging prior to transfer is to determine suitability for endovascular or open repair. This, combined with consideration of the availability of requisite personnel, equipment, and surgeon expertise, will determine the venue the patient should be transferred to. Given the value that a venue suitable for operative repair brings in case of REVAR failure, or that imaging brings to the open repair patient who gets aortic balloon occlusion, it is clear that a hybrid suite that offers both imaging and open surgical capabilities is the most desirable. Absent this type of suite, pre-arrival review of the imaging will determine if the patient is going to go to the operating room for open repair or the endovascular suite for REVAR. Although REVAR can be performed with portable fluoroscopy, it is the opinion of these authors that the compromised image quality, acquisition fluidity, and image processing render it an undesirable limitation and one that could preclude offering REVAR to all but the most straightforward of cases.

Even more so than for open repair, the setup of the endovascular room can be complicated, needing to accommodate anesthesia teams and equipment, the radiographic unit, monitors, power injectors, IVUS drivers, and disposables galore. Standardization of the room layout and instrumentation for all EVARs will translate, in the emergency setting, to efficient utilization of time as operator attention can be focused on pre-procedural planning while the room and patient are being prepared per protocol by others in the team. We have developed room layout maps for positioning of all equipment and personnel to simplify preparation of the room and to get it done prior to the patient's arrival. While many leave the radiographic unit off to the side until the REVAR begins, once the patient is positioned on the table, we generally position the radiographic unit over their mid abdomen, out of the way of anesthesia's efforts to insert lines and any groin access, yet available to guide placement of central lines or aortic occlusion balloons. Whether the patient is destined for open or endovascular repair, an aortic occlusion balloon can be positioned under fluoroscopic guidance to be inflated if or when needed. If needed, this can usually be accomplished under local anesthesia, while venous access and arterial monitoring lines are being placed by the anesthesia team.

Most standard integrated suites have a floor- or ceiling-mounted angiographic system and a "sliding" radiolucent table to allow for easy patient positioning under fluoroscopy. A control panel is also typically attached tableside under a transparent drape in order to allow the operator to control the table position, radiographic gantry, and fluoroscopic and radiographic settings. A surgeon who is facile with operation of the radiographic equipment can often more expeditiously select desired options and positions than when working through a middleman, the radiology technician, thereby reducing radiation and procedural time. In some setups, the control panel is separated from the tabletop to decrease the clutter around the patient and improve the accessibility that the surgeon has to the patient. While a radiology technician knowledgeable in imaging acquisition and processing software is required in either case, the operator of separated controls cannot be the surgeon or part of the sterile team. Given the emergency nature of REVAR, and the a la carte nature of endovascular procedures in general, it is imperative that there be a person available to fetch supplies. Not only should they be knowledgeable about elective EVAR but also the extra devices and maneuvers that might be required for REVAR. Furthermore, they need to be familiar with inventory and placement of catheters, stents, endografts, and other equipment in the room so that they can be obtained and ready to use on a short notice. Rails are also placed on the side of the moveable radiolucent table to serve as attachment sites for table-mounted retractor systems should the operation be converted to an open procedure.

Observational studies used to assess integrating surgery and radiology in one suite have revealed increased workflow times involving preparation and anesthesia ranging from as little as 18 min to as long as 120 min. [19] Due to the amount of equipment and personnel involved in such cases, it may be helpful to have a designated team that is familiar with the procedure and the equipment used for aortic aneurysm repairs. Centers with simulation suites may help prepare personnel to reduce workflow times and potentially improve patient outcomes. This will be discussed in a later section.

Inventory

For elective EVAR, it is not uncommon for an endograft representative to bring devices to the case rather than relying on a hospital's inventory. In the ruptured scenario, however, there will rarely be sufficient time to rely on a representative so a critical factor in determining whether a hospital can provide REVAR on a routine basis is their willingness to stock a wide variety of sizes of aortic endografts and endograft components, as well as the sheaths, guidewires, catheters, stents, and balloons which may be needed to complete a repair. While not commonly used in elective practice, aorto-uni-iliac (AUI) devices offer some advantages in the ruptured AAA situation, most notably a reasonable degree of hemostasis at the time of initial endograft deployment without having to cannulate the docking junction and deploy the contralateral limb to attain it, though complete hemostasis still requires iliac occluder placement and femoral-femoral bypass grafting. Although an unusual occurrence, AUI endografts have also been employed to cover the contralateral limb of a bifurcate body when the docking junction cannot be successfully cannulated, converting the case to the AUI with femoral-femoral bypass configuration, with iliac occlusion, as needed [20, 21]. Large bore sheaths are typically required (18–24 F) to deliver most aortic stent grafts so these need to be kept in inventory. Critical to the use of aortic occlusion balloons, as described in greater detail in an upcoming chapter, is the availability of two 12Fr × 55–65 cm sheaths to allow endograft deployment over an occlusion balloon with subsequent balloon extraction. In addition, it is important to have a variety of guidewires available with varying tip characteristics to be able to negotiate a variety of vascular anatomies and varying degrees of stiffness to facilitate device tracking through tortuous anatomy.

Given the potential for conversion to open repair, a laparotomy instrument tray and a variety of vascular clamps should be available, which will also come in handy if open femoral access is chosen. Recently, the off-label use of the Perclose ProGlide Suture-Mediated Closure System (Abbott Vascular, Santa Clara, CA) in the "preclose" configuration of two cross deployed ProGlide devices to permit percutaneous EVAR has gained popularity for its increased speed and reduced wound complications. While something one should begin with electively, in the hands of an experienced operator the deployments of these devices are feasible and can be performed in a rapid fashion, consistent with the urgency of a ruptured AAA [22]. Other devices that may be helpful to have in stock include a variety of peripheral and visceral bare metal or covered stent grafts. The 510 series Palmaz stents can be used as a bailout strategy to treat type Ia endoleaks, while short balloon expandable stents or endografts may be needed to preserve the renal arteries in case of accidental coverage by the main aortic stent graft.

The question often arises as to which of the available aortic endografts is best for the ruptured aneurysm situation, to which we would unquestionably respond that it would be the endograft you are most familiar and comfortable with. That being said, considering the differences in aortic aneurysm morphology and access vessel size and tortuosity, and that different endografts have different performance characteristics and available sizes, it make sense for any center seeing any volume of ruptured aneurysms to consider stocking two complementary endograft systems, including a broad array of their sizes and components. Most of the aortic endograft systems are of the modular bifurcated design, with either one or two docking limbs, which work well for most situations. In certain anatomic situations, such as with a narrow distal aorta or a ruptured common iliac aneurysm, a unibody bifurcated or aorto-uni-iliac design may be advantageous, the latter of these also being valuable when there is a unilateral iliac occlusion. Regardless of the endografts chosen to be stocked, it is incumbent on the surgeon/interventionist to become familiar with each device's IFUs prior to using it in the emergent setting. Lack of familiarity with device sizing and operation of the deployment system are serious potential pitfalls that can lead to increased fluoroscopy and procedural times and, potentially, REVAR failure leading to conversion to open surgical repair or suboptimal endovascular bailout strategies.

As with elective EVARs, approximately two thirds of ruptured aortic aneurysms have suitable anatomy for on-label REVAR. The overwhelming number of exclusions or anatomic challenges pertains to the aortic neck, be it due to its shortness, angulation, or both. Although fenestrated endografts (Zenith Fenestrated Z-Link ™) have the potential to tackle these cases in the elective setting, they are custom made and require more time than typically available in the ruptured AAA setting. While some high-volume centers have had experience creating customized fenestrations at the time of the procedure by modifying currently marketed endografts, this is an off-label use and cannot be recommended outside of an investigator-sponsored investigational device exemption. Furthermore, performing fenestrated endografting (FEVAR) has been shown to be a time-consuming process, both for planning and deployment, which makes it impractical, at least for most operators, in the ruptured setting [23]. Alternatively, though still procedurally more complicated, stable patients with ruptured juxtarenal aneurysms who have contraindications for open repair, such as a hostile abdomen, can be treated with chimney or snorkel grafts, provided suitable devices and experience are available.

Creation of an Acute Aortic Treatment Program

Arguably, the most important factor in a rAAA patient's outcome is not the type of repair they undergo, open or REVAR, but the coordination of care they receive from presentation through diagnosis, transfer, and ultimate treatment, all of which should be expedited in order to minimize mortality rates. This is what distinguishes an acute aortic "program," something designed around process improvements in the care of rAAA patients, from an acute aortic "center," which is really more of a marketing concept. Programmatic changes in clinical practice brought about through education and the introduction of acute care pathways have led to more rapid diagnosis of patients with rAAA, while coordination of transfer to appropriate facilities for definitive therapy, and the delivery thereof, is more a matter of resource management but a critical element of the program nonetheless. Davies et al. published a report on the creation of an acute aortic treatment center that placed a goal on treating patients from "door to intervention time in under 90 min" with the belief that this would reduce both mortality and morbidity from acute aortic syndromes including rAAA [24]. Other centers have instituted a multidisciplinary approach that included emergency department physicians, operating room staff, radiology technicians, and anesthesiologists. Mehta et al. demonstrated that after instituting a standardized protocol, they were able to reduce mortality rates to 18 % with REVAR [8]. Implementation of these protocols in tertiary high-volume regional centers has led to process improvements resulting in both a decrease in perioperative complications and lower morbidity and mortality.

While the present driver for the development of acute aortic programs is at the physician and hospital level, based on the desire to improve patient outcomes and perhaps to invigorate a lackluster service line, healthcare policy makers have their eye on them to see if they can reduce costs as well. Healthcare quality initiatives such as the Leapfrog Group have proposed creating "evidence-based hospital" referral criteria for centers that perform elective AAA repair which would require, among other things, an annual AAA volume exceeding 50 cases and having intensive care units run by board-certified intensivists [25]. However, it has been reported that this regional center strategy leads to longer times for patients to get to the operating room as well as a potential increase in ICU days used, but it has not been shown to affect mortality, patient compliance with follow-up, or graft-related morbidity [26]. Reaching a different conclusion, with specific focus on transfer of patients, Vogel et al. showed that patients who were not transferred had a significantly higher mortality within 24 h of surgery when compared to those patients who were transferred to specialized centers [27]. As healthcare policy changes focus more on quality-driven outcomes, it is clear that implementation of clinical pathways and protocols will increase over the next decade in an effort to improve patient care while limiting morbidity and mortality rates but mostly to reduce costs. Establishing a multidisciplinary approach and acute aortic treatment center will allow for increased patient accessibility, reduction in time to definitive treatment, and ultimately better outcomes. The winners will be those therapies that prove to be most cost effective and those healthcare systems that can deliver them the most efficaciously in each region.

The Role for Simulation

True care coordination does not occur by simply writing a memo, policy, or protocol but by instituting changes in the way we operate. Surgical simulation, or more appropriately surgical skills training, has become a required element of surgical residencies but only teaches the performance of a procedure. Simulation has been defined as a device or exercise that allows active participants to undergo conditions that are likely to occur in real life [28]. And what condition are you more likely to encounter in real life than the need to coordinate your care with that of others on the team? While most studies on simulation centers have focused on improving endovascular and open skills for surgical residents [29], some are shifting toward improving nontechnical skills such as communication, teamwork, judgment, and leadership for other healthcare personnel [30]. In addition, by providing a simulated environment, observations and immediate feedback can be given so that the participants can then apply what they've learned to real life.

The operating room is a complex working environment, especially in the setting of a life-threatening emergency such as an acute aortic aneurysm rupture. A multitude of healthcare personnel must be mobilized and coordinated to deliver optimal care. While early REVAR protocols focused on the procedure itself, many institutionalized protocols at tertiary centers (especially those which have defined themselves as an acute aortic treatment center) have been broadened to address issues of care all along the patient's path, from presentation to treatment. As such, multidisciplinary simulation exercises would seem a reasonable approach to improve outcomes and decrease morbidity and mortality. Mehta and colleagues considered that and prior to implementing their own protocol for endovascular treatment of rAAA they had healthcare personnel undergo a series of a simulations in which patients with known asymptomatic AAAs presented to the emergency department with symptoms of rupture [8]. By doing this they were able to enhance the knowledge of all personnel who may be involved such as anesthesiologists, the operating room staff, radiology technicians, and emergency physicians and nurses. Although their study did not specifically look at the relationship of this simulation training to their overall performance, it is clear that they thought it was important to do this prior to implementing endovascular repair of ruptured aortic aneurysms at their institution.

Simulation exercises can be of two different varieties: procedural simulation (skills training, Fig. 9.2) and scenario simulation (team training). Both can play a role in the preparation for initiation of a REVAR program. While participating

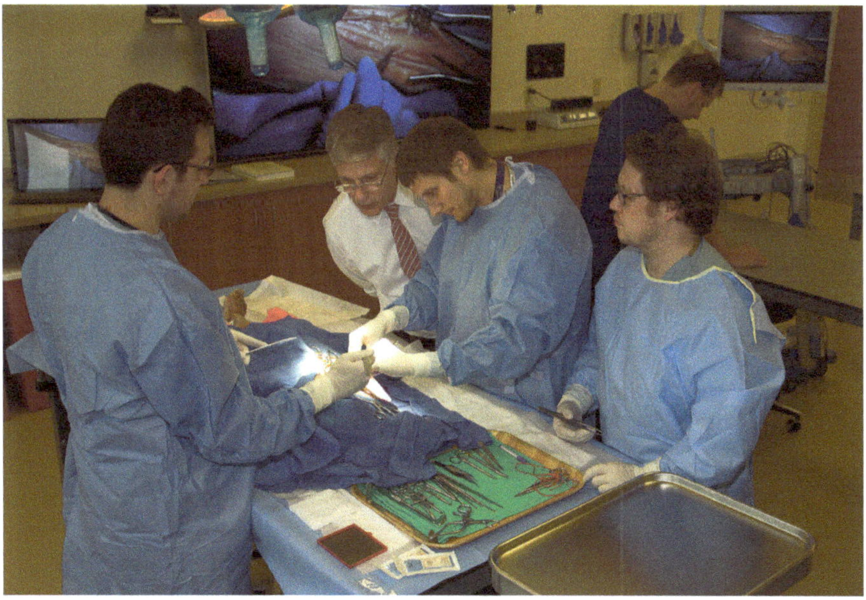

Fig. 9.2 Traditional surgical skills training focuses on an individual's performance of a procedure or component thereof

surgeons would be expected to be competent in performance of elective EVAR, REVAR simulation allows them to learn and practice the maneuvers necessary for EVAR deployment over aortic balloon occlusion, for difficult contralateral gate cannulations and for the use of percutaneous closure devices. More importantly, simulation can help prepare the trainee for what to do when something goes wrong. The second facet of simulation involves team training and performance, as assessed by direct observation and evaluation of individual and team procedural preparation, interaction, communication, and vigilance. Simulated operative experiences have been shown to provide a realistic representation of crisis scenarios that allow a team to perform their duties in a safe and controlled environment, with the added advantage of receiving constructive feedback in both technical and nontechnical skills. Applying this to a rAAA scenario should enhance preparedness, allow for better utilization of resources, improve multidisciplinary care, and help identify and reduce the number of adverse events [30] by allowing teams of healthcare providers to identify lapses of care, real or potential, in their preparation for instituting a REVAR program. Ideally, scenario simulations will include all providers in the pathway, from EMS personnel picking up and transporting patients to ED nurses and physicians rendering initial care and diagnosis, all the way through to the delivery of definitive treatment. As such, our recently opened Center for Learning and Innovation includes simulated patient domiciles (complete with robotic pets; Fig. 9.3a), an actual ambulance which pitches and rocks (Fig. 9.3b), simulated ED rooms (Fig. 9.3c), ORs (Fig. 9.3d), and endovascular suites. In addition to the inherent value of bringing the team together in the first place, all facets of the patient's simulation can be broken down into components, measured, and analyzed for opportunities for improvement. Such outcomes improvement initiatives are expected to play an ever increasing role in the delivery of healthcare in the years to come.

Summary

Incorporating REVAR into your practice involves more than just learning the techniques of the procedure. If optimal outcomes are to be obtained, the entire process of care for patients with ruptured AAAs needs to be coordinated, from initial evaluation at presentation through transport and treatment. This involves both education and standardization of care through implementation of clinical pathways and protocols. Regardless of the ultimate therapy employed, REVAR or open aneurysm repair, all patients will benefit from better coordination of the healthcare teams responsible for their care.

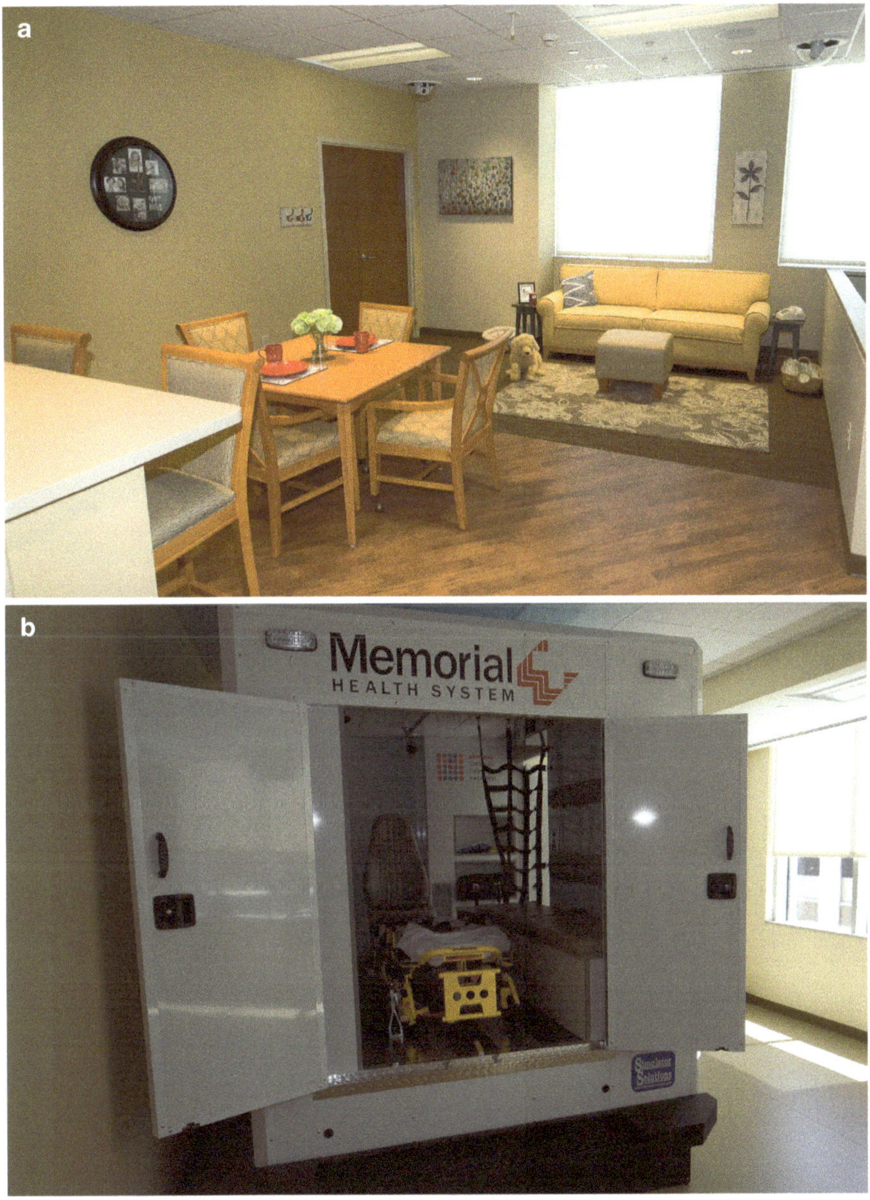

Fig. 9.3 (**a**) Simulated patient living room, with mechanical distracting dog, in a simulated patient home that includes a full bedroom, bathroom, kitchen, and living room, all outfitted with cameras for observation. (**b**) Simulated ambulance bay on a mechanized chassis to roll and pitch for simulated patient transport and en route management. (**c**) Simulated emergency room bay with X-ray (control room on right) and a variety of equipment and cameras. (**d**) Simulated operating room complete with full anesthetic equipment and case-specific anatomic models for team training of procedures

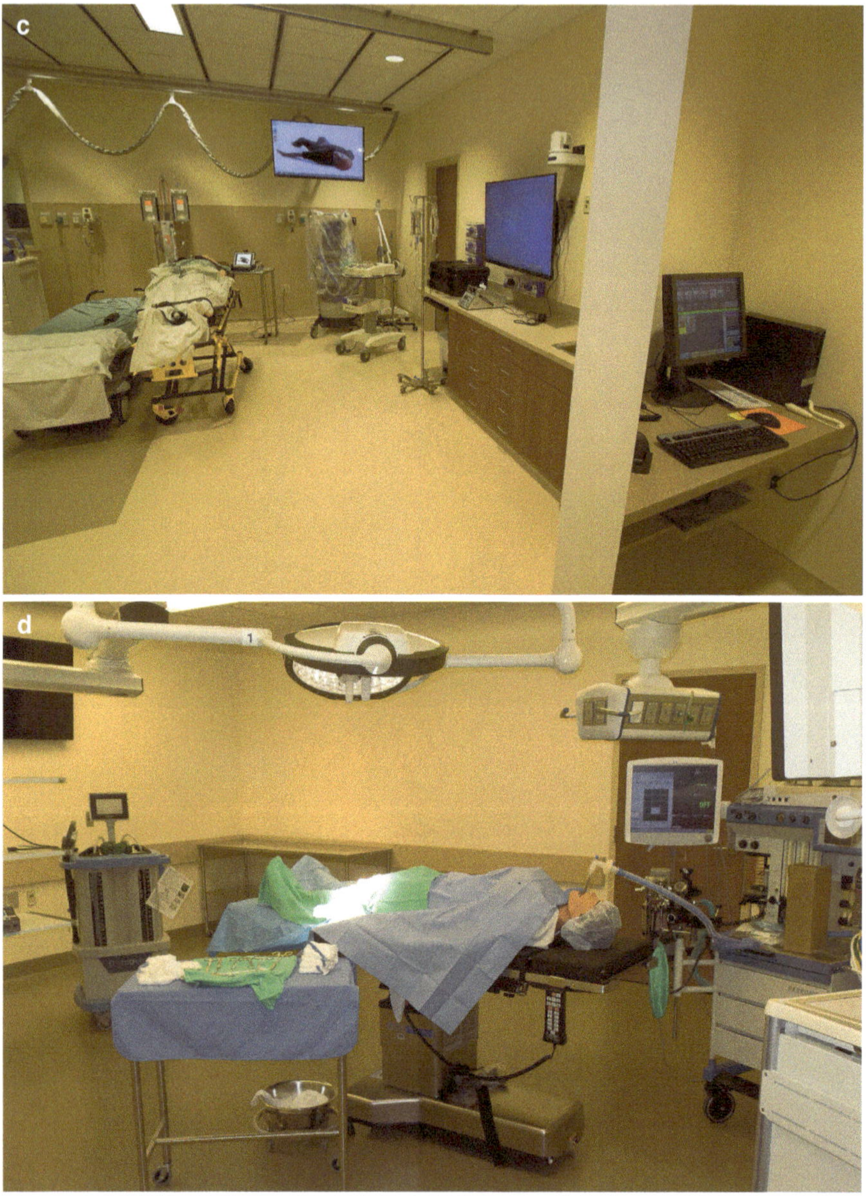

Fig. 9.3 (continued)

References

1. Talledo O, Livesay J. Endovascular aneurysm repair is Not the treatment of choice in most patients with ruptured abdominal aortic aneurysm. Tex Heart Inst J. 2013;40(5):556–9.
2. Giles K, Hamdan A, Pomposelli F, et al. Population-based outcomes following endovascular and open repair of ruptured abdominal aortic aneurysms. J Endovasc Ther. 2009;16(5):554–64.

3. Noel AA, Gloviczki P, Cherry KJ, et al. Ruptured abdominal aortic aneurysms: the excessive mortality rate of conventional repair. J Vasc Surg. 2001;34:41–6.
4. Sah D, Ozsvath K, Sternbach Y. Establishing a protocol for endovascular treatment of ruptured abdominal aortic aneurysms: outcomes of a prospective analysis. J Vasc Surg. 2007;44:1–8.
5. The IMPROVE Trial Invetigators. Endovascular or open repair strategy for ruptured abdominal aortic aneurysm: 30 day outcomes from IMPROVE randomised trial. BMJ. 2014;348.
6. Veith FJ, Rockman CB. Randomized trials show EVAR is the best option for ruptured AAAs. Endovasc Today. 2015; 65–70, and The recent randomized trials of EVAR versus open repair for ruptured abdominal aortic aneurysms are misleading. Vasc 2015;23:217–9.
7. Hodgson KJ. EVAR for ruptured aneurysms: Are the data complete? Semin Vasc Surg. 2012;25:217–26.
8. Manish Mehta MD, MPH. Endovascular aneurysm repair for ruptured abdominal aortic aneurysm: the Albany vascular group approach. J Vasc Surg. 2010;52:1706–12.
9. Boyle JR, Gibbs PJ, Kruger A, Shearman CP, Raptis S, Phillips MJ. Existing delays following the presentation of ruptured abdominal aortic aneurysm allow sufficient time to assess patients for endovascular repair. Eur J Vasc Endovasc Surg. 2005;29:505–9.
10. Hoshina K, Kato M, Miyahara T, et al. A retrospective study of intravascular ultrasound use in patients undergoing endovascular aneurysm repair: its usefulness and a description of the procedure. Eur J Vasc Endovasc Surg. 2010;40(5):559–63.
11. Jordan Jr WD, Pearce BJ. Using IVUS during EVAR and TEVAR: improving patient outcomes. Semin Vasc Surg. 2009;22(3):172–80.
12. Criado E, Kabbani L, Cho K. Catheter-less angiography for endovascular aortic aneurysm repair: a new application of carbon dioxide as a contrast agent. J Vasc Surg. 2008;48(3):527–34.
13. Mehta M, Taggert J, Darling 3rd RC, Chang BB, Kreienberg PB, Paty PS, Roddy SP, Sternbach Y, Ozsvath KJ, Shah DM. Establishing a protocol for endovascular treatment of ruptured abdominal aortic aneurysms: outcomes of a prospective analysis.asc. J Vasc Surg. 2006;44:1–8.
14. Raux M, Marzelle J, Kobeiter H. Endovascular balloon occlusion is associated with reduced intraoperative mortality of unstable patients with ruptured abdominal aortic aneurysm but fails to improve other outcomes. J Vasc Surg. 2015;61:304–8.
15. Saito N, Matsumoto H, Yagi T, et al. Evaluation of the safety and feasibility of resuscitative endovascular balloon occlusion of the aorta. J Trauma Acute Care Surg. 2015;78(5): 897–903.
16. The IMPROVE Trial Investigators. Observations from the IMPROVE trial concerning the clinical care of patients with ruptured abdominal aortic aneurysm. Br J Surg. 2014;101:216–24.
17. Dick F, Erdoes G, Opfermann P, Eberle B, Schmidli J, von Allmen RS. Delayed volume resuscitation during initial management of ruptured abdominal aortic aneurysm. J Vasc Surg. 2013;57:943–50.
18. van der Vliet JA, van Aalst DL, Schultze Kppl LJ, Wever JJ, Blankensteijn JD. Hypotensive hemostatis (permissive hypotension) for ruptured abdominal aortic aneurysm: are we really in control? Vascular. 2007;15:197–200.
19. Lothert M, Pearce B, McKinsey K, et al. Integrating surgery and radiology in one suite. A multicenter study. J Vasc Surg. 2004;30:494–9.
20. Kiguchi MM, Forbes TL, Teijink JA, et al. Clinical application and early outcomes of the aortouni-iliac configuration for endovascular aneurysm repair. J Vasc Surg. 2014;60(6): 1452–9.
21. Smit JG, van Marle J. Repair of abdominal aortic aneurysms with aorto-uni-iliac stent graft and femoro-femoral bypass. S Afr J Surg. 2012;50(2):33–6.
22. Torsello GB, Kasprazak B, Klenk E, Tessarek J, et al. Endovascular suture versus cutdown for endovascular aneurysm repair: a prospective randomized pilot study. J Vasc Surg. 2003;38(1): 78–82.
23. McNally M, Scali S, Freezor RJ, et al. Three-dimensional fusion computed tomography decreases radiation exposure, procedure time, and contrast use during fenestrated endovascular aortic repair. J Vasc Surg. 2015;61(2):309–16.
24. Davies M, Younes H, Harris P, et al. Outcomes before and after initiation of an acute aortic treatment center. J Vasc Surg. 2010;52:1478–85.

25. Brooke BS, Perler BA, Dominici F, Makary MA, Pronovost PJ. Reduction of in-hospital mortality among California hospitals meeting Leap- frog evidence-based standards for abdominal aortic aneurysm repair. J Vasc Surg. 2008;47:1155–64.
26. Sarangarm D, Knepper J, Marek J, et al. Post-endovascular aneurysm repair patient outcomes and follow-up are not adversely impacted by long travel distance to tertiary vascular surgery centers. Ann Vasc Surg. 2010;24(8):1075–81.
27. Vogel TR, Nackman GB, Brevetti LS, et al. Resource utilization and outcomes: effect of transfer on patients with ruptured abdominal aortic aneurysms. Ann Vasc Surg. 2005;19(2): 140–53.
28. Krummel TM. Surgical simulation and virtual reality; the coming revolution. Ann Surg. 1998;228:635–7.
29. Robinson W, Baril D, Taha O, et al. Simulation-based training to teach open abdominal aortic aneurysm repair to surgical residents requires dedicated faculty instruction. J Vasc Surg. 2013;58:247–53.
30. Aggarwal A, Undre S, Moorthy K. The simulated operating theatre: comprehensive training for surgical teams. Qual Saf Health Care. 2004;13 Suppl 1:i27–32.

Chapter 10
Guidelines for Transfer to Specialized Centers

Matthew Mell

Introduction

Ruptured abdominal aortic aneurysm remains a highly time-sensitive condition where if left untreated 25 % of patients die within 2–4 h [1] (Fig. 10.1). However, many patients remain stable enough in the immediate short time following rupture to allow potential to achieve definitive treatment. Prompt treatment is often not possible at the presenting center and transfer to specialized care is necessary. As such, it is imperative that transfer is expedited to provide the greatest chance for a favorable outcome. In considering the appropriate patient for transfer, a number of questions often arise including suitability for treatment, need for definitive imaging prior to transfer, mode of transportation, which facility to transfer to, clinical management principles during transfer, and feasibility of transfer in the anticipated time interval of stability. Presently, few sending and receiving hospitals have systems in place to expediently transfer, and professional standards are yet to achieve widespread implementation.

M. Mell, MD, MS
Division of Vascular Surgery, Stanford University School of Medicine,
300 Pasteur Drive, Stanford, CA H3600, USA
e-mail: mwmell@stanford.edu

B.W. Starnes et al. (eds.), *Ruptured Abdominal Aortic Aneurysm*,
DOI 10.1007/978-3-319-23844-9_10

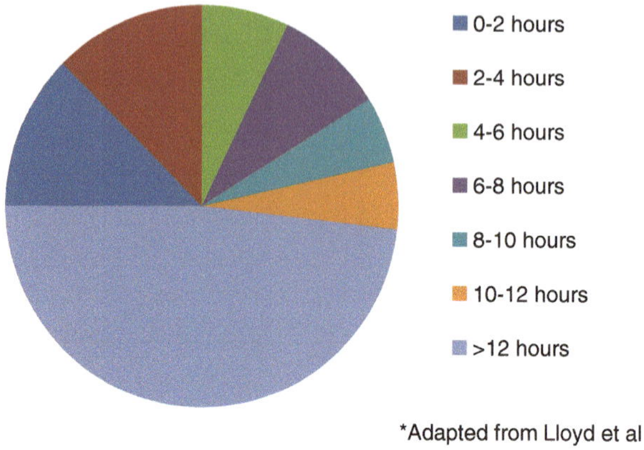

Fig. 10.1 Time from admission to death for untreated ruptured abdominal aortic aneurysms (Adapted from Lloyd et al. [1])

Current State

Emergency Department Deaths for Ruptured Abdominal Aortic Aneurysm

One of the perceived limitations in achieving a successful outcome for a patient requiring transfer is the potential opportunity cost of awaiting transfer. When no organized system of care exists specifically for the care of ruptured abdominal aortic aneurysm, emergency department (ED) death can occur when local treatment is unavailable. Although some of these ED deaths encompass those who arrive in extremis, a percentage of these deaths also reflect those who deteriorate while awaiting definitive care [2]. A recent study using the Nationwide Emergency Department Sample (NEDS) data found 7 % of patients died in the ED and another 6 % admitted to the presenting hospital died without treatment. It is not possible from the NEDS dataset to determine exactly why patients died in the ED or were not offered transfer; however, one can hypothesize that these patients were either in extremis on presentation precluding transfer or worsened while awaiting transfer. The study suggests that the later explanation may be a larger factor as those more likely to have an ED death included those who were older and who presented to nonmetropolitan hospitals (Table 10.1). Nonmetropolitan hospitals were also most likely to transfer patients. The high ED death rate and transfer rate may imply that these facilities were not able to provide local care. Without a rapid and reliable transfer process, a percentage of these deaths are likely preventable with better regional systems of care.

The need for predefined transfer plans may be even more important in geographic regions where the land mass to hospital facility ratio is greatest. The NEDS study also identified differences in ED death by region. The West had almost double the ED death rate even after adjusting for demographic and hospital factors. Further underscoring the difficulties with transfer across larger geographic constraints, the

Table 10.1 Predictors of ED death for ruptured abdominal aortic aneurysm

Factor		Adjusted OR[a]	95 % CI	*P*-value
Rural vs. urban teaching hospital		1.9	1.2–2.9	0.001
Rural vs. urban nonteaching hospital		1.4	0.9–2.1	0.12
Low-volume ED		1.3	0.8–2.2	0.25
Moderate-volume ED		1.0	0.7–1.4	0.92
High-volume ED		1.0	Referent	
Region	East	0.5	0.3–0.8	0.008
	South	0.4	0.3–0.7	0.001
	Midwest	0.6	0.4–0.9	0.02
	West	1.0	Referent	
Trauma designation		0.9	0.5–1.4	0.54
Age (per decade)		1.9	1.6–2.2	<0.0001
Male gender		0.7	0.5–0.9	0.008

[a]Adjusted for comorbidity and insurance status

West was also the least likely to transfer patients. As the Western Region of the United States has approximately 25 % of the US population but 50 % of the land mass, our findings suggest that patients who have greater travel distances and travel times to the initial ED may be more likely to become clinically unstable upon arrival or before transfer can be arranged (REF).

Transfer for Treatment of Ruptured Abdominal Aortic Aneurysm

In the current era of publically reported outcomes, many centers remain concerned about the implications on overall institutional mortality when accepting high-risk patient transfers. In the case of ruptured abdominal aortic aneurysms, single-center studies have reported equivalent outcomes for treatment of ruptured abdominal aortic aneurysm after transfer [3–7]. However, in these studies only those receiving treatment for their aneurysm were included. Thus, those transferred who did not undergo treatment or who died prior to reaching the receiving hospital were not captured These studies suffer from survivor bias given that patients had to survive transfer and be stable enough for treatment on arrival.

This limitation was addressed in a follow-up study using an intent-to-treat analysis linking State Inpatient Databases and Emergency Department Databases for New York, California, and Florida to compare outcomes for ruptured abdominal aortic aneurysm between those transferred for care with those treated at the presenting institution [8]. Almost 20 % of patients were transferred for definitive care (REF). Most patients were transferred a short distance (median, 27 miles), and few (<8 %) traveled great distances defined as >100 miles. The study found equivalent mortality rates for those transferred (45 %) patients to those treated without transfer

Table 10.2 Inter-facility transfer and ruptured abdominal aortic aneurysm mortality

	Adjusted odds ratio[a]	95 % CI	*P*-value
Nonoperative deaths excluded	0.81	0.68–0.97	0.02
Nonoperative deaths included	1.30	1.05–1.60	0.01

[a]Adjusted for age, gender, weekend presentation, admission year, state, comorbidity, and insurance status

(43 %). Unfortunately, among those transferred, 17 % still died without receiving treatment. When accounting for these patients in the intent-to-treat analysis, transfer was actually associated with an increased mortality (Table 10.2).

Although transfers were more common on weekends, mortality was independent of time of presentation. One of the interesting findings was the annual increase in transfer rates over time from 15 % in 2005 to 24 % in 2010. Transferred patients had fewer comorbid medical conditions and were more likely to present to smaller non-teaching hospitals. These findings further support the hypothesis that those most likely to benefit from transfer are those that are stable enough to receive an operation when they arrive at the receiving facility. Establishing transfer guidelines is unlikely to benefit those who are in extremis at the initial treating facility, but likely will have the greatest impact on those patients who are harmed by delays in care that convert them from stable to potentially unstable while awaiting transfer. The key finding thus far is that the benefits of the current de facto transfer process seen on a population level could be interpreted that transfer is associated with a higher mortality; the alternative and likely more accurate summation is that attention should be focused on improving the transfer process to increase the likelihood of clinical stability during transfer and consequently improve overall survival [9].

Patient Selection

Although under the development by the Western Vascular Society, no current guidelines or standards exist in the United States for selecting the ruptured abdominal aortic aneurysm patient suitable for repair, especially when inter-facility transfer is needed. Clinical algorithms [10–15] for predicting death have been reported, but clinical utility is still questioned. Hospitals and clinicians considering the acceptance of transferred patients are often faced with patients who are not hemodynamically stable or have a large burden of preexisting comorbidities making survival from repair even more challenging. Prior studies have hypothesized that transferred patients who die without a repair were either not candidates for repair or were those who would have been candidates but decline during the transfer process. Included in the unsuitable repair group are patients that have forgone prior elective repair often due to extensive comorbidities. Not uncommonly, these patients request repair when presented with the life-threatening realization that they are dying from a ruptured aneurysm.

Electing to proceed with transfer of these types of patients including the unstable patient is a difficult decision point for both the clinicians and the patient where the default is often to initiate transfer. A recent survey of vascular surgeons in the Western United States revealed that most had few if any exclusion criteria for accepting transfers for ruptured abdominal aortic aneurysm [16]. Specifically, age was not a consideration. Only 7 % reported age greater than 90 years as preclusion for transfer. Similarly, 19 % did not consider transfer for those with severe underlying systemic disease and 34 % for those unable to perform activities of daily living [2].

The approach of US vascular surgeons is in stark contrast to those that practice in a socialized medical system with a recent survey of the United Kingdom providers citing underlying health and lifestyle considerations as major factors in the decision-making process [17]. Both groups identified cardiac arrest requiring CPR as a contraindication to transfer, but hypotension requiring inotropic support was not.

Without established guidelines for patient selection, current transfer decisions vary across institutions, regions, and on a case-by-case basis. This likely increases time delay as the request for clinical evaluation, diagnostic laboratory tests, or radiographic imaging may be extensive, time intensive, and ultimately unnecessary. For example, respondents in the US study were far more likely to require evaluation by a surgeon or a CT scan prior to transfer compared with the UK respondents [16]. In summary, there is a growing need as transfer has become more common to provide guidance on who clearly will not benefit, while maintaining liberal criteria for those in whom transfer would be advantageous when combined with an efficient and efficacious overall approach to treatment.

Key Components to Regionalization of Care

With an organized regional system of care, operative repair can be performed in over 95 % of transferred ruptured abdominal aortic aneurysm patients, with 67 % survival [18]. Optimum transfer is dependent upon proper coordination between the sending facility and the receiving facility. Sending facilities should develop processes to streamline diagnosis, build relationships to predetermine the preferred transfer facility, have a standard communication method, and have a reliable provider for transport. It is also imperative to insure that any imaging is transmitted judiciously either by disc or electronically to the receiving center. Prompt and effective communication at the receiving center is a core component of a successful regional transfer plan. This includes rapid connectivity between providers, guidelines on patient management during transfer, and a streamlined process to efficiently achieve operative repair. Many centers have one uniform access phone number that includes administrative oversight of the phone calls to insure available resources are immediately available at the receiving center. Once the transfer is accepted, this should initiate a process that readies the operating room, catheterization lab, and hospital bed resources, as appropriate, in preparation for patient arrival. Mobilization of these resources allows for more rapid access to definitive repair.

There is no single model of regionalization that is known to be superior to others. For some regions, a single receiving facility or a hub-and-spokes model is optimum. For this to work, there needs to be a "no-denial" policy as the system would fail if the hub often could not accept transfers secondary to resource limitations. In contrast, when beds or resources are frequently limited in tertiary care regional centers, a network model works better. Ideally, in either system, the receiving hospital should strive to achieve a "no-denial" policy for appropriate transfer patients to avoid the need for referring facilities to simultaneously call multiple hospitals seeking an accepting location. If such a policy is not feasible, required resources should be known at the potentially receiving facility to achieve a denial as rapidly as possible to avoid added delays in care. The mode of transportation that provides the most rapid transport should be utilized, which may depend on distance, traffic, weather, and availability.

Optimizing Care During Transfer

Although patient selection and an organized regional transfer plan are important in improving outcome for patients suffering ruptured abdominal aortic aneurysms, how a patient is actually rendered care during the physical transfer is also important. There are little data to guide the best approach during this critical time period. Avoiding hypertension to prevent conversion to frank rupture is important. Patients should receive intravenous nitroglycerin, esmolol, sodium nitroprusside, and pain medication as necessary to minimize risk of hypertension and tachycardia. For those presenting with hypotension, permissive hypotension and limitation of crystalloid is commonly utilized to achieve a systolic blood pressure between 70 and 100 mmHg. Borrowing from the improved mortality found in trauma patients resuscitated with a blood product-rich resuscitation, blood products are preferred to treat hypotension [6]. However, it is not recommended to delay transfer to await blood products if not readily available.

While patients are in the transfer process, the receiving facility should be coordinating an organized and standard treatment approach. In fact, an organized treatment algorithm for ruptured abdominal aortic aneurysm has led to improved operative survival, approaching 75 % in some single-institution studies [3, 4, 19]. The treatment algorithm should include trained physicians, operating room, and radiology personnel, immediate availability of blood products and a standard resuscitation protocol, rapid access to endovascular inventory. and a predefined treatment algorithm including guidelines for converting endovascular to open repairs. These elements should be in place such that at the time of patient arrival, a rapid assessment can occur followed by quick movement toward the definitive treatment area. The goal is to eliminate time delay in each phase of care to maximize the likelihood of optimum patient outcome.

The Potential Role for Best-Practice Guidelines

At present, a minority number of centers that accept transfers have a formal protocol for doing so. Recent data shows that in the Western Region of the United States, 60 % of physicians who accept ruptured abdominal aortic aneurysm transfers do not have a formal protocol for treatment, and 70 % do not use a transfer protocol or clinical guidelines [16]. The absence of data definitively demonstrating the advantage of such protocols has hampered the widespread adoption of transfer guidelines. In the absence of data, the development of best-practice guidelines targeted to reduce variation and improve transfer efficiency may provide a framework to address key components of an effective transfer process. The goal should be to eliminate unnecessary steps at each step in the evaluation and treatment process. Reduction of time delay increases the chances that a patient will arrive clinically stable and remain a repair candidate. Improving the proportion of transferred patients who arrive in condition to receive AAA repair will increase the overall ruptured abdominal aortic aneurysm survival [9].

The utilization of transfer for the patient with ruptured abdominal aortic aneurysm has increased yearly since 2005, as has the utilization of transfer for rural patients with ruptured abdominal aortic aneurysm [8, 20]. As specialized centers for treatment of acute aortic conditions expand, there is risk of reduction in case volume and diminished expertise of local facilities [21]. This may be the underlying etiology of the steady rise in transfer volumes as it parallels the increase in operative repairs for ruptured aneurysms treated with an endovascular approach. Another potential contributing factor may be the increasing cost of providing a complete vascular device inventory, as well as the changing patterns of providing vascular care. Recent general surgeon graduates who are practicing as community surgeons have much less vascular experience than in the past. Thus, many are not qualified upon graduation to provide the breadth of vascular care that their predecessors reaching retirement age have historically done. The net effect is a reduction in facilities that have resources and case volumes to treat the most complex vascular cases including ruptured abdominal aortic aneurysms. Thus, transfer is becoming an increasingly common practice and the need for standardization of approach to transfer is needed.

Future Directions

Although no best-practice guidelines currently exist in the United States for transfer of ruptured abdominal aortic aneurysms, criteria are under development by the Western Vascular Society (WVS). The WVS guidelines will focus on elements common to practice in the United States and will borrow some from the guidelines currently used in the United Kingdom (UK). Those guidelines are endorsed by the Vascular Society of Great Britain and Ireland, The Royal College of Emergency Medicine, and The Royal College of Radiologists [22] (Table 10.3). The impact of

Table 10.3 Best-practice guidelines for the management and transfer of patients with a diagnosis of ruptured abdominal aortic aneurysm to a specialist vascular center [22]

1. A clinical diagnosis of ruptured abdominal aortic aneurysm (ruptured abdominal aortic aneurysm) should be considered:
In patients over the age of 50 years presenting with abdominal/back pain AND hypotension
In patients with a known AAA and symptoms of either abdominal/back pain OR hypotension/collapse
In patients where an alternative diagnosis is considered more likely on clinical grounds, ruptured abdominal aortic aneurysm still must be excluded, with radiological confirmation made prior to referral. *Level 3, strong recommendation*
2. Permissive hypotension is advocated for patients with a clinical diagnosis of ruptured abdominal aortic aneurysm to maintain an alert patient and systolic blood pressure >70 mm Hg is acceptable. *Level 4, strong*
3. If a specialist vascular service cannot be provided on-site, the patient requires transfer to a center with appropriate facilities and expertise. Transfer agreements with the local ambulance service should be in place. *Level 4, strong recommendation*
4. Rapid and coordinated transfer can reduce delays in the patient journey and improve outcome. *Level 3, strong.* To expedite transfer the most senior doctor available should lead and be actively involved the care of any patient with suspected ruptured abdominal aortic aneurysm. Outgoing referrals should go to a senior vascular trainee or consultant
Items 5–18 below are all Level 5, with strong recommendation
5. All patients with a clinical or radiological diagnosis of ruptured abdominal aortic aneurysm should be assessed as to their current clinical state AND premorbid level of function to determine suitability for transfer
6. Patients aged <85 with no/mild/moderate systemic disease should be referred to the receiving hospital's on-call vascular service without delay
7. Patients age >85 or with severe systemic disease will benefit from a consultant*–consultant discussion prior to transfer to a vascular unit
8. Impaired mental capacity is not a contraindication to assessment and transfer
9. Patients who have been previously turned down for elective surgery should still be discussed via a consultant–consultant referral
10. Contraindications to transfer are restricted to those with cardiac arrest in the current admission and intubated patients. Such patients are unlikely to survive transfer and surgery
11. There are no ESSENTIAL investigations required prior to transfer. However, a blood gas and an emergency department ultrasound are considered useful, if these incur no delay
12. Investigations including FBC, U&E, amylase, X-match, and CT scans MUST not delay transfer to a center that can provide definitive care. If an alternative diagnosis is more likely, or the investigation can be performed without causing delay, it is reasonable to perform these investigations before transfer
13. Patients should be treated, if necessary, with both analgesia (according to the College of Emergency Medicine [CEM] guidelines) and fluids before and during transfer. Blood products and inotropes may be required, their use should be supervised by a ST4 or above, trainee or equivalent, or consultant
14. A time-critical transfer in a 999 ambulance, preferably with a paramedic crew, is required, although this is not essential
15. Patients requiring inotropic support will need a suitably experienced and trained medical escort for transfer

Table 10.3 (continued)

16. The facility to transfer CT images electronically must be in place to ensure all images are transferred to the receiving hospital. If electronic transfer is not possible, a CD or DVD of DICOM files must accompany the patient
17. Patients should not travel with blood products, unless transfusion already commenced
18. Patients who remain cardiovascularly stable should be transferred to either an emergency department resuscitation bed or local equivalent. Patients who are unstable may need rapid transfer to theaters
19. Transfer to a specialist vascular center should occur within 30 min of diagnosis

the UK guidelines on patient outcome has not been studied. With implementation of the WVS recommendations, investigators hope to be able to evaluate the impact on reducing variation in care, increasing the utilization of operative repair, and improving survival.

As care is streamlined, it provides additional opportunity to further study the critical factors that may offer further survival benefit. There still exist many knowledge gaps in optimizing the care for the patient with ruptured abdominal aortic aneurysm who requires inter-facility transfer for definitive care. This includes what factors important in transfer increase the likelihood of meaningful survival, the minimal diagnostic evaluation required before transfer, and the best resuscitative method during transfer. Furthermore, refinements in communication between facilities to coordinate data and information sharing could be enhanced. Finally, paramedic triage in the field analogous to trauma field triage may facilitate initial transport to hospitals equipped with ruptured abdominal aneurysm expertise and bypass less skilled centers. For example, paramedics or emergency medical technicians may be able make the diagnosis of ruptured abdominal aortic aneurysm in the field using standardized approaches and triage criteria. With these and other theoretic advances, population-level outcomes could translate to additional survival for those suffering ruptured abdominal aortic aneurysms.

References

1. Lloyd GM, Bown MJ, Norwood MG, et al. Feasibility of preoperative computer tomography in patients with ruptured abdominal aortic aneurysm: a time-to-death study in patients without operation. J Vasc Surg. 2004;39(4):788–91.
2. Mell MW, Callcut RA, Bech F, et al. Predictors of emergency department death for patients presenting with ruptured abdominal aortic aneurysms. J Vasc Surg. 2012;56(3):651–5.
3. Mell MW, O'Neil AS, Callcut RA, et al. Effect of early plasma transfusion on mortality in patients with ruptured abdominal aortic aneurysm. Surgery. 2010;148(5):955–62.
4. Starnes BW, Quiroga E, Hutter C, et al. Management of ruptured abdominal aortic aneurysm in the endovascular era. J Vasc Surg. 2010;51(1):9–17; discussion 17–8.
5. Vogel TR, Nackman GB, Brevetti LS, et al. Resource utilization and outcomes: effect of transfer on patients with ruptured abdominal aortic aneurysms. Ann Vasc Surg. 2005;19(2):149–53.
6. Hames H, Forbes TL, Harris JR, Lawlor DK, DeRose G, Harris KA. The effect of patient transfer on outcomes after rupture of an abdominal aortic aneurysm. Can J Surg. 2007;50(1): 43–7.

7. Azizzadeh A, Miller 3rd CC, Villa MA, et al. Effect of patient transfer on outcomes after open repair of ruptured abdominal aortic aneurysms. Vascular. 2009;17(1):9–14.
8. Mell MW, Wang NE, Morrison DE, Hernandez-Boussard T. Interfacility transfer and mortality for patients with ruptured abdominal aortic aneurysm. J Vasc Surg. 2014;60(3):553–7.
9. Karthikesalingam A, Holt PJ, Vidal-Diez A, et al. Mortality from ruptured abdominal aortic aneurysms: clinical lessons from a comparison of outcomes in England and the USA. Lancet. 2014;383(9921):963–9.
10. Antonello M, Frigatti P, Maturi C, et al. Open repair for ruptured abdominal aortic aneurysm: is it possible to predict survival? Ann Vasc Surg. 2009;23(2):159–66.
11. Chen JC, Hildebrand HD, Salvian AJ, et al. Predictors of death in nonruptured and ruptured abdominal aortic aneurysms. J Vasc Surg. 1996;24(4):614–20. discussion 621–613.
12. Hardman DT, Fisher CM, Patel MI, et al. Ruptured abdominal aortic aneurysms: who should be offered surgery? J Vasc Surg. 1996;23(1):123–9.
13. Samy AK, Murray G, MacBain G. Glasgow aneurysm score. Cardiovasc Surg. 1994;2(1): 41–4.
14. Samy AK, Murray G, MacBain G. Prospective evaluation of the Glasgow Aneurysm Score. J R Coll Surg Edinb. 1996;41(2):105–7.
15. Tambyraja A, Murie J, Chalmers R. Predictors of outcome after abdominal aortic aneurysm rupture: Edinburgh Ruptured Aneurysm Score. World J Surg. 2007;31(11):2243–7.
16. Mell MW, Schneider PA, Starnes BW. Variability in transfer criteria for patients with ruptured abdominal aortic aneurysm in the western United States. J Vasc Surg. 2015.
17. Hinchliffe RJ, Ribbons T, Ulug P, Powell JT. Transfer of patients with ruptured abdominal aortic aneurysm from general hospitals to specialist vascular centres: results of a Delphi consensus study. Emerg Med J. 2013;30(6):483–6.
18. Haveman JW, Karliczek A, Verhoeven EL, et al. Results of streamlined regional ambulance transport and subsequent treatment of acute abdominal aortic aneurysms. Emerg Med J. 2006;23(10):807–10.
19. Mehta M, Taggert J, Darling 3rd RC, et al. Establishing a protocol for endovascular treatment of ruptured abdominal aortic aneurysms: outcomes of a prospective analysis. J Vasc Surg. 2006;44(1):1–8; discussion 8.
20. Maybury RS, Chang DC, Freischlag JA. Rural hospitals face a higher burden of ruptured abdominal aortic aneurysm and are more likely to transfer patients for emergent repair. J Am Coll Surg. 2011;212(6):1061–7.
21. Davies MG, Younes HK, Harris PW, et al. Outcomes before and after initiation of an acute aortic treatment center. J Vasc Surg. 2010;52(6):1478–85.
22. Vascular Society, College of Emergency Medicine, Royal College of Radiologists. Best practice guidelines for the management and transfer of patients with a diagnosis of ruptured abdominal aortic aneurysm to a specialist vascular centre. London: VSGBI, CEM, RCR; 2012. http://www.collemergencymed.ac.uk/Shop-Floor/Clinical%20Guidelines/default.asp. Cited June 2015.

Chapter 11
Hypotensive Hemostasis in Patients Presenting with Ruptured Aortic Aneurysm

Felice Pecoraro, Bernard Krüger, Johnny Steuer, Neal Cayne, Zoran Rancic, Frank J. Veith, and Mario Lachat

Introduction

In contrast to peripheral vascular injury, which may be controlled with a tourniquet or manual compression to stabilize the patient before definitive repair, in the ruptured intrathoracic and intra-abdominal aorta or its branches, external compression is rarely an alternative. Acute and severe blood loss leads to hypotension and cardiovascular shock, resulting in multisystem organ failure and eventual death. However, aggressive fluid resuscitation in these patients can be detrimental as large-volume infusion may lead to further blood loss, hemodilution [1], dilutional

F. Pecoraro
Clinic for Cardiovascular Surgery, University Hospital, Zurich, Switzerland

Institute for Cardiovascular Anesthesia, University Hospital, Zurich, Switzerland

B. Krüger
Vascular Surgery Unit, University of Palermo, University Hospital 'P. Giaccone', Palermo, Italy

J. Steuer
Clinic for Cardiovascular Surgery, University Hospital, Zurich, Switzerland

Department of Surgery, Section for Vascular Surgery, South Hospital, Stockholm, Sweden

N. Cayne
New York University Medical Center, New York, NY, USA

Z. Rancic • M. Lachat (✉)
Clinic for Cardiovascular Surgery, University Hospital, Zurich, Switzerland
e-mail: mario.lachat@usz.ch

F.J. Veith
Clinic for Cardiovascular Surgery, University Hospital, Zurich, Switzerland

New York University Medical Center, New York, NY, USA

B.W. Starnes et al. (eds.), *Ruptured Abdominal Aortic Aneurysm*,
DOI 10.1007/978-3-319-23844-9_11

coagulopathy, and hypothermia [2]. Moreover, in ruptured abdominal aortic aneurysm (rAAA), massive retroperitoneal bleeding contributes to the development of intra-abdominal hypertension (IAH) and ultimately to abdominal compartment syndrome (ACS) with a high risk of severe complications and death [3]. Finally, massive transfusion of red blood cells, thrombocytes, and/or coagulation factors may be accompanied by severe immunologic reaction and transfusion-related acute lung injury (TRALI) [4]. To avoid these scenarios and/or complications, hypotensive hemostasis is advocated.

From a historical point of view, in 1949 Andresen et al. reported their experience in the management of gastric hemorrhage suggesting that "No transfusion should be given in the first days except for evidence of severe anoxia. Then try 1 or 2 transfusions of 150–200 CC of citrated blood" [5]. This original experience first advised a switch from resuscitation with high amount of fluids to achieve a neo-physiological blood pressure to the concept of *hypotensive hemostasis*, limiting the resuscitation fluids in cases of massive blood loss. In 1981, Akins showed in an observational single-center study that in patients with blunt aortic injury, the use of beta-blockers and antihypertensive therapy permitted stabilizing the patient to allow delayed aortic repair until extracorporeal circulation with the use of a heart-lung machine could be initiated, which was often a necessity in the era preceding the current use of endovascular aneurysm repair (EVAR) [6]. In 1991 Crawford [7] advocated, in patients presenting with rAAA, the use of small volumes of whole blood or crystalloid to maintain blood pressure around 50–70 mmHg until cross-clamping of the aorta was accomplished. A similar fluid restriction scheme was reported in 2002 by Veith and Ohki [8] for EVAR in rAAA. Controlled hypotension using vasodilators to lower the blood pressure to <100 mmHg was reported first by our group in 2002 and later by Yilmaz et al. [9]. In 2007 Blankensteijn confirmed in a prospective (nonrandomized) study the feasibility of controlled hypotension in candidates for open surgery and endovascular repair. However, to date, there is no prospective randomized controlled trial demonstrating the advantage of hypotensive hemostasis over standard resuscitation management [10].

Resuscitation is generally initiated when aortic rupture is confirmed by ultrasound and/or CTA. In analogy to trauma patients, reducing the time from the initial event to having the bleeding under control in rAAA may increase the chance of survival [11]. Based on a Cochrane meta-analysis, there is no clear evidence on which type of fluid should be employed (crystalloids or colloids) in patients presenting with hemorrhagic shock. However, the lack of outcome differences made the authors advise the use of crystalloids for economic reasons [12]. If fluid administration is not sufficient to restore the arterial blood pressure or undesirable such as in the presence of a large retroperitoneal hematoma, vasopressor drugs may be employed in order to reduce the risk of tissue hypoperfusion. However, the use of vasopressors is justified only transiently and just to reach systolic arterial pressures of 80–90 mmHg [13]. If cardiac function is depressed, an inotropic agent should be utilized [14]. Control of corporeal temperature is another relevant measure that can influence not only arterial pressure but also acid-base status and coagulation.

Hypothermia (<35°) is associated with higher mortality and morbidity in patients presenting with hypotension in association with hemorrhagic shock [15]. In 1965 Shaftan et al. reported that "Blood loss from an arterial injury is greatest in quantity and prolonged when fluids or vasopressors are given and least and shortest when either resuscitation is withheld or vasodilators are administrated" [16]. In fact, general anesthesia, necessary for the open approach in rAAA, and the resulting vasoplegia following its induction require a high volume of fluids to achieve an adequate volume balance and blood pressure. This fluid load increases the risk of hemorrhage, hypothermia and coagulation disorders, and abdominal compartment syndrome. Moreover, general anesthesia with the use of myorelaxation decreases the abdominal wall tone and therefore may contribute to the transition from a contained to a frank aortic aneurysm rupture [17, 18].

Hypotensive Hemostasis Protocol and Experience at the University Hospital Zurich (USZ)

The hypotensive hemostasis protocol at USZ is based on *permissive hypovolemia* and *controlled hypotension*. Permissive hypovolemia consists in minimizing the administration of fluids (crystalloids and/or colloids), whereas controlled hypotension implies active lowering of the blood pressure with vasodilators and/or betablockers in normotensive or hypertensive patients to a target systolic blood pressure <90 mmHg. In such patients, fluid infusion is restricted to a minimum just to keep the intravenous lines open.

In patients presenting with low blood pressure but who are otherwise hemodynamically stable, some fluids (100–500 ml) may be administered to maintain a target systolic blood pressure of ≥70 mmHg. We define "stable" as a systolic blood pressure of any value that does not require an increase in the amount of fluids or vasoactive pressors/dilators to remain constant over a longer period of time (>5 min). In patients who are critically hypotensive or who are unstable or who get unconscious, a bolus of 250 ml of fluid (colloid or crystalloid or blood) may be infused. In addition, vasoactive pressors may eventually be required to restore and/or maintain the systolic blood pressure around 70 mmHg. Even under such low blood pressure circumstances, conversion to general anesthesia is not necessary as long as the patient maintains intact airway reflexes. Transfusion of blood cells, coagulation factors, and platelets is based on the respective guidelines. Briefly, hematocrit is maintained over 24 %, and transfusion of coagulation factors and/or platelets is based on blood samples and rotational thromboelastometry (ROTEM).

The pressure-lowering effects of vasodilators are often more pronounced in patients with hypovolemia. Drugs must therefore be titrated carefully to the desired effect. Short-acting vasoactive drugs have a limited effect with regard to time. In case of inadvertent over-dosage or intentional termination of the permissive hypotension after achieving sufficient hemostasis, the hypotensive effect of the drugs will fade rapidly.

Vasoactive Drugs

Esmolol, a short-acting and selective adrenergic β1-receptor antagonist, decreases heart rate and contractility, is metabolized by red blood cell esterases, and has an elimination half-life of approximately 9 min. It can be titrated to effect by repetitive i.v. bolus doses of 100 μg/kg up to a dose of 500 μg/kg followed by continuous i.v. infusion up to 125 μg/kg/min. The target range of the heart rate is 60–80 bpm.

Glyceryl trinitrate (nitroglycerin), a vasodilator with more prominent effects on peripheral veins than on arteries, decreases the preload of the heart by pooling of blood in the venous system. The elimination half-life is 2–3 min. Onset of action is immediate by relaxation of smooth muscle cells following an increase of intracellular concentrations of cyclic guanosine monophosphate (cGMP). Titration to effect is done by repetitive i.v. bolus doses of 25 μg up to 75–100 μg/min followed by a continuous i.v. infusion of up to 300 μg/min. Reflex tachycardia is a physiological response to decreased preload and can be counteracted by esmolol i.v.

After control of bleeding has been achieved in the operating room, all pressure-lowering drugs are discontinued, and hypovolemia is corrected as necessary. Appropriate fluid resuscitation is the base for vasoactive drugs to sufficiently raise systemic blood pressure to the desired level. Norepinephrine, acting primarily as a vasopressor, *is the first choice*, followed by epinephrine as second choice in case of profound shock and/or in order to enhance the cardiac contractility.

Norepinephrine (noradrenaline), a stimulator of both adrenergic α1/2-receptors and β1-receptors, raises the systemic blood pressure primarily by arterial vasoconstriction to a lower extent by its positive inotropic and chronotropic effects. It has an immediate onset of action and a half-life of 2–3 min. An i.v. bolus of 0.1 μg/kg is repetitively given followed by a continuous i.v. infusion of 0.01–0.3 μg/kg/min (0.8–24 μg/min for an 80 kg patient).

In cases of persisting clinical and laboratory signs of arterial hypoperfusion after appropriate correction of hypovolemia and vasopressor support with norepinephrine 0.3 μg/kg/min, impaired cardiac function may be the underlying cause, and epinephrine should be considered to improve cardiac inotropy.

Epinephrine (adrenaline) stimulates adrenergic β1/2-receptors with a resulting increase in cardiac chrono- and inotropy at lower dosage (0.01–0.1 μg/kg/min i.v.) and adrenergic α1/2-receptors with progressive peripheral arterial vasoconstriction at higher dosage (0.1–0.3 μg/kg/min i.v.). It has an immediate onset of action and a half-life of 2–3 min. *If epinephrine is needed as a bolus (0.1–0.2 μg/kg i.v.), cardiopulmonary resuscitation is usually imminent.*

Hypovolemia must be repeatedly ruled out or corrected if high doses of noradrenaline are infused, particularly if combined with epinephrine, since hypovolemic vasoconstriction may cause profound tissue ischemia and necrosis. Simple use of a central line pressure or wedge pressure measurement from a Swan-Ganz catheter can help determine if the patient needs additional volume or pressor medications (Table 11.1).

Table 11.1 Vasoactive substances

Substance and pharmacokinetic mechanism of action	Primary pharmacodynamic mechanism of action	Half-life	Dosage repetitive i.v. bolus	Dosage of continuous i.v. infusion
Esmolol-specific antagonist at adrenergic β1-receptor	Decrease of cardiac chrono- and inotropy	9 min	100 μg/kg up to cumulative 500 μg/kg/min	Up to 125 μg/kg/min
Glyceryl trinitrate increase of intracellular cGMP by nitric oxide	Vasodilation (venous > arterial) with resulting reduction in cardiac preload	2–3 min	25 μg up to cumulative 75–100 μg/min	Up to 300 μg/min
Norepinephrine agonist at adrenergic α1/2- and β1-receptors	1. Vasoconstriction (α1/2)	2–3 min	0.1–0.15 μg/kg	0.01–0.3 μg/kg/min
Epinephrine agonist at adrenergic α1/2-and β1/2-receptors	1. Increase of cardiac ino- and chronotropy (β1) 2. Vasoconstriction (α1/2)	2–3 min	0.1–0.15 μg/kg	0.01–0.1 μg/kg/min: increase of heart rate and contractility 0.1–0.3 mcg/kg/min: vasoconstriction

Intra-aortic Balloon

Endoclamping of the aorta with a large-size compliant balloon such as Reliant® (Medtronic) or the Coda (Cook) has been shown to be useful in patients with unstable hemodynamics and/or those patients unresponsive to fluids and catecholamines (Fig. 11.1). Endoclamping can be used for both the endovascular and the surgical approach. In stable low-pressure patients, especially when a large retroperitoneal hematoma has been identified preoperatively, it can also be used during the EVAR procedure to avoid further volume increase of the hematoma. The balloon can be placed under local anesthesia, utilizing a long (preferably ≥40 cm) sheath for prevention of caudal migration during and after inflation. To avoid balloon-related complications, the inflation site should be free of major atherosclerotic aortic disease or aneurysm. Moreover, as the balloon is placed superior to the major branches of the abdominal aorta, the duration of the balloon inflation should be kept as short as possible, since inflation brings about temporary renovisceral ischemia.

Discussion

Based on the early positive experience and subsequent systematic follow-up of the patients at our center, we have routinely applied the principles of hypotensive hemostasis for nearly 20 years. The feasibility of EVAR in rAAA using hypotensive hemostasis, including permissive hypovolemia, controlled hypotension, and local anesthesia, was reported by our group in 2001 [19]. In this series of 21 patients, restricted volumes of fluids and erythrocyte transfusions were enough to maintain hemodynamic stability prior to the completion of EVAR (Fig. 11.2).

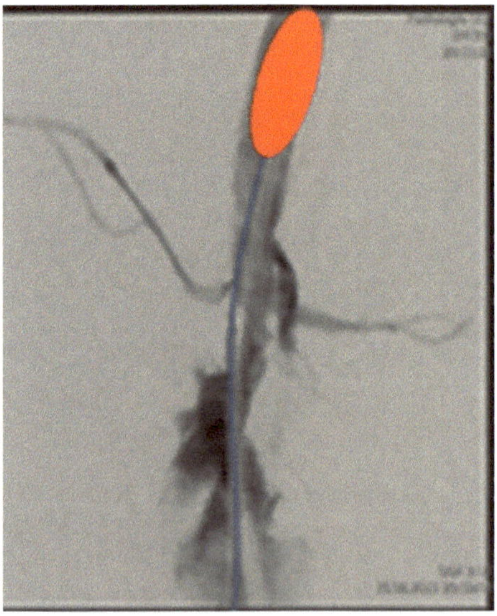

Fig. 11.1 Intraoperative angiogram. After placing a guide wire, an aortic balloon is delivered and inflated suprarenal (here supraceliac) to achieve proximal hemorrhage control

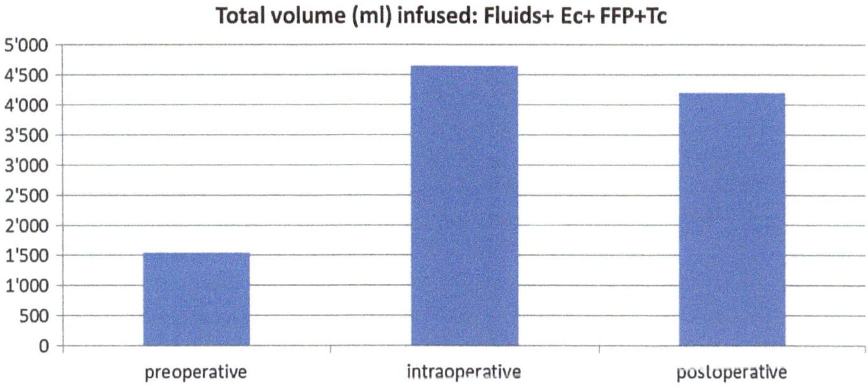

Fig. 11.2 Total amount of fluids and transfusions given preoperatively, intraoperatively, and postoperatively. *Fluids* crystalloids and/or colloids, *Ec* erythrocytes, *FFP* fresh frozen plasma, *Tc* thrombocytes, (Modified from Lachet et al. [19])

Generally, most patients remain stable with preserved mental function at a systolic blood pressure of 70–90 mmHg. To achieve stable hemodynamics at this blood pressure level, very limited amounts of fluids and vasoactive pressors are necessary during EVAR under local anesthesia. As a first step, analgesia is optimized to decrease the sympathomimetic activity. Low dosages of opioids are used and titrated to the desired effect. In patients undergoing interventions under local anesthesia, special care must be taken not to abolish consciousness and risk compromising spontaneous breathing and the protective airway reflexes. Advantages of local anesthesia include the preservation of sympathetic tone, yielding improved hemodynamic stability, preservation of muscle tone, and thereby the possibility to better contain the bleeding, and, in addition, any procedure under local anesthesia offers the best neurological monitoring. The main disadvantages are related to eventual acute loss of consciousness and an uncontrolled airway, suboptimal pain control, and the patient not lying still. Conversely, general anesthesia has the advantages of a controlled airway and optimal pain control. However, by using general anesthesia, most of the advantages of local anesthesia are lost, and it is more time-consuming when compared to local. If general anesthesia is required for an open operation, the patient should be fully prepped and draped prior to induction, and, ideally, an aortic occlusion balloon should first be placed under local anesthesia so that it can be inflated in cases of severe hypotension at any point prior to or during the procedure.

The use of hypotensive hemostasis was advocated by the clinical practice guidelines of the European Society for Vascular Surgery as it "might have a beneficial effect on the survival in cases of abdominal aortic aneurysm rupture." To maintain blood pressure in a range of 50–100 mmHg was recommended [20]. Limitations of hypotensive hemostasis are related mainly to brain, heart, and kidney perfusion. The brain perfusion is self-regulated within the systolic blood pressure range of 50–100 mmHg. The risk of cerebral hypoperfusion and thus ischemic stroke especially in patients with concomitant cerebrovascular disease should always be acknowledged. If the operation is conducted under local anesthesia, initial signs of cerebral hypoperfusion can be realized early, and cerebral perfusion is usually satisfactory if the patient responds adequately to neurological stimuli and is communicating verbally. Also, coronary perfusion may be at risk with low blood pressure. In patients with known coronary artery disease undergoing the procedure under local anesthesia, electrocardiographic and clinical signs of myocardial ischemia should be analyzed, whereas in patients operated under general anesthesia, transesophageal echocardiography should be considered. The kidneys generally have a fairly good tolerance of temporary ischemia. However, concurrent insults, such as contrast medium injection, increase the risk of renal injury. Urine output is a valid tool in the monitoring of the renal function.

In summary, aggressive fluid resuscitation in aorta rupture patients can be detrimental, as large-volume infusion can lead to further blood loss and hemodilution, coagulopathy, and hypothermia. Moreover, massive retroperitoneal bleeding may result in abdominal compartment syndrome with a high risk of further severe complications and death. Finally, extensive transfusion of blood cells, thrombocytes, and/or coagulation factors may be accompanied by transfusion-related acute lung injury. To avoid such scenarios and/or complications, hypotensive hemostasis, including permissive hypovolemia and controlled hypotension, is advocated.

References

1. Morrison CA, Carrick MM, Norman MA, Scott BG, Welsh FJ, Tsai P, et al. Hypotensive resuscitation strategy reduces transfusion requirements and severe postoperative coagulopathy in trauma patients with hemorrhagic shock: preliminary results of a randomized controlled trial. J Trauma. 2011;70(3):652–63.
2. Bougle A, Harrois A, Duranteau J. Resuscitative strategies in traumatic hemorrhagic shock. Ann Intensive Care. 2013;3(1):1.
3. Mayer D, Rancic Z, Veith FJ, Pecoraro F, Pfammatter T, Lachat M. How to diagnose and treat abdominal compartment syndrome after endovascular and open repair of ruptured abdominal aortic aneurysms. J Cardiovasc Surg. 2014;55(2):179–92.
4. Vlaar AP, Hofstra JJ, Determann RM, Veelo DP, Paulus F, Kulik W, et al. The incidence, risk factors, and outcome of transfusion-related acute lung injury in a cohort of cardiac surgery patients: a prospective nested case–control study. Blood. 2011;117(16):4218–25.
5. Andresen AF. Management of gastric hemorrhage. Modern Med. 1949;17(20):72–5.
6. Akins CW, Buckley MJ, Daggett W, McIlduff JB, Austen WG. Acute traumatic disruption of the thoracic aorta: a ten-year experience. Ann Thorac Surg. 1981;31(4):305–9.
7. Crawford ES. Ruptured abdominal aortic aneurysm. J Vasc Surg. 1991;13(2):348–50.
8. Veith FJ, Ohki T. Endovascular approaches to ruptured infrarenal aorto-iliac aneurysms. J Cardiovasc Surg. 2002;43(3):369–78.
9. Yilmaz N, Peppelenbosch N, Cuypers PW, Tielbeek AV, Duijm LE, Buth J. Emergency treatment of symptomatic or ruptured abdominal aortic aneurysms: the role of endovascular repair. J Endovasc Ther. An Official Journal of the International Society of Endovascular Specialists. 2002;9(4):449–57.
10. van der Vliet JA, van Aalst DL, Schultze Kool LJ, Wever JJ, Blankensteijn JD. Hypotensive hemostatis (permissive hypotension) for ruptured abdominal aortic aneurysm: are we really in control? Vascular. 2007;15(4):197–200.

11. Cothren CC, Moore EE, Hedegaard HB, Meng K. Epidemiology of urban trauma deaths: a comprehensive reassessment 10 years later. World J Surg. 2007;31(7):1507–11.
12. Perel P, Roberts I. Colloids versus crystalloids for fluid resuscitation in critically ill patients. Cochrane Database Syst Rev. 2011(3):CD000567
13. Dellinger RP, Levy MM, Carlet JM, Bion J, Parker MM, Jaeschke R, et al. Surviving Sepsis Campaign: international guidelines for management of severe sepsis and septic shock: 2008. Crit Care Med. 2008;36(1):296–327.
14. Kaye P, O'Sullivan I. Myocardial contusion: emergency investigation and diagnosis. Emerg Med J. 2002;19(1):8–10.
15. Hoey BA, Schwab CW. Damage control surgery. Scand J Surg. SJS Official organ for the Finnish Surgical Society and the Scandinavian Surgical Society. 2002;91(1):92–103.
16. Shaftan GW, Chiu CJ, Dennis C, Harris B. Fundamentals of physiologic control of arterial hemorrhage. Surgery. 1965;58(5):851–6.
17. Kozek-Langenecker SA, Afshari A, Albaladejo P, Santullano CA, De Robertis E, Filipescu DC, et al. Management of severe perioperative bleeding: guidelines from the European Society of Anaesthesiology. Eur J Anaesthesiol. 2013;30(6):270–382.
18. Bettex DA, Lachat M, Pfammatter T, Schmidlin D, Turina MI, Schmid ER. To compare general, epidural and local anaesthesia for endovascular aneurysm repair (EVAR). Eur J Vasc Endovasc Surg. The Official Journal of the European Society for Vascular Surgery. 2001;21(2):179–84.
19. Lachat ML, Pfammatter T, Witzke HJ, Bettex D, Kunzli A, Wolfensberger U, et al. Endovascular repair with bifurcated stent-grafts under local anaesthesia to improve outcome of ruptured aortoiliac aneurysms. Eur J Vasc Endovasc Surg. The Official Journal of the European Society for Vascular Surgery. 2002;23(6):528–36.
20. Moll FL, Powell JT, Fraedrich G, Verzini F, Haulon S, Waltham M, et al. Management of abdominal aortic aneurysms clinical practice guidelines of the European society for vascular surgery. Eur J Vasc Endovasc Surg. The Official Journal of the European Society for Vascular Surgery. 2011;41 Suppl 1:S1–58.

Chapter 12
Ruptured Abdominal Aortic Aneurysms: Aortic Occlusion Balloons

Zachary M. Arthurs

> **Key Points**
> - Endovascular proximal aortic occlusion can support both open and endovascular repair of ruptured abdominal aortic aneurysms.
> - Aortic occlusion balloon deployment requires radiographic guidance.
> - Aortic occlusion provides a rapid method to limit ongoing hemorrhage; the key to good outcomes remains to be rapid aneurysm exclusion.
> - Technical success requires clinical expertise, an aortic occlusion balloon set, and operative team training.

Introduction

In 1950, Lieutenant Colonel Carl W. Hughes first attempted transfemoral aortic occlusion during the Korean War for traumatic cases of abdominal hemorrhage [1]. In a hostile environment, he utilized a Foley catheter inserted through the aorta to achieve thoracic aorta occlusion; three patients with massive blood loss were treated in this fashion. Over the past 60 years, balloon technology and surgeon expertise has evolved dramatically. Today, the majority of abdominal aortic aneurysms are treated with endovascular stent grafts, and mirroring the treatment paradigm of this disease, endovascular therapies compromise 60–80 % of most vascular surgeons' practices. One of the most dramatic advances in endovascular therapy has been the treatment of ruptured abdominal aortic aneurysms (RAAA). Endovascular aortic occlusion provides proximal aortic control to support aneurysm repair for both open and

Z.M. Arthurs, MD, RPVI, FACS
Department of Vascular Surgery, San Antonio Military Medical Center, San Antonio, TX, USA
e-mail: arthursz@mac.com

B.W. Starnes et al. (eds.), *Ruptured Abdominal Aortic Aneurysm*,
DOI 10.1007/978-3-319-23844-9_12

endovascular methods. The advantages are immediate placement under local anesthesia, ability to position at multiple levels in the aorta, rapid hemodynamic improvement, and reduction of hemorrhage.

RAAA Protocols

Specific RAAA protocols are outlined in this text. It is imperative that prior to treating RAAAs, the hospital and surgeon team has a predetermined protocol. Within the protocol, aortic occlusion balloons can be utilized for proximal aortic control. The choice of open repair or endovascular repair is often a critical step in the protocol. Surgeon preference, endograft availability, endovascular resources, and patient anatomy all factor into whether open or endovascular repair is employed. Within both of these treatments, proximal aortic occlusion can support hemodynamic stability.

Empiric Aortic Occlusion Balloon Placement The aortic occlusion balloon is positioned as the first step for treating all RAAAs. Once the patient has been diagnosed with RAAA and transferred to the operative suite, the aortic occlusion balloon (AOB) is positioned prior to hemodynamic instability and prior to aneurysm repair. The patient is positioned in the operative suite on an imaging table, prepped and draped, and the AOB set is utilized to percutaneously position the balloon in the supraceliac aorta. Once in position, the balloon can be selectively inflated based on hemodynamic status [2, 3].

Having proximal control with this approach offers several advantages. It can be used to support induction of general anesthesia, which is the most common time point for hemodynamic collapse to occur. Immediate proximal control affords the operative team time to plan for the procedure. This allows the surgeon to review CTA findings and make final endograft selections. Anesthesia providers may be obtaining IV access, handling blood products, and preparing cardiac medications. Subjectively, proximal control settles the operative time, and it allows the operative team a moment to review the operative plan and ensure a successful procedure.

The advantages far outweigh the disadvantages, but there are barriers to implementing this technique. If a predetermined protocol is not in place or the AOB set is not readily available, this technique could delay proximal control. In most centers that utilize this technique, the AOB can be positioned in 3–5 min. Time is a barrier to this technique that can be overcome with appropriate preparation prior to treating RAAAs. If open repair is chosen, the femoral access site will need to be addressed at the end of the procedure; this will add time at the end of the procedure to close the arteriotomy. In the case of endovascular repair, the access site is needed for the repair and adds no additional time.

Selective Aortic Occlusion Balloon Placement With this approach, the balloon is not positioned preemptively, but instead placed at the surgeon's discretion. Advocates for this approach site the added benefits of rapid EVAR without the delay of placing an AOB [4]. Loss of mentation and hemodynamic collapse are the two most common criteria prompting AOB placement. The AOB set is opened and prepared; if the patient worsens, the AOB is positioned emergently. If general anesthesia with open or endovascular repair is chosen, there is very little benefit to selective placement. Hemodynamic collapse with general anesthesia, loss of sympathetic drive, and loss of abdominal domain is generally profound. Once it occurs, 3–5 min required to place an AOB or secure an aortic clamp can be the difference between survival and death. When utilizing endovascular repair, the added steps of sheath placement and balloon positioning are negligible. If stiff wire access is obtained in the thoracic aorta, sheath placement and balloon placement can be performed in less than 60 s.

Technique

Femoral Arterial Access The access site for AOB is chosen based on the planned contralateral limb placement for endovascular repair. When utilizing as an adjunct to open repair, the iliac vessel with the largest external iliac diameter, minimal tortuosity, and the side with low atherosclerotic burden is chosen. Femoral cutdown can be utilized in this setting, but it will require more time to achieve proximal control. In addition, the femoral cutdown will require more local anesthetic to achieve access. If electrocautery is utilized, this can be stimulating and require additional medications to treat pain, which may reduce cardiac output and decrease vascular tone. For these reasons, percutaneous access is the preferred approach with this technique. Ultrasound-guided access affords the surgeon direct visualization of the femoral artery and reduces the time for femoral cannulation. In addition, the technique reduces the risks of retroperitoneal access. Often, the retroperitoneal hematoma and hemoperitoneum associated with RAAA distort inguinal anatomy, making access based on landmarks difficult. Hypotension further challenges the surgeon's ability to achieve access based on palpation of the femoral pulse. Routine ultrasound utilization eliminates the challenges of access in this setting.

The surgeon may choose an 18-gauge access needle or an echogenic tip micro-introducer kit for initial cannulation. Once wire access is achieved, a 5Fr sheath is placed. A 0.035′ angled tip floppy or stiff glidewire (Terumo) can be used to cross the iliac artery anatomy and aortic aneurysm. Iliac tortuosity and aneurysm angulation may require a selective catheter to cannulate the supraceliac aorta. A 5 Fr Kumpe catheter (Cook Medical, IN), 65 cm, can direct the wire appropriately into the supraceliac aorta and thoracic aorta. With the catheter tip in the thoracic aorta, a 5–10 cc contrast injection can confirm true lumen access and appropriate position. A 0.035′ Lunderquist wire (Cook, Bloomington, IN), 260 cm, is placed.

Balloon and Sheath Selection The chosen balloon should be included in the AOB set. Table 12.1 shows characteristics of currently available aortic balloons. The two primary models are the Cook CODA balloon and Medtronic Reliant balloon. Both

Table 12.1 Commercially available aortic molding balloons in the USA

Product	Maximum inflation diameter	Sheath size	Shaft size	Shaft length
Coda	32, 40 mm	14 F	10 F	120 cm
Reliant	46 mm	12 F	8 F	100 cm
Equalizer	20, 27, 33, 40 mm	14–16 F	7 F	65, 110 cm
Q50 Plus	50 mm	12 F	–	65, 100 cm

balloons are semi-complaint aortic balloons that were designed for endograft molding. The CODA balloon is available in two different sizes; the 32 mm diameter is generally acceptable for proximal control. The Reliant balloon spans all sizes up to 46 mm. In addition, the Reliant balloon can be removed through a 12 F sheath and has a smaller shaft size, 8 F, compared to the CODA balloon. Either balloon will successfully oppose the aortic lumen and create occlusion in this setting. The smaller sheath size may be utilized if a totally percutaneous technique is performed. In addition, the smaller shaft size may be advantageous if the surgeon plans to perform additional technical steps from the same sheath as the CODA balloon; this will be described further.

A 12–14 F sheath, 45–60 cm, can be utilized to achieve aortic occlusion. For open repair, this will be adequate. When utilizing EVAR with a bifurcated device, the CODA balloon is positioned on the side of the planned contralateral limb. Imaging can be performed through the central wire lumen or through the side arm of the sheath (Fig. 12.1a). Once the endograft main body is deployed, the AOB can then be placed on the ipsilateral side while gate cannulation and limb extensions are performed (Fig. 12.1b–d). Most patients will tolerate temporary deflation of the AOB for endograft deployment at the proximal seal zone followed by placement of the AOB within the main body of the endograft. Placing an 18–20 F sheath allows room for double access next to the occlusion balloon and placement of an imaging catheter near the renal vessels. Iliac occlusive disease can be detrimental if the sheath is unable to be passed through the iliac vessels. Once the endograft main body is deployed, the AOB can then be placed on the ipsilateral side while gate cannulation and limb extensions are performed. When Endologix AFX is utilized (Endologix, CA) for EVAR, a 18–20 F contralateral sheath allows room to place the snare alongside the balloon shaft. This eliminates the need to deflate the occlusion balloon if the patient is unstable. The surgeon's choice of sheath will be based on the balloon chosen and their planned approach for RAAA repair.

Balloon Positioning and Inflation Under fluoroscopic guidance, the balloon is directed to the thoracic aorta. The balloon should be positioned above the aortic aneurysm between the pararenal and retrocardiac aorta. The quality of aorta should also be appreciated on preoperative axial imaging to avoid areas with thrombus, plaque, and calcification. Placing the balloon in the thoracic aorta at the level of the 12th vertebral body will allow working room for imaging below the balloon and it will facilitate delivery of the main endograft from the ipsilateral side. Even with this position, the balloon may require partial deflation to allow the nose cone on the

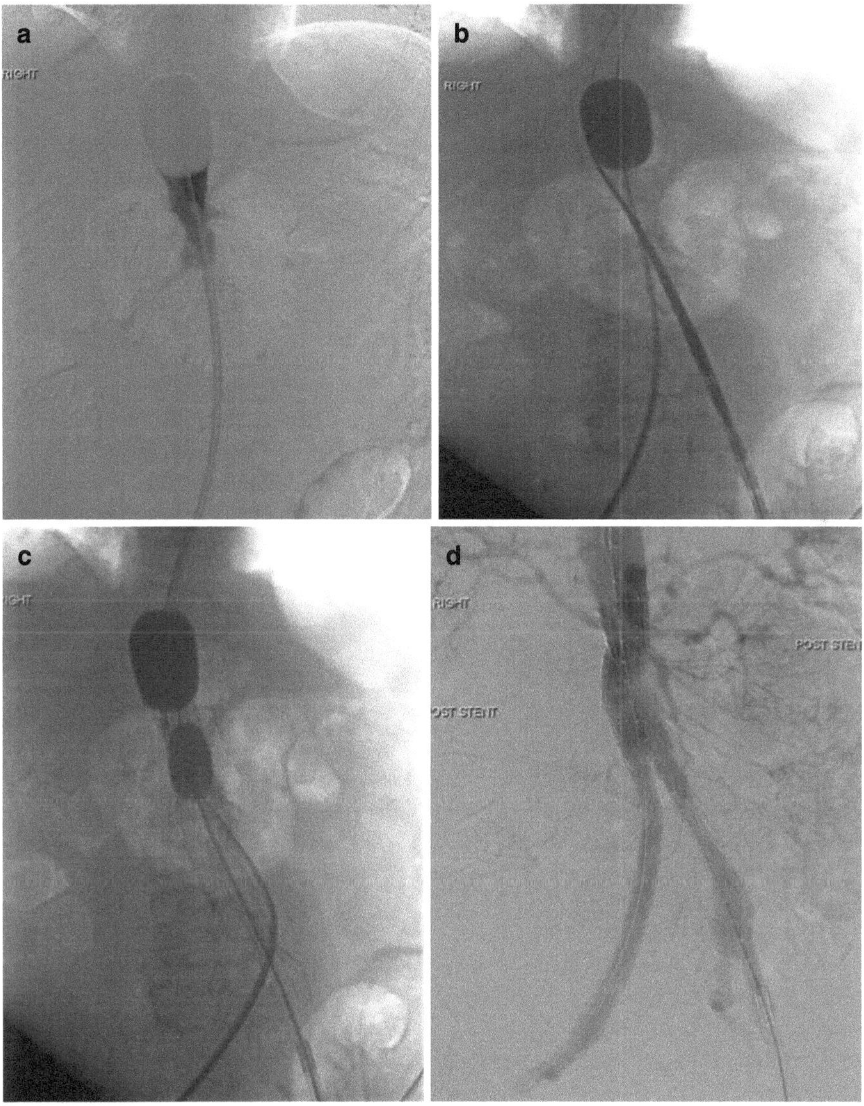

Fig. 12.1 Intraoperative placement aortic occlusion balloon during EVAR for hemodynamically unstable RAAA. Images provided by Dr. Benjamin W. Starnes, University of Washington. (**a**) The AOB is positioned at the level of the 12th rib. The renal arteries are marked below the AOB. (**b**) The stent graft is positioned with the AOB inflated. Partial AOB deflation allows positioning of the stent graft below the renal arteries. (**c**) The stent graft is deployed with the AOB inflated. The ipsilateral limb is completed, achieving seal within the common iliac artery. A second aortic occlusion balloon is then positioned within the stent graft seal zone from the ipsilateral side. (**d**) The contralateral limb is completed, and the completion angiogram demonstrates RAAA exclusion without endoleak

endograft to pass. A 60 cc syringe with contrast is used to inflate the balloon under direct visualization. The volume of contrast required to achieve aortic apposition is marked. During test inflation, it is also important to support the back of the balloon with the sheath to avoid balloon displacement down the aorta (Fig. 12.2). When this occurs, the balloon is not fully opposed to the aortic wall, and downward pressure causes the balloon to drag down the aortic wall. This can result in aortic plaque embolization. Once test inflation and positioning is complete, the balloon is deflated. The position of the balloon is marked on the table with a sterile marker, the sheath is also marked or sutured in place, and the volume of contrast used to create aortic occlusion is recorded. Balloon inflation is then reserved for hemodynamic support. At this step, the surgeon may proceed with open or endovascular repair.

Open RAAA Repair With open surgery, proximal aortic occlusion may be required to support anesthesia induction and laparotomy. Aortic occlusion provides afterload needed to support cerebral and coronary perfusion; this will reduce the amount of cardiac pressors and fluid administered for induction. In addition, optimizing coronary perfusion will improve cardiac output. The surgeon primary goal is to place an infrarenal clamp at the infrarenal location. Once infrarenal control and distal control are obtained, the balloon can be deflated and then pull back through the infrarenal neck. At this stage, the surgeon can digitally control the aorta and feel the balloon and wire pass through this point. Aortic clamps can then be positioned for open repair.

Endovascular Aneurysm Repair for RAAA When general anesthesia is chosen, the aortic occlusion balloon provides the same advantages described for open repair. If the balloon is not required, the stent graft can be deployed in a standard fashion. If the balloon is required to support hemodynamics, the main body of a bifurcated device can be deployed below the balloon in an infrarenal location. If the patient can tolerate balloon deflation, pulling the balloon down into the aneurysm sac just prior to proximal stent graft deployment avoids trapping the balloon beyond the stent graft and proximal stents. If the proximal AOB must remain inflated due to patient condition, it is my preference to ensure the contralateral sheath is well above the stent graft seal zone. This allows the AOB to be re-sheathed in the proximal aorta, and then the sheath and balloon can be pulled caudally between the stent graft and the aortic wall. The goal is to avoid stent graft displacement. Once the bifurcated system has been deployed, the AOB can be placed from the ipsilateral approach while the contralateral limbs are deployed.

The AFX device (Endologix, Irvine, CA) deserves mention due to technical considerations with deployment. The contralateral wire can be snared from the same iliac limb that contains the AOB. If the patient is unstable and requires AOB inflation, both the AFX bifurcated piece and the supporting proximal extensions can be deployed over the AOB. The AOB can then be deflated and removed within a sheath as described above. This technique allows complete aneurysm exclusion with the balloon in position.

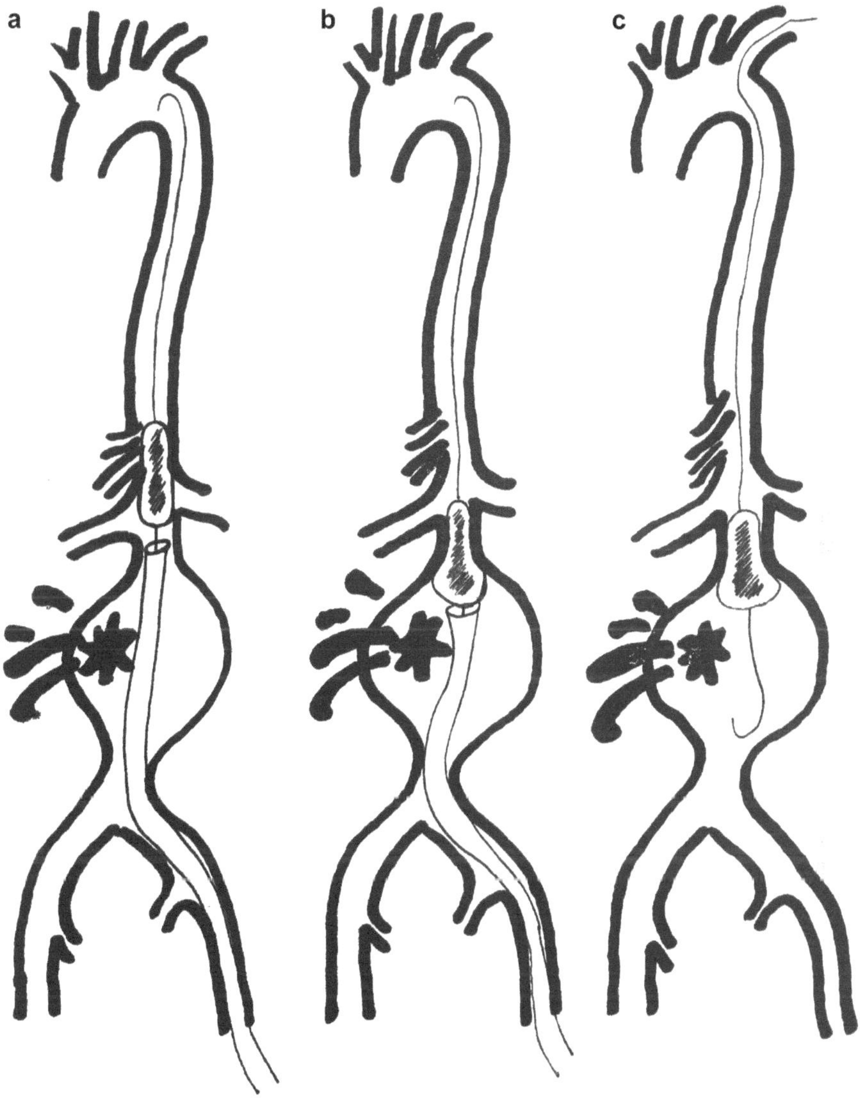

Fig. 12.2 Aortic occlusion balloon position for proximal control. (**a**) The support sheath is positioned beneath the occlusion balloon in the paravisceral segment. In this example, the balloon is situated in parallel aorta but is occluding the renal and visceral arteries. (**b**) The occlusion balloon is wedged at the infrarenal aortic neck. This position will require directed forward pressure on the sheath to ensure occlusion. This will allow perfusion of the viscera and both kidneys. (**c**) This illustrates occlusion balloon deployment from the left brachial or axillary approach

Table 12.2 Aortic occlusion balloon set for RAAA

Devices	Description	Size	Length
Micropuncture kit	Echogenic tip, 21 g introducer needle, 0.018′wire	5 F	11 cm
Wires	Angled tip, glide wire (Terumo) Lunderquist wire (Cook Medical)	0.035′	260 cm
Catheters	Kumpe catheter	5 F	65 cm
Sheaths	Support sheath	12–20 F	45–60 cm
Balloon	Occlusion balloon	12–16 F	65–120 cm

Sheath Removal The final step after either open or endovascular repair requires sheath removal. If large sheath percutaneous closure was utilized, the pre-placed sutures can be secured after sheath removal; otherwise, femoral cutdown will be required to close the arteriotomy.

AOB Set

Table 12.2 provides an example AOB set. All of the devices listed can be substituted for other items that are functionally similar. This is meant to augment the institution's basic endovascular set. Having this set prearranged with the operative case-cart can save critical time when treating RAAA.

Technical Considerations

While deployment of an AOB is a simple and rapid task, there are challenges maintaining complete aortic occlusion in unstable patients while performing EVAR with devices available in the USA. Ideally, an AOB catheter could be positioned to arrest hemorrhage, imaging could be performed above and below the catheter, and the stent graft system could be deployed over the same catheter system. With technology currently available in the USA, aortic occlusion balloon placement requires a separate sheath and wire; this requires a separate access point dedicated to AOB control.

Several surgeons have utilized upper extremity access for AOB placement. The clear advantage of this technique is that it allows both femoral access points to be utilized for EVAR. Surgeons in favor of this approach utilize aortic flow to float the occlusion balloon from the origin of the left subclavian artery to the infrarenal aneurysm (Fig. 12.1) [5]. Balloon stability is improved from this position as the balloon can be wedged at the aortic neck. However, there are several pitfalls to this technique. The brachial artery is often not able to accommodate a rigid 12 F sheath. Thrombotic complications and cerebral embolization can occur with arch manipulation. This requires a third access point in addition to both femoral access points. In addition, arch and descending thoracic aortic catheterization increases the complexity of AOB placement in an after-hours environment; this may increase the time to achieve hemorrhage control. For these reasons, femoral access is the preferred approach by many experts [6–8].

Balloon positioning also deserves special consideration. Ideally, aortic control is achieved at the lowest possible position to arrest hemorrhage while maximizing spine, visceral, and renal perfusion. Once a stiff wire is positioned in the thoracic aorta, it is possible to place the AOB in an infrarenal position or pararenal position, which spares paravisceral perfusion. This should be considered if a delay in EVAR is anticipated. Occluding the aorta in the thoracic aorta causes spinal and visceral malperfusion. This can result in overwhelming visceral ischemia, which is a secondary insult to ongoing hypotensive shock. The ensuing hepatic reperfusion can result in profound coagulopathy, continued blood loss, abdominal compartment syndrome, and multisystem organ failure. Hepatic ischemia in a shock model occurs after 10–15 min of aortic occlusion; therefore, AOB times should be recorded and noted every 3–5 min. Temporarily positioning the AOB in the descending thoracic aorta allows room to image the renal vessels and deploy the stent graft system.

Aortic Rupture and Embolization AOBs can cause severe damage to the aortic wall. Iatrogenic aortic rupture is the most catastrophic event with this technique. Performing this technique with radiographic guidance should eliminate this risk. The AOB may increase aortic embolization if there is significant manipulation in regions of thrombus and debris. If the aortic wall has intraluminal thrombus at or above the paravisceral segment, it is best to avoid this region. Embolization into the visceral arteries could result in mesenteric ischemia. Renal artery embolization can hasten renal failure. Distal embolization into the legs can typically be treated with thromboembolectomy from the femoral arteries.

Clinical Results

Doctors Starnes, Mehta, and Veith pioneered this technique in the USA. All three have reported their experience with various evolutions in technique, and currently, all three utilize AOBs in their RAAA protocols [3, 9]. Individually, they have reported the utility of AOB placement, and typically, 25 % of patients will require aortic occlusion balloon inflation to support hemodynamic compromise [10]. With balloon inflation, restoration of hemodynamic stability is achieved in 90–95 %, but most importantly, intraoperative mortality is dramatically reduced by 20 % when compared against open aortic cross clamp [11]. Retrospective series have attempted to examine the impact of AOB utilization on 30-day and in-hospital mortality; however, abdominal compartment syndrome, blood transfusions, hypotension, and multi-organ system failure account for the variability in overall outcome [12]. It is logical that early arrest of hemorrhage for AOB placement reduces these fatal postoperative events.

Conclusion

Proximal aortic balloon occlusion is a fundamental technique that can limit hemorrhage during RAAA treatment. Having a protocol and aortic occlusion balloon set in place will dramatically improve the time required for placement. Proximal aortic control with remote aortic occlusion augments both open surgical therapy and endovascular therapy. There are many possible modifications to this technique; practitioners should adopt the procedure that they are accustomed to and comfortable performing in an expeditious manner.

References

1. Hughes CW. Use of an intra-aortic balloon catheter tamponade for controlling intra-abdominal hemorrhage in man. Surgery. 1954;36(1):65–8.
2. Arthurs Z, Starnes B, See C, Andersen C. Clamp before you cut: proximal control of ruptured abdominal aortic aneurysms using endovascular balloon occlusion--case reports. Vasc Endovascular Surg. 2006;40(2):149–55.
3. Starnes BW, Quiroga E, Hutter C, Tran NT, Hatsukami T, Meissner M, et al. Management of ruptured abdominal aortic aneurysm in the endovascular era. J Vasc Surg. 2010;51(1):9–17; discussion 8.
4. Hinchliffe RJ, Braithwaite BD, Hopkinson BR. The endovascular management of ruptured abdominal aortic aneurysms. Eur J Vasc Endovasc Surg. 2003;25(3):191–201.
5. Matsuda H, Tanaka Y, Hino Y, Matsukawa R, Ozaki N, Okada K, et al. Transbrachial arterial insertion of aortic occlusion balloon catheter in patients with shock from ruptured abdominal aortic aneurysm. J Vasc Surg. 2003;38(6):1293–6.
6. O'Donnell ME, Badger SA, Makar RR, Loan W, Lee B, Soong CV. Techniques in occluding the aorta during endovascular repair of ruptured abdominal aortic aneurysms. J Vasc Surg. 2006;44(1):211–5.
7. Arthurs ZM, Sohn VY, Starnes BW. Ruptured abdominal aortic aneurysms: remote aortic occlusion for the general surgeon. Surg Clin North Am. 2007;87(5):1035–45, viii.
8. Mehta M. Endovascular aneurysm repair for ruptured abdominal aortic aneurysm: the Albany vascular group approach. J Vasc Surg. 2010;52(6):1706–12.
9. Mehta M, Taggert J, Darling 3rd RC, Chang BB, Kreienberg PB, Paty PS, et al. Establishing a protocol for endovascular treatment of ruptured abdominal aortic aneurysms: outcomes of a prospective analysis. J Vasc Surg. 2006;44(1):1–8; discussion.
10. Mehta M, Byrne J, Darling 3rd RC, Paty PS, Roddy SP, Kreienberg PB, et al. Endovascular repair of ruptured infrarenal abdominal aortic aneurysm is associated with lower 30-day mortality and better 5-year survival rates than open surgical repair. J Vasc Surg. 2013;57(2):368–75.
11. Raux M, Marzelle J, Kobeiter H, Dhonneur G, Allaire E, Cochennec F, et al. Endovascular balloon occlusion is associated with reduced intraoperative mortality of unstable patients with ruptured abdominal aortic aneurysm but fails to improve other outcomes. J Vasc Surg. 2015;61(2):304–8.
12. Mehta M, Darling 3rd RC, Roddy SP, Fecteau S, Ozsvath KJ, Kreienberg PB, et al. Factors associated with abdominal compartment syndrome complicating endovascular repair of ruptured abdominal aortic aneurysms. J Vasc Surg. 2005;42(6):1047–51.

Chapter 13
Operative Strategies

Marlin Wayne Causey, Niten Singh, Philip S.K. Paty, Manish Mehta, Ruth A. Benson, S. Bahia, R.J. Hinchliffe, I.M. Loftus, Benjamin W. Starnes, Andrew Holden, Kaj H. Johansen, Matthew J. Eagleton, Jarrad Rowse, Sira M. Duson, Edward Y. Woo, and Sean P. Lyden

M.W. Causey, MD
University of California-San Francisco, 400 Parnassus Avenue,
San Francisco, CA 94143, USA
e-mail: mwcausey@msn.com

N. Singh, MD (✉)
University of Washington, Box 359908, 325 Ninth Avenue, Seattle, WA 98104, USA
e-mail: singhn@uw.edu

P.S.K. Paty, MD (✉)
Surgery, Albany Medical College, Albany, NY, USA
e-mail: Patyp@albanyvascular.com

M. Mehta, MD, MPH
Vascular Surgery, Vascular Health Partners of Community Care Physicians,
Albany, PC, NY, USA
e-mail: MMehta@VascularHealthPartners.com

R.A. Benson
Department of Vascular Surgery, University Hospitals Coventry and
Warwickshire NHS Trust, Coventry, UK
e-mail: ruth.benson@gmail.com

S. Bahia
St. Georges University Hospitals NHS Trust, St. Georges University of London,
London, UK
e-mail: bahia_sandeep@yahoo.co.uk

R.J. Hinchliffe
Bristol Centre for Surgical Research, University of Bristol,
Bristol, UK
e-mail: robhinchliffe@gmail.com

I.M. Loftus
St. Georges University Hospitals NHS Trust, St. Georges University of London,
London, UK
e-mail: ian.loftus@stgeorges.nhs.uk

B.W. Starnes et al. (eds.), *Ruptured Abdominal Aortic Aneurysm*,
DOI 10.1007/978-3-319-23844-9_13

B.W. Starnes, MD (✉)
Division of Vascular Surgery, Department of Surgery, Regional Vascular Center at Harborview Medical Center, University of Washington,
325 9th Ave, Box 359908, Seattle, WA 98104, USA
e-mail: starnes@uw.edu

A. Holden, MBChB (✉)
Department of Interventional Radiology, Auckland Hospital, Auckland, New Zealand
e-mail: andrewh@adhb.govt.nz

K.H. Johansen, MD, PhD, FACS (✉)
Vascular Surgery, Swedish Medical Center, University of Washington School of Medicine, Seattle, WA, USA
e-mail: Kaj.Johansen@swedish.org

M.J. Eagleton, MD (✉) • J. Rowse, MD
Department of Vascular Surgery, H32, Cleveland Clinic Lerner College of Medicine-CWRU, 9500 Euclid Avenue, Cleveland, OH 44195, USA
e-mail: eagletm@ccf.org

S.M. Duson, MD • E.Y. Woo, MD (✉)
MedStar Health Vascular Surgery, MedStar Vascular Program, Department of Vascular Surgery, Georgetown University, Washington, DC, USA
e-mail: Edward.y.woo@medstar.net

S.P. Lyden, MD (✉)
Department of Vascular Surgery, The Cleveland Clinic Foundation,
9500 Euclid Avenue, Cleveland, OH 44195, USA
e-mail: Lydens@ccf.org

Transabdominal Repair of Ruptured Abdominal Aortic Aneurysms

Marlin Wayne Causey and Niten Singh

History of Transabdominal Repair of Ruptured Abdominal Aortic Aneurysms

The first accounts of abdominal aortic aneurysm repair date back to Egyptian, Greek, and Byzantine surgeons. These early techniques were further developed for elective repairs by others, such as Pare and Hunter [1]. Credit for the first open treatment of a ruptured retroperitoneal aneurysm is typically given to Astley Cooper, who in 1817 ligated the aorta at the bifurcation for a ruptured left iliac artery aneurysm [2]. However, none of these early treatments using aortic ligation were successful. In 1923, Rudolph Matas successfully ligated a ruptured abdominal aortic aneurysm that occurred from a syphilitic infection [3]. These early treatments for ruptured aneurysms were almost universally fatal, and in 1953 Henry Bahnson reported the first successful ruptured aortic aneurysm repair with a homograft [4]. In 1954, Cooley and DeBakey had improved survival to 50 % in a report of six patients [5]. In years to follow increasing reports were published of the successes encountered with open repair of abdominal aortic aneurysms [6, 7]. These advances and more widespread training led to widespread utilization and technical refinements in open aortic surgery at other centers. Formal training in aortic repair first began in 1962 through the American Board of Surgery with pioneers such as Edwin Wiley, Wiley Barker, William Blaisdale, and many others [8]. These surgeons at vascular training centers helped establish surgical mentorship, formalization of vascular care, and standardization of open aortic repair paving the way for a more widespread and successful management of ruptured aortic aneurysms.

Modern Evolution of Open Rupture AAA Repair

Open repair of abdominal aortic aneurysm has evolved significantly over the past decade with the introduction of aortic occlusion balloons for proximal supraceliac aortic control prior to laparotomy [9–11]. In the past, the patient was placed on the operative table with an incision made upon the induction of general anesthesia so as to maximize the tamponade effect of truncal muscle tone. Trainees were taught to rapidly enter the abdomen and quickly obtain proximal vascular control at the supraceliac aortic level. However, the utilization of endovascular aortic occlusion balloons via transfemoral access has allowed proximal supraceliac aortic control prior to midline laparotomy to be a relatively straightforward procedure, should open repair be necessary in the marginally compensated patient. Resuscitation was covered in previous chapters, but the modern vascular surgeon should be trained in the placement of aortic occlusion balloons from preferably a transfemoral or if needed a transbrachial approach [10, 11]. The use of endovascular occlusion balloons will allow for supraceliac aortic control while the patient is under local anesthesia, maintaining their truncal tone, and in parallel to other necessary anesthetic procedures.

Endovascular Aortic Balloon Occlusion During Open Repair

The supraceliac aortic balloon occlusion technique was covered previously; however, there are several important aspects that are essential when placing the balloon prior to open surgical repair. There are several larger semi-compliant balloon catheters that are currently available and can be used for aortic occlusion and should be placed in a manner that ensures it will remain secure once inflated throughout the open repair. The placement of the balloon is facilitated by percutaneous femoral access and advancing an appropriately sized sheath in regard to diameter (12–14 Fr.) and length (45–55 cm), up to the aortic neck. To prevent occlusion balloon prolapse into the aneurysm, the sheath hub should be sutured in place to the patient at the skin entry site; the occlusion balloon should also be marked with in indelible marker at the sheath exit site and also secured in position; one could use an adherent drape to ensure no movement. Positioning the balloon in a section of the supraceliac aorta that is above the diaphragm allows application of a conventional clamp without having to lose occlusion balloon control, should conventional proximal control with a clamp be preferred or necessary. Finally, if the use of a transfemoral approach cannot be performed, a transbrachial approach is a less commonly used alternative

[10]. Patients with highly tortuous aortoiliac anatomy or with iliac stenosis or occlusions may be best served by using a transbrachial approach or rapid open surgical approach to proximal aortic control.

Patient Preparation, Positioning, Incision Planning, and Operative Adjuncts

Once the time has come for open surgical transabdominal repair, with or without proximal aortic endovascular balloon control, conventional wisdom and techniques are paramount. The patient should be widely prepped and draped (from the clavicle to the knees) while still awake. Positioning of the patient follows standard elective cases, but two caveats may be necessary. If access or monitoring is an issue, the right arm may need to be placed on an arm board for the anesthetic team, and the left arm should be tucked by the patient's side, which will facilitate movement of the angiographic table during fluoroscopy. Once positioning, surgical cleansing, and placement of endovascular aortic occlusion balloon are accomplished, induction of general anesthesia should occur simultaneously with the abdominal incision. Often it is during induction of anesthesia that the patient will become hypotensive and might require inflation of the aortic occlusion balloon. Clear communication should occur between the surgeon and anesthesia team to ensure that the anesthesia team is aware of the events that are transpiring in the operative field. The anesthesia team should also place a nasogastric tube early in the process for gastric decompression and esophageal identification; however, this should be performed only after the airway is secure, especially since oral intake status is commonly unknown. The choice of incision is often based on surgical preference, and a proximally placed midline incision below the xiphoid process may facilitate surgical exposure of the supraceliac aorta and provide extensive abdominal exposure. The xiphoid process can even be excised for additional exposure. A conventional midline laparotomy incision allows for added exposure of deep pelvic structures, particularly in patients with a larger habitus or with long ovoid abdominal anatomy. The use of intraoperative cell salvage (i.e., Cell Saver/Haemonetics, Braintree, MA) to gather suctioned blood will also minimize the amount of transfused banked blood necessary. In one series, the use of this modality reduced the transfusion requirement by almost 400 mL in elective cases where the average blood loss was 1140 mL [12]. Overall, cell salvage technology commonly permits collection of approximately 1/3 the volume of the intraoperative blood loss.

Technical Aspects of Proximal Control

Once the abdomen is opened, a systematic approach should be undertaken. Importantly, if at any point the patient becomes hemodynamically unstable, swift proximal aortic control is paramount. This may be done using either the prepositioned endovascular aortic occlusion balloon or surgical control. If an aortic occlusion balloon could not be placed, there are several nuances to successful transperitoneal exposure of the supraceliac aorta. With hemodynamic instability, rapid control of the aorta may be performed manually with minimal operative dissection by tracing the plane between the stomach and liver (gastrohepatic ligament), manually separating the crural fibers with blunt dissection, and separating the periadvential plane down to the spine and either performing manual compression or applying a surgical clamp. During the era of open rupture repair, aortic compressor devices existed for this very purpose. A nasogastric tube is very helpful when performing a rapid exposure as it will help avoid inadvertent clamping of the esophagus and facilitate aortic identification in the unstable hypotensive patient. Should time and patient factors allow for a more elegant dissection, this should be accomplished as it will minimize any iatrogenic injury and minimize raw surface irritation and bleeding in patients that are at high risk of coagulopathy. After entering the abdomen, the left triangular ligament and fibrous liver appendix connecting the top surface of the liver to the diaphragm should be divided to minimize any tearing of the liver and allow right-sided mobilization of the left lobe of the liver. Next, the abdominal wall should be retracted and this is often facilitated by utilizing a Vascular Omni-Flex System (Omni-Tract Surgical; St. Paul, MN) to set up appropriate retraction [13]. Once appropriate initial exposure is obtained, this system can greatly facilitate the

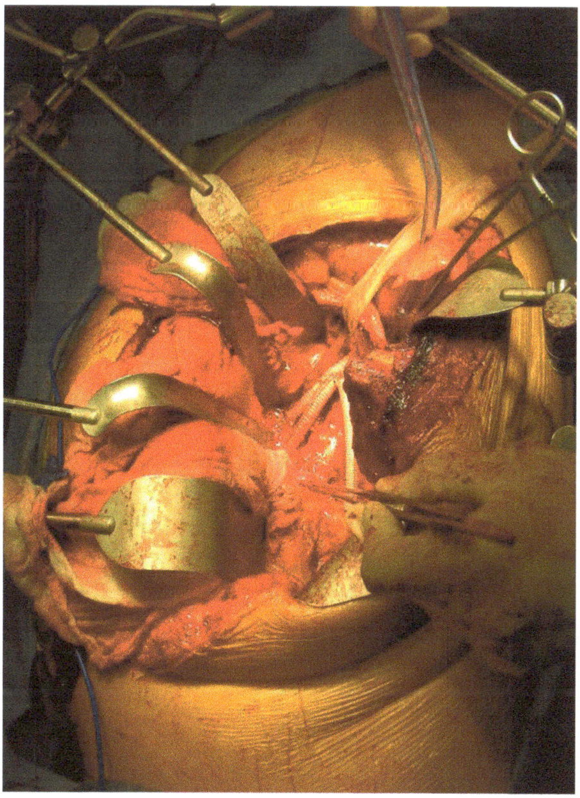

Fig. 13.1 Exposure with Vascular Omni-Flex System (Omni-Tract Surgical; St.Paul, MN) retractor for aortic exposure

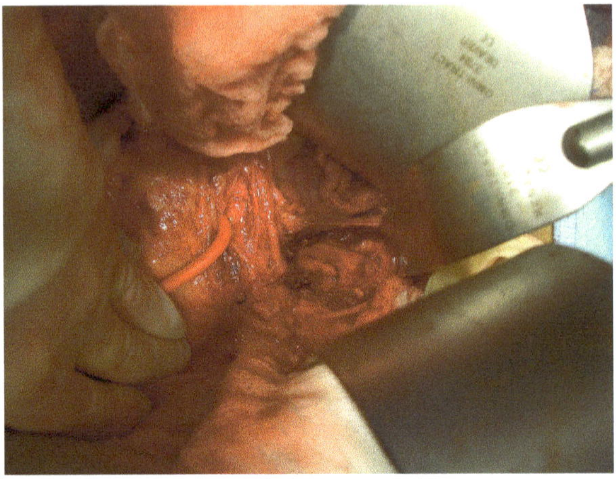

Fig. 13.2 Division of crural fibers transversely allows identification of the anterior surface of the supraceliac aorta

procedure (Fig. 13.1). Should a bilateral subcostal incision be used, the lower abdominal wall should also be retracted with heavy suture to the inferior abdominal wall. Next, the operator should feel that the gastric tube is in the body of the stomach so as to ensure that the esophagus may be easily identified and to allow for stomach decompression. The gastrohepatic ligament is divided slightly away from the liver (to avoid tearing or injury) and the caudate lobe is identified and protected. Renal vein retractors are often helpful at this point to laterally displace the liver and an assistant to identify and protect the esophagus. At this point, the diaphragmatic crus is divided. In cases of ruptured aneurysms, this is most rapidly performed by dividing the crural fibers transversely and identifying the anterior surface of the supraceliac aorta (Fig. 13.2). Once identified, the crural fibers on either side of the aorta should be divided and the aorta dissected down to the spine. Circumferential exposure is not necessary, but manual palpation for intercostal branches should be carefully done in order to identify an appropriate site for clamping, avoid intercostal branch injury, and ensure that the clamp tips are on the spine allowing for complete aortic clamping. Aortic clamping is necessary for hemodynamic instability, and if the patient is maintaining a blood pressure, the clamp could be prepositioned and secured in place with a silastic vessel loop and covered with a towel (to avoid being dislodged) (Fig. 13.3).

For the more experienced surgeon, assessment of the location of the retroperitoneal hematoma may also help guide operative exposure and proximal control. Often these patients will present with a CT scan that can provide valuable information regarding the site of rupture and anatomy. While supraceliac control is an important surgical maneuver, identification of the involvement of the retroperitoneal hematoma may clue the surgeon to the possibility of obtaining proximal control below the renal arteries. When the retroperitoneal hematoma has not obscured or distorted the duodenum, the retroperitoneum may be incised and rapid control of the infrarenal neck obtained through manual palpation, oftentimes through the superior aspect of the hematoma [14]. The hematoma, often, will dissect the surrounding tissue

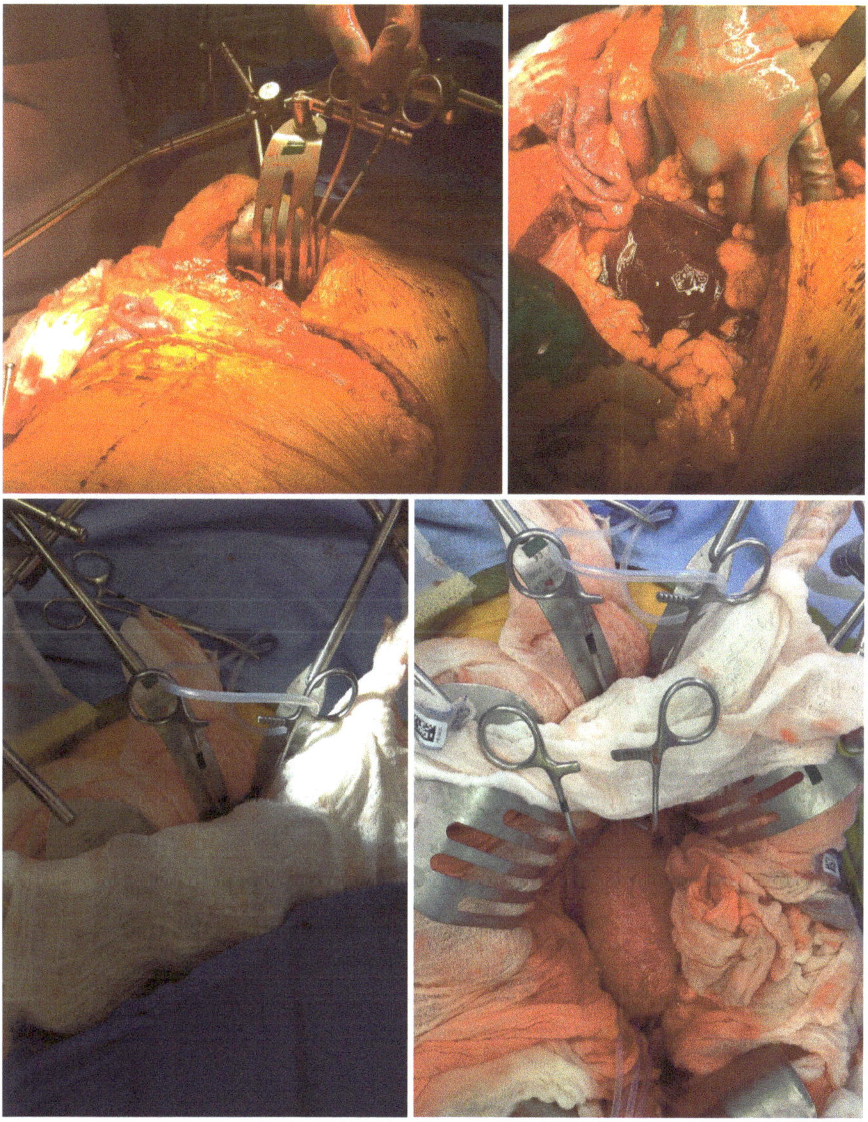

Fig. 13.3 Adequate aortic exposure requires appropriate use of retractors, and aortic clamp positions

away from the neck and control can be obtained. The key points with this technique is to be cautious with the inferior mesenteric vein and left renal vein. Iatrogenic injury of the left renal vein, in particular, can lead to additional hemorrhage. While it is a more advanced technique, direct infrarenal aortic clamping with a supraceliac aortic occlusion balloon in place to provide a secondary means of proximal control is becoming a more modern practice.

Distal Control

The location of the distal clamp is largely determined by the extent of the aneurysm, and, oftentimes, much of the retroperitoneal dissection has been done by the periaortic hematoma. In this scenario, the clamps are placed over the identified common iliac arteries. If the patient is stable after proximal clamping or has common iliac aneurysms, minimal dissection of the retroperitoneal aorta is performed by getting control of the bilateral external iliac arteries, followed by the internal iliac arteries. The clamps may then be moved to a more proximal location once the extent of repair is better defined. In order to obtain control of the right external iliac artery, the cecum and terminal ileum and retroperitoneal attachments are divided along the white line (the fusion plane between the peritoneum and retroperitoneum), which is a relatively safe dissection plane. The external iliac artery is usually easily controlled circumferentially, and if the internal iliac artery proves difficult for circumferential dissection, direct clamping using a hypogastric clamp is typically feasible. For identification and control of the left iliac arteries, the sigmoid colon is retracted medially and the white line divided. Once the external iliac artery is identified, similar maneuvers are performed to circumferentially isolate it and dissect the internal iliac artery to the extent necessary to place a clamp. When more expeditious distal control is required, the iliac arteries can be controlled by balloon occlusion after opening the aortic sac to visualize the bifurcation [14].

In instances that require inflation of an aortic occlusion balloon, once proximal clamp control is obtained, the balloon may be removed and the sheath withdrawn into the external iliac artery and a smaller balloon placed to control the iliac artery. With this maneuver, the contralateral iliac artery is the remaining vessel that requires control, which can be obtained with the maneuvers listed previously. This particular sequence may provide benefit in most circumstances as it minimizes the need to reposition the retractors during definitive repair. One particular situation deserves special attention, which is in circumstances when clamping or occlusion of the supraceliac aorta is necessary in an unstable patient. In this situation, the added time for the iliac artery dissection will lead to prolonged bowel and liver ischemia time that will certainly worsen the acidosis and coagulopathy. It is beneficial to be able to move the proximal clamp to either the infrarenal or suprarenal position to allow for visceral perfusion. Since this will require opening the retroperitoneal hematoma, the surgeon should be prepared to obtain balloon control of the iliac arteries from inside the aneurysm should distal clamping prove to be difficult.

Aortic Exposure Near the Aneurysm

When exposing the infrarenal aorta from a transabdominal approach, most aneurysms may be repaired from an infracolic approach. To perform this approach, the transverse colon is retracted superiorly, between moist laparotomy pads to expose the

Fig. 13.4 Important anatomic relationships when analyzing a preoperative CT scan for open repair

- Diameter of the supraceliac aorta
- Aortic disease (calcium and thrombus) at the supraceliac level and juxtarenal neck (as to adequacy for clamping)
- Relationship of left renal vein to the aorta (anterior, retroaortic, circumaortic)
- Relationship of the renal arteries to the left renal vein (an identification of accessory arteries)
- Tortuosity and stenosis of the iliac arteries (when performing an open repair with balloon occlusion the less diseased an tortuous iliac system should be utilized; significant iliac disease should be bypassed with a bifurcated graft)
- Size of the aneurysm and concomitant iliac artery aneurysms (tube graft or bifurcated graft)

root of the mesentery. The small bowel is gathered to the patient's right and controlled with either moist laparotomy pads or wrapped in a moist towel. The duodenum is mobilized away from the aorta with careful attention paid to avoid injury to the inferior mesenteric vein. The duodenum should be sufficiently dissected away from the aorta so that a large slotted or fence-type retractor may be easily placed for rightward displacement of the small bowel. To aid in bowel retraction, duodenal and retroperitoneal mobilization should be performed prior to applying static retraction. For cases of rupture, this process is largely facilitated by the dissection performed by the periaortic hematoma. Once this process is complete, the next task is to identify the left renal vein. One of the key preoperative tasks when a CT scan is obtained is to determine the anatomic relationships of the mesenteric vessels, renal arteries, and especially the left renal vein (3.2 % will be retroaortic, 1.6 % circumaortic, 0.2 % with a left-sided IVC, 0.4 % with a duplicated IVC, and 0.4 % with a horseshoe kidney) [15]. Figure 13.4 lists important anatomic factors for open repair when looking at the preoperative CT scan. Once the left renal vein is identified, it should be mobilized. Depending on the location of the aneurysm, the vein is commonly spared, and there are four tributaries that are commonly ligated in an elective setting to minimize injury to the vein as it is retracted (left inferior phrenic vein, left suprarenal vein, left gonadal vein, left second lumbar vein). In the setting of a ruptured AAA, the left gonadal vein and lumbar vein are generally all that is required for cephalad retraction of the left renal vein. The next step is identification of the renal arteries. Another key preoperative task when CT scanning is available is to understand the relationship of the renal arteries to one another and in relationship to the aneurysm. The renal arteries should be identified to avoid clamp injury and the relationship to the aortic neck analyzed. Unfortunately, due to the expanded use, improved technology, and operator proficiency, most open repairs for rupture are done when there is an inadequate infrarenal aortic neck. When this is encountered, the aorta above the renal arteries should be dissected with care taken to identify the superior mesenteric artery, particularly as the dissection proceeds cephalad. If necessary for proximal exposure, the left renal vein may be ligated with the preferred technique to perform the ligation close to the inferior vena cava and no ligation of the left renal vein tributaries to allow for collateral drainage. The left renal vein can also be divided between two vascular clamps for additional exposure and repaired at the conclusion of the case. Other important preoperative tasks are to identify whether there is one or multiple renal arteries and their origin since they have segmental embryologic development, giving rise to frequent anomalous origins or accessory renal arteries.

Aneurysm Repair

Once proximal aortic control (either clamping or balloon occlusion) is achieved, the aortic neck has been established, and distal control has been obtained, consideration should quickly be made for possible repositioning of proximal aortic control to a desired location preferably below the renal arteries but if needed below the SMA. Either position of the clamp is possible, but there will be more back bleeding from uncontrolled lumbar arteries and collaterals when the clamp is further from the proximal anastomotic site. Once the aneurysm is clamped and ready for repair, the aneurysm is opened along the anterior surface and all thrombus removed from the aneurysm sac. The aneurysm is tailored to the proximal neck and often a self-retaining retractor helps keep the aneurysm sac open. Any large back-bleeding lumbar arteries should be quickly oversewn. A helpful technique in avoiding excessive lumbar back bleeding is to place hemoclips on the lumbar arteries after gaining proximal and distal aortic control and prior to opening the aneurysm sac. The aorta is sized and a tightly woven Dacron or GORE-TEX graft is sutured to the aortic neck and either designed as a tube graft or bifurcated graft. In cases where it is necessary to perform an aortic endarterectomy or the proximal neck is friable, a felt strip is useful in reinforcing the aortic wall suture line. The suture line should be performed with a large needle that allows a deep-seated continuous suture line. Once the proximal anastomosis is completed, the proximal clamp may be moved down to the graft to allow perfusion of the visceral and renal arteries, if required. The distal anastomosis, if sewing a tube graft to the aortic bifurcation, is performed in a similar manner after clamp control of the common iliac arteries is established (by replacement when necessary of the distal balloon control). Should a bifurcated graft be required, suitable anastomotic sites are identified along the iliac arteries, and an end-to-end (common iliac) or end-to-side anastomotic technique (external iliac) is preferred to preserve pelvic circulation unless there is concomitant aneurysmal disease. Care needs to be taken to ensure that the graft is passed under the ureters.

Reimplantation of the inferior mesenteric artery (IMA) was a topic of discussion in the past with ruptured AAAs. In the elective setting if there is adequate back bleeding from the IMA or no bleeding signifying occlusion, it can routinely be ligated. However, if the back bleeding is poor, it should be reimplanted. Numerous studies found that routine reimplantation of the IMA provides no benefit over maintaining adequate organ perfusion in the perioperative setting [16]. Others have advocated selective ligation and reimplantation based on clinical bowel inspection. Unlike in elective aortic reconstruction, detailed knowledge of colonic collateral circulation is difficult to obtain for all patients undergoing a ruptured AAA repair. Our approach is to inspect the IMA and if possible based on the stability of the patient reimplant the IMA.

Removal of Transfemoral or Transbrachial Sheath and Bowel Assessment

Aortic retractors should be left in place at this point, and if an inferior bar on the Omni retractor is used, this should be removed to allow easy access to the femoral sheath, if necessary. The sheath should be left in place and the femoral artery exposed proximally and distally to allow control during the arteriotomy repair. Interrupted sutures are beneficial in minimizing any narrowing of the arteriotomy repair. Similar repair for a transbrachial sheath should also be performed if used. If used, heparinization is reversed at this point to ensure adequate hemostasis of the repair. Once the aneurysm repair is completed, the aneurysm sac is closed along with the retroperitoneum to ensure no exposed graft may touch the small bowel to avoid future aortoenteric fistula. Often, in the setting of a large retroperitoneal hematoma, the retroperitoneum cannot be re-approximated. In this setting, an opening is created in the gastrocolic ligament, and the omentum can be mobilized and passed through this opening to cover the graft so that it is separated from the small bowel. The small bowel is returned to its anatomic position and assessment of bowel viability should be performed. Areas of questionable bowel should be assessed by means of Doppler on the antimesenteric border, fluorescein wood's lamp with injection of methylene blue, or planned re-exploration.

With the sheath in place if an aortic occlusion balloon was utilized, an arteriogram can easily be performed if there is concern about lower extremity perfusion prior to removing it. If a preclose technique for the percutaneous access was utilized, the sutures can be tied at this point [17]. Otherwise, a femoral incision with femoral artery repair is relatively rapid and easy to perform, and if needed, proximal control from an intra-abdominal approach can be obtained, in the setting of a high puncture of the femoral artery.

Assessment for Intra-abdominal Hypertension and Abdominal Compartment Syndrome

Prior to fascial closure, intra-abdominal hypertension assessment is necessary. Elevated abdominal pressures (above 20 mmHg) are common following repair (50 % of patients) with around 20 % developing the abdominal compartment syndrome and its association with increased mortality [18, 19]. Factors predictive of patients who are at increased likelihood for abdominal compartment syndrome are those who receive unbalanced blood product resuscitation (less than one unit of plasma for every 2 units of red blood cells) or significant early postoperative resuscitation with crystalloids [20, 21]. Though data establishing patients that will need increased postoperative resuscitation requirements are not available, factors associated with increased risk of ischemia-reperfusion insult are preoperative hypotension, 6 or more liters of blood loss, and intraoperative resuscitation with 12 or more liters [22]. A useful intraoperative technical assessment is to obtain a baseline peak airway pressure with the abdomen completely open. Clamps may then be placed on the fascia and the fascia approximated with assessment of any change in peak airway pressure. An airway pressure over 30 mmHg or significant increase should prompt concern for compartment syndrome and the need for delayed abdominal closure. Any clinical concern for abdominal hypertension or the subsequent development of compartment syndrome should prompt delayed fascial closure. Significant acidosis, coagulopathy, and hypothermia should also prompt delayed closure as it is rapid and will facilitate more rapid lethal triad correction by minimizing additional operative time. Temporary abdominal closure is easily obtained using a system designed for open abdominal drainage, such as the ABThera open abdomen negative pressure therapy system for temporary abdominal wall closure (KCI; San Antonio, TX). This and other negative pressure systems are tailored and placed onto the gutters to ensure adequate peritoneal drainage. With the ABThera system, there is a fenestrated visceral protective layer that may be customized to the patient's body habitus with the goal to have the edges reach well into the paracolic gutters and pelvis so as to optimize peritoneal fluid drainage (Fig. 13.5). Over top of this, placed is a fenestrated piece of foam to approximate the abdominal wall and centralize the drainage process to the canister. This is then sealed with the provided clear drape over the abdominal wall with drape adherence improved by ensuring the skin is dry and using an adhesive skin protective barrier, such as mastisol (Eloquest Healthcare; Ferndale, MI). The drape is then cut with the open abdomen tubing set then placed directly over the clear drape and connected to the 1 L canister and negative pressure therapy unit. The negative pressure unit may provide 100–150 mmHg of negative pressure with 125 mmHg being a common setting. Other methods have been described such as simple coverage of the abdomen with an iodine impregnated drape, but these may not optimize peritoneal drainage. Temporary abdominal closure technique in patients with suspicion of abdominal compartment syndrome is maintained with re-exploration occurring every 24–48 h with closure performed as soon as possible to avoid the loss of abdominal wall domain and the need for complex abdominal wall closure. It is important to note that the patient needs continuous intubation while the abdominal wall is temporarily closed. Early abdominal closure is optimal, though not always possible due to the significant volume resuscitation and substantial bowel edema caused by systemic inflammatory response in the first 24–48 h following ruptured aneurysm repair. Median closure time is 6 days and may often be achieved with primary fascial closure when open abdomen times are short [23].

Conclusion

Open repair of abdominal aortic aneurysms has evolved significantly over the past decade, particularly with the increased use of endovascular aortic balloon occlusion and delayed abdominal wall closure. The fundamental tenants of the repair though haven't changed – avoidance of general anesthetic until prepared for rapid

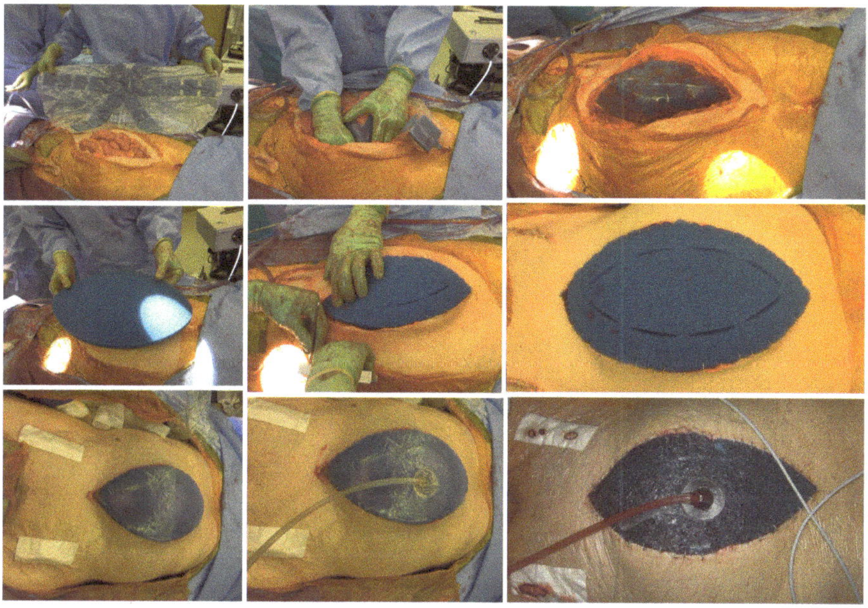

Fig. 13.5 Placement of an abdominal wound vac following repair of a ruptured abdominal aortic aneurysm. Demonstrated the technique of temporary abdominal closure is easily obtained using a system designed for open abdominal drainage, such as the ABThera open abdomen negative pressure therapy system for temporary abdominal wall closure (KCI; San Antonio, TX). In the top row there is a there is a fenestrated visceral protective layer that may be customized to the patient's body habitus with the goal to have the edges reach well into the paracolic gutters and pelvis so as to optimize peritoneal fluid drainage. The *middle row* demonstrates a piece of foam to approximate the abdominal wall and centralize the drainage process to the canister. Notice that this layer is best secured by using staples to secure the foam to the wound edges. The *bottom row* demonstrates sealing of the AbThera with the provided clear drape over the abdominal wall. Drape adherence improved by ensuring the skin is dry and using an adhesive skin protective barrier, such as mastisol (Eloquest Healthcare; Ferndale, MI). The drape is then cut with the open abdomen tubing set then placed directly over the clear drape and connected to the 1L canister and negative pressure therapy unit. The negative pressure unit may provide 100-150mmHg of negative pressure with 125mmHg being a common setting

proximal aortic control, rapid acquisition of proximal control, distal control with hemodynamic stability, aneurysm repair, and cautious closure with low threshold for delayed abdominal wall closure. Ruptured aneurysm repair may also be associated with significant coagulopathy, acidosis, and hypothermia requiring significant resuscitation. This resuscitation may predispose the patient to intrabdominal hypertension and ultimately abdominal compartment syndrome requiring abdominal decompression which may be avoided with temporary abdominal wall closure in the initial postoperative period. Aggressive but balanced resuscitation is essential with hypovolemia and the systemic inflammatory response driving the initial resuscitation. Overall systematic and focused repair will maximize results of open repair for ruptured abdominal aortic aneurysms understanding that even with modern medical advances, there remains significant mortality when open repair is required.

Open Repair: Retroperitoneal

Philip S.K. Paty and Manish Mehta

History and Perspective

Although the usual technique to perform open repair of ruptured AAA has been through a transperitoneal approach, there is a logical thought process that underlies a vascular surgeon's use of a retroperitoneal exposure. First, the aorta is a retroperitoneal structure. There is, therefore, no need to directly manipulate or avoid bowel or other intraperitoneal structures in order to expose the aorta. Second, exposure of the entire abdominal aorta from the level of the diaphragm to the iliac bifurcation is easily obtained. The surgeon has facile exposure of the paravisceral aortic segment for supraceliac aortic control, clamp placement, and visceral branch reconstruction as necessary. Lastly, there is less physiologic insult to the patient as compared to the transperitoneal approach. This has been debated but is apparent in terms of the duration of postoperative ileus, fluid requirements, and overall length of hospital stay [24].

Initial attempts by surgeons to perform aortic surgery utilized the retroperitoneal approach. Frer and Cooper in 1806 and 1836, respectively, emergently ligated iliac aneurysms using a retroperitoneal exposure [25]. The modern era of aortic replacement was ushered in by Dubost, who performed the first elective aortic homograft replacement of an abdominal aortic aneurysm in 1952 through a retroperitoneal approach [26].

The technique that evolved from this point was mainly an anterolateral exposure as championed by Sir Charles Rob, which was unwieldy for AAA rupture due to difficulty exposing the supraceliac aorta and was largely abandoned during the 1960s and 1970s in favor of transperitoneal exposure [27]. In 1980, Williams reported his use of an extended posterolateral approach for treatment of occlusive and aneurysmal disease of the abdominal aorta [28]. It was this seminal paper that allowed the extensive exposure of the aorta necessary for its use in repair of ruptured AAA.

Surgical Approach

Preoperative Patient Preparation

In general, the prehospitalization and preoperative preparation for the patient with a ruptured AAA is no different for the patient whether a retroperitoneal or transperitoneal exposure is used for repair. Large-bore IV line placement and permissive hypotension are recommended for access and to reduce over resuscitation and operative mortality, respectively. Well-coordinated systems of transfer and communication between emergency field personnel, emergency department, and vascular surgical teams allow the best opportunity for a successful patient outcome. Unless there is a known history of AAA, a preoperative CT scan or Emergency Department FAST ultrasound study is necessary to have a diagnosis of ruptured AAA before utilizing the retroperitoneal technique.

Left Posterolateral Retroperitoneal Approach

Positioning A suction bean bag (Olympic Vac-Pac) is placed on the operating table before the patient is brought into the operating suite. The patient is initially placed supine on the bean bag. If the patient is hemodynamically stable, large-bore central venous access and peripheral arterial lines are placed prior to induction of anesthesia. Regardless of hemodynamic stability, preoperative antibiotics are given. After the induction of general anesthesia, the patient is rotated into a modified right lateral decubitus position. The patient is positioned with the table break 5–10 cm cephalad to the left iliac crest. The patient's torso is shifted toward the left and rotated until the left shoulder is elevated 45–60° from the horizontal position while the pelvis is rotated 15–30° to allow access to both groins [29]. The left upper extremity is brought across the chest and supported by blankets, a sling, or a stand. The left thigh is elevated above the horizontal plane to relax the ipsilateral iliopsoas muscle. This maneuver improves access to the distal aorta and left iliac arteries. To open the space between the iliac crest and the costal margin, the table is flexed at the table break (Fig. 13.6). At this point, the operating table should be tilted in a slight reverse Trendelenburg positioning so that the plane of the planned retroperitoneal incision is level.

Incision The patient is prepped and draped from the mid chest to the mid thighs bilaterally. Ideally, a self-retaining retractor (Buchwalter) is anchored to the left rail of the operating table. The incision is made sharply from the lateral edge of the ipsilateral rectus muscle between the umbilicus and pubic symphysis in an oblique fashion posteriorly and superiorly through the 10th interspace to the posterior axillary line. The use of this higher incision allows exposure of the paravisceral and supraceliac portions of the aorta.

Initial Exposure and Clamp Placement The muscle layers of the lateral abdominal wall are divided to the lateral border of the rectus abdominis (incision of the anterior sheath of the rectus allows medial retraction and later exposure of the distal right common iliac artery if needed). The deepest layer, the transversus abdominis, is initially divided laterally and then medially to facilitate separation of the anterior abdominal wall from the peritoneum, which is usually thicker and more discrete laterally. The intercostal muscles are divided on the superior margin of the underlying rib. This incision is carried to the posterior axillary line. Entrance into the pleural cavity is not an issue and can be repaired at the end of the procedure.

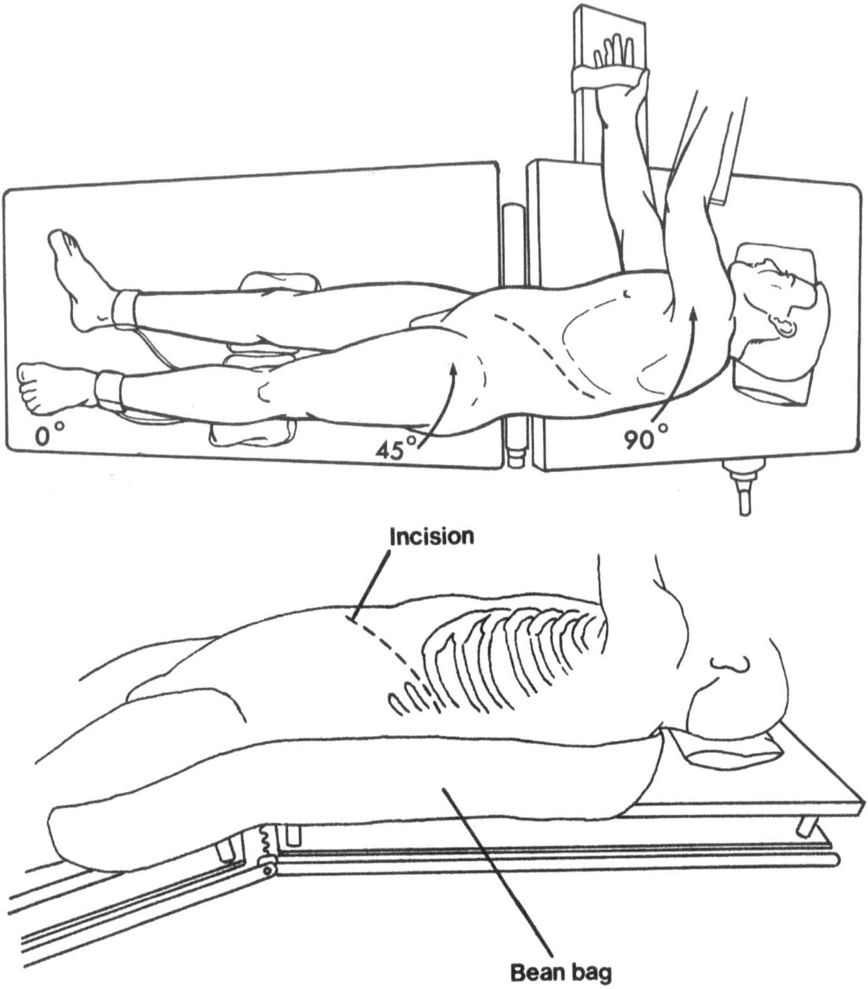

Fig. 13.6 (**a**) Position of patient on operating table. (**b**) Location of tenth interspace incision (With permission from Darling et al. [35])

In the setting of rupture, the hematoma may have already created the retroperitoneal dissection plane. The initial exposure is performed laterally and posterosuperior to the left kidney so as to avoid manipulation and inadvertent entrance into the cavity of the aneurysm rupture and hemodynamic collapse. The surgeon's left hand palmar surface is placed on the left psoas muscle and directed cephalad to the posteromedial diaphragm and crus thereby bluntly elevating the peritoneum off the diaphragm. The surgeon should be careful to not violate the fascia overlying the psoas major muscle in order to minimize dissection-related bleeding and cutaneous and genitofemoral nerve injury. The blunt dissection is complete when the supraceliac aorta is palpable beneath the diaphragmatic crus directly on the distal thoracic vertebrae.

At this point, the prime consideration is the placement of the proximal supraceliac aortic clamp. If a self-retaining retractor (Buchwalter) has been placed, the deepest Richardson-type blade is padded with a laparotomy pad and placed to medially retract the peritoneum and its contents so that the diaphragmatic crus is visible. Alternatively, a large deep handheld Deaver retractor is used to obtain the same exposure. Care must be taken to avoid vigorous retraction of the anterior and cephalad margin of the incision as this may result in splenic or renal injury

The initial maneuver to control the supraceliac aorta is to compress it posteriorly with the tips of the fingers of the left hand against the anterior portion of the thoracic vertebrae [29] (Fig. 13.7). The crural fibers are then snipped transversely with a scissors to expose and directly visualize the distal thoracic aorta for clamp placement. A Fogarty clamp should be used as it is relatively less traumatic than a Debakey Aneurysm clamp. The patient should not be heparinized. With experience, the time from skin incision to clamp placement is less than 5 min.

At this point, the self-retaining retractor should be placed to allow more stable retraction. The retroperitoneum is widely exposed at this point, and the left kidney is retracted medially and cephalad. All blades used for retraction (rigid or malleable) should be padded to minimize the risk of traction injuries to underlying organs. Care must also be taken by the surgeon to identify the course of the left ureter and thereby avoid the potential for avulsion type injuries.

The surgeon's attention should be directed to identifying the aortic neck so as to minimize renal and visceral ischemia from the supraceliac clamp. In over 90 % of patients, the aneurysm will originate below the level of the renal arteries. The landmarks for the infrarenal neck of the aortic aneurysm are the origin of the left crus of the diaphragm, the lumbar branch of the left renal vein, and the left renal artery. The lumbar branch of the left renal vein, which crosses the aorta in a posterior and perpendicular fashion and caudad to the left renal artery, should be secureły ligated (Fig. 13.8). The lympho-areolar tissue is dissected to expose the proximal infrarenal aorta.

A working knowledge of vena caval and renal venous anomalies is important as one of the major causes of mortality in these cases is due to iatrogenic venous injuries. Failure to appreciate aberrant renal venous anatomy such as retro aortic renal veins or circumaortic renal venous collars or more rarely left-sided or duplicated caval systems may result in significant blood loss. Preoperative CT imaging may identify these types of variant anatomy. If recognized, planned division of the anterior or posterior collar divisions or an approach anterolateral to the aorta may avert catastrophe. Also, the course of the inferior vena cava is such that the separation between it and the aorta is less as it courses in a caudal direction. Thus, injuries to the IVC may occur from the medal extent of the transverse placement of the aortic clamp. Direct injury to the IVC and iliac veins may again be averted with careful dissection on the adventitial surface of the aorta and subsequent clamp placement under direct vision.

Once the neck is identified and dissected free on its lateral anterior and posterior surfaces, the clamp should be placed here but not clamped. The supraceliac clamp should be opened briefly and then the aorta is clamped distally. This will allow any

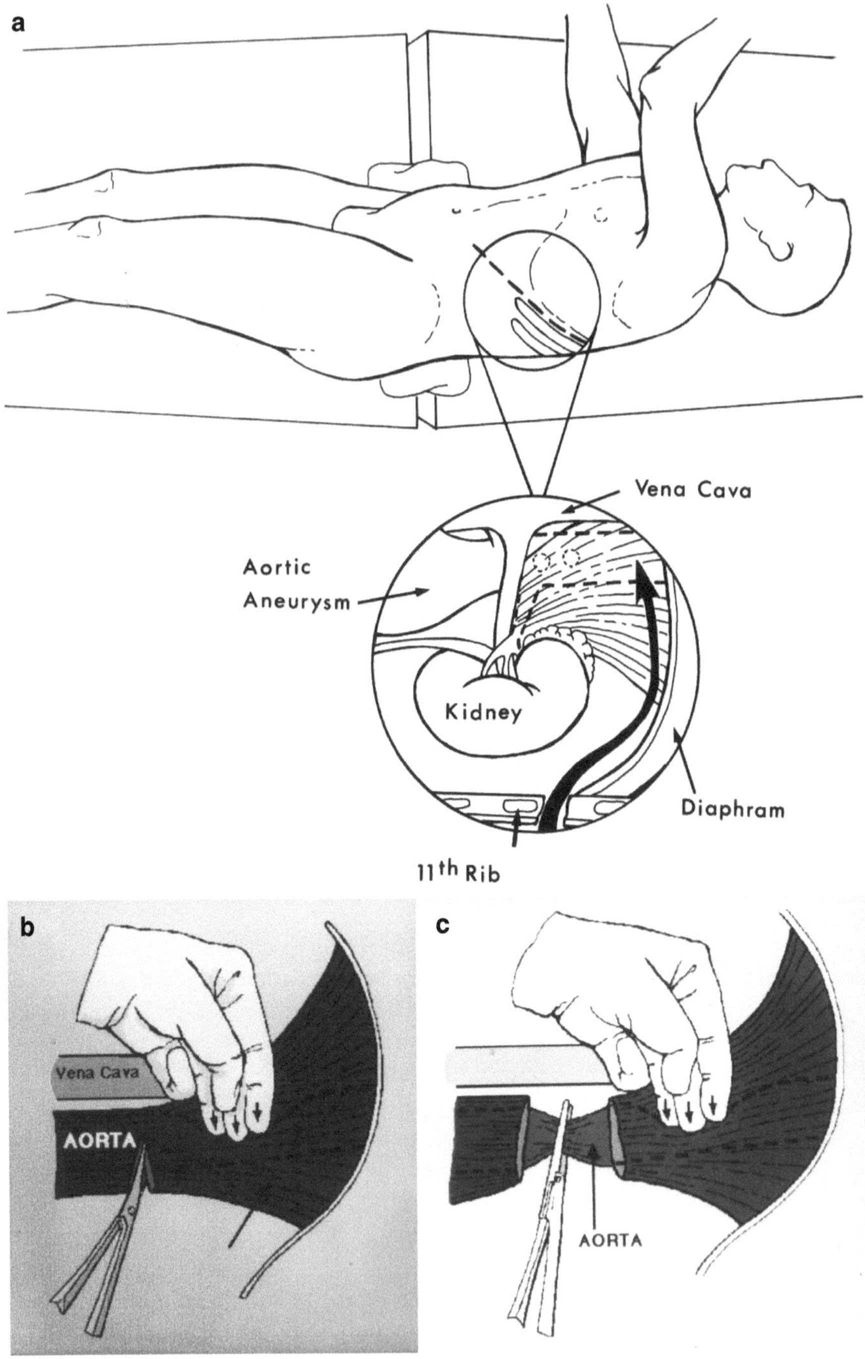

Fig. 13.7 (**a**) Left retroperitoneal entry for supraceliac aortic control (With permission from Chang et al. [36]). (**b**) Manual compression of supraceliac aorta and transverse division of diaphragmatic crus (With permission as above). (**c**) Supraceliac aortic clamp placement (With permission as above)

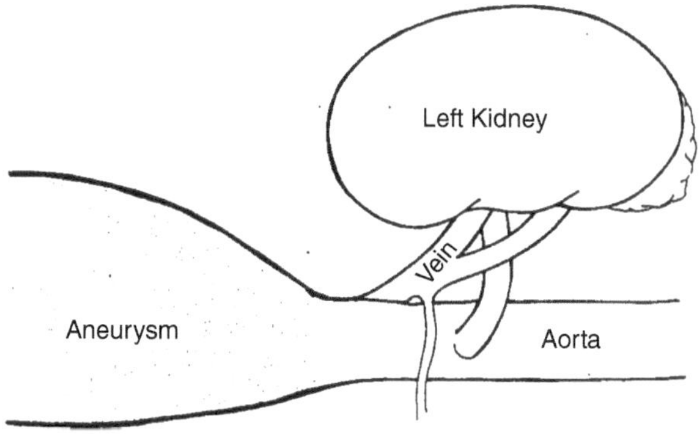

Fig. 13.8 Lumbar branch of Left renal vein (With permission from Leather et al. [37])

stasis clot proximal to the supraceliac clamp to flush distally and not into the renal and visceral arteries.

If there is no infrarenal aortic neck, the surgeon needs to make a decision whether to perform further dissection of the paravisceral aortic segment along with the renal and visceral arterial branches or to leave the supraceliac clamp in place. My preference is to leave the supraceliac clamp in place and control the celiac, superior mesenteric, and renal arteries.

Distal arterial control is obtained next. The distal aorta, proximal right common iliac artery, and entire left iliac system can be exposed and clamped through the left extended retroperitoneal exposure. If there is significant distal involvement of the distal right common or external iliac arteries, then a small suprainguinal counter incision can be made on the right by a second surgeon to obtain extraperitoneal exposure of the external iliac artery. Alternatively, right iliac artery control can also be obtained with a balloon occlusion catheter through the left flank incision at the time the aneurysm is opened. Additionally, vertical groin incisions can be made to expose the femoral arteries for distal arterial control and anastomosis. As the patient is not systemically heparinized, flushing the outflow arteries with local heparin prior to clamp placement may prevent distal arterial thrombosis due to stasis.

Aortic Reconstruction The lumbar arteries and the inferior mesenteric artery if they can be identified can be controlled from outside the sac with clips. The sac is then opened with electrocautery, and residual back-bleeding vessels are ligated with 3-0 polypropylene transfixion sutures. The aneurysm neck may be transected completely or partially with the posterior medial wall remaining intact. My preference is to completely transect the aorta to allow precise suture placement through the full aortic wall thickness, thus minimizing later development of pseudoaneurysm. When creating the neck with scissor dissection, the key is to perform the dissection from lateral to medial along the anterior and posterior walls. The surgeon can thus precisely identify the adventitial layer allowing a secure anastomosis.

The type of graft material used is per surgeon's preference. My preference is to use a tube or bifurcated polytetrafluroethylene graft. The proximal graft anastomosis is performed using a parachuted anastomotic technique with a continuous 3-0 polypropylene suture. The anastomosis starts medially at the 9 o'clock position and is parachuted anteriorly to the 12 o'clock position. At this point, the graft is loosely retracted up anteriorly to allow visualization of the medial and posterior aspect of the aorta to which the graft is sewn next to the 6 o'clock position. The anastomosis is then tightened and the remainder of the anastomosis is completed. Once the suture line is tested, the graft is bled to rid the aorta of any stasis clot, and the clamp is replace on the proximal graft, which is then flushed with heparinized saline.

If an infrarenal anastomosis is not possible, a beveled proximal anastomosis with branch grafts to the involved renal vessels may be necessary. Though the extended left retroperitoneal approach, the entire left renal artery is easily visualized. With further division of the left crus, the lateral pararenal/visceral aorta is well visualized. The right renal artery is best exposed once the aorta has been divided. The right renal artery can be exposed up to its transverse portion beneath the inferior vena. Control of the left renal artery is best obtained with Yasargil-type neurosurgical clamps. The right renal artery is best controlled with "C"-shaped curved Cooley clamp.

If possible, it is best to bevel the visceral segment and reconstruct the renal vessel(s) with separate 6–8 mm end-to-end anastomoses, which are pre-sewn onto the main body of the aortic graft. The proximal aortic anastomosis to the paravisceral aortic segment is performed first. The aortic clamp is then repositioned from the native aorta to the proximal graft after flushing the graft as previously detailed to allow perfusion of the visceral and renal arteries. The anastomosis to the renal arteries is performed next in a spatulated end-to-end fashion with 6-0 continuous polypropylene sutures. Once this is completed, the aortic graft is clamped below the lower most renal graft limb.

Next the distal aortic, iliac, or femoral anastomoses are completed. The distal graft limbs of the graft are tunneled anatomically along the axis of the vessels. On occasion, this may not be possible for limbs tunneled from within the left flank incision to distal exposure of right iliac or femoral arteries due to inflammation or prior surgery. In this situation, the right limb graft limb can be tunneled via the preperitoneal prevesical space of Retzius. Prior to performing distal anastomoses, embolectomy catheters should be passed distally intra-arterially to retrieve any stasis thrombus, 4 French for iliac and 3 French for femoral arteries. The distal arteries should then be flushed with heparinized saline and re-clamped. Once the distal anastomoses are completed, the clamps are removed and Doppler interrogation is performed.

If there is any concern regarding intestinal viability or traction injury to the spleen, the peritoneum can be purposefully incised to allow for direct inspection of the intra-abdominal contents. At this point, any defects in the peritoneum are repaired. If entrance into the pleural cavity does occur, it should be fixed directly upon incision closure by sewing the cut diaphragmatic edge to the next highest rib while catheter suction is maintained in the pleural cavity. Alternatively, tube thoracostomy can be placed. The abdominal wall musculature is closed in layers followed by closure of the subcutaneous tissue and skin. Closure of the wound is made easier by taking the flex out of the table, which allows a tension free repair.

Retroperitoneal Exposure for Secondary Rupture After EVAR

Surgical conversions following EVAR have been described by a few centers, all utilizing the standard transperitoneal approach via midline laparotomy [30, 31]. The retroperitoneal approach to the abdominal aorta as described for open repair of ruptured AAA can be easily utilized for secondary AAA rupture after an EVAR with explant of the endovascular graft. A surgeon's familiarity with the extended left retroperitoneal exposure in elective situations involving infrarenal, juxtarenal, and pararenal abdominal aortic aneurysms may allow one to extend the use of this approach to more complex clinical scenarios. The same attributes of the left retroperitoneal exposure that facilitate repair in ruptured aneurysm, such as the ability to control the entire abdominal aorta from the distal thoracic segment to the iliac bifurcation, apply to open repair in patients with rupture after failed endovascular repair [32].

The positioning, incision, and exposure are identical to the technique for repair of ruptured AAA detailed previously. The degree of difficulty in exposing the operative field in the retroperitoneum in the setting of a previously deployed aortic endograft varies depending upon the amount of inflammation present, which is due either to the mere presence of the endograft within the aorta or a reactive response to prior attempts at translumbar coil embolization of persistent type I or II endoleaks. The appearance may resemble that of an inflammatory aneurysm; therefore, maneuvers to minimize injury to adjacent structures (duodenum and renal veins), such as maintaining the dissection within the retroperitoneum as posterior as possible, and attempts to identify the ureter early with or without the use of preoperatively placed stents may facilitate the procedure. The supraceliac aortic dissection is usually free of inflammation, whereas the infra- and juxtarenal portions of the aorta are often significantly inflamed rendering the dissection hazardous. The safest method is to approach the lateral and posterior aspect after initial clamp placement. Another alternative is to obtain control with an intra-aortic balloon directed from one of the femoral arteries and inflated at the supraceliac aortic level.

If further dissection of the aortic neck cannot be safely performed, the initial supraceliac aortic clamp is left in place, distal clamps are placed, and the aneurysm sac is opened. If information is available regarding the previously deployed endograft in terms of suprarenal versus infrarenal fixation, this may help plan subsequent control and clamping of the distal aorta. In patients with a known suprarenal fixation, it is often preferable to leave the aortic cross clamp on the supraceliac aorta. With a known infrarenal device, assuming the aorta can be accurately dissected, is minimally diseased and has no significant aneurysmal component, the cross clamp can be moved to the infrarenal aorta.

The single most important factor in deciding between partial and complete stent graft explant is whether the endograft can be completely removed without destroying the aortic wall (Fig. 13.9). The surgeon needs to remember that the goal is to control bleeding and reconstruct in line flow as expeditiously as possible. Other considerations include the type of stent graft fixation (suprarenal versus infrarenal and active with hooks/barbs vs. passive with self-expanding stent only), as this may influence the site of aortic clamping and the possible adjunctive need for visceral endarterectomy and/or revascularization with complete stent graft explant. Infrarenal aortic clamping with only partial stent graft explant might be a significantly less morbid procedure when compared with supraceliac aortic clamp and complete stent graft explant, with possible visceral reconstructions, particularly in the patient with aneurysm rupture [33]. In cases of rupture secondary to a type IA endoleak, the proximal endograft may slide out easily. Lastly, some endografts with suprarenal fixation can be "captured with a cut syringe barrel, thereby facilitating explant [34].

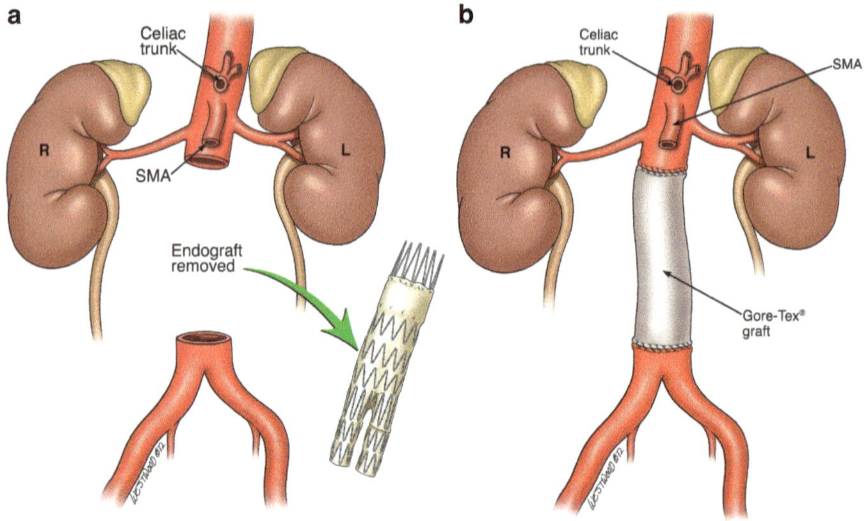

Fig. 13.9 (**a**) Complete endograft explant. (**b**) Infrarenal aortic replacement with prosthetic graft

In AAA rupture patients with infrarenal stent grafts, the proximal aortic clamp is placed at the suprarenal level, the aneurysm sac is opened, the entire infrarenal stent graft can be explanted including the iliac limbs, and aortoiliac reconstruction is performed as needed (Fig. 13.9). In AAA rupture patients with suprarenal self-expanding stents for fixation, aortic control is obtained by placing a supraceliac aortic clamp. In these cases, partial stent graft explant with transaction of the stent graft within the proximal aortic neck is performed. In AAA rupture patients with stent grafts that have had placement of proximal Palmaz stents, aortic control is obtained via a supraceliac aortic clamp, or an aortic occlusion balloon, with partial or complete stent graft explant. When the proximal aortic stent graft is partially explanted, the proximal graft is sewn to the composite endograft/proximal aorta with or without pledgets depending on the friability of the aortic wall (Fig. 13.10). Renal arterial reconstruction may be necessary as previously detailed depending upon the wall integrity and extent of the proximal aortic aneurysm (Fig. 13.11).

If the entire distal portion of the endograft can be removed, the aortic graft is sewn to the aorta, iliac, or femoral arteries depending on the extent of aneurysmal and occlusive disease. In instances when the iliac limbs cannot be explanted due to scarring, either the distal anastomosis is constructed beyond the iliac stent grafts or the aortic bifurcation is then oversewn (Fig. 13.12), or the limbs are transected at the aortic bifurcation, and the aortic tube graft is sutured directly to the distal aortic bifurcation, and the stent graft limbs are incorporated within the anastomosis. Alternatively, the limbs of a bifurcated graft can be sewn individually to the remaining endograft limbs or the distal body of the endograft (Fig. 13.13). Interrupted 5-0 polypropylene sutures are then used to secure the native distal iliac arteries to the distal portion of the remaining EVAR limbs.

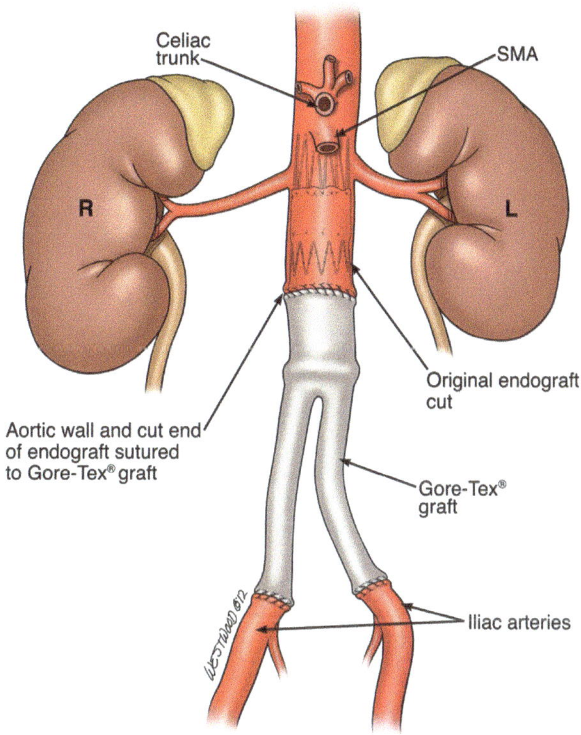

Fig. 13.10 Partial proximal endograft explant after aortic reconstruction

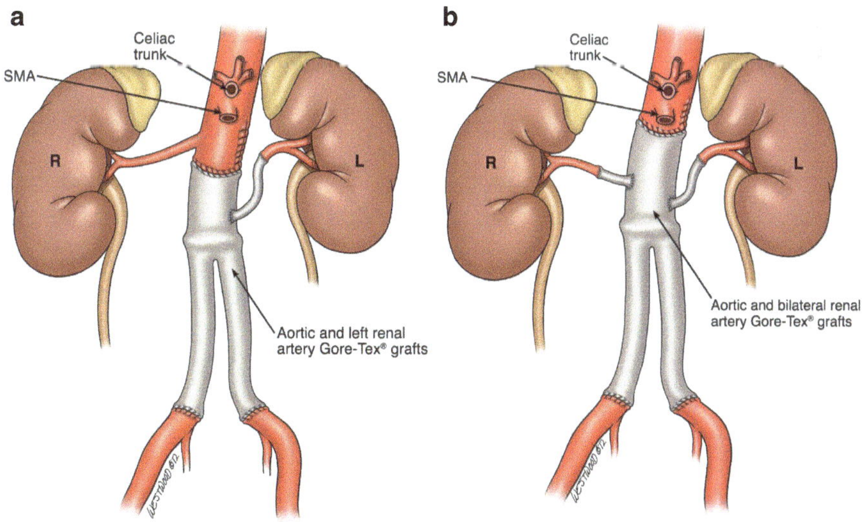

Fig. 13.11 (**a**) Complete endograft explant and left renal artery bypass. (**b**) Complete endograft explant and bilateral renal artery bypass (Note: renal grafts offset to allow sequential renal reperfusion)

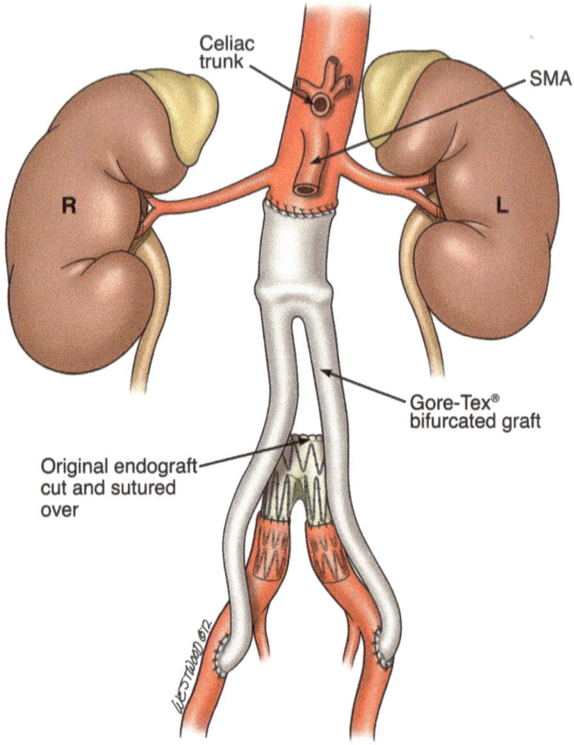

Fig. 13.12 Partial distal endograft explant with end-to-side distal reconstruction

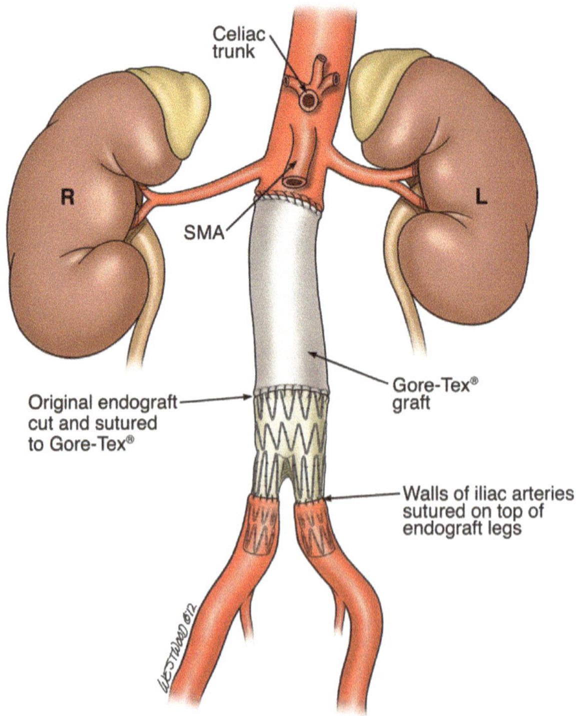

Fig. 13.13 Partial distal endograft explant with anastomosis to residual endograft (Note: interrupted sutures to secure iliac limbs to native iliac arteries)

Conclusion

The extended left retroperitoneal approach can be used to perform open repair of de novo ruptured AAA or after delayed rupture of the AAA sac after EVAR. The ideal method to incorporate the technique is through experience with elective repair. The ability to directly deal with the aortic reconstruction without the need to pay attention to intraperitoneal structures is the principle advantage of this technique.

Rupture EVAR Using Bifurcated Stent Grafts

Manish Mehta and Philip S.K. Paty

Introduction

The metamorphosis of rAAA treatment from open surgical repair to EVAR has evolved significantly over the past two decades from being performed selectively by a few centers in hemodynamically stable patients only to being performed by most endovascular specialists in many centers in patients with varying degrees of hemodynamic instability [38–40]. Collectively, worldwide experience demonstrates that an increasing number of rEVAR procedures are being performed yearly. The endovascular approach is less invasive, eliminates laparotomy, eliminates aortic cross clamping, decreases surgical bleeding and possibly general anesthesia, and has been shown to decrease the mortality of rAAA repair with fewer complications, shorter hospital length of stay, and more patients being able to return home rather than going to institutional care after these emergent procedures [41, 42]. Factors that influence institutions ability to offer rEVAR to patients include not only established infrastructures that can provide comprehensive care for rAAA patients but also well-trained surgeons/interventionists that can perform complex endovascular aortic procedures in emergent circumstances using currently available devices. This chapter will focus attention on the use of modular bifurcated stent grafts for managing patients with rAAA.

Approach to Ruptured EVAR

Introduction of EVAR for rAAA has forced us to reevaluate protocols that facilitate expeditious patient transfer to the operating rooms for EVAR or open surgical repair. Today, the question is not whether patients with rAAA should undergo EVAR rather how to develop systems that allow for broader utilization of these complex procedures that have shown great benefit in high-risk patients with aneurysm rupture.

This chapter focuses on the use of modular bifurcated stent grafts for rEVAR; there are several additional aspects that merit discussion as they have an impact on procedure technical aspects, including standardized protocol-based approach to rAAA, anatomic suitability for rEVAR, choice of anesthesia, percutaneous vs. femoral cutdown approach, bifurcated vs. aorto-uni-iliac stent grafts, and the implications of using aortic occlusion balloon during rEVAR.

There remain several fundamental concerns regarding EVAR for rAAA that include the anatomical suitability for EVAR, the availability of dedicated staff and equipment to perform emergent EVAR at all hours, the feasibility of treating hemodynamically stable and unstable patients by EVAR, and the surgeon/interventionists' ability to manage unexpected scenarios under emergent circumstances [43, 44]. Many of the high-volume institutions have adopted a standardized protocol-based approach to managing rAAA patients [45]. The hemodynamic status of the rAAA patient generally dictates the need for a preoperative CT scan, and although while planning for this emergent open surgical repair, a preoperative CT is not considered a necessity, while planning an emergent EVAR, most would agree that we would like to have a CT scan for evaluating the feasibility of EVAR as well as for stent graft sizing. So the question is whether one has the time to get an emergent CT scan prior to EVAR, and if not are there other tools available that might help us manage these hemodynamically unstable patients by endovascular means? Published data on the feasibility of preoperative CT in patient with rAAA would indicate that 88 % (49 of 56) of the patients died >2 h after admission with the diagnosis of ruptured AAA, the median time interval from the onset of symptoms to admission to the hospital was 2.5 h, and the interval between hospital admission with the diagnosis of ruptured AAA and death was 10.5 h [46]. This data would clearly suggest that majority of the patients with ruptured AAA have the time to undergo an emergent CT scan, particularly if there is an established protocol that facilitates early diagnosis and transfer of patient from the ER to the OR.

The proportion of rAAA patients that are suitable for EVAR is variable and on the basis of two meta-analysis ranges from 47 to 67 %. What has also been reported is that when compared to elective AAA, rAAAs have larger infrarenal aortic diameters and shorter neck lengths. These differences in AAA morphology likely have an effect on the ability to perform rEVAR, and it is likely that institutions that treat a higher proportion of rAAA by EVAR expand on the stent graft indications for use of these high-risk patients [47]. Several institutions including ours have tried to identify the impact of rEVAR in patients with favorable versus unfavorable aortic neck morphology [48, 49]. We further analyzed aortic neck morphology via CT scans in 180 consecutive patients with rAAA that underwent rEVAR (74, 41 %) or OSR (106, 59 %) [50]. Based on EVAR device-specific favorable versus hostile aortic neck morphology, we identified that only 34 % of patients with rAAA had neck morphology that would meet the "indication for use" for available stent grafts. The rEVAR patients with hostile aortic necks had a significantly higher incidence of female gender (32 % vs. 19 %, $p<0.01$), mean maximum AAA diameter (7.4 cm vs. 5.5 cm, $p<0.01$), abdominal compartment syndrome (20 % vs. 4 %, $p<0.01$), type I endoleaks (16 % vs. 4 %), and the need for all secondary interventions (77 % vs. 40 %, $p<0.01$) during long-term follow-up. The 30-day mortality was the lowest in rEVAR patients with favorable aortic necks and the highest in the OSR patients (favorable 8 %, hostile 23 %, OSR 43.4 %, $p < 0.01$), and both favorable and hostile rEVAR patients had a better cumulative 3-year survival than OSR (favorable 64 %, hostile 67 %, OSR 44 %, $p < 0.01$). Mayer et.al. reported their experience of 473 rAAA patients where over time they transitioned to rEVAR in 100 % of patients with rAAA [51]. This was the first study to address the outcomes of complete replacement of all rAAA to be treated from open surgical repair to rEVAR. Their findings suggested that nearly all patients with rAAA can undergo rEVAR with a low mortality of 24 % and a low turndown rate of 4 %. However, with transition to rEVAR for all patients, surgeons/interventionists and institutions also need to have the ability to manage more challenging anatomy and comfortably utilize adjunctive endovascular techniques in managing the hostile proximal landing zones.

Depending on one's comfort level and the logistics, EVAR for rupture can be performed under local anesthesia via percutaneous approach to general anesthesia and femoral artery cutdown. The potential benefit of local anesthesia/conscious sedation and percutaneous approach is that it might avoid the loss of "sympathetic tone" in the compromised ruptured AAA patients. One has to be comfortable with obtaining percutaneous access and using closure devices in patients that might be hemodynamically unstable with difficult to palpate femoral pulses. Although the advantage may be significant, it must be balanced by the potential difficulties encountered during these emergent procedures, as the patient might not be coherent and cooperative enough to lie still. The potential advantages of using modular bifurcated stent grafts over aorto-uni-iliac devices are that it allows for cases to be done via percutaneous approach with local anesthesia and femorofemoral bypass is not needed.

Endovascular Setup and Techniques

Adequate resuscitation of patients with ruptured AAA is vital to a successful outcome. As long as the patients maintain a measurable blood pressure, the techniques of "hypotensive hemostasis" by limiting the resuscitation to maintain a detectable blood pressure can help minimize ongoing hemorrhage. The patient is prepped and draped in supine position, and via a percutaneous or femoral artery cutdown, ipsilateral access is obtained using a needle, floppy guidewire, and a guiding catheter. The floppy guidewire is exchanged for a super-stiff wire that can be used to place a large sheath (12–14 Fr × 45 cm length) in the ipsilateral femoral artery and the sheath advanced up to the juxtarenal abdominal aorta so it is ready to be used to deliver and support the aortic occlusion balloon if needed. A compliant occlusion balloon should always be available in these procedures, and in hemodynamically unstable patients, the occlusion balloon is advanced through the ipsilateral sheath over the super-stiff wire into the supraceliac abdominal aorta under fluoroscopic guidance, and the balloon is inflated as needed [52]. For detailed discussion on aortic occlusion balloon use, see Chap. 12. Contralateral femoral access is subsequently obtained via percutaneous or cutdown approach in a similar fashion and a "marker flush catheter" advanced to the juxtarenal aorta for an arteriogram.

Ruptured EVAR Using Bifurcated Stent Grafts

As expected, the emergence of EVAR has also resulted in the evolution of stent graft design. A detailed discussion on stent graft design is well beyond the scope of this chapter, but one has to consider the various stent graft configurations available when performing rEVAR. The stent graft best suited for managing rAAA is likely the one the operator is most comfortable using in elective circumstances. With that said, there are several implications of stent graft design that might impact rEVAR under emergent circumstances, and since there is no evidence in literature evaluating the validity of one stent graft over another in managing rAAA, maybe it is best to understand some of these nuances that might have advantages under emergent circumstances. Bifurcated stent grafts can be divided into several categories based on their fixation (suprarenal vs. infrarenal), modularity (one docking limb vs. two docking limbs), and sealing mechanism (stent + graft vs. polymer + graft). Regardless of the design and improvements in lower profile delivery systems, controlled deployment mechanisms, and active fixation methods, it is also clear that bifurcated stent grafts perform significantly better when they are used to treat anatomy within its "indications for use" (IFU) [53]. Unfortunately, high-risk patients with rAAA require quick response to stop the hemorrhage, and operators are sometimes forced to perform emergent rEVAR under unfavorable circumstances and sometimes require the use of aortic occlusion balloon. In such conditions, factors to consider should include the implications of need for aortic occlusion balloon with (1) suprarenal vs. infrarenal fixation stent grafts and proximal aortic neck angulation and morphology, (2) aorto-uni-iliac vs. modular bifurcated stent grafts with one or two docking limbs, (3) polymer-based devices and the time requirements for polymers to cure and seal the aortic neck, and (4) the need for adjunctive procedures including single or multiple chimneys for visceral arteries, the use of Palmaz stent or EndoAnchors for proximal seal, femorofemoral bypass, and the need for iliac artery occlusions depending on the planned procedure.

The decision to use a particular stent graft type is determined by the patient's aortoiliac morphology, and there are several factors to consider regarding the use bifurcated vs. aorto-uni-iliac stent grafts for rAAA: (1) inability to access the contralateral gate expeditiously and (2) inability to access the contralateral iliac artery due to significant occlusive disease and/or tortuosity. The use of aorto-uni-iliac devices during elective or emergent EVAR does require interruption of flow from the contralateral common iliac artery into the AAA via a placement of an occluder device and a femorofemoral bypass. Several studies have documented the use of aorto-uni-iliac devices for rEVAR with outcomes similar to the use of bifurcated stent grafts. It is likely that the use of aorto-uni-iliac devices might expand on the applicability for rEVAR [54, 55]. For more on the use of aorto-uni-iliac stent grafts for rEVAR, please see the next chapter by Ian Loftus.

The placement of the stent graft main body is planned based on the aortoiliac morphology that is best suited for rEVAR. Unless prohibited, in hemodynamically stable patients, following the initial arteriogram, the aortic occlusion balloon is removed from the initial ipsilateral side and the stent graft main body advanced under fluoroscopic guidance; this limits the number of catheter exchanges. In hemodynamically unstable patients that require inflation of the aortic occlusion balloon, the "marker flush catheter" is exchanged for the stent graft main body which is delivered up to the aortic neck. An arteriogram is done via the sheath that is used to support the aortic occlusion balloon, the tip of the stent graft main body is aligned with the lowermost renal artery, the occlusion balloon is subsequently deflated and withdrawn back with the delivery sheath into the AAA, and the stent graft main body is deployed. In the rare instance when patient's hemodynamic status is extremely compromised and the aortic occlusion balloon cannot be deflated, there are several alternatives to consider. The sheath housing the aortic occlusion balloon should be advanced to a level above the renal arteries and the stent graft deployed at the infrarenal level. This maneuver allows for the occlusion balloon to be deflated and retrieved into the sheath without compromising the proximal stent graft fixation and seal. In these particular situations, one needs to consider the use of aorto-uni-iliac stent grafts or the conversion of bifurcated devices to aorto-uni-iliac to avoid further delays in obtaining proximal stent graft seal while cannulating the bifurcated stent graft contralateral gate. The alternative is to communicate with the anesthesiologist so they can manage the patient's hemodynamics, deflate and withdraw the aortic occlusion balloon, and deploy the main body-bifurcated stent graft. Then expeditiously from the main body ipsilateral side advances the aortic occlusion balloon over the wire up to the aortic neck and inflate. This maneuver allows for the seal of the stent graft at the proximal aortic neck while reestablishing proximal occlusion at the aortic neck within seconds. This temporary deflation of the aortic occlusion balloon rarely results in hemodynamic collapse and usually is of little consequence. Of importance is to recognize that once the occlusion balloon is reinflated within the bifurcated main body, it requires gentle forward traction to counteract the downward traction from forces of the systolic blood pressure which if left to itself could result in prolapse of the main body stent graft distally into the AAA. The exact steps here might vary depending on the use of bifurcated stent grafts with suprarenal vs. infrarenal fixation and modular components that have a single docking vs. two docking limbs. Depending on what particular bifurcated device one is comfortable using, one needs to rehearse the steps and plan accordingly. Finally, the occlusion balloon inflated and secured within the proximal bifurcated main body creates a more hemodynamic stable environment for the patient and allows us to move onto the next steps which include contralateral gate cannulation. The remainder of the rEVAR procedure is performed similar to as in elective circumstances; following contralateral gate cannulation, appropriately sized iliac stent graft extensions are advanced and deployed as needed to obtain complete aneurysm exclusion.

Expanding the Proximal Stent Graft Landing Zone for Ruptured Pararenal AAA

In addition to treating ruptured infrarenal AAA, bifurcated stent grafts have also been used for managing ruptured pararenal AAA with the addition of adjunctive chimney procedures – EVAR [51, 56]. Currently published data is limited and would suggest that adjunctive chimney techniques with the use of bifurcated stent grafts likely allows a higher percentage of rAAA patients to be treated by endovascular means, but it is also likely that the resultant type I endoleaks and overall mortality will also be higher. When planning these emergent procedures, we need to be vigilant in understanding some of the nuances of the available evidence and in planning these complex procedures.

Rupture After EVAR

The goal of AAA repair is to reduce the risks for aneurysm rupture and death. However, none of the currently available stent grafts is completely effective in preventing aneurysm rupture after EVAR, and lifelong surveillance is needed. We evaluated our experience of delayed AAA rupture after EVAR and found that the most common risk factors contributing to rupture included type I endoleaks with stent graft migration (63 %), type I endoleaks without stent graft migration (11 %), type II endoleaks (19 %), and undetermined etiology (7 %). In this series, 41 % of patients with rAAA after EVAR underwent another EVAR procedure with an operative mortality of 9 %, whereas 55 % required conversion to surgical repair with an operative mortality of 20 % [57].

Although bifurcated stent grafts might have a role in managing rupture after EVAR, stent graft migration from proximal fixation sites and type I endoleaks remain the most common cause of rupture after EVAR [58]. In these circumstances, bifurcated stent grafts are infrequently needed, and most patients require proximal stent graft extensions with or without chimney or fenestrated stent graft use to lengthen the proximal stent graft seal zone. If bifurcated stent grafts are the only available devices in such emergent circumstances, they can be utilized to advance the proximal landing zone and convert the original bifurcated stent graft into aorto-uni-iliac configuration, as needed (Figs. 13.14 and 13.15)

Conclusions

Endovascular repair of rAAA is evolving and offers the potential for improved patient survival. Unlike elective EVAR, during emergent EVAR, the time for preoperative planning is limited, and often the preoperative imaging is less than ideal; under these circumstances, one often has to get creative and utilize more of a "problem-solving approach" to address challenging issues that might arise during these emergent circumstances. A standardized multidisciplinary approach can be instrumental in organizing pathways that can accommodate individual practices and hospital infrastructure and facilitate a seamless transition of these often hemodynamically unstable patients from the time of diagnosis to successful rEVAR. There are several important technical aspects including the choice of anesthesia, percutaneous vs. femoral cutdown approach, use of aortic occlusion balloons, use of bifurcated vs. aorto-uni-iliac stent grafts, and adjunctive procedures that need to be well understood as one embarks on performing these procedures.

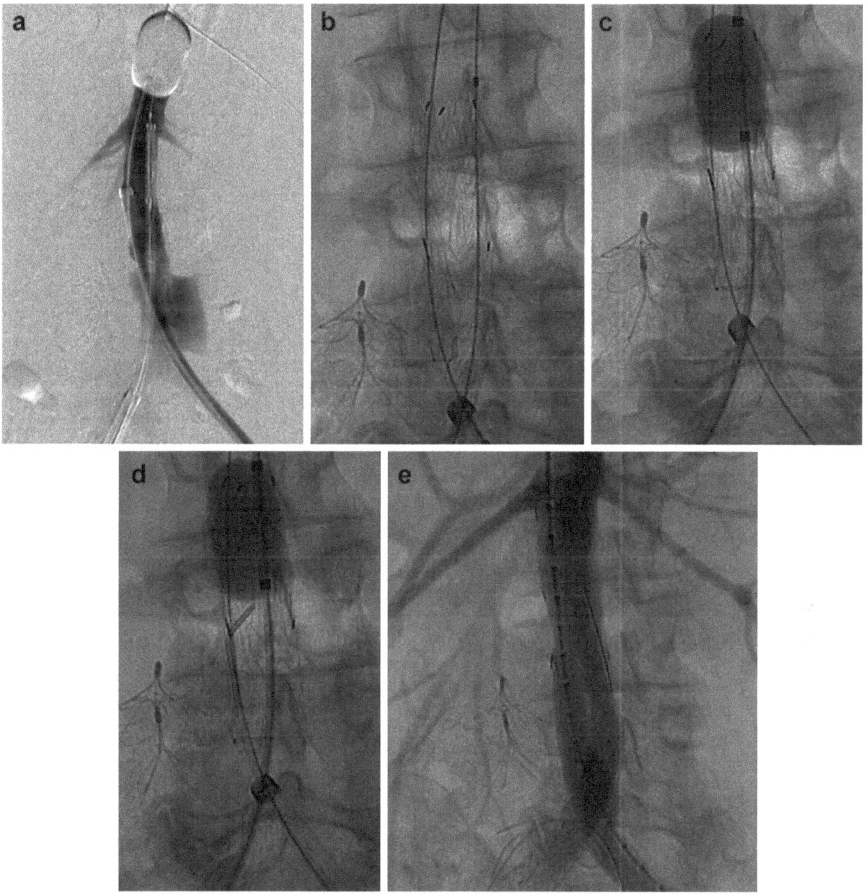

Fig. 13.14 Bifurcated stent grafts for ruptured EVAR and use of aortic occlusion balloon (AOB). (**a**) Bifurcated stent graft advanced to the level of the lowermost renal arteries, and occlusion balloon advanced from contralateral side and inflated at supraceliac aorta. (**b**) Deflate and retrieve the AOB and deploy the bifurcated stent graft. (**c**) Advance the AOB from within the stent graft main body and inflate at the level of the aortic neck. (**d**) Cannulate bifurcated stent graft contralateral limb with occlusion balloon maintaining aortic occlusion and apply forward traction on AOB catheter to prevent AOB and stent graft prolapse into the aneurysm. (**e**) Completion arteriogram following ruptured EVAR with bifurcated stent graft

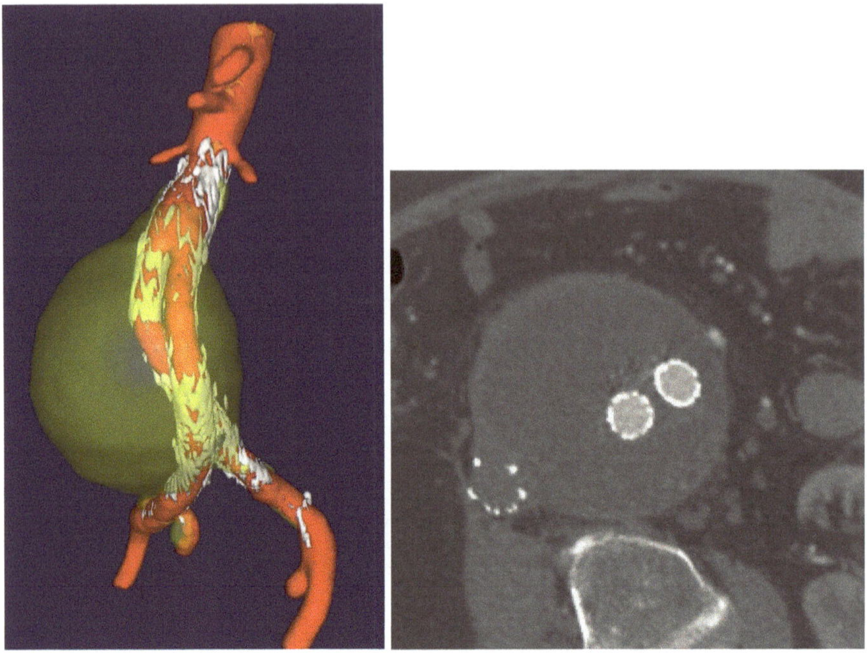

Fig. 13.15 Post-op CTA following ruptured EVAR with bifurcated stent graft

EVAR-AUI: The European Experience

Ruth A. Benson, S. Bahia, R.J. Hinchliffe, and I.M. Loftus

Introduction: The Origins of the AUI Graft

The first English language report into the use of a balloon expandable aorto-uni-ilac (AUI) stent for AAA management was published in 1991 [73] (Fig. 13.16), although it had already been reported in the Russian literature in 1988 [82]. Parodi's novel method described the use of a balloon expandable stent loaded onto a deployment device and inserted into the aneurysmal aorta via retrograde femoral artery access. This was accompanied by contralateral iliac occlusion and a femorofemoral crossover graft. Designed to exclude the aneurysm, they described initial clinical success in 5 patients, all of whom had been denied open repair due to significant comorbidity.

Encouraged by this early experience, surgeons in Europe began to create their own versions of the graft. Published results of small UK-based series followed. The Leicester group reported their initial experiences in 1997 [79], with a refined method

Fig. 13.16 The Parodi-Palmaz device. The Palmaz stent was sutured to a dilated PTFE graft [70]

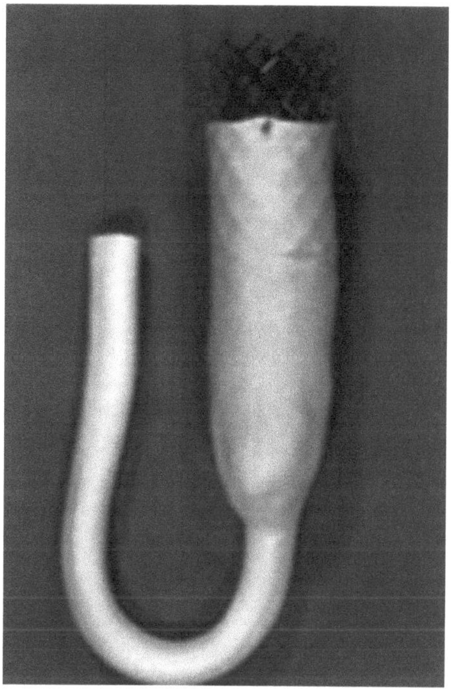

using an 8-mm pre-dilated PTFE tube graft with the addition of a proximal Palmaz stent, mounted onto a 30-mm balloon. They described successful deployment in 20 patients, providing clear accounts of the complications they encountered. Initial results were positive, but long-term efficacy was yet to be proven.

Results from larger UK and European cohorts followed, all supporting the feasibility of endovascular AUI aneurysm repair. Survival in elective patients was reported as 90 % at 4 months, even among high-risk patients. Overall, the merits of the AUI graft were becoming increasingly apparent [64]. They were readily custom-made by the surgeon. Access and deployment were simple, using preexisting technology and equipment. It was becoming apparent that there was an emerging role in the treatment of patients with significant comorbidity for whom open repair was not an option. It was suitable for AAA where anatomy was more complex or where there were tortuous or unilaterally occluded iliac arteries.

Initially as bifurcated devices were designed, the AUI technique maintained superiority, the perceived advantage being the range of patients in whom it could be implanted. In a review of 154 AAA CT scans, Armon et al. found 55 % of patients were suitable for implantation of an AUI graft, compared to only 10 % for an early bifurcated endograft [60]. Investigators in the Amsterdam Acute Aneurysm Trial found that 45.8 % of patients presenting with ruptured AAA (rAAA) were suitable for AUI, while others found only 20 % of ruptures were suitable for bifurcated grafts [70, 76]. These data was applicable to the endografts available to the authors at the time and would not be representative of the range of devices now available.

The European Experience: Graft Complications

An increase in the number of surgeons adopting AUI was followed by the identification of novel complications linked both to the learning curve and to the specifics of the grafts themselves. Ivancev's report of his group's experiences in 45 patients detailed a variety of complications. Early issues included insertion of endografts that were too short (necessitating conversion to open repair), iatrogenic renal artery occlusions, graft kinking, iatrogenic iliac dissection, and type 2 endoleaks [71]. Mortality remained high, as these were patients selected because their comorbidity precluded open repair (OR). At 1 year, surveillance identified significant stent migration in 5 patients and the presence of type 2 endoleaks in 3 requiring embolization.

Despite routine femorofemoral crossover graft, some patients developed significant buttock claudication [72]. Indeed the requirement for a crossover graft raised the most doubts about the longevity of AUI as a procedure despite evidence suggesting better durability in aneurysmal compared to occlusive disease [84].

Relatively favorable rates of early complications of femorofemoral crossover bypass grafts were documented in a study of 136 elective patients treated with AUI in Nottingham [83, 84]. Frequency of groin or graft infection was found to be equivalent to bifurcated devices. Further publication of a larger cohort, an 8-year experience in 231 patients, demonstrated an infection rate of 11 %, a cumulative 3-year patency rate of 91 %, and 5-year patency of 83 % [67]. Importantly, their large case series enabled them to identify factors promoting graft occlusion, mostly related to technical issues with the AUI. However, patency rates remained comparable with those reported following OR and bifurcated grafts.

"Peri-graft Extravasation": The Risk of the Endoleak and Surveillance

First proposed by White, the terminology now used when classifying endoleaks has become ubiquitous in the setting of endovascular AAA repair [85]. Endoleaks remain the most common indication for reintervention following EVAR, and the early adopters of AUI began to address the design of surveillance programs. Initially, CT imaging was the only established method for identifying stent migration or leak, but valid concerns regarding mounting costs and risks of cumulative radiation exposure were raised. In their prospective study of aneurysm morphology and radiological and ultrasound appearances following AUI repair, the Leicester group compared the ability to identify AAA migration or peri-graft extravasation (endoleak) 6 weeks postimplantation using CT and duplex ultrasound. They found duplex to be comparable, and in some cases superior, due to its less invasive nature, lower cost, and greater effectiveness in identifying the site of endoleak [80]. Attempts to predict the risk of endoleak preoperatively based on CT imaging were unsuccessful, with a lack of correlation between the number of patent lumbar or inferior mesenteric arteries and risk of endoleak [83, 84]. The need for postoperative surveillance was firmly established.

AUI and the Ruptured AAA: A Victim of Its Own Success

The success of AUI in patients with poor physiological status meant that progression to its use for rAAA was inevitable. Successful deployment was first published by Yusuf et al. in 1994 [87]. This group published early results of their surgeon-manufactured endografts in 30 patients including a further 2 rAAA using a modified Gianturco (self-expanding) stent, Dacron graft, and Wallstent [86]. The graft was preloaded onto either the Chuter (18 F, 5/30) or the Ivancev delivery system (20 F, 25/30 cases).

In a setting where mortality for rAAA had been persistently high for decades, endovascular repair with the AUI technique offered hope for radically increasing patients' chances of short-term survival [59]. One particular advantage was seen as the AUI's ability to gain rapid hemostasis without laparotomy and anatomic applicability over a relatively large proportion of patients. The technique was thought to create far less of a physiological insult, although much like EVAR today, selection bias toward more frail patients meant that outcomes were not as positive as some had predicted [64].

AUI Devices/Occluders/Technique

A number of AUI devices have been used to treat aneurysmal aortic disease over the years (Table 13.1); however, the technique for intervention remains broadly similar, i.e., insertion of an occlusive aortic balloons depending on the hemodynamic state of the patient, followed by deployment of the AUI device (Fig. 13.17), and insertion of an occluder for a patent contralateral iliac system and a crossover graft [68]. Several occluder devices have been utilized in the literature, including the Talent device (Medtronic, nitinol, woven polyester, 8–24 mm distal diameter, 31–35 mm stent length, 17.5 F delivery system), the Zenith iliac plug (Cook, 14–24 mm diameter, 30 mm length, 14–16 F delivery system), as well as AMPLATZER plugs (St. Jude Medical, 3–22 mm, 7 F) for particularly small iliac vessels [63].

Alsac's group in France published outcomes for 37 consecutive patients presenting with rAAA over a 4-year period [59]. From a cohort of 17 patients treated with EVAR, 8 were managed with AUI (a mix of Cook and Medtronic grafts). Patients were not randomized – EVAR was attempted if possible, but in those

Table 13.1 Aorto-uni-iliac grafts used in European centers performing endovascular AAA repair

Stent graft	Construction	Proximal diameter (main body)	Distal diameter (main body)	Sheath size	Comments
Endofit (LeMaitre vascular)	Self-expanding, nitinol, PTFE, 2 layers	20–36 mm	12–20 mm	18 or 22 F, hydrophilic	10–20 cm length
Talent (Medtronic)	Self-expanding, nitinol, polyester fabric	22–36 mm	14–16 mm	22 or 24 F	Bare-spring proximally (if >22 mm) to pararenal placement
Endurant (I/II) (Medtronic)	Self-expanding, nitinol, suprarenal fixation	23–36 mm	14 mm	18 F or 20 F	102–5 mm of graft covered
Zenith (Cook)	Self-expanding, stainless steel and nitinol, braided polyester, suprarenal fixation	24–36 mm	12 mm	20 F	Distal components 12–24 mm diameter

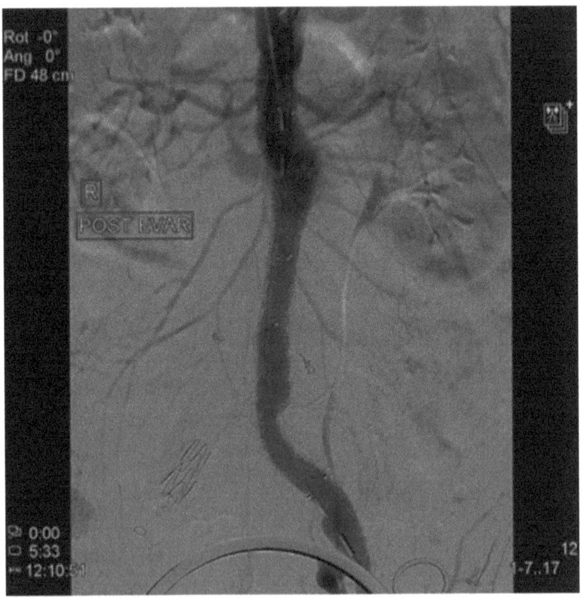

Fig. 13.17 Post-EVAR digital subtraction angiogram with contralateral common iliac artery occluder [74]

with hemodynamic instability, open repair (OR) appeared to be the first choice. Overall, operating time was significantly less in the combined EVAR group, with reduced blood loss and length of intensive care stay. Interestingly, on retrospective analysis, 73 % of the patients who were treated with OR due to "unfavorable anatomy" were actually suitable for EVAR. The 30-day mortality following EVAR was also lower at 23.5 % vs. 50 %, although this narrowly missed reaching statistical significance.

Several interesting points were raised by this study. By 2005, the ability to perform bifurcated EVAR under local anesthetic was well established, and the authors confirmed that their own experience had begun with bifurcated grafts. Their use of AUI followed a change in practice for those patients requiring extremely quick hemorrhage control or those with complex anatomy. They noted that the need for crossover grafts necessitated a conversion to general anesthesia after aneurysm sealing, with associated additional risks and often prolonging surgery beyond that of bifurcated stents.

Attempts to run randomized studies followed soon after. The Nottingham-based pilot study comparing AUI (two-part Gianturco stents with uncovered suprarenal component) with OR was designed to include a cohort who were considered fit for either form of repair in an attempt to reduce patient selection bias [66]. Their technique allowed for the initial procedure to be performed under local anesthetic, after which patients were fully anesthetized prior to stent deployment (Fig. 13.18). This followed experiences with severe ischemic pain from the occluded limb. The contralateral iliac artery was occluded with the Zip plug (Cook Europe, Copenhagen, Denmark or Endomed, Arizona, USA). In total, 103 patients were admitted with suspected ruptured AAA, but selection criteria meant that only 11 completed AUI and 12 OR. Results were similar for both in terms of complication rates, median hospital stay, and time from admission to surgery. The authors expressed disappointment that AUI didn't seem to confer significant improvement. However, their success in piloting one of the first pragmatic randomized trials for management of rAAA was laudable.

The BiFab study investigated the use of a modular AUI stent graft using off-the-shelf stock of four body and four limb sizes (compared to over 600 various components making up bifurcated kits) [69]. Sixty-five patients presenting with either symptomatic or ruptured infrarenal AAA were recruited from seven European centers [69]. Aneurysm exclusion was complete in a median time of 40 min, with a blood loss of only 200–800 ml. Despite this, perioperative mortality remained high at 40 %, and overall procedure time was longer than reported times for bifurcated grafts. The authors highlighted that other techniques such as aortic balloon occlusion allow for more rapid hemostatic control, after which there is more time for either technique to be used. They also encountered several operator-specific complications such as overstenting of the renal arteries and catching of the graft on the sheath, although this did not appear to translate to increased need for reintervention at 1-year follow-up.

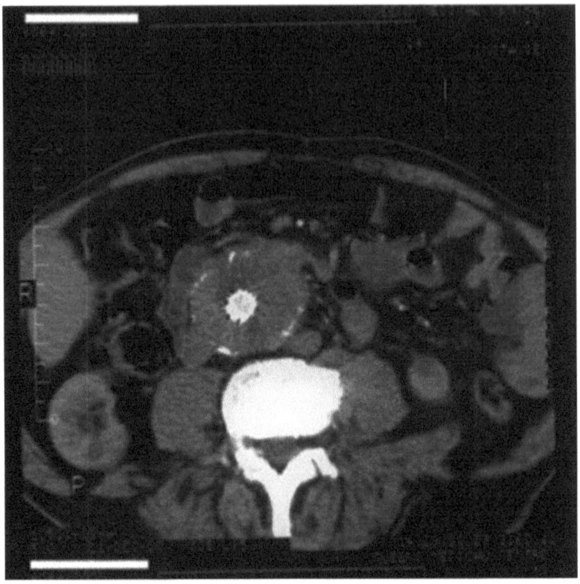

Fig. 13.18 Successfully excluded rAAA with AUI [65]

Other trials comparing EVAR with OR in rAAA included both bifurcated grafts and AUI, which indicated the direction of trends for endovascular repair. The French ERA trial included 150 patients in its EVAR arm, with a variety of procedures and grafts used [61], although the trial did not demonstrate any significant differences between EVAR and OR even for EVAR patients stratified as low or intermediate risk for OR.

Another earlier multicenter study evaluating outcomes in 26 patients undergoing EVAR vs. 29 undergoing OR demonstrated a similar 30-day mortality and complication rate, a pattern that persisted to 1 year [81]. These authors specifically stated a preference for bifurcated grafts, unless anatomy dictated an AUI, and this only applied to one out of 26 patients.

Despite the clear rise in user preference for bifurcated grafts as first-line EVAR in ruptures, European trials testing various AUI devices for rAAA continued. The ERA trial enrolled 100 consecutive patients across 10 institutions (49 AUI and 51 OR) [74]. As in previous trials, authors commented that there was no difference between preoperative comorbidity and hemodynamic status between the two groups, to refute any suggestion of selection bias. As with previous studies, AUI led to less blood loss and shorter duration of stay in intensive care. Despite this, differences in in-hospital/30-day mortality (35 and 39 % respectively) and 3-month mortality (40 % and 42 % respectively) were equivocal. One of the significant findings of the study was the fact that AUI was suitable in at least 50 % of patients presenting with rAAA. The Amsterdam Acute Aneurysm Trial collaborators, in another randomized control trial, reported a 30-day mortality of 21 % for AUI and only 25 % for OR [75]. Although there still didn't appear to be a significant difference between the two surgical modalities, relative improvements in early outcomes following all ruptures demonstrated the benefits of dedicated vascular centers providing a 24-h endovascular and specialist vascular service.

The more recent IMPROVE trial confirmed these ongoing short-term improvements in outcome, but did not report on differences in results between patients having AUI and bifurcated grafts [65].

Bifurcated Grafts Versus the AUI

There are few studies directly comparing results of bifurcated and AUI grafts, perhaps due to the now clear preference for the bifurcated graft among endovascular specialists. The benefits of AUI, namely, quicker exclusion of the aneurysm sac, often led to its use in more unstable patients with unfavorable anatomy, thus skewing results and deterring surgeons from using it as a first-line graft. Carrafiello observed higher mortality following AUI for rAAA, but also demonstrated that poor hemodynamic state had the greatest negative effect on survival and suggested that AUI was used preferentially in this group to get rapid hemostasis [61].

Results from the ENGAGE registry looking at outcomes for elective AAA reviewed outcomes in 1172 patents, in which only 7.1 % were treated with AUI [78]. The authors noted a higher rate of cardiopulmonary disease in the AUI group, with increased frequency of postoperative complications and longer hospital stays. Despite this, at 30 days and 1 year, the incidence of reintervention and all-cause mortality was equivalent between the two groups.

Conclusion

The global success of EVAR following its initial incarnation cannot be overestimated. The AUI technique paved the way for successful treatment of a cohort previously considered inoperable. However, with the development and continued improvements of bifurcated devices, along with increasing endovascular skills, AUI has fallen from favor. This largely relates to the need for a crossover grafts rather than concerns about the AUI device in isolation. Although AUI has evolved into the variety of bifurcated grafts now available, it still plays a significant role in the treatment of anatomically challenging AAA and for patients requiring speedy aneurysm exclusion. Its use in rAAA has been successfully explored and championed by the European vascular surgery community. Many still maintain a stock AUI on the shelf, available as part of their endovascular armamentarium.

Physician-Modified Endovascular Grafts for Treating Ruptured Abdominal Aortic Aneurysms

Benjamin W. Starnes

Key Points

- Physician-modified endovascular grafts have been successfully used to treat patients presenting with rAAA who are not candidates for standard EVAR.
- These procedures are off-label in nature and require the umbrella of an FDA-approved investigational device exemption (IDE) clinical trial in order to be reimbursed.
- These grafts may be manufactured prior to the arrival of the patient from the transferring facility.

Introduction

The purpose of this chapter is to introduce the concept of custom fenestrated EVAR for managing ruptured abdominal aortic aneurysms (rAAA). Fenestrated endovascular repair was first performed in 1999 by the late John L. Anderson of Adelaide, Australia, and involves the preoperative placement of "fenestra" or windows, in precise locations on an endograft in order to treat juxtarenal AAA [88]. Currently in the United States, there is only one manufacturer of an FDA-approved fenestrated endograft, and these custom-designed grafts require a minimum of 4 weeks to arrive at the implanting facility after the graft has been meticulously planned and the order has been placed. Thus, many believe that custom-designed devices cannot be used in a rupture situation. We will demonstrate that this is not true.

Vascular surgeons have long been known to innovate to meet the needs of their patients. At the University of Washington, we initiated a protocol for managing rAAA with an endovascular first strategy in 2007 and reduced our 30-day mortality from 58 to 32 % overall with those patients harboring anatomy suitable for EVAR experiencing an 18 % mortality risk at 30 days [89]. We quickly learned that reasons for ineligibility for EVAR revolved around inadequate, often short, infrarenal aortic necks. We thus began customizing our own devices in an off-label fashion to create single, double, and even triple fenestration endografts to treat this subset of patients who could not wait the lengthy duration to receive the custom-made graft and/or were too sick to undergo open repair [90, 91]. In this chapter, we describe the technique of physician-modified endografting to treat asymptomatic, symptomatic, or even ruptured AAA.

Technique

Device Preparation

All operative procedures are performed concurrently with back table device modification while the patient is being prepared for surgery. In urgent situations, temporary aortic balloon occlusion can be performed to bide time, especially with single and double fenestration cases where graft manufacture time is less than 30 min. The device is chosen according to standard instructions for use in sizing guidelines, and a routine aortic oversizing of 10–15 % for the main body graft is utilized. The bifurcated graft is unsheathed on a separate table, and a sterile marking pen is used to mark the location of the fenestrations based on both length and clock face and arc-length measurements that had been previously determined with reconstruction imaging software. Minor adjustments are made in localization of the fenestrations to allow for maximum usage of strut-free fenestrations when possible. When this is not possible and multiple fenestrations are required, struts within fenestrations are preferentially avoided for the renal arteries. An ophthalmic Bovie cautery device (Medtronic, Minneapolis, Minn) is used to carefully burn the Dacron fabric to create all fenestrations and thus avoid fabric fraying and allow for heat sealing. Gold, 15-mm Amplatz Gooseneck Snares (EV3 Endovascular Inc., Plymouth, Minn) are then used to reinforce all fenestrations. These are handsewn into place using 4-0 Prolene suture in a 720° running fashion (Fig. 13.19). A typical final PMEG device is depicted in Fig. 13.20.

When time permits, diameter-reducing ties are then used to constrain the device along its posterior border (opposite the superior mesenteric artery [SMA] and/or celiac fenestration at 6 o'clock) by rerouting the existing proximal trigger wire through and through the graft material at the midportion of each of the top two Z stents. This is facilitated using a micropuncture needle from inside the graft. The constraining ties are then tied down into place over the trigger wire. The bare stent is then reconstrained in the top cap, and the entire graft wetted with heparinized saline and then reloaded into the existing sheath.

PMEG Procedural Details

The majority of these procedures are performed in a modern hybrid operating room utilizing a Siemens Artis Q Zeego System (Siemens, Munich, Germany). Common femoral access is almost always achieved in a standard percutaneous fashion and the stent graft delivered up into position near the visceral vessels. A contrast aortogram with 20 mL of dilute contrast injected at 10 mL/s is performed with the PMEG in place to mark the visceral vessels (Fig. 13.21). Proper orientation of the graft (SMA anterior) is confirmed by rotating the graft clockwise under fluoroscopy and

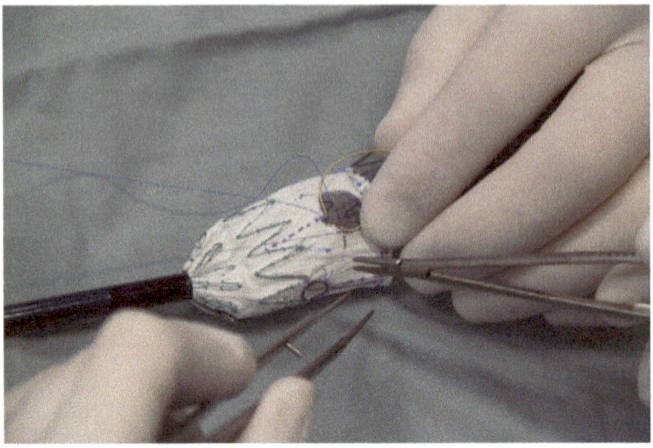

Fig. 13.19 Gold, 15-mm Amplatz Gooseneck Snares (EV3, Plymouth, Minn) were then used to reinforce all fenestrations. These were handsewn into place using 4-0 Prolene suture in a 720° running fashion

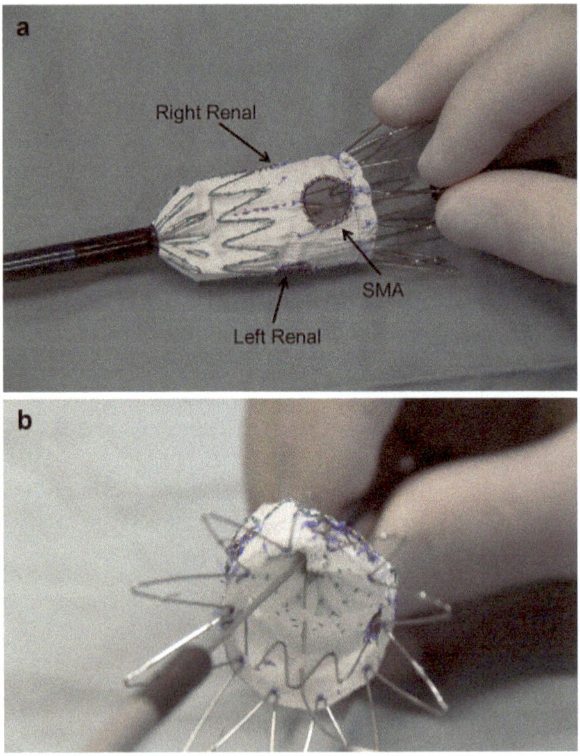

Fig. 13.20 A typical physician-modified endovascular graft (PMEG) prior to device repackaging (**a**). Fenestrations for the superior mesenteric artery (*SMA*) (*struts present*) and left and right renal arteries (*strut-free*) were created for this particular patient. (**b**) Rerouting of the trigger wire to allow for placement of graft constraining ties

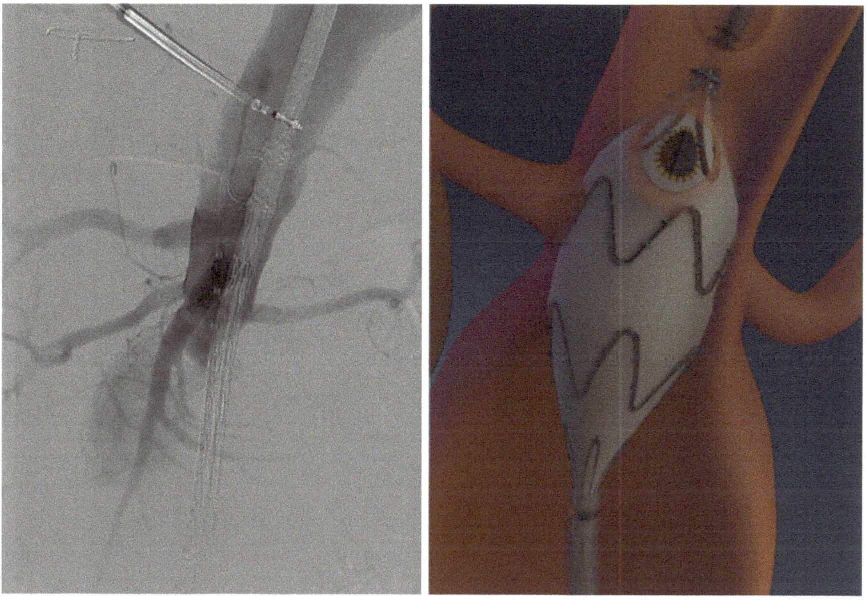

Fig. 13.21 Contrast aortography and cartoon demonstrating the origins of all four visceral vessels with the physician-modified endovascular graft (PMEG) device in situ prior to and after deployment

confirming that the SMA fenestration moves from left to right instead of right to left, which would denote a posterior orientation of the SMA fenestration (Fig. 13.22). The graft is then carefully deployed down to the opening of the contralateral limb. The contralateral limb is then selected, and, typically, an 18–20 Fr DrySeal sheath (W.L. Gore, Flagstaff, AZ) is inserted into the contralateral limb over a stiff wire under direct fluoroscopic visualization. It is important to hub the DrySeal sheath to create a stable working platform. Double 6 or 7 Fr Ansel sheaths (Cook Inc.) are used directly through the end of the DrySeal sheath to individually select the renal arteries while maintaining stability of the PMEG device. Once the renal arteries are completely selected with each 6 or 7 Fr sheath, diameter-reducing ties are freed by pulling the proximal trigger wire out, and then the top cap is released and the main body deployed. At this time, the remainder of the main body device is deployed, the top cap is retrieved, and a CODA balloon (Cook Inc.) is used to seat the proximal portion of the graft in the zone of the visceral aortic stent graft segment (Fig. 13.23). The renal arteries are then individually stented with appropriately sized iCAST stents (Atrium USA, Hudson, NH), and the stents are flared proximally into the aortic stent graft using 9–12 mm standard angioplasty balloons (Fig. 13.24). The remainder of the procedure involves standard placement of docking limbs to the level of each iliac bifurcation and seating of the stent graft overlap and seal zones with a molding balloon (CODA, Cook Inc.). A completion aortogram is performed at the completion of each procedure (Fig. 13.25).

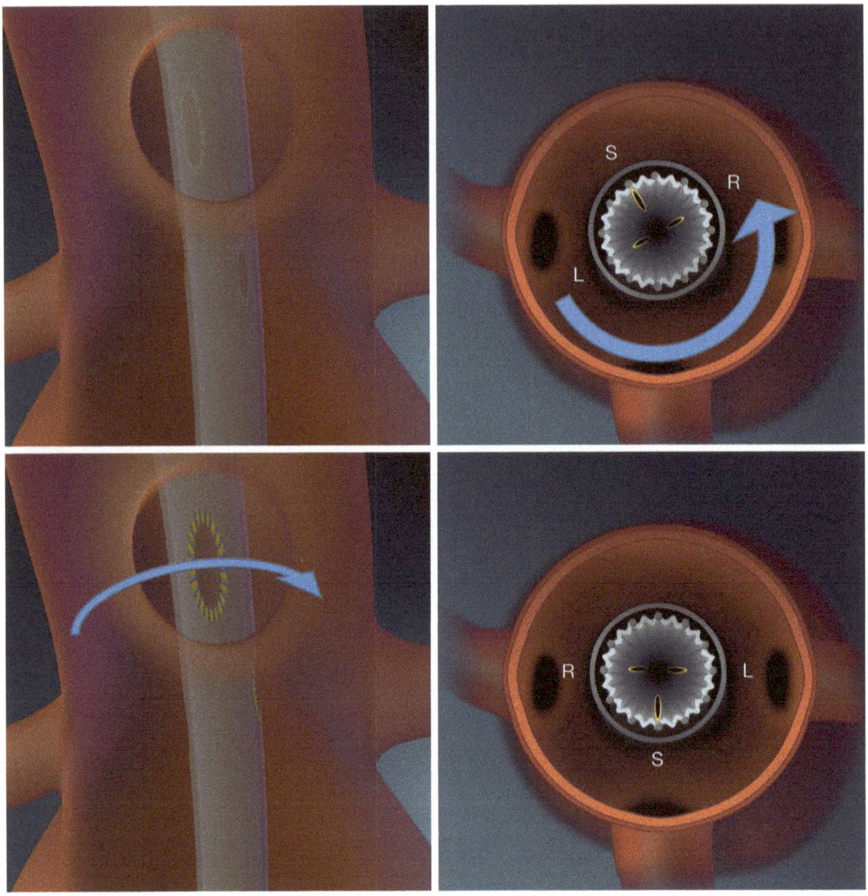

Fig. 13.22 Proper orientation of the graft is confirmed by rotation of the graft clockwise and viewing the SMA fenestration move from left to right on the screen

Other devices from other manufacturers have been successfully modified to include Medtronic Endurant (Medtronic, Minneapolis, MN), Bolton Relay (Bolton, Sunrise, FL), and Gore Excluder (W.L. Gore, Flagstaff, AZ). It is important to know how to successfully reload each of these devices prior to embarking on a surgeon-modified repair of a ruptured abdominal aortic aneurysm.

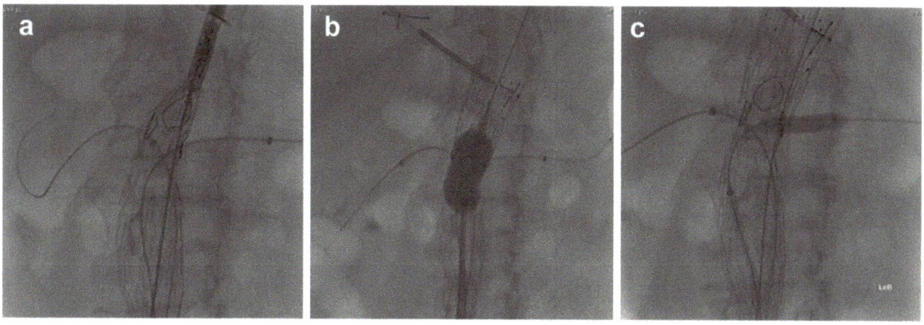

Fig. 13.23 Physician-modified endovascular graft (PMEG) procedure. (**a**) Both renal arteries have been selected through the renal fenestrations and a sheath advanced into the left renal artery. (**b**) Seating of the proximal graft with the renal sheaths securely in place. (**c**) Stent grafting and subsequent flaring of the renal artery stents

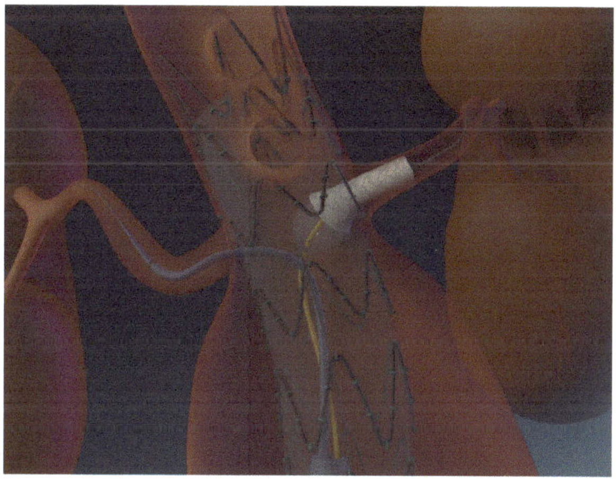

Fig. 13.24 Flaring of the renal stents with appropriately oversized balloons

Conclusions

Custom-designed and manufactured devices can be used to successfully repair ruptured abdominal aortic aneurysms. In the future, more patients harboring ruptured abdominal aortic aneurysms will benefit from technological improvements and a "kit" type of off-the-shelf tools and devices to personalize therapy for each patient.

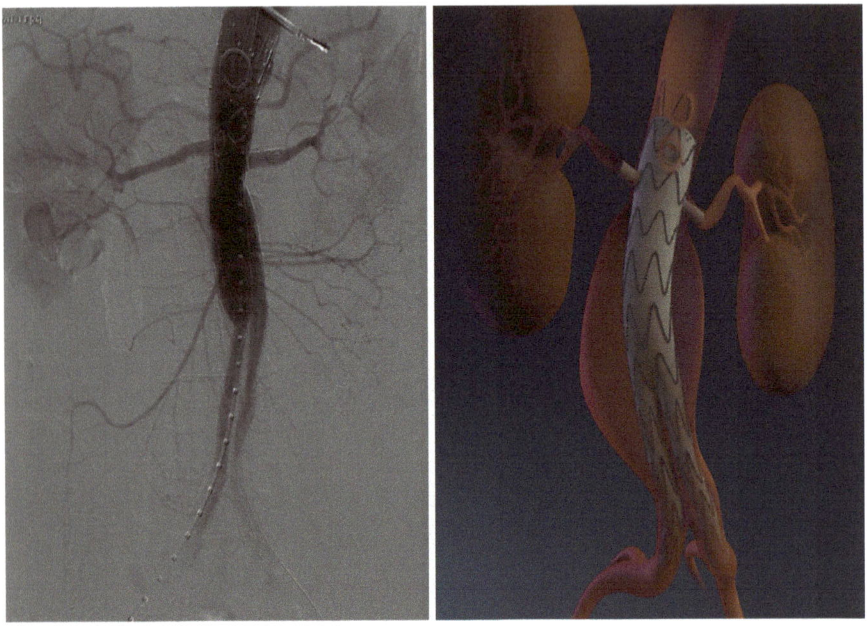

Fig. 13.25 Completion aortogram and cartoon demonstrating absence of endoleak and good alignment of all three visceral vessel fenestrations

Endovascular Aneurysm Sealing for Ruptured Abdominal Aortic Aneurysm

Andrew Holden

Key Points

- Endovascular aneurysm sealing can potentially treat a broad range of ruptured abdominal aortic aneurysms with minimal inventory
- Full aneurysm sealing with endobags provides rapid tamponade of bleeding as well as minimizing the risk of endoleak
- The procedure is still in evolution and more experience is required

Introduction

The concept of endovascular aneurysm sealing has been developed in recent years to address some of the recognized deficiencies of conventional endovascular aneurysm repair (EVAR) for abdominal aortic aneurysm (AAA). Endovascular aneurysm sealing

(EVAS) using the Nellix® endovascular system (Endologix, Irvine, CA, USA) seals the entire aneurysm sac with polymer-filled endobags. This sac sealing strategy has the potential to significantly reduce the incidence of endoleak, migration, and reintervention. Early clinical data are encouraging in the elective AAA setting [92–94].

The role of EVAR in the ruptured AAA (rAAA) setting is extensively discussed elsewhere in this publication. Most publications to date have failed to show an early survival advantage for EVAR over open surgical repair [95–98]. However, recent publications have shown a consistent but nonsignificant trend for lower mortality for EVAR [99] as well as faster hospital discharge and better quality of life [100]. There are number of potential advantages and limitations in using Nellix® EVAS in the rAAA setting – these will be discussed as well as a review of the limited evidence currently available.

Nellix® EVAS Procedure

The Nellix® EVAS procedure in the elective AAA repair setting has been previously described [94, 101]. Each Nellix® device consists of a chromium cobalt balloon expandable stent, covered in expanded polytetrafluoroethylene (ePTFE) and surrounded by a polyurethane endobag. The stents are mounted on 10 mm diameter minimally compliant angioplasty balloons. Devices are introduced from each common femoral artery. Device lengths are selected to land immediately below the lowermost renal artery and above the iliac artery bifurcation on each side. The stents are deployed at the same infrarenal level proximally, and the angioplasty balloons are usually then deflated to maintain perfusion to the lower body. The endobags are "prefilled" with saline via endobag fill tubes, usually until a pressure within the endobags of 180 mmHg is reached. The endobag fill pressure is sufficiently above the patient's systolic pressure to allow complete displacement of the blood lumen in the aneurysm sac and proximal and distal sealing zones without risking arterial injury. Angiography is possible through the nose cone of the Nellix® delivery system, and this is performed to confirm aneurysm exclusion. The prefill step provides an accurate estimate of polymer fill volume and assesses device stability during endobag filling. There is also some ability to reposition the stents after the prefilled saline has been aspirated. After saline aspiration, the endobags are filled with a matching volume of polymer until a fill pressure of at least 180 mmHg is reached. The polymer is a polyethylene glycol (PEG) diacrylate, provided in a two-part solution that cross-links or cures when mixed in 3–5 min to form a solid hydrogel. While the hydrogel is curing, the angioplasty balloons are inflated to maintain a smooth blood flow lumen. Completion nose cone angiography is used to confirm complete aneurysm seal. If there are any concerns regarding complete seal, a secondary polymer fill via an outer endobag fill tube is possible. The final repair consists of two covered stent flow lumens to maintain perfusion to the pelvis and lower limbs as well as endobags that both fixate and seal the aneurysm, minimizing the risk of endoleak or migration (Fig. 13.26).

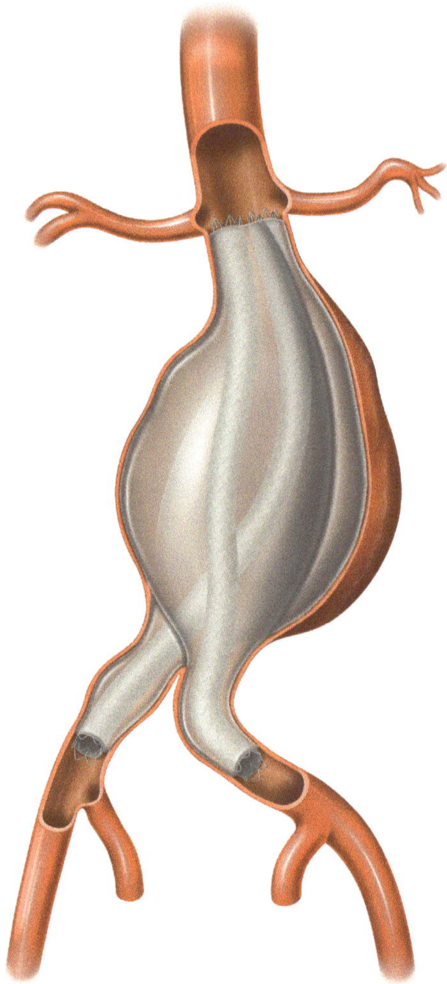

Fig. 13.26 The Nellix® endovascular system. Note the paired covered stents with surrounding endobags that seal the entire aneurysm sac (Image courtesy of Endologix Inc.)

There are some significant alterations to the standard Nellix® EVAS procedure in the rAAA setting [102–104]. As with many EVAR cases performed in the rAAA setting, Nellix® EVAS cases have often been performed under local anesthesia with permissive hypotension (Fig. 13.27). Percutaneous femoral artery access is usually obtained with the low profile (17 F OD) and hydrophilic coating of the delivery system being advantageous. Once the devices are introduced and positioned, the stents are deployed. The angioplasty balloons may be left inflated during the procedure – this can improve device stability in challenging anatomy but may also provide some reduction in flow to the aneurysm rupture site. In rAAA cases, it is common to add iodinated contrast to the saline used to prefill the endobags (usually 20–30 % contrast). This allows direct fluoroscopic visualization of the endobags as they fill. Because the aortic wall is not intact within the aneurysm, the endobags

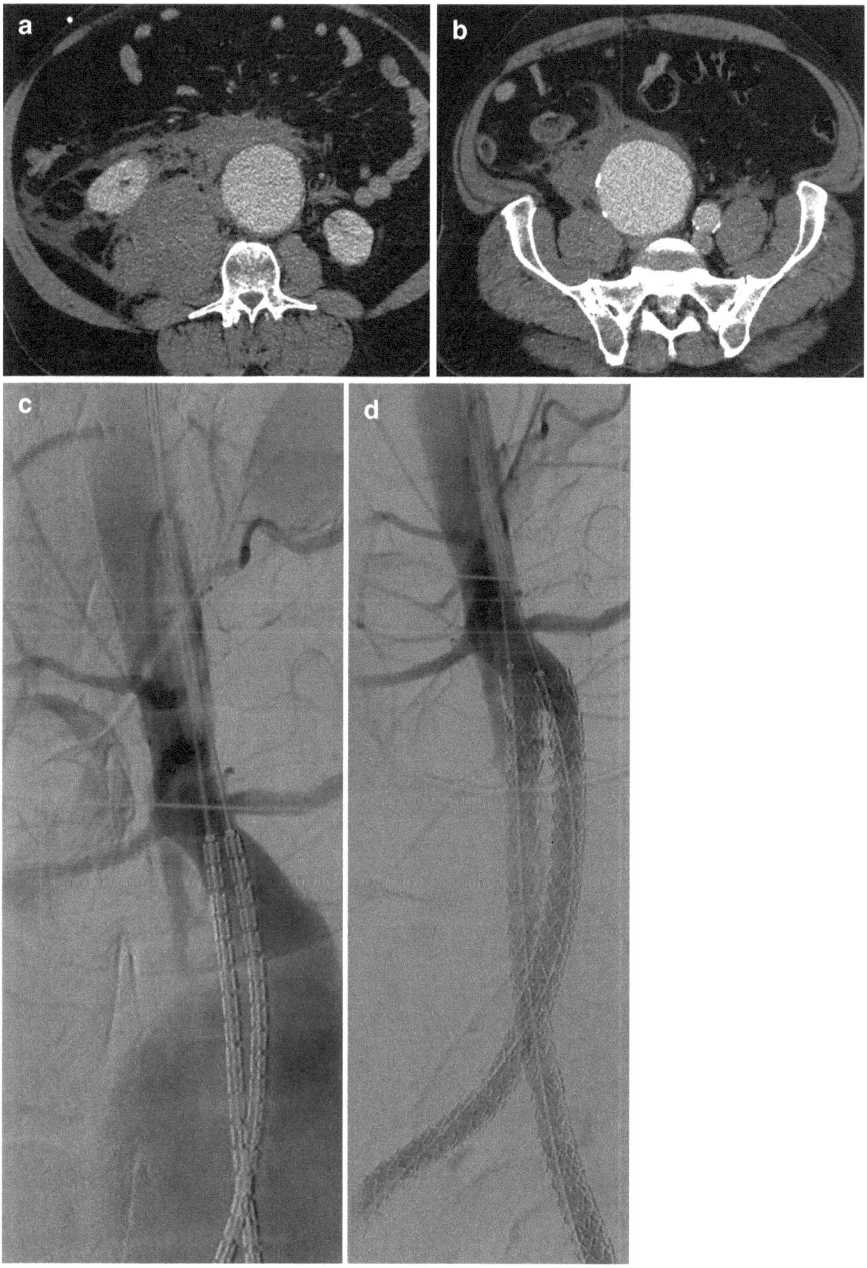

Fig. 13.27 Treatment of an rAAA with the Nellix® endovascular system. (**a**) Ruptured AAA. (**b**) Concomitant right common iliac artery aneurysm in the same patient. (**c**) Positioning of the Nellix stents in the infrarenal aortic neck. (**d**) Completion angiography after EVAS showing complete exclusion of the aneurysm. (**e**) Follow-up CT showing exclusion of both abdominal and iliac artery aneurysms. A covered stent was used to extend into the right external iliac artery

Fig. 13.27 Continued

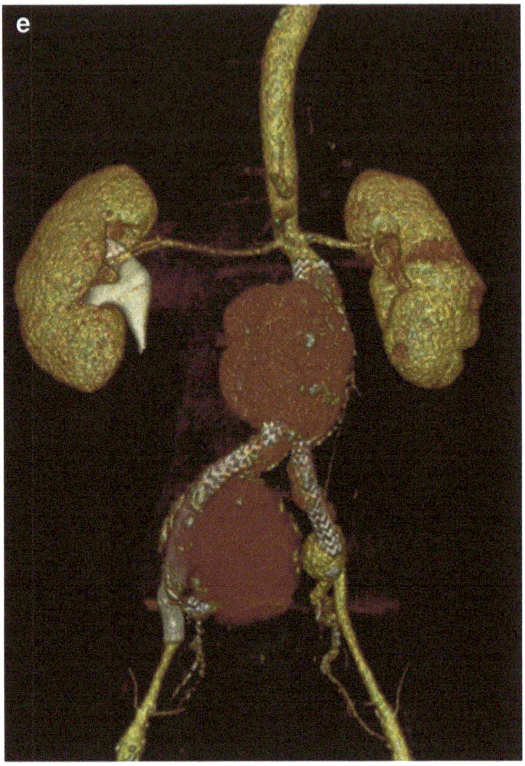

may bulge through the aortic defect, and the usual pressure threshold of 180 mmHg may not be reached. Prefill is halted if focal endobag bulging is observed or endobag pressure reaches 180 mmHg and angiography performed to confirm aneurysm exclusion. The saline is then aspirated and rapidly replaced with the same volume of polymer. Completion angiography is again performed. If there is any ongoing perfusion of the aneurysm, secondary fill can be performed via outer fill tubes. A secondary prefill can be performed with dilute contrast to confirm the endobags are filling in the sealing zones. This can then be aspirated and exchanged for more polymer to achieve an optimized aneurysm seal.

In both elective and ruptured aneurysm treatment with Nellix, parallel grafts can be used in the renal and mesenteric arteries to improve seal [102, 105, 106]. This allows the Nellix devices to be deployed more proximally in the aorta and is important in patients with hostile infrarenal neck anatomy. However, chimney Nellix EVAS does involve increased procedural time and complexity as well as upper limb arterial access for the parallel grafts. It has been reported that parallel graft techniques can also positively impact on the technical success of EVAR in rAAA [107].

Imaging Surveillance After Nellix® EVAS Procedure

The components of the Nellix device are well visualized on post-procedural CT, including the endobags and stents. A periaortic hematoma is typically seen on early postoperative studies, but this usually resolves with time (Fig. 13.28).

Advantages of Nellix® EVAS in rAAA

The potential advantages of Nellix EVAS over conventional EVAR when treating ruptured AAAs are listed in Table 13.2. EVAS appears to be able to treat a wider range of patient anatomies than EVAR while still remaining within company instructions for use [108]. Cases are simple to plan as all Nellix stents are 10 mm in diameter with the current length range from 100 to 180 mm at 10 mm increments. If a pre-procedural CT is performed, the infrarenal aortic and common iliac artery lengths are all that are required to facilitate device selection. Inventory is limited to

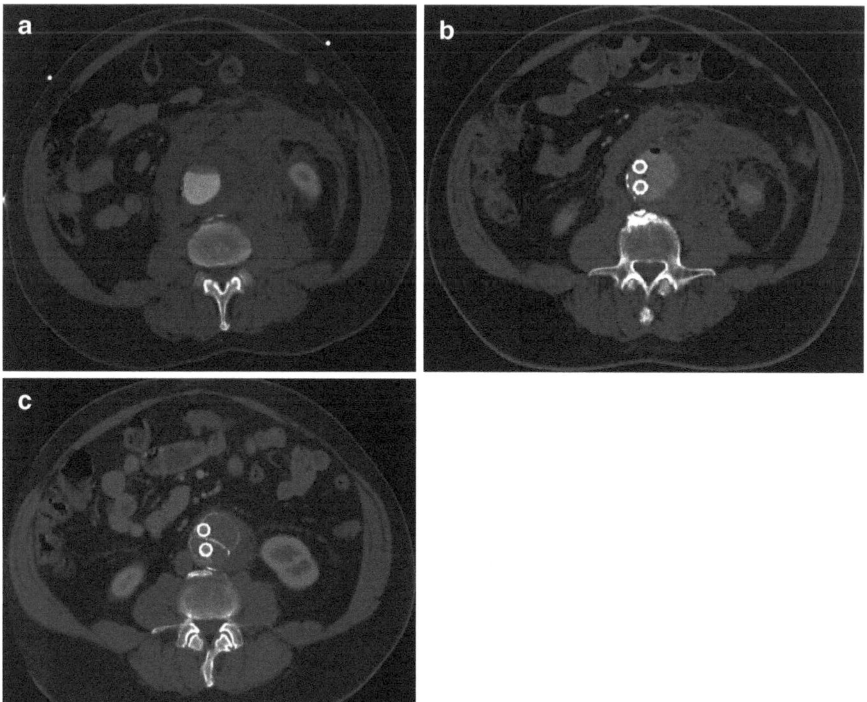

Fig. 13.28 Follow-up after repair of a rAAA with the Nellix® endovascular system. (**a**) Ruptured AAA with large retroperitoneal hematoma. (**b**) CT performed after Nellix EVAS showing the endobags filled with polymer including low-density contrast. Flow is present in the Nellix stent lumens. (**c**) CT at 6 months after EVAS repair showing resolution of the retroperitoneal hematoma

Table 13.2 Potential advantages of Nellix EVAS in rAAAs

Ability to treat a wider range of aortic anatomies
Simplicity of procedural planning
Limited inventory to be held to provide a ruptured aneurysm EVAS service
Procedural simplicity
Early tamponade of the rupture by prefilling the endobags
Prevention of type 2 endoleaks

treat a wide range of patients, and this means it is a viable proposition for many institutions to carry sufficient inventory to offer a ruptured AAA EVAS service.

The procedure is simple without the need for cannulation of an endograft contralateral short limb. Procedural times have been relatively short and predictable [94]. Prefill of the endobags with saline provides rapid tamponade of the aneurysm and hemodynamic stability without the need for a temporary aortic occlusion balloon. While rapid endovascular balloon occlusion (REBO) is an important adjunct to EVAR in unstable rAAA patients [109], this procedural does add complexity and the potential for complications [110]. Nellix EVAS has demonstrated effectiveness at preventing endoleaks, especially type 2 endoleaks [92, 94]. Following ruptured AAA repair with EVAR, persistent type 2 endoleaks may produce ongoing retroperitoneal bleeding [111]. This can be avoided by complete aneurysm sealing.

Disadvantages of Nellix® EVAS in rAAA

There are potential disadvantages in using Nellix EVAS to treat ruptured aneurysms. As previously discussed, the endobag may not be constrained by the aneurysm wall in the area of rupture and even bulge through the wall defect. In this situation, normal endobag fill pressure may not be achieved and the endobag may aggravate the aortic wall injury. The lack of constraint could also result in incomplete endobag sealing with an endoleak. Fortunately, in the limited experience to date, this scenario appears uncommon with both endobag prefill and polymer fill occurring in an identical manner to elective aneurysm repair. It should be noted that some bulging of the endobag through an aortic defect may not be of any hemodynamic significance because the aneurysm is excluded.

Evidence Behind Nellix® EVAS in rAAA

The available evidence to date is limited to case reports and limited single-center series [102–104]. There were some ruptured aneurysms treated in the Global FORWARD EVAS Registry, but these cases have not been fully analyzed. In most reported cases, aneurysm morphology was outside of instructions for use guidelines for current EVAR devices and also Nellix EVAS. Despite this, the rate of technical success has been high. In almost all cases, endobag filling has been identical to elective repair with no problems reaching endobag fill pressures of at least 180 mmHg. However, much more experience is required to understand the real potential of this exciting new technique.

Conclusions

Endovascular aneurysm sealing (EVAS) using the Nellix® endovascular system for ruptured abdominal aortic aneurysms offers potential advantages over conventional EVAR including an ability to treat a broader range of aortic anatomies with a limited product inventory. Hemodynamic stability can be achieved quickly by the filling of endobags, and resultant endoleaks appear to be very uncommon. However, experience is still limited and the optimum EVAS technique is still to be defined.

Aortocaval Fistula

Kaj H. Johansen

Background

The vast majority of aortic aneurysms rupture into the surrounding retroperitoneum or, uncommonly, directly into the peritoneal cavity, thus automatically constituting a surgical emergency. However, on rare occasions, an aortic aneurysm may erode into surrounding venous structures, most commonly the inferior vena cava, thereby forming an *aortocaval fistula*. Preoperative recognition of this rare entity may be problematic: unlike the abdominal, flank, or back pain and cardiovascular collapse that almost always attend the "usual" presentation of aneurysm rupture, patients with an aortocaval fistula may display delayed or subtle symptomatology or sometimes none at all.

Epidemiology

Aortocaval fistula is extremely rare, historically often becoming evident only at open operation for aneurysm repair or at postmortem examination. Accordingly, an accurate assessment of its prevalence has been relatively unavailable. It is thought to accompany aortic aneurysm in 0.3–1 % of cases: it appears to be more common – 2 to 3 % of cases – when patients present with aortic aneurysmal rupture. Because in contemporary practice, the overwhelming majority of aneurysm patients are managed by endovascular means, an intrinsic diagnostic component of which includes ultrasound, CT, MR, or aortographic imaging of the aneurysm, an accurate determination of the prevalence of aortocaval fistula associated with abdominal aortic aneurysm should now be possible. Perhaps as a more useful guide, during the author's 40-year vascular surgical career (of which a substantial part has been devoted to the open management of aortic aneurysms), he has managed only four patients with an aortocaval fistula.

Risk factors for the development of aortocaval fistula include not only the presence of a contiguous aortic aneurysm but marked aneurysm sac enlargement as well: in one series of patients with an aortocaval fistula, the average aneurysm diameter was 11 cm [112]. Upon extremely rare occasions, mycotic aortic aneurysmal infection may be associated with aortocaval fistula development [113]. An aortocaval communication may develop in the absence of an aortic aneurysm, usually on a congenital basis [114] or due to penetrating trauma [115]: iatrogenic injury resulting in an aortocaval communication, most notoriously during lumbar discectomy [116], has occurred. These scenarios are extremely rare and discussion of them is beyond the scope of this chapter.

Anatomy and Pathophysiology

Erosion of an aortic aneurysm into the inferior vena cava is facilitated, of course, by the fact that the two vessels are contiguous in the upper retroperitoneal midline. As a consequence, an aortocaval fistula will generally be located in the right posterolateral aspect of the aneurysm sac. And, as also noted, increased aneurysm diameter, signifying greater compression of the nearby vena cava, and for a longer period of time, is associated with a higher likelihood of fistula formation [112]. A few cases of erosion of an aortic aneurysm into the left renal vein, almost always when it is in a retroaortic position, have been reported [117]. Erosion of an aortoiliac aneurysm into a common iliac vein has also been reported [118]. The pathophysiology and clinical presentation in such circumstances does not otherwise differ from a "standard" aortocaval fistula].

As noted above, certain aortocaval fistulas may be asymptomatic and thus an unexpected finding at the time of aneurysm imaging (Fig. 13.29) or open repair. In other circumstances, patients may present with symptoms consistent with what is, in essence, a large central arteriovenous fistula resulting in increased cardiac preload and high-output physiology, i.e., elevated cardiac output, an increased pulse pressure, diminished peripheral resistance, and tachycardia.

Because aortic aneurysms almost always occur in the context of advanced age and, not infrequently, chronic cardiac dysfunction, the resultant increase in cardiac preload associated with a large aortocaval fistula often results in high-output congestive heart failure, upon occasion lethal if not identified and treated urgently [119, 120]. The predictable onset of congestive heart failure following development of an aortocaval fistula has in fact resulted in a well-validated animal model for studying the pathophysiology of congestive heart failure [121].

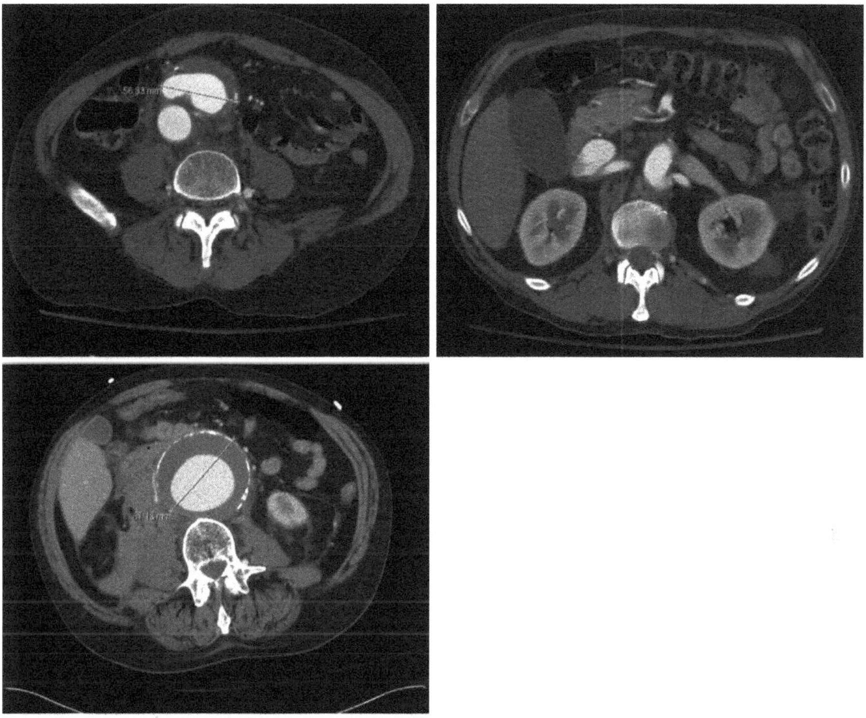

Fig. 13.29 Abdominal CTA shows contrast flow from the AAA lumen into a crescentic, mostly effaced IVC. Note substantially increased aneurysm diameter, a risk factor for the development of aortocaval fistula [112]

Clinical Presentation and Diagnosis

As noted, the essence of the presentation of an aortocaval fistula is the development of a large central arteriovenous fistula. Clinically, turbulent fistula flow may produce an audible epigastric bruit, and upon occasion, abdominal wall venous collaterals can be observed. Markedly elevated inferior vena caval pressures may result in lower body anasarca, and elevated renal venous pressures may be associated with hematuria [122]. The aortic aneurysm itself may be not only pulsatile, but a midabdominal thrill may be palpable.

Imaging studies will not uncommonly demonstrate evidence for a central arteriovenous communication, predominantly on the basis of early venous filling on CT scan (Fig. 13.30) or MRA [123, 124]. Retroperitoneal and/or abdominal wall venous collateral opacification may be evident. During duplex scanning of an aortic aneurysm, a focal high velocity signal on the right side of the aneurysm may be indicative of an aortocaval fistula [125, 126].

As previously noted, in contemporary practice, an aortocaval fistula will generally be identified during the detailed contrast-enhanced imaging that always attends endovascular aneurysm repair or upon aortography preparatory to EVAR placement (Fig. 13.31). Historically, an aortocaval fistula might only be

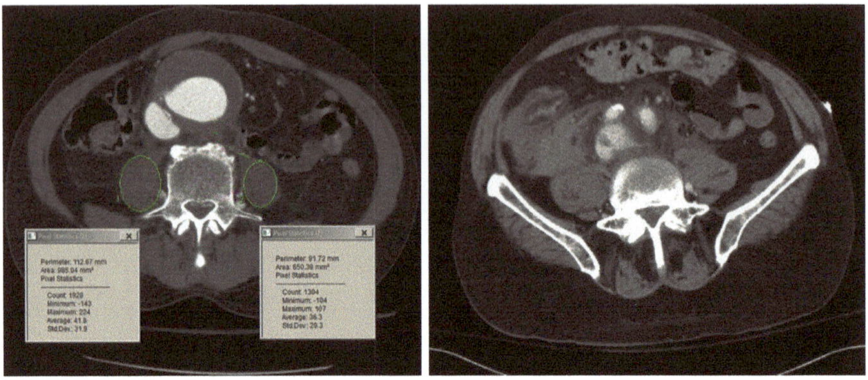

Fig. 13.30 Early venous filling, as seen in this abdominal CTA, is diagnostic of arteriovenous fistulization in general and aortocaval fistula in particular

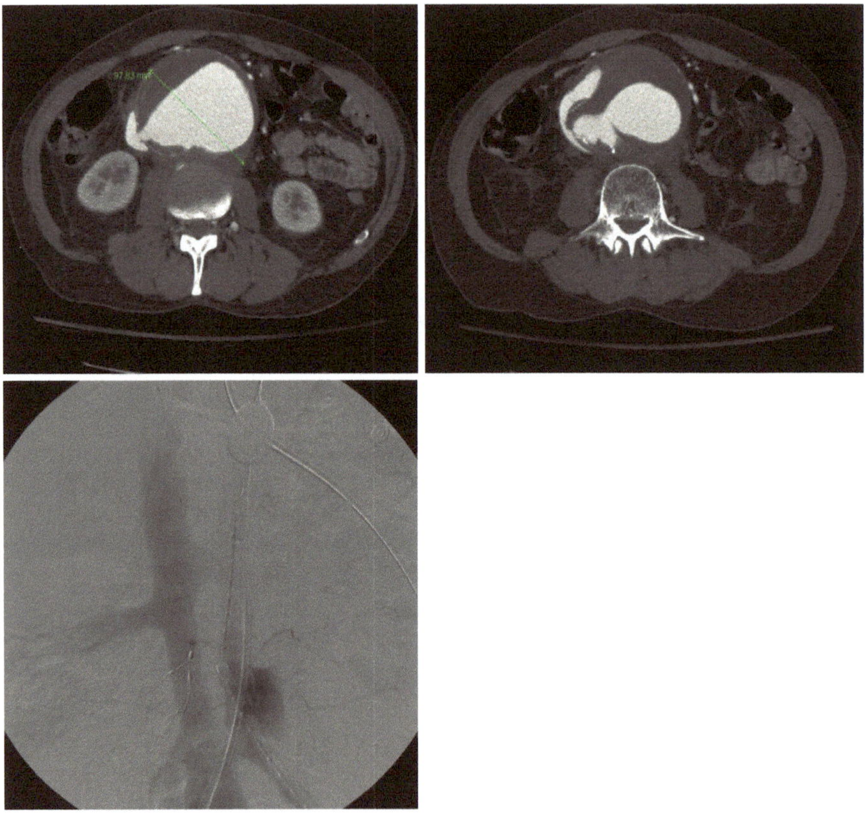

Fig. 13.31 Aortic aneurysm sac contrast injection preparatory to EVAR placement for ruptured AAA (Note aortic occlusion balloon) displays IVC opacification and "uncovers" a previously undiagnosed aortocaval fistula

diagnosed upon torrential venous bleeding occurring at the moment of incision of the aneurysm sac during open aneurysm repair.

Management

Aortocaval fistula, once developed, is a morbid and potentially lethal problem, predominantly because of its effect on central cardiopulmonary hemodynamics. Such patients are at elevated operative risk because of their cardiac dysfunction. If the diagnosis is made preoperatively, repair is urgent.

Currently, the vast majority of aortic aneurysms are repaired by percutaneous endovascular means. Endovascular stent graft (EVAR) decompression of the aortic aneurysm sac and resultant aneurysm sac thrombosis should be expected to halt any significant flow through the aortocaval fistula [127, 128]. The presence of any one of the various types of post-EVAR endoleak might be expected to result in persistent aortocaval fistula flow; successful endoleak management generally should be curative, although upon unusual occasions, covered stent placement within the inferior vena cava to halt flow through a persistent aortocaval fistula has been required [129].

Open repair of aortic aneurysm is now uncommonly performed, usually obligated because of perirenal aortic "neck" anatomy deemed unfavorable for EVAR. Accordingly, only a vanishingly small number of aneurysms complicated by aortocaval fistula will be managed by open techniques. If such an uncommon circumstance presents itself, the dilemma is that what was initially an elective (or, at worst, urgent) open aneurysm repair may be converted, at the time the aneurysm sac is opened, into potentially catastrophic venous back bleeding from the uncontrolled inferior vena cava. Optimal operative strategy at the time should include the use of an autotransfuser, digital, and/or sponge-stick control of venous bleeding (if the fistula has been diagnosed preoperatively, positioning of a large occlusion balloon in the inferior vena cava may provide substantial hemostatic control [130], avoidance of attempts to dissect and control the friable inferior vena cava, and fistula closure with large deep monofilament suture bites of the site of venous back bleeding [131]). Care must be taken at this time that mural thrombus from within the aneurysm sac not be translocated into the inferior vena cava, whence it might then embolize into the pulmonary circulation [132].

Patients who have had a long-standing aortocaval fistula may require careful postoperative volume management, since the excess extracellular volume they have accumulated will need to be cleared via the kidneys and heart which have been in varying degrees of failure for weeks or months. Aggressive dialysis or CRRT may be required.

Outcomes

A large majority of patients with aortic aneurysm associated with an aortocaval fistula should achieve satisfactory management of this problem following EVAR placement, and if the original aortocaval fistula was small, it may well not even be evident that it has been repaired. A substantial proportion of patients so managed should experience improved cardiopulmonary and renal function after repair of the aortocaval fistula because such treatment has resolved the patient's preexisting central arteriovenous fistula and its resulting hyperdynamic, hypervolemic state [133].

Dealing with Ruptured Common Iliac Artery Aneurysms

Matthew J. Eagleton and Jarrad Rowse

Introduction

Common iliac artery aneurysms can occur in isolation or in association with abdominal aortic aneurysms (AAA). Most asymptomatic iliac artery aneurysms are discovered incidentally as a result of the widespread use of abdominal ultrasonography and computed tomography (CT); however, their natural history remains largely ill-defined. Common iliac artery aneurysms are defined as greater than 1.85 cm in men and 1.5 cm in women with the rate of rupture increasing significantly once the aneurysms are greater than 3.0 cm [134, 135]. Endovascular repair has enabled a safer approach to elective surgery, but the rate of mortality with rupture of iliac artery aneurysms remains relatively high. In addition, the presence of an iliac artery aneurysm can alter the treatment algorithm for those patients presenting with an AAA. This may have even greater consequences if the patient presents with a ruptured AAA or a ruptured iliac artery aneurysm.

Incidence and Etiology

Iliac artery aneurysms are the most common aneurysm following aortic aneurysms; however, in isolation, they only constitute 2 % of all aneurysms with an estimated 0.05 % prevalence in the general population [136]. Common iliac artery aneurysms represent the majority (70–90 %) of isolated iliac artery aneurysms with the remainder being hypogastric artery aneurysms (10–30 %). External iliac artery aneurysms have been rarely reported in isolation, and they even more rarely present with rupture [137, 138]. Typically, iliac artery aneurysms are found in men in their seventh–eighth decade of life [134, 137]. Most iliac artery aneurysms are due to atherosclerotic degeneration and are associated with risk factors not unlike those seen in aortic aneurysms, in particular male gender, advanced age, white race, smoking history, and hypertension [139]. Less commonly, iliac artery aneurysms may be pseudoaneurysms secondary to penetrating trauma or from iatrogenic injury during pelvic, hip, or spine surgery [140, 141]. Less than 20 % are inflammatory aneurysms related to Behcet's disease or arise secondary to dissections, fibromuscular dysplasia, Takayasu's arteritis, other connective tissue disorders, or infection [137, 142].

Common iliac artery aneurysms are more commonly seen in conjunction with other aneurysms in particular abdominal aortic aneurysms (AAA). Fifteen to 40 % of common iliac artery aneurysms are associated with an AAA, and approximately half of common iliac artery aneurysms are bilateral. About two-thirds of patients with iliac artery aneurysms have involvement of more than one segment of the iliac artery tree [137]. It is not uncommon to observe a common iliac artery aneurysm with an associated hypogastric artery aneurysm, and in particular as these aneurysms progress in size, there is a tendency to involve the hypogastric artery [143].

Clinical Presentation

The clinical presentation of solitary common iliac artery aneurysms is quite variable and often obscure. While these aneurysms can present with vague lower abdominal and flank pain as the only symptom, approximately 50 % are incidentally found on pelvic imaging. The average size of CIAAs at diagnosis is between 4 and 5 cm, and as the aneurysm increases in size, the patient may describe urinary obstruction, pain on defecation secondary to rectal compression, paresthesias of the lower extremity owing to pelvic nerve compression, arterial thrombosis, emboli, and fistulae [137, 144]. Clinical signs of rupture include hypotension and abdominal, groin, or thigh pain. Retroperitoneal rupture may be contained, but intraperitoneal rupture can be catastrophic with eminent death [137, 143].

Rupture of an associated AAA can occur in up to 50 % of patients with an iliac artery aneurysm [135]. Rupture of the common iliac artery aneurysms into the iliac vein or inferior vena cava has been described, and this scenario results in a massive arteriovenous fistula [145]. Some of these, without retroperitoneal hemorrhage, occasionally remain hemodynamically stable for days or even weeks. These patients can present with lower limb swelling, a continuous abdominal bruit, abdominal pain, decreased lower extremity pulses on physical exam, heart failure, and renal dysfunction [135]. Rupture into the adjacent sigmoid colon has also been described, with patients presenting with profuse gastrointestinal hemorrhage [146].

If rupture or symptomatic aneurysm is suspected, workup should first include a detailed history with special attention to current risk factors for aneurysm development followed by a physical examination including abdominal examination, rectal examination, and complete vascular examination. Up to 70 % of patients with iliac artery aneurysms will have a pulsatile mass on physical exam [137]. Imaging should promptly follow history and examination with computed tomography angiography (CTA) of the abdomen and pelvis as the first choice for quick and accurate diagnosis. Ultrasound may be useful for evaluation particularly if contraindications to CT angiography are present. Vascular surgery should be promptly consulted along with initiation of resuscitation [137, 138].

Elective Repair and Incidence of Rupture

Preventing the mortality associated with common iliac artery aneurysms hinges on identifying those patients with significant risk of rupture and providing prophylactic repair [144]. Like most aneurysms, the risk of rupture of common iliac artery aneurysms increases with increasing size; however, no ruptures of these aneurysms when they are less than 3 cm have been reported [134, 135, 137, 139]. For aneurysms between 3 and 4 cm, the risk of rupture is estimated to be 5–9 % over 5 years [147, 148]. Once these aneurysms reach 6 cm, the rates of rupture have been reported in the literature from 14 to 70 % and mortality as high as 60 % [137, 139]. In contrast, mortality as low as 5 % has been reported in open elective repair and even lower approximately 1 % in endovascular repair [134, 135, 139].

Recommendations for elective repair continue to evolve as we learn more about the progression and natural history of common iliac artery aneurysms. Elective repair has traditionally been recommended for iliac aneurysms of at least 3 cm, but more recently, several studies have advocated 3.5 cm as the mark for elective repair. Aneurysm expansion appears to accelerate after 3 cm, and aneurysms between 3 and 5 cm expand at 0.26–0.29 cm/year in two studies [134, 135]. These studies recommend serial follow-up for aneurysms less than 3.5 cm, while repair in high-risk patients can be delayed until the aneurysm has reached 4 cm. All symptomatic aneurysms or those larger than 5 cm should be repaired expeditiously. Furthermore, if a coexisting AAA is present with indicated repair, an IAA that is less than 3 cm should be considered for concomitant repair particularly due to the risk of peri-graft degeneration and subsequent development of type 1b endoleaks [137, 149, 150].

Surgical Approaches

The approach to open surgical and endovascular treatment of elective and ruptured iliac artery aneurysms is dependent on the morphology of the aneurysm. These can be broken into five broad categories: common iliac artery aneurysms (CIAA) with proximal and distal neck adequate for open or endovascular repair, isolated CIAA with adequate proximal neck and disease that extends to the common iliac bifurcation, CIAA with adequate proximal neck and disease extending past the common iliac bifurcation, CIAA with inadequate proximal neck due to either proximal extension of the iliac disease or concomitant AAA, and bilateral CIAA [151]. Other classification systems based on the ability to treat aneurysm with endovascular therapy have been developed [152]. Hypogastric artery aneurysms represent an additional anatomic challenge, but will not be addressed in detail within this chapter. Those patients with compromised proximal common iliac arteries will require open or endovascular repair that extends onto the aorta. The same is true for those with bilateral common iliac artery aneurysms. In many cases, aneurysmal disease that extends down to the level of the common iliac artery bifurcation can have preservation of pelvic flow with preservation of the hypogastric artery utilizing open repair, but this becomes much more challenging with an endovascular approach.

Open Surgical Repair

Open repair of ruptured common iliac artery aneurysms are frequently managed in the same manner as ruptured AAA. Open repair of isolated iliac artery aneurysms can be approached from transperitoneal or retroperitoneal approaches based on patient anatomy and surgeon's preference. If there is suitable proximal non-aneurysmal iliac artery, the common iliac artery aneurysm may be repaired with a simple interposition graft (Fig. 13.32). When the entire iliac artery is involved, however, more proximal aortic control with a graft sutured to the infrarenal aorta performed. Management of the distal aspect, during open repair, can be managed with surgical control of both the hypogastric artery and external iliac artery. This can be accomplished with surgical clamps or placement of occlusion balloons. The limb of the graft can be fashioned so that it is anastomosed directly to the common iliac bifurcation incorporating the ostia of both branch vessels (Fig. 13.33). If there is significant splaying of the two branches, they can be incorporated into individually utilizing a side branch sutured to the iliac limb creating a bifurcated-type system (Fig. 13.34), thus preserving pelvic flow. Even in elective repair, incorporation of the internal iliac artery may not be possible in up to 30 % of patients, thus resulting in the need to ligate this vessel [135]. In instances of hypogastric artery aneurysm or patient instability, it may be necessary to sacrifice the internal iliac artery with suture ligation of its origin or its branches. A further discussion of hypogastric artery sacrifice and its complications is discussed in more detail below.

Endovascular Repair

Proximal Landing Zone Management

Endovascular repair of common iliac artery aneurysms requires a suitable proximal and distal fixation and seal. As with open repair, isolated iliac artery aneurysms with suitable proximal diameter and length may be treated with endovascular repair constrained to the iliac artery (Fig. 13.35). With the availability of covered self-expanding stent graft systems such was the Fluency stent graft (Bard, Tempe, AZ), Gore Viabahn (Gore Medical, Flagstaff, AZ), and the Wallgraft (Boston Scientific, Marlborough, MA), endovascular repair has become more readily accessible [153–155]. In addition, the isolated use of iliac limbs from EVAR devices has allowed for treatment of elective and ruptured common iliac artery aneurysms. The limitations of these devices, however, are their proximal diameter and assuring that this allows for adequate oversizing in the proximal common iliac artery in order to provide a durable seal and fixation. In the setting in which the proximal common iliac artery is too large, consideration for use of a conventional EVAR device in the proximal location should be given.

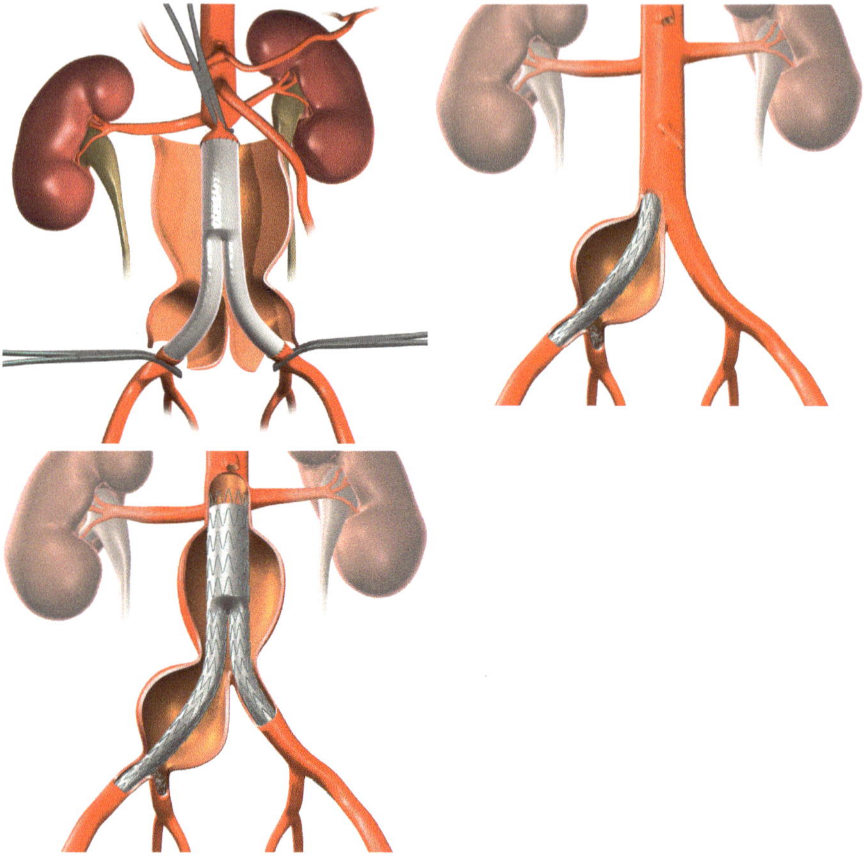

Figs. 13.32, 33 and 34 Illustrations demonstrating open repairs of iliac artery aneurysm that allows for preservation of both the external and internal iliac artery

Distal Landing Zone Management

Hypogastric Artery Preservation

Distal fixation depends on the diameter, length, and aneurysmal involvement of the distal common iliac artery. Current stent graft iliac limbs allow for incorporation of distal seal zones with a diameter of 25 mm (with use of a 28 mm distal iliac limb). This is frequently referred to as the "bell-bottom" technique, which allows for sealing in a larger iliac artery and preservation of antegrade flow into the internal iliac artery [156]. This can also be accomplished by mating a proximal aortic cuff with an iliac limb in order to obtain a distal seal [157]. These techniques have shown early technical success, but given the large size of the iliac artery, patients undergoing these types of procedures require close, long-term follow-up due to the potential for continued expansion and ultimate failure with the development of a type Ib endoleak. If the diameter is larger, or the aneurysm extends into the origins of the external or internal iliac arteries, sacrifice of the hypogastric artery may be necessary with extension of the distal landing zone into the external iliac artery.

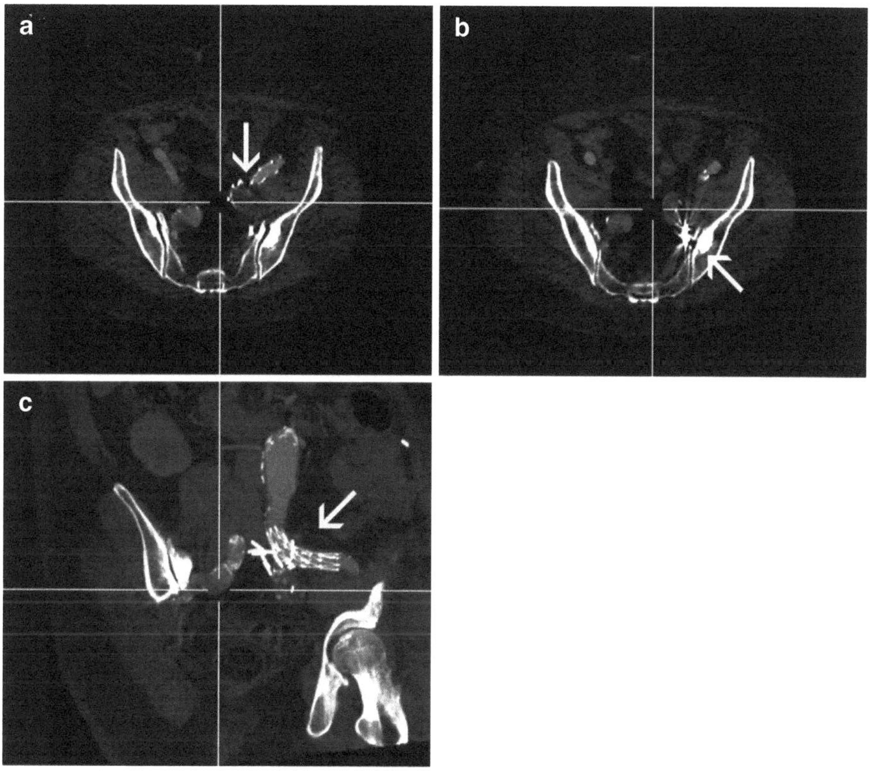

Fig. 13.35 Postoperative computed tomography (CT) scan from a patient who underwent endovascular therapy for ruptured right common iliac artery and hypogastric artery aneurysms. (**a**) The residual aneurysm sac is visible (*arrow*). (**b**) To exclude the aneurysms, it was necessary to coil embolize the branches of the hypogastric artery aneurysm individually (*arrow*). (**c**) There was sufficiently sized common iliac artery length and diameter that the limb of an endograft was used to obtain a proximal seal within the common iliac artery and distal seal within the external iliac artery (*arrow*). Postoperatively, the patient had no complaints of buttock claudication

In the elective setting, it has been estimated that nearly one-quarter of EVAR cannot be performed without addressing an internal iliac artery [158, 159]. If it is felt that preservation of the internal iliac artery is mandatory and a distal seal cannot be obtained using conventional endovascular devices, alternate methods are employed in an attempt to preserve hypogastric patency. One option is to utilize hybrid procedures using open techniques to preserve hypogastric perfusion. This can include relocation of the hypogastric artery to the ipsilateral external iliac artery directly [160]. Alternately bypasses to the internal iliac artery can be performed either arising from the external iliac artery or in a retrograde fashion arising from the femoral artery [161, 162]. When the clinical situation does not allow for this increased complexity, such as with a ruptured aneurysm, more creative approaches have been described such as aorto-uni-iliac endovascular repair combined with femorofemoral arterial bypass and endovascular preservation of external to internal iliac artery flow using stent grafts (Fig. 13.36).

Alternate endovascular techniques have been developed to allow for preservation of both internal iliac artery and external iliac artery flow while excluding the com-

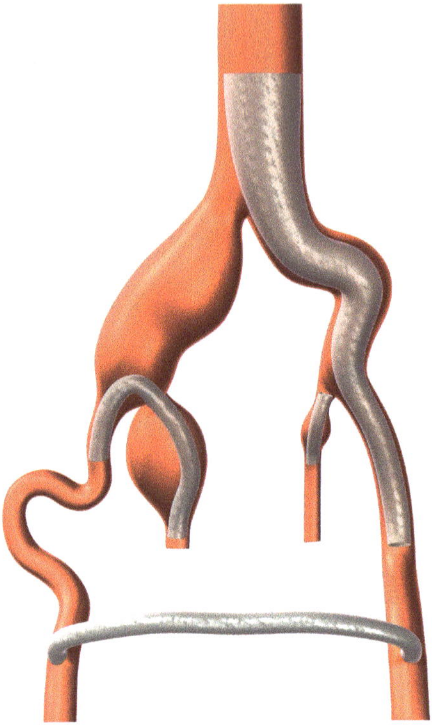

Fig. 13.36 Illustration demonstrating an aorto-uni-iliac device, femorofemoral bypass, and external to internal iliac artery stent grafting

mon iliac artery aneurysm. The majority of these techniques have been described in the elective setting, but they can be easily transferred into the emergent setting if necessary. One of the most commonly described techniques is the use of parallel graft techniques, also known as double-barrel, chimney-graft, or sandwich techniques. In most cases, an EVAR is placed in the proximal aorta. In some instances, a large iliac limb is utilized with two additional stent grafts placed next to each other within this limb – one preserving flow into the external iliac artery and one into the internal iliac artery (Fig. 13.37). This approach requires that stent graft supplying the internal iliac artery be advanced from a more proximal approach such as the brachial or axillary artery. Alternately, the graft supplying the internal iliac artery can run parallel to the aortic graft and extend up to the level of the renal arteries. These approaches have demonstrated to have excellent initial technical success in the elective setting, but there is no significant data on their use in the emergent treatment of ruptured iliac artery aneurysms [163–167]. While initial use appears to be successful, long-term outcome assessments are not available. One of the biggest advantages of these techniques is that the procedure can be performed with currently available commercial products.

Endovascular technology is rapidly advancing, and these techniques will likely be replaced with the use of anatomy-specific devices designed for branching into the internal iliac artery with iliac-branch devices (Fig. 13.38). These devices have a branch incorporated into the main common iliac artery limb, with delivery systems designed to allow for easy cannulation of this additional branch. In the United States, these devices are currently under clinical evaluation and not commercially available, and their use in emergent settings has not been reported. In the elective setting, however, their use has excellent technical success with outstanding mid- and long-term patency rates, even in complex anatomy [168, 169].

Hypogastric Artery Sacrifice

In some instances and in cases in which time to exclusion of a ruptured aneurysm requires rapid intervention, occlusion of the internal iliac artery is necessary. This may occur in both endovascular surgery and open surgery (as discussed above). Coverage of a stent graft into the external iliac artery and resultant hypogastric artery occlusion can be necessary in order to obtain a durable distal fixation and seal. There are several options for hypogastric artery management in this setting which depend on specific patient anatomy. In situation in which there is at least 5 mm of parallel iliac artery proximal to the hypogastric origin and 15 mm distal, simple coverage of the origin of the hypogastric artery can suffice, without any additional intervention necessary [170]. This technique assumes 10–15 % oversizing of the iliac limb or stent graft.

When the sealing zone is not adequate near the origin of the hypogastric artery, further efforts must be made to occlude that vessel in order to prevent a type 2 endoleak. The origin of the hypogastric artery, if it is not aneurysmal, can be occluded with either coils (Fig. 13.37) or occluder/plug devices. These procedures provide the ability to completely seal the iliac artery aneurysm on that side. In the setting of aneurysmal hypogastric artery aneurysms, occlusion of this vessel near its origin may not be possible, and in these cases, each of its subsequent branches needs to be selectively occluded prior to placement of the endovascular stent graft (Fig. 13.35). Failure to occlude these branches can result in continued perfusion of the aneurysm and ongoing hemorrhage in the emergent setting of a ruptured aneurysm.

While sometimes necessary, occlusion of the hypogastric artery should not be considered an innocuous procedure. Ischemic complications following hypogastric artery occlusion are not uncommon and can range in severity from mild buttock claudication to colonic and rectal ischemia requiring resection. Given this, if possible, attempts at preservation of at least one hypogastric artery should be attempted if possible in this emergent setting. It has been suggested that interruption of the internal iliac arteries at its origin only that preserves the deep pelvic collaterals, and preservation of ipsilateral and iliac and femoral circumflex arteries are critical in limiting pelvic ischemic complications and obtaining best outcomes [171] Studies not focusing on preserving pelvic collateral circulation, however, have reported pelvic ischemic complication rates approaching 40 % in patients who have undergone bilateral hypogastric artery occlusions [158, 172, 173]. The most common complication of hypogastric artery occlusion is the development of buttock claudication ranging from 10 to 60 % of the cases, with higher rates in those patients requiring

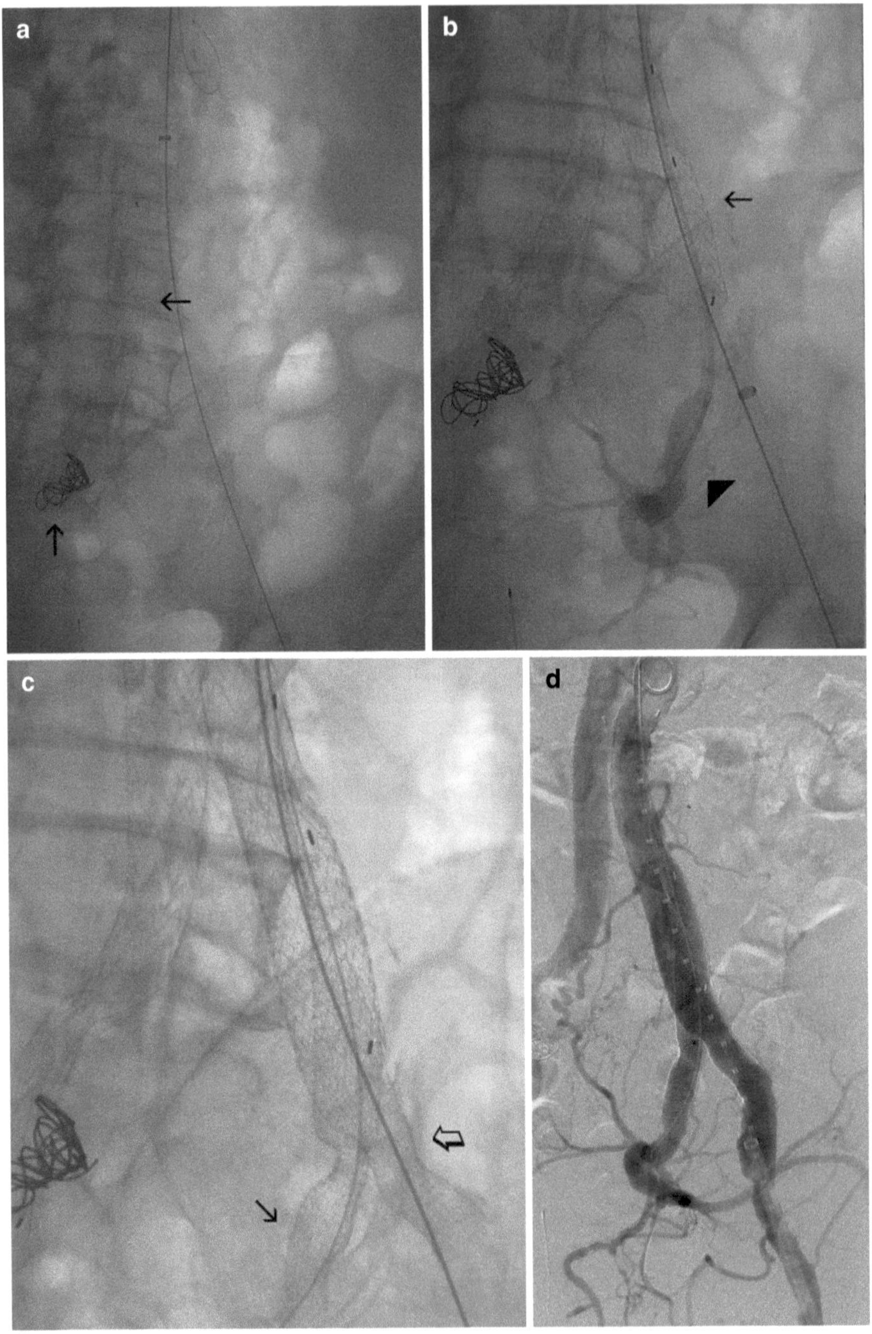
a
b
c
d

bilateral occlusions [158, 162, 171–182]. In a meta-analysis assessing outcomes from hypogastric occlusion during EVAR report, the overall incidence of buttock claudication is approximately 28 %, with an incidence of 31 % in those undergoing unilateral embolization and 35 % in those undergoing bilateral embolization ($p = 0.46$) [159]. This insignificant difference between unilateral and bilateral hypogastric artery embolization likely highlights the importance of ipsilateral iliac and femoral circumflex arteries in maintaining pelvic collateral flow [178, 193]. In addition, the need for embolization in the more distal branches of the hypogastric artery is also associated with an increased incidence of complications [180]. Buttock claudication does improve in up to 50 % of patients over time, but in those in whom it is persistent, it severely affects their quality of life [183]. Another complication of concern is the development of new-onset erectile dysfunction which ranges from 9 to 43 % [171, 172, 176, 178, 184], with an overall incidence on meta-analysis of 17 %, with a nonsignificant but slightly higher rates in those undergoing bilateral embolization (15 % versus 18 %) [159]. Several studies have described some of the rare complications after elective hypogastric artery occlusion including sciatic nerve palsy, paraplegia, gluteal necrosis, and colonic ischemia, although patients included in many of these studies had embolization of deep internal iliac branches which has a significantly higher incidence of pelvic ischemia [180, 183–186, 192].

Outcomes of Emergent Repair

Outcomes of elective endovascular repair of common iliac artery aneurysms are excellent and are associated with low mortality rates. The outcomes for treatment of ruptured iliac artery aneurysms are few in number and are largely reported in small

Fig. 13.37 Serial imaging from a patient that underwent elective endovascular repair of bilateral common iliac artery aneurysms that developed distal to an aorto-bi-iliac artery graft. (**a**) On the right side, the patient had previously undergone coil embolization (arrow) of the origin of the hypogastric artery and stent graft exclusion of the common iliac artery aneurysm with extension from the surgical graft to the external iliac artery. (**b**) When the patient subsequently underwent repair of the left common iliac artery, attempts were made to preserve hypogastric artery flow. In order to achieve hypogastric preservation, initially a large Gore Excluder graft (Gore Medical, Flagstaff, AZ) was placed in the left limb of the surgical graft and extended to just above the iliac bifurcation (arrow). Through an axillary artery exposure, antegrade access was obtained through this graft and into the hypogastric artery (triangle). (**c**) Two Viabahn stent grafts were delivered from below through the femoral artery and from above through the axillary artery and extended from the Excluder above into the external iliac artery (open arrow) and internal iliac artery (solid arrow), together creating a seal within the Excluder graft proximally. (**d**) This allowed for exclusion of the common iliac artery aneurysm with preservation of both of its branches

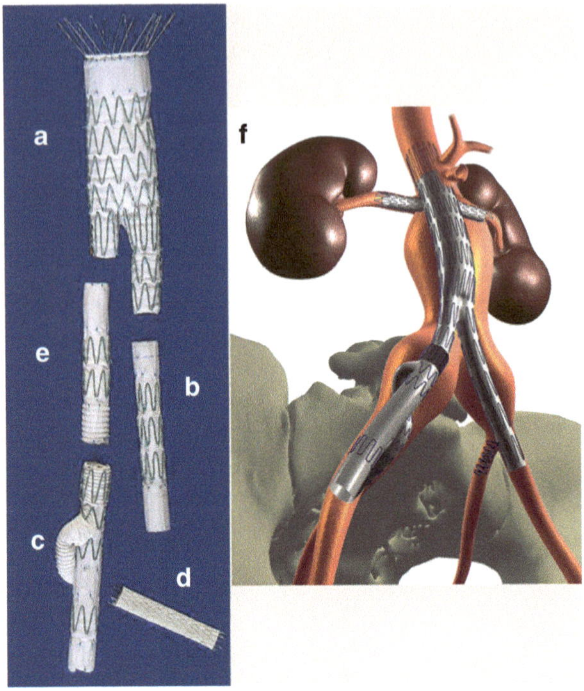

Fig. 13.38 An example of a hypogastric branched endograft system made by Cook Medical (Cook Medical, Bloomington, IN). The device is made to mate with a standard infrarenal aortic endograft main body component (**a**). The hypogastric branched endograft (**c**) is placed first and mated with the internal iliac artery with a branch extension (**d**) which is either a balloon expandable stent graft or self-expanding stent graft. Once completed, the main body bifurcate component is placed and the contralateral iliac artery sealed with a standard iliac component (**b**). The hypogastric branched endograft is mated with the bifurcate component with a bridging segment (**e**). Ultimately these components are interlocked to allow for proximal and distal seal above and below aortoiliac aneurysms providing for preservation of flow to at least one internal iliac artery (**f**). Different configurations of this design from different companies are currently under clinical evaluation

case series or single-incident case reports [146, 187–189]. There is limited information specifically evaluated outcomes from larger case series. In an analysis of 31, 161 patients undergoing elective and emergent isolated iliac artery aneurysm repair from 1988 to 2011 from the National Inpatient Sample, endovascular aneurysm repair has increased steadily over time, surpassing open repair in 2003 [190]. The overall rate of repair increased after the introduction of endovascular repair from 28 to 71 repairs per 10 million in the US population. In addition, total deaths decreased from 4.4 to 2.3 deaths per 10 million of the US population after the introduction of endovascular repair. Interestingly, of all the deaths in 2011, 73 % were after open repair despite the fact that open repair comprised only 20 % of total isolated iliac artery aneurysm repairs performed in 2011. Overall operative mortality for elective and urgent repairs decreased from 13.4 to 2.4 % during this period. The number of urgent repairs, however, has remained stable at approximately 15 procedures per 10 million of the US population. For patients undergoing urgent procedures, the in-hospital mortality was 7.5 % for open repair versus 1.1 % for endovascular repair ($P<0.001$).

Huang et al. evaluated the outcomes from the Mayo Clinic for 715 patient undergoing elective and emergent repair of common iliac artery aneurysms using either open surgery ($N=394$, 90 %) or endovascular repair ($N=44$, 10 %) [135]. While not specifically focusing on the treatment of ruptured iliac artery aneurysms, it is the largest series of both elective and urgent/emergent iliac artery aneurysm repairs reported. Mortality rates were greater in those patients undergoing emergent repair (3 % versus 27 %, $P<0.001$). Major complications occurred in 23 % of patients and were more common after emergent repair. Primary and secondary patency rates of the iliac limb were 99 % and 100 %, respectively, and did not differ between open and endovascular repair. For those undergoing endovascular repair, 31 % of patients had an endoleak diagnosed at discharge – but this represented a 90 % freedom from type 1 endoleak. Five-year survival was better in those patients undergoing elective repair compared to emergency surgery (68 ± 3 % versus 34 ± 8 %, $P<0.001$). Three-year survival was similar between those undergoing open and endovascular repair (both elective and emergent repairs combined), and rupture was the best predictor of decreased survival ($P<0.001$).

Five-year patency rates after open repair were higher after elective (97 ± 1 %) compared with emergency repair (73 ± 12 %, $P=0.03$). At 3 years, there was no difference in patency rates for combined open and elective repair when comparing open and endovascular results. For the whole group, there was a trend toward higher rates of reintervention for those undergoing endovascular repair (9 % versus 18 %, $P=0.06$), with a 5-year freedom from reintervention of 79 % ± 2 %. Freedom from reintervention was higher in those undergoing elective open repair (87 % ± 2 %) compared with those undergoing emergent open repair (72 ± 8 %, $P=0.002$). After both elective and emergent repair, the incidence of buttock claudication survivors was higher in those undergoing endovascular repair (34 % versus 5 %, $P=0.001$). Buttock claudication was associated with hypogastric artery occlusion and occurred in 27 % of patients after open repair who underwent internal iliac artery ligation and 45 % of those after endovascular repair who had internal iliac artery embolization – this did not differ significantly.

Chaer and colleagues presented outcomes of 71 patients undergoing open ($N=19$) or endovascular ($N=52$) repair of iliac artery aneurysms [191]. Fifteen (21 %) patients in this series were symptomatic: 7 in the open group and 8 in the endovascular group. Symptomatology included flank pain, claudication, distal embolization, and ureteral obstruction. Of these, only 7 patients presented with acute rupture (4 with open repair and 3 with endovascular repair). In those presenting with rupture, the mortality rate was 50 % in those undergoing open repair and 33 % in those undergoing endovascular repair. Similarly, Patel et al. report on a series of 56 patients treated with open ($N=24$) or endovascular ($N=32$) repair of iliac artery aneurysms [139]. In this series, only 7 patients were treated for rupture, with the majority ($N=6$) being repaired with open surgery. Postoperative morbidity was observed in this group with two patients suffering ureteral injury: 1 patient with an open abdomen and 1 patient with postoperative hemorrhage requiring a return to the operating room. No morbidity was observed in the one patient that underwent emergent endovascular repair. Thirty-day mortality for those undergoing open, emergent repair was 17 %. There was a trend toward longer hospital stays for those undergoing emergent open repair versus endovascular repair (22 days versus 9 days, $P=0.26$). Overall, long-term patency rates of the iliac limbs were similar between the two groups and approached 98 % at 5 years.

Conclusions

Common iliac artery aneurysms remain an ill-defined medical condition that we are continuing to develop an understanding of with regard to their natural history and timing of intervention. Common iliac artery aneurysm rupture is similar to AAA rupture with regard to clinical presentation and outcomes. Open repair remains a viable treatment option for these patients, but is rapidly being replaced by a variety of endovascular technologies. Outcomes for these techniques, both acute and long-term, may hinge on the ability to preserve at least on internal iliac artery. With advancements in technology, this will become increasingly easy with improved short- and long-term outcomes. These approaches will be readily applied to the emergent settings and may dramatically improve outcomes.

Management of Ruptured Abdominal Aortic Aneurysms in Association with Aortic Dissection

Sira M. Duson and Edward Y. Woo

Introduction

Abdominal aortic aneurysm (AAA) rupture and aortic dissection combined are the most common cause of aortic death in the United States [194]. AAA rupture is the 15th leading cause of death overall and 10th in men greater than 55 years of age [195]. Thirty to 50 % of these patients die before reaching the hospital. Another 30–40 % die after reaching the hospital without ever having surgery. The operative mortality rate is 30–50 % and the overall mortality rate approaches 80–90 % [196]. There are 9,000 new cases of descending thoracic aortic dissections (TBAD) reported per year in the United States with an incidence of 0.5–4 cases per 100,000 per year [196]. Uncomplicated TBAD treated with best medical management have survival rates of 85 %, 71 %, 38 %, and 20 % at 1, 5, 10, and 15 years, respectively [197].

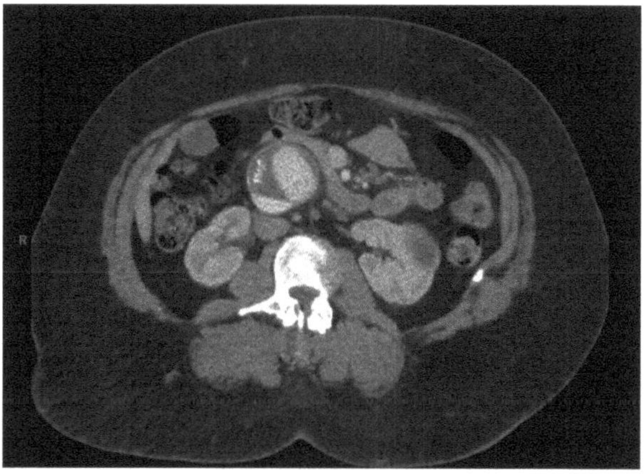

Fig. 13.39 Simultaneous abdominal aortic aneurysm and dissection

These aortic pathologies are independently devastating. Together, ruptured abdominal aortic aneurysm in association with aortic dissection (rdAAA) presents an especially challenging situation. Principles of aneurysm and dissection management must both be considered, in order to facilitate effective and durable intervention.

The purpose of this chapter is to present potential management options for an rdAAA. As mentioned, this condition is especially challenging to treat since adequate repair of the dissection and ruptured aneurysm must be achieved. Dissection results from a tear in the intimal layer of the aorta, permitting blood flow within the medial layer [194, 195]. A false lumen is created in the intramural space as a result of thc clcavagc planc that dcvclops bctwccn thc laycrs of thc intima and mcdia [198]. Meanwhile, aneurysm formation involves a complex process of destruction of the aortic media and supporting lamina through degradation of elastin and collagen [199]. This leads to a decrease in tensile strength in the aortic wall, which can then lead to aneurysm formation and potential rupture [199]. In addition, aneurysmal degeneration can occur in aortic dissections due to the weak wall of the false lumen. In the case of rupture, the goal is to control hemorrhage by sealing the rupture and/or replacing the injured aorta.

Concurrent aortic dissection and AAA was once thought to be rare [200] (Fig. 13.39).

Recent studies reveal a subset of patients with type B aortic dissection, at an increased risk for later development of AAA and thus eventual potential rupture. The patients at highest risk include those with COPD and those 69 years of age or older [201]. Male gender, history of smoking, and chronic dissection were also associated with AAA, but to a lesser degree [201]. Other studies have determined predictors of aortic growth in the setting of acute thoracic dissection; however, these studies are not limited to abdominal aortic growth. It may be important to be aware of these predictors of aortic growth, since the abdominal aorta may also be affected. Van Bogerijen et al. [202] conducted a systemic literature review and summarized several predictors of aortic growth in uncomplicated acute type B aortic dissection. These factors include age <60year, white race, Marfan syndrome, fibrinogen-fibrin degradation product level ≥20 ug/mL at admission, aortic diameter ≥40 mm on initial imaging, proximal descending thoracic aorta false lumen (FL) diameter ≥22 mm, elliptic formation of the true lumen, patent FL, partially thrombosed FL, saccular formation of the FL, presence of one entry tear, large entry tear ≥10 mm located in the proximal part of the dissection, FL located at the inner aortic curvature, fusiform dilated proximal descending aorta, and areas with ulcer-like projections [202]. Perhaps the patients with these aforementioned characteristics warrant more intense serial observation to monitor for aortic growth.

Several studies have demonstrated that endovascular repair of standard abdominal aortic aneurysms has more promising outcomes [198, 203]. Although, open and endovascular approaches can be utilized in treating a ruptured abdominal aortic aneurysm in association with dissection, the focus of this chapter will primarily be endovascular management.

Diagnosis

Imaging modalities available to evaluate rdAAA include CT, MRI, and ultrasound. CT angiogram can be quickly obtained and useful in planning an endovascular aortic intervention. MR angiography also provides information about the rdAAA, but in the setting of an aortic rupture, MRA is a lengthy exam to undertake. Furthermore, MR offers little information on calcification and thrombus which is important especially for endovascular repair. Ultrasound is a quick screening tool that can be used at the bedside to help reveal the presence of a rupture. However, it does not offer the specific information that is seen on axial imaging. Intraoperatively, intravascular ultrasound (IVUS) is even more helpful. IVUS is able to differentiate the true and false lumens, demonstrating the proximal and distal extent of the dissection flap, in addition to offering information on the aortic anatomy.

Preoperative Management

Similar principles of preoperative management should apply to rdAAA as in a ruptured abdominal aneurysm without dissection. If the patient is slightly hypotensive, without clinical signs of end organ ischemia, there is no need for aggressive hydration. Elevating the blood pressure increases chance of hemorrhage by overcoming the tamponade created during the initial rupture [204]. If there is evidence of decreased perfusion such as altered mental status or oliguria, resuscitation with blood is preferable to crystalloid fluid. Excessive isotonic fluid dilutes the blood volume leading to a decrease in red blood cells, platelets, clotting factors, and overall coagulation [205].

Open Surgical Management

Open repair of rAAA follows the tenets for standard open repair. However, if the dissection flap extends proximally or distally beyond the aneurysm, surgical fenestration is required. Proximally, supraceliac control of the aorta should be obtained. The aortotomy still only involves the aneurysm sac, but resection of the dissection flap is performed with long scissors extending proximally. This then allows for sewing the proximal anastomosis to one lumen. The fragile nature of the freshly dissected aortic wall may require suture buttressing in the form of Teflon pledgets. Similarly, the distal anastomoses are treated in the same manner. Often, a bifurcated graft is needed to allow for the surgical fenestrations to be extended into each iliac artery distally. It is important to remember that the clamps need to be placed in a location far enough away from the planned anastomosis to allow for the fenestration to be performed.

Endovascular Management

Endovascular management of rdAAA involves repairing the ruptured abdominal aortic aneurysm and working around a dissection flap. If the dissection is isolated to the aneurysm, then treatment is essentially the same as treating a standard AAA. When the dissection involves the sealing zones in the normal aorta and/or iliacs, treatment becomes more complicated (Fig. 13.40a, b). Standard procedures, such as balloon occlusion, for treating a rAAA should be implemented as needed.

Optimal planning is necessary to ensure appropriate exclusion of the aneurysm. Groin access with open surgical exposure is especially useful if the dissection extends to the distal external iliac arteries or common femoral arteries (Fig. 13.41). Intravascular ultrasound (IVUS) can be very helpful in differentiating the true and false lumens and confirming that access is within the true lumen (Fig. 13.42). It is also helpful in preventing the wire from traversing in and out of the true and false lumens during passage up the aorta. Deploying a stent graft within the false lumen of the aorta and/or iliac vessels could have devastating consequences. For this reason, IVUS should be utilized, if possible, to confirm true lumen placement.

Choosing the type of stent graft is partially based upon individual experience and partially based upon anatomic considerations. Suprarenal fixation may or may not be desired depending on the dissection flap. In addition, utilization of a unibody versus a modular device versus an aorto-uni-iliac device should be determined by the extent of the dissection and how difficult management of the contralateral limb will be due to the dissection.

One of the most challenging aspects of treating rdAAA is obtaining a seal if the dissection extends beyond the aneurysm sac. In either situation, the flap prevents apposition of the endograft to the full aortic wall allowing for continued perfusion of the sac and rupture. Resolution of this issue can be approached from many different means.

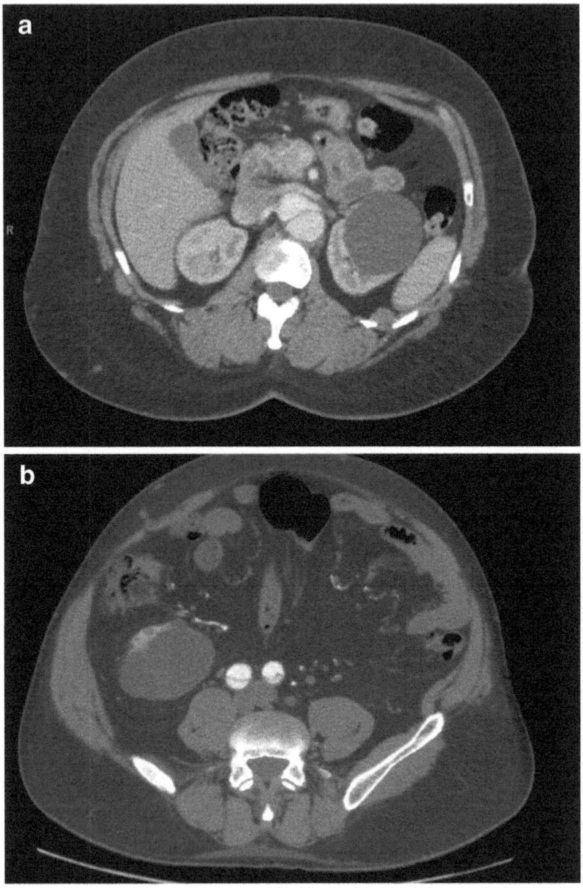

Fig. 13.40 An aortic dissection extending to the proximal (**a**) and distal (**b**) endovascular seal zones

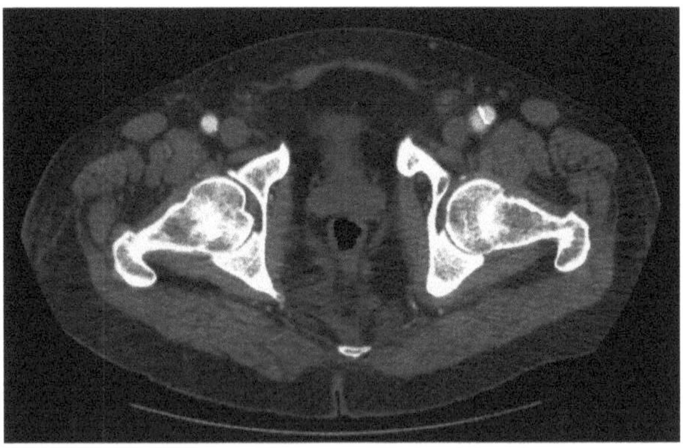

Fig. 13.41 A dissection flap extending into the left common femoral artery

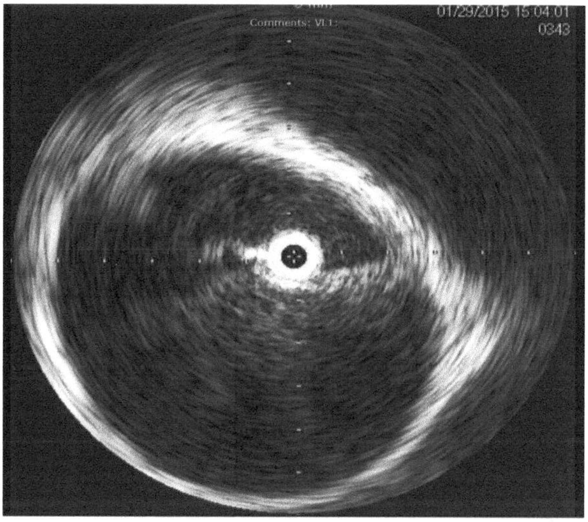

Fig. 13.42 Intravascular ultrasound of the aorta demonstrating an aortic dissection. Note the wire and IVUS probe in the true lumen

In an acute setting with a type B dissection, the flap may still be mobile. As a result, TEVAR to treat the dissection and entry tear with extension to the celiac artery in combination with EVAR to treat the infrarenal aneurysm could lend enough radial force to fully expand the true lumen and exclude the false lumen by shifting the flap completely. Uncovered balloon expandable stents can also be used, especially over the renovisceral segment, to maximize true lumen expansion. However, abdominal aortic aneurysmal formation and subsequent rupture is rare in the acute setting of a type B dissection. More commonly, patients will have a chronic dissection with chronic aneurysmal degeneration. In these circumstances, the flap is more fibrotic and immobile.

Under these circumstances, the goal is to achieve complete exclusion of the false lumen, and the extent of the dissection will mandate treatment. Proximally, if the dissection extends above the renovisceral segment, flow must be maintained to these branches (Fig. 13.43). Complete thoracoabdominal repair with branched or fenestrated devices is an option if available. The proximal and distal seal zones are obtained in the non-dissected vessels, and the remainder of the aorta is excluded with perfusion to the renovisceral segment via the branches/fenestrations [206]. Alternatively, parallel graft construction can be used to maintain perfusion and exclude the rdAAA, but significant concern must be given to potential gutter leaks that can lead to continued hemorrhage in a ruptured situation [207].

Exclusion of the false lumen can also be achieved by covering all fenestrations between the true and false lumens. This entails aortic endografting in the thoracic and abdominal aorta to cover all aortic fenestrations. Covered stent grafts are also utilized in the branch vessels to eliminate true and false lumen connections (Fig. 13.44). If there are fenestrations in the aortic segment around the renal and visceral vessels, then this technique is not viable unless these fenestrations can also

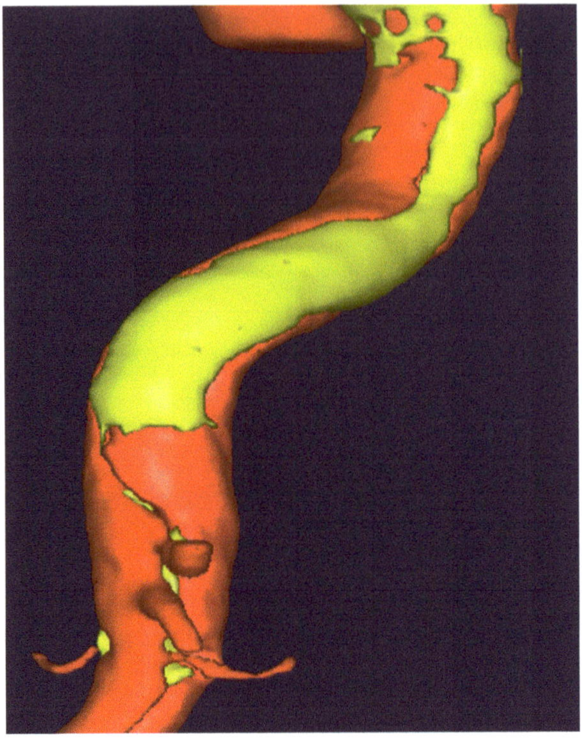

Fig. 13.43 An aortic dissection extending above and involving the renovisceral segment

be sealed. Furthermore, because this is a rupture, allowing for progressive false lumen thrombosis is not an option. Thus, immediate seal and exclusion must be achieved or one risks continued hemorrhage from the rdAAA.

Another technique to treat rdAAA is to eliminate the dissection flap and allow for endograft apposition to the full aortic wall. Tashiro et al. [208] proposed the "cheese wire" technique. Bilateral common femoral artery access is obtained and a wire is advanced into the true lumen on one side under IVUS and fluoroscopic guidance. A catheter is advanced over the wire to the dissection flap. The wire is exchanged for a 16-gauge Ross Modified Colapinto needle [208]. A large compliant balloon is advanced into the false lumen from the opposite femoral artery and inflated. The needle is oriented toward the balloon and advanced until it punctures the balloon. This confirms that the needle is within the false lumen. A glide wire is placed through the needle and snared from the opposite side. Both ends of the wire are pulled inferiorly using a sawing motion to shear the intimal flap to a level 2 cm proximal to the aortic bifurcation. An endograft can then be placed in the single lumen aorta. It should be noted, however, that massive embolization of the dissection flap may result necessitating open surgical conversion.

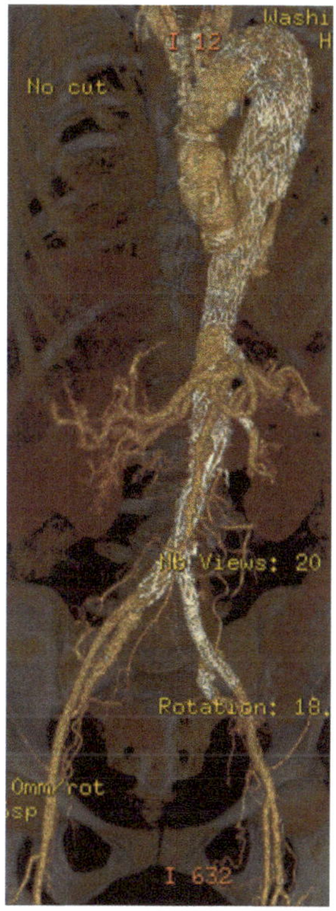

Fig. 13.44 Placement of covered stent grafts into the celiac and left renal arteries to seal fenestrations between the true and false lumens

It is important to note that internal iliac artery can serve as a significant contributor of flow to the false lumen. Under circumstances where the dissection extends to the external iliac artery, hypogastric flow to the false lumen must be halted. Embolization with a large plug is optimal to induce immediate thrombosis. Access to the internal iliac artery can sometimes be challenging. In some situations, this can only be obtained by entering the false lumen first (Fig. 13.45).

Complete exclusion of the false lumen is ideal for treating rdAAA. However, as described above, this may be difficult to perform. As a result, false lumen embolization to promote thrombosis may be useful. In addition, this may be helpful to prevent any residual bleeding secondary to a type II endoleak. Norberto et al. [209] described entering the false lumen and depositing coils to induce thrombosis. Others have described using various glues as well [209]. Another technique described by Idrees et al. [210] involves the deploying an occlusion plug. In this case, the occlusion plug is deployed into the false lumen through a distal fenestration [210, 211]. Ultimately, complete thrombosis of the false lumen is necessary for successful treatment in the setting of an rdAAA.

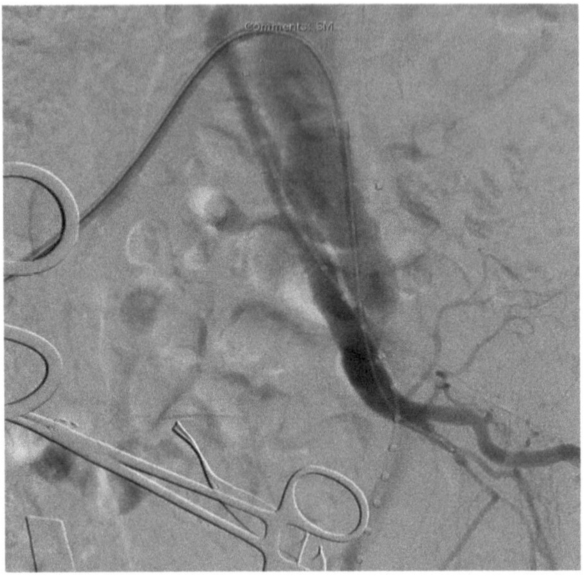

Fig. 13.45 Accessing the internal iliac artery by entering the false lumen

Conclusion

A ruptured abdominal aortic aneurysm in association with aortic dissection is a rare condition. Treatment can be quite complex and difficult. Ultimately, open repair may offer the simplest solution to achieving hemostasis. However, this may be poorly tolerated in many patients. Endovascular solutions are evolving but must be tailored to the patient and the particular anatomy. Ultimately, false lumen exclusion is mandatory.

Surgical Conversion for Rupture After EVAR

Sean P. Lyden

Key Points

- EVAR failure is growing in incidence.
- Identification of device features influences removal technique.
- Reason for failure influences repair type.
- Hybrid repairs lessen the surgical time when endograft is well incorporated.

Endovascular abdominal aneurysm repair (EVAR) is now used in the vast majority of infrarenal aortic aneurysm repairs yearly in the United States [212]. Studies on anatomic criteria suggest that less than 60 % of patients have anatomy amenable for EVAR within approved device anatomic limitations [213]. This often forces physicians to perform EVAR in patients outside the stent graft indications for use (IFU) [214, 215]. While successful in many instances, devices that are placed outside of the IFU have a higher risk of aneurysm growth and failure [215–218]. Although some EVAR failures are salvageable by endovascular methods [219–221], many of these failures will require open conversion [222, 223]. A 2015 study of Medicare patients who had EVAR between 2001 and 2008 found a 5.4 % risk of ruptured aneurysm through 8 years [224]. With increased utilization of EVAR, specially outside the IFUs, the likelihood of a surgeon emergently treating a ruptured aneurysm from a failed EVAR is growing as well. When converting ruptured EVARs to open repair, the ultimate goal is to fix the area of rupture, stop the bleeding, and have the patient survive.

Preoperative Considerations

Identification of the type of endograft and the mode of failure is of critical importance when planning open surgical conversion after EVAR. The type of endograft may be discovered in patient's medical record on a patient's implant wallet card. In the absence of that, it is most accurately determined by plain abdominal x-ray. Plain film radiography can also be the best imaging modality to identify component separation (type IIIb endoleak) or the previous use of Heli-FX EndoAnchors (Aptus, Sunnyvale, CA). When component separation is identified, endovascular repair with limb or cuff extension should be considered as a first-line repair (Fig. 13.46). The scout image or three-dimensional curved planar reconstruction from computerized tomographic (CT) imaging can also be used but may be more difficult to discern the metal structure of the device. Some EVAR devices have active fixation, some have suprarenal fixation, and some have the stents on the outside of the device, while others on the inside. The presence of these various features should be noted as they may impact the approach or conduct of the repair (Table 13.3). Devices with active fixation can be more difficult to remove and may require cutting of the stent struts to allow removal without damaging the aortic wall. Suprarenal fixation is now common to many devices. The height of the stent strut above the fabric varies between devices from 11 to 35 mm. The higher the device extends into the visceral aortic segment will affect potential clamp positions and ability to remove the entire stent. The location of the stents on the outside of the fabric, especially on the limbs, can make removal of the device more difficult.

When possible CT imaging with intravenous contrast obtained with arterial and delayed imaging usually will allow identification of the cause of endograft failure.

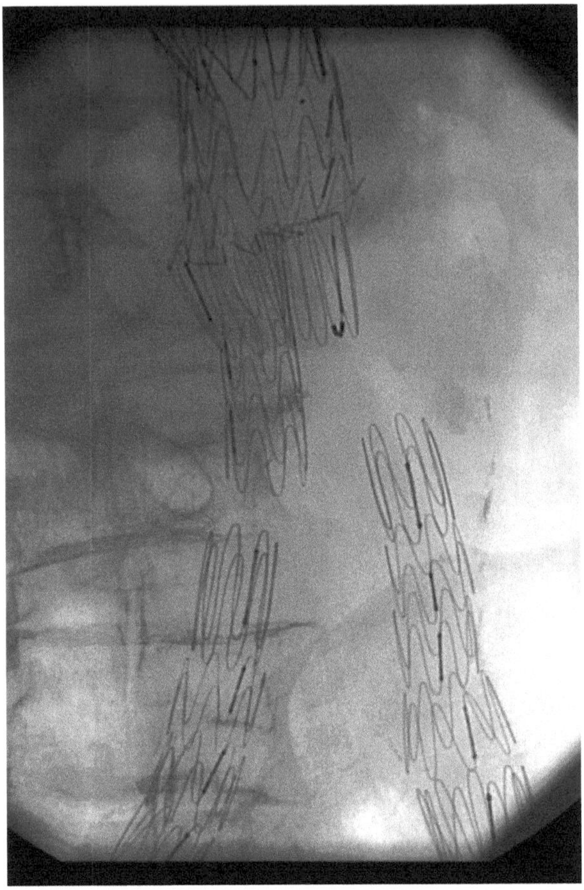

Fig. 13.46 Cook Zenith Endograft with bilateral limb separation on plain film radiograph

Table 13.3 Fixation features of FDA-approved endografts

Guidant Ancure[a]	Infrarenal Elgiloy stent with hooks
Medtronic AneuRx[b]	Infrarenal radial force stents outside fabric
Gore Excluder/C3[c]	Infrarenal nitinol stent with anchors
Cook Zenith/Flex[d]	Stainless steel suprarenal stent with barbs
Endologix Powerlink/AFX[e]	Infrarenal or suprarenal nitinol stent without anchors
Medtronic Talent[b]	Suprarenal nitinol stent without anchors
Medtronic Endurant[b]	Suprarenal nitinol stent with anchors
Trivascular Ovation Prime[f]	Suprarenal nitinol stent with anchors
Lombard Aorfix[g]	Infrarenal nitinol stent with hooks

[a]Guidant, Menlo Park, CA
[b]Medtronic, Santa Rosa, CA
[c]W.L. Gore Flagstaff, AZ
[d]Cook, Bloomington, IN
[e]Endologix, Irvine CA
[f]Trivascular, Santa Rosa, CA
[g]Lombard Medical, Irvine, CA (Note: Ancure, AneuRx, and Talent are no longer sold in the United States)

Close evaluation should be done for aneurysmal degeneration of the sealing zones, proximal or distal migration, component separation, presence and type of endoleak, and graft infection. The reason for failure may significantly alter the surgical approach, clamping positions, and reconstruction options including the ability to leave functioning components behind. Partial explanting of EVAR devices may limit the operative insult and can be successful in accomplishing repair [217, 223]. In a series of 100 patients treated with conversion, 22 stent grafts were not completely removed due to aneurysmal progression of the suprarenal segment with AAA exclusion and good distal fixation, difficulty removing a well-incorporated endograft both proximally and distally, or isolated limb problem with good proximal fixation [217].

Operative Approach

The surgical exposure can be done through retroperitoneal, thoraco-retroperitoneal, midline, and transverse abdominal incisions. All approaches can be effective with the key being the anticipated proximal clamp location and reason for rupture and conversion. The surgeon's expertise should be the strongest influence on the approach taken. When comfortable with all approaches, the thoraco-retroperitoneal approach offers the most flexibility in options for proximal control. This flexibility is more likely to be needed in cases with proximal failures from aneurysmal degeneration of the pararenal segment and repairs with proximal failures of suprarenal fixation devices. The exposure of the paravisceral aorta allows proximal extension of the aortotomy above the device to facilitate removal.

A midline approach can be better when imaging identifies distal seal failures or patients with large iliac aneurysms. This approach will allow better distal control of both iliac arteries. When a distal failure is identified in self-expanding EVAR devices and the proximal EVAR device remains securely attached in a long neck, the aortic neck can be clamped and the proximal portion left in situ.

Technical Challenges

Case series documenting outcomes removing endografts stent grafts have identified several technical challenges encountered during removal of endografts including periaortic inflammation; removal of suprarenal components; removal of hooks, barbs, or endostaples; and endothelialization of uncovered stents [225–227].

Inflammation of the tissues around the endograft is found sporadically and can increase the difficulty of the exposure both proximally and distally. The etiology for this inflammation is not understood and has been identified with all graft types including grafts with active and passive fixation and internal and external stents. This finding is unpredictable and not always present and can be similar to the inflammation found occasionally when dissecting out chronically occluded arteries. The presence of EndoAnchors may also lead to inflammation as they extend through the aortic wall as well. Simple palpation of the aortic wall is adequate to identify the location and extent of the endograft components in most cases, but preoperative identification on axial imaging in relation to the renal, visceral, and iliac vessels is helpful. Devices with active fixation or EndoAnchors may be found to penetrate the aortic wall, and care should be taken not to injure one's self on these barbs and hooks.

Proximal control and limiting bleeding is the first objective. Endoluminal proximal balloon occlusion can be helpful to stabilize the hypotensive patient and can be very useful prior to the induction of anesthesia. For endoluminal femoral balloon occlusion to be successful, support with a large diameter long sheath is critical to avoid distal migration of the balloon. A 12 French 40 cm sheath should be long enough to reach the level of the celiac artery and large enough to allow for placement of any occlusion balloon.

When endoluminal control has not been used, proximal exposure should be obtained away from the area of rupture and above the endograft. The risk of inadvertent injury to adjacent structures is lessened in this fashion. Supraceliac control is most commonly used as none of the current iterations of infrarenal aortic endografts with suprarenal fixation have stents long enough that they should extend above the celiac artery.

Midline supraceliac control requires ligation and takedown of the falciform ligament, division of the left triangular ligament, and retraction laterally of the medial lobe of the liver. This is followed by opening of the gastrohepatic ligament and lateral retraction of the esophagus. A nasogastric tube is helpful in identifying and retracting the esophagus. Sharp dissection of the division of the lateral diaphragmatic crura exposes the aorta. Dissection of the aortic wall will help avoid the clamp from sliding off the aorta during the remainder of the operation. Retroperitoneal supraceliac control requires transection of the crus of the diaphragm. Relocation of the clamp position to a more distal location should be done once the hemorrhage is controlled, the proximal endograft is removed or the infrarenal aortic neck is no longer an issue. This can help limit renal and visceral ischemic time.

Distal exposure may require the ability to access the external and internal iliac arteries especially if the entire device is to be removed. An alternative distal control strategy is to clamp the endograft limbs once the aorta is opened or to use balloon occlusion of the endograft limbs once the graft is transected.

In the setting of rupture, after the proximal aorta is clamped, the infrarenal aortic wall should be opened and thrombus evacuated. If the patient is hemodynamically stable, a brief examination for securely fixed areas of the graft and the presence of type II and III endoleaks should be performed as this can alter how much of the device needs to be removed. Important factors when deciding when not to remove the entire endograft include location of endograft problem (proximal or distal), extent of problem, and prevention of native tissue injury. When the exact location of failure cannot be determined, the goal should be to remove as much of the device as possible.

Device Removal

Some devices with uncovered suprarenal stents and devices that have had a giant balloon expandable stent placed across the proximal fixation into the native aorta can become covered with neointimal hyperplasia, which will require endarterectomy of that portion of the aorta to allow removal. Collapse of self-expanding stents will help facilitate removal as well as clamping above the entire device. Many times stepwise removal is best. Wire cutters are useful tools to transect the stents allowing partial or stepwise removal.

The most commonly used maneuver to assist in successful removal of the aortic stent graft is a traditional "clamp and pull" method. This works well for all devices without suprarenal or active fixation. In aortic stent grafts with active fixation, the approach should be individualized. The Ancure ([212] Guidant, Menlo Park, CA) device hooks are commonly seen to extend through the entire aortic wall, and traction on the device can lead to aortic wall injury. Transection of the sealing stent with heavy scissors or metal cutters can facilitate removal of the stent with the hooks allowing the device to be peeled out. Extension of the aortotomy on the sealing stent has also been helpful. The barbs on the Excluder (WL Gore & Ass., Flagstaff, Az) device do not deeply penetrate the aortic wall and can usually be remove with simple traction alone. For Zenith devices (Cook Inc., Bloomington, IN), many have adopted the technique described by Koning which involves collapsing the device into a transected 20 ml syringe [227]. By cutting off the closed end of a syringe, the syringe cylinder can be then used as a sheath to recapture the proximal stent from the aortic wall. The device is collapsed sequentially from distal to proximal with constraining ties allowing advancement of the syringe and collapse of the device. The suprarenal portion is oftentimes covered with endothelium and advancing the sheath while applying traction on the endograft will perform an endarterectomy as the stents and barbs pull free from the aortic wall. A more recent publication advocated using a disposable rigid proctoscope instead of modifying a syringe [228]. The Endurant (Medtronic, Santa Rosa, CA) and Ovation Prime (Trivascular, Santa Rosa, CA) devices have much more robust suprarenal fixation and anchors, and I have not found that either device will collapse using a modified syringe. Staged partial removal of the suprarenal components using wire cutters is required (Fig. 13.47). In patients who have large balloon expandable stainless steel stents within the aortic neck, these stents can be crushed with a clamp to facilitate removal. When intima is removed with suprarenal components, care should be taken to assess for patency of the renal and visceral vessels after restoration of flow to this segment of the aorta. Devices with EndoAnchors used in the repair may transverse the entire aortic wall. When transaortic fixation of EndoAnchors is present, they could be unscrewed and extracted from the device and aortic wall or left intact as the situation warrants.

When the proximal stent graft fixation is secure and the aortic neck intact and of adequate length, partial device explant might be the best option. A new proximal anastomosis can be performed with the stent graft transected flush within the aortic wall and new surgical graft sutured together [217]. This provides permanent fixation to the native aorta, endograft, and surgical graft. This can be done with an aortic clamp on the infrarenal neck for self-expanding devices.

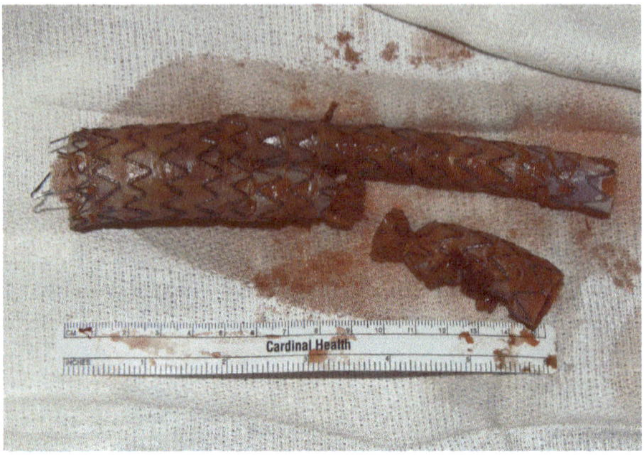

Fig. 13.47 Endurant endograft removed after wire cutter used to cut away incorporated suprarenal fixation

Limb Removal

Removal of endograft limbs is generally done with gentle traction on the limb. Some features of the device that seem to influence the ease or difficulty of removal include the material composition, diameter of the iliac vessel, and location of the stents relative to the fabric. In general, the farther an endograft limb extends into normal diameter iliac arteries, the harder it becomes to remove. The ePTFE (expanded polytetrafluoroethylene) stent grafts tend to pull out easier that polyester fabric stent grafts. Designs with stents on the outside of the fabric also tend to be more difficult to remove.

When the iliac artery is easily exposed distal to the end of the endograft, transection of the artery and sewing to the native vessel can be a simple solution. When the limbs are not easily removable and extend far down into the normal iliac arteries, it is often easier to transect them at the aortic bifurcation and sutured to the repair (Figs. 13.48 and 13.49). Leaving behind limbs that are well-incorporated graft may potentially improve outcomes and by limiting the time needed to obtain more extensive exposure and reducing blood loss. When possible, the remaining endograft portions should be suture fixed to the native vessels to reduce the risk of late migration.

Hybrid Reconstructions

When portions of an endograft have been incorporated into the repair, closure of the aortic sac around the device may minimize potential device movement. Patients that have in situ retention of a portion of the endograft still require lifelong CT surveillance as future complications of the remaining EVAR elements are possible. Late failure of hybrid repairs using transected endografts has been reported [222].

Treating the endoleaks as a cause of ruptured aneurysm without graft explantation is reasonable when patients will not tolerate removal. Transaortic graft sutures for fixation of type I endoleaks has been successfully performed as well as suturing through and through the proximal sealing stent and aortic wall with circumferential felt pledget reinforcement. Type II endoleaks have been treated with ligation of lumbar arteries or

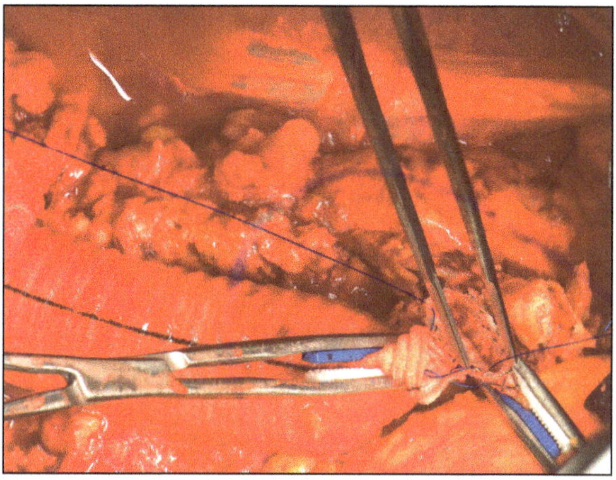

Fig. 13.48 Operative photograph of suturing bifurcated aortic graft to AneuRx endograft limbs at the origin of normal iliac arteries

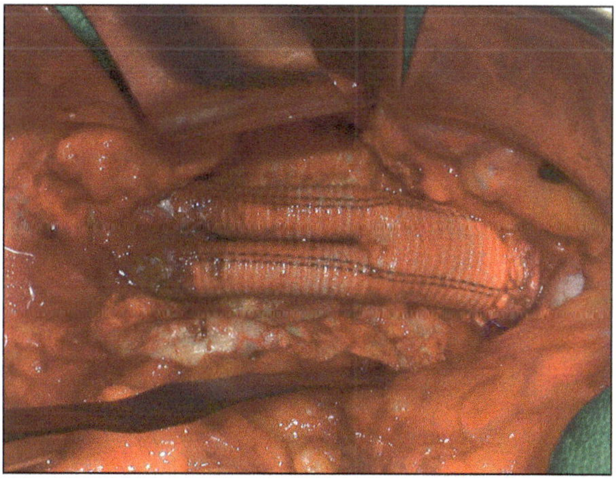

Fig. 13.49 Completed bifurcated aortic repair to iliac limbs of Excluder endograft

inferior mesenteric arteries [222]. Unfortunately, there are also reports of failures of these methods with proximal migration as well as development of new endoleaks [222].

Outcomes

The outcomes of stent graft explant and surgical reconstructions are dependent of the underlying indications for failure. Elective removal of aortic endografts has been shown to be performed with similar risk to open repair [223]. A series of 41 explants noted an elective conversion 30-day mortality of 3.3 %. However, later data from the same group noted a higher elective mortality of 9.9 % attributing the increased risk to more aggressive treatments [217]. Both reports noted the influence of urgent and emergent repairs contributing to increasing mortality risk. Ruptures were found in 9 of 100 failed EVARs and had a 55 % 30-day mortality. Mehta et al. reported a series of 1721 EVAR patients, in which 27 patients present with rupture after EVAR; 58 % underwent open surgical repair, and 42 % had redo EVAR with an overall mortality of 15 % [221]. Chaer and colleagues noted conversion for rupture in 12 patients with a 33 % mortality, performing a complete explant in only five patients [222]. A large series from 17 US medical centers identified 15 late ruptures from 1736 patients who underwent EVAR. For patients who underwent repair for delayed rupture, mortality at 30 days and 1 year were 44.4 % and 66.7 %, respectively [229]. A recent review of the world literature found only 152 ruptures after 16,974 EVAR procedures. Open surgical treatment was undertaken in 61 % (95 % CI 53–68) of the patients who underwent treatment. The pooled estimate for perioperative mortality was 32 % (95 % CI 24–41). A significantly lower mortality was found with endovascular treatment than open surgical management ($p=0.027$) [230]. The risk of late rupture is undoubtedly under reported in the literature as evidenced by the 5.4 % risk of late rupture seen in a recent publication of Medicare patients [224]. As more ruptured EVAR conversions are reported the optimal techniques for repair will be better defined.

Conclusions

EVAR has revolutionized the approach to aortic surgery with markedly lower early risk than open repair. Although rare, the risk of late rupture from EVAR persists and surgeons need to be familiar with techniques for stent graft explant and surgical reconstructions. The type of device and location of failure leading to rupture influence the approach taken. Partial removal can facilitate quicker repair in select circumstances. Overall mortality for conversion to open repair after rupture remains high.

References

Transabdominal Repair of Ruptured Abdominal Aortic Aneurysms

1. Livesay JJ, Messner GN, Vaughn WK. Milestones in the treatment of aortic aneurysm: Denton A. Cooley, MD, and the Texas Heart Institute. Tex Heart Inst J. 2005;32(2):130–4.
2. Brock RC. The life and work of Sir Astley Cooper. Guy's Hospital Reports. 1968;117(3): 147–168.
3. Matas R. Ligation of the abdominal aorta: report of the ultimate result, One year, five months and nine days after ligation of the abdominal aorta for aneurism at the bifurcation. Ann Surg. 1925;81(2):457–64.

4. Bahnson HT. Treatment of abdominal aortic aneurysm by excision and replacement by homograft. Circulation. 1954;9(4):494–503.
5. Cooley DA, Debakey ME. Ruptured aneurysms of abdominal aorta; excision and homograft replacement. Postgrad Med. 1954;16(4):334–42.
6. Farrar T, Adson MA, Kirklin JW, Martin WJ, Barker NW. Surgical treatment of acute rupture of abdominal aortic aneurysms: report of two cases. Proceedings of the staff meetings. Mayo Clinic. May 16 1956;31(10):299–304.
7. Javid H, Dye WS, Grove WJ, Julian OC. Resection of ruptured aneurysms of the abdominal aorta. Ann Surg. 1955;142(4):613–21; discussion, 621–613.
8. Mills Sr JL. Vascular surgery training in the United States: a half-century of evolution. J Vasc Surg. 2008;48(6 Suppl):90S–7; discussion 97S.
9. Arthurs ZM, Sohn VY, Starnes BW. Ruptured abdominal aortic aneurysms: remote aortic occlusion for the general surgeon. Surg Clin North Am. 2007;87(5):1035–45, viii.
10. Matsuda H, Tanaka Y, Hino Y, Matsukawa R, Ozaki N, Okada K, et al. Transbrachial arterial insertion of aortic occlusion balloon catheter in patients with shock from ruptured abdominal aortic aneurysm. J Vasc Surg. 2003;38(6):1293–6.
11. O'Donnell ME, Badger SA, Makar RR, Loan W, Lee B, Soong CV. Techniques in occluding the aorta during endovascular repair of ruptured abdominal aortic aneurysms. J Vasc Surg. 2006;44(1):211–5.
12. Huber TS, Carlton LC, Irwin PB, Flug RR, Harward TR, Flynn TC, et al. Intraoperative autologous transfusion during elective infrarenal aortic reconstruction. J Surg Res. 1997;67(1):14–20.
13. Ramos TK, Stoney RJ. The medial visceral rotation approach to the proximal abdominal aorta: how to assemble and use the omni-tract(R) retractor system. Surg Technol Int. 1993;2:299–302.
14. Zarins CK, Gewertz BL, editors. Atlas of vascular surgery. 2nd ed. Philadelphia: Elsevier; 2005.
15. Aljabri B, MacDonald PS, Satin R, Stein LS, Obrand DI, Steinmetz OK. Incidence of major venous and renal anomalies relevant to aortoiliac surgery as demonstrated by computed tomography. Ann Vasc Surg. 2001;15(6):615–8.
16. Desikan S, Singh N, Tran N, Quiroga E, Garland BT, Starnes BW. The incidence of ischemic colitis after repair of ruptured abdominal aneurysms is decreasing in the endovascular era. Ann Vasc Surg. 2015;29(4):624–5.
17. Lee WA, Brown MP, Nelson PR, Huber TS. Total percutaneous access for endovascular aortic aneurysm repair ("Preclose" technique). J Vasc Surg. 2007;45(6):1095–101.
18. Djavani K, Wanhainen A, Bjorck M. Intra-abdominal hypertension and abdominal compartment syndrome following surgery for ruptured abdominal aortic aneurysm. Eur J Vasc Endovasc Surg Off J Eur Soc Vasc Surg. 2006;31(6):581–4.
19. Mehta M, Darling 3rd RC, Roddy SP, Fecteau S, Ozsvath KJ, Kreienberg PB, et al. Factors associated with abdominal compartment syndrome complicating endovascular repair of ruptured abdominal aortic aneurysms. J Vasc Surg. 2005;42(6):1047–51.
20. Rubenstein C, Bietz G, Davenport DL, Winkler M, Endean ED. Abdominal compartment syndrome associated with endovascular and open repair of ruptured abdominal aortic aneurysms. J Vasc Surg. 2015;61(3):648–54.
21. Mell MW, O'Neil AS, Callcut RA, Acher CW, Hoch JR, Tefera G, et al. Effect of early plasma transfusion on mortality in patients with ruptured abdominal aortic aneurysm. Surgery. 2010;148(5):955–62.
22. Kimball EJ, Adams DM, Kinikini DV, Mone MC, Alder SC. Delayed abdominal closure in the management of ruptured abdominal aortic aneurysm. Vascular. 2009;17(6):309–15.
23. Mayer D, Rancic Z, Meier C, Pfammatter T, Veith FJ, Lachat M. Open abdomen treatment following endovascular repair of ruptured abdominal aortic aneurysms. J Vasc Surg. 2009; 50(1):1–7.

Open Repair-Retroperitoneal

24. Sicard GA, Reilly JM, Rubin BG, et al. Transabdominal retroperitoneal incision for abdominal aortic surgery: report of a prospective randomized trial. J Vasc Surg. 1995;21:174–81.
25. Patel J. Chirurgie de la Fourche Aortique. La Presse Med. 1950;58:214–7.
26. Dubost C, Allary M, Oeconomos N. Resection of an aneurysm of the abdominal aorta. Arch Surg. 1952;64:405–8.
27. Rob C. Extraperitoneal approach to the abdominal aorta. Surgery. 1963;53:87–9.
28. Williams GM, Ricotta J, Zinner M, et al. The extended retroperitoneal approach for treatment of extensive atherosclerosis of the aorta and renal vessels. Surgery. 1980;88:846–55.
29. Chang BB, Shah DM, Paty PSK, et al. Can the retroperitoneal approach be used for ruptured abdominal aortic aneurysms? J Vasc Surg. 1990;11:326–30.
30. Lyden SP, McNamara JM, Sternbach Y, Illig KA, Waldman DL, Green RM. Technical consideration for late removal of aortic endografts. J Vasc Surg. 2002;36:674–8.
31. Kelso RL, Lyden SP, Butler B, Greenberg RK, Eagleton MJ, Clair DG. Late conversion of aortic stentgrafts. J Vasc Surg. 2009;49:589–95.
32. Mehta M, Paty PSK, Roddy SP, Taggert JB, Sternbach Y, Kreienberg PB, Chang BB, Darling III RC. Treatment options for delayed AAA rupture following endovascular repair. J Vasc Surg. 2011;53:14–20.
33. Lipsitz EC, Ohki T, Veith FJ, Suggs WD, Wain RA, Rhee SJ, et al. Delayed open conversion following endovascular aortoiliac aneurysm repair: partial (or complete) endograft preservation as a useful adjunct. J Vasc Surg. 2003;38:1191–8.
34. Kong OH, Hinnen JW, Baalen JM. Technique for safe removal of an aortic endograft with suprarenal fixation. J Vasc Surg. 2006;43:855–7.
35. Mehta M, Paty PS, Roddy SP, Taggert JB, Sternbach Y, Kreienberg PB, et al. Treatment options for delayed AAA rupture following endovascular repair. Vasc Surg. 2011;53(1): 14–20.
36. Chang BB, Paty PK, Shah DM, Leather RP. Selective use of retroperitoneal aortic exposure in the emergency treatment of ruptured and symptomatic abdominal aortic aneurysms. Am J Surg. 1988;156:108–10.
37. Leather RP, Shah DM, Kaufman JL, Fitzgerald KM, Chang BB, Feustel PJ. Comparative analysis of retroperitoneal and transperitoneal aortic replacement for aneurysm. Surg Gynecol Obstet. 1989;168:387–93.

Rupture EVAR Using Bifurcated Stentgrafts

38. Yusuf SW, Whitaker SC, Chuter TA, et al. Emergency endovascular repair of leaking aortic aneurysms. Lancet. 1994;344:1645.
39. Marin ML, Veith FJ, Cynamon J, et al. Initial experience with transluminally placed endovascular grafts for the treatment of complex vascular lesions. Ann Surg. 1995;222(4): 449–65.
40. Veith FJ, Lachat M, Mayer D, Malina M, Holst J, Mehta M. Collected world and single center experience with endovascular treatment of ruptured abdominal aortic aneurysms. Ann Surg. 2009;250(5):818–24.
41. Sadat U, Boyle JR, Walsh SR, Tang T, Varty K, Hayes PD. Endovascular vs open repair of acute abdominal aortic aneurysms – A systemic review and meta-analysis. Speicher PJ, Barbas AS, Mureebe L. Open versus endovascular repair of ruptured abdominal aortic aneurysms. Ann Vasc Surg 2014;28(5):1249–57.

42. Edwards ST, Schermerhorn ML, O'Malley AJ, Bensley RP, Hurks R, Cotterill P, et al. Comparative effectiveness of endovascular versus open repair of ruptured abdominal aortic aneurysms in the Medicare population. J Vasc Surg. 2014;59(3):575–82.
43. Coppi G, Silingardi R, Gennai S, Saitta G, Ciardullo AV. A single center experience in open and endovascular treatment of hemodynamically unstable and stable patients with ruptured abdominal aortic aneurysms. J Vasc Surg. 2006;44:1140–7.
44. Mehta M, Paty PS, Byrne J, Roddy SP, Taggert JB, Sternbach Y, et al. Hemodynamic status impacts outcomes of endovascular aneurysm repair for rupture. J Vasc Surg. 2013;57: 1255–60.
45. Starnes BW, Quiroga E, Hutter C, Tran NT, Hatsukami T, Meissner M, et al. Management of ruptured abdominal aortic aneurysm in the endovascular era. J Vasc Surg. 2010;51:9–18.
46. Lloyd GM, Brown MJ, Norwood MGA, et al. Feasibility of preoperative computed tomography in patients with ruptured AAA; A time to death study in patients without operation. J Vasc Surg. 2004;39:788–91.
47. Mehta M, Byrne J, Darling III RC, Paty PSK, Roddy SP, Kreienberg PB, et al. Endovascular repair of ruptured infrarenal abdominal aortic aneurysm is associated with lower 30-day mortality and better 5-year survival rates than open surgical repair. J Vasc Surg. 2013;57: 368–75.
48. Slater BJ, Harris EJ, Lee JT, et al. Anatomic suitability of ruptured abdominal aortic aneurysms for endovascular repair. Ann Vasc Surg. 2008;22(6):716–22.
49. Richards T, Goode SD, Hinchliffe R, et al. The importance of anatomical suitability and fitness for the outcome of endovascular repair of ruptured abdominal aortic aneurysms. Eur J Vasc Endovasc Surg. 2009;38(3):285–90.
50. Mehta M, Burton B, Byrne J, Paty PSK, Taggert JB, Roddy SP, et al. The impact of favorable and hostile aortic neck morphology on the outcomes of endovascular repair of ruptured abdominal aortic aneurysms. J Vasc Surg. 2013;57(5):88S–9.
51. Mayer D, Aeschbacher S, Pfammatter T, Veith FJ, Norgren L, Magnuson A, et al. Complete replacement of open repair for ruptured abdominal aortic aneurysms by endovascular aneurysm repair: a two-center 14-year experience. Ann Surg. 2012;256(5):688–95.
52. Berland TL, Veith FJ, Cayne NS, Manish M, Dieter M, Mario L. Technique of supraceliac balloon control of the aorta during endovascular repair of ruptured abdominal aortic aneurysms. J Vasc Surg. 2013;57:272–5.
53. Antoniou GA, Georgiadis GS, Antoniou SA, Duhan G, Murray D. A meta-analysis of outcomes of endovascular abdominal aortic aneurysm repair in patients with hostile and friendly neck anatomy. J Vasc Surg. 2013;57(2):527–38.
54. Hinchliffe RJ, Braithwaite BD, European Bifab Study Collaborators. A modular aortouniiliac endovascular stent-graft is a useful device for the treatment of symptomatic and ruptured infrarenal abdominal aortic aneurysms: one-year results from a multicentre study. Eur J Vasc Endovasc Surg. 2007;34(3):291–8.
55. Peppelenbosch N, Geelkerken RH, Soong C, Cao P, Steinmetz OK, Teijink JA, Lepäntalo M, et al. Endograft treatment of ruptured abdominal aortic aneurysms using the Talent aortouniiliac system: an international multicenter study. J Vasc Surg. 2006;43(6):1111–23; discussion 1123.
56. Dias NV, Bin JA, Sveinsson M, Bjorses K, Malina M, Kristmundsson T. Impact of renal chimney grafts on anatomical suitability for endovascular repair in ruptured abdominal aortic aneurysms. J Endovasc Ther. 2015;22(1):105–9.
57. Mehta M, Paty PS, Roddy SPR, Taggert JB, Sternbach Y, Kreienberg PB, et al. Treatment options for delayed AAA rupture following endovascular repair. J Vasc Surg. 2011;53: 14–20.
58. Schlösser FJ, Gusberg RJ, Dardik A, Lin PH, Verhagen HJ, Moll FL, et al. Aneurysm rupture after EVAR: can the ultimate failure be predicted? Eur J Vasc Endovasc Surg. 2009; 37:15–22.

EVAR-AUI The European Experience

59. Alsac JM, et al. Emergency endovascular repair for ruptured abdominal aortic aneurysms: feasibility and comparison of early results with conventional open repair. Eur J Vasc Endovasc Surg. 2005;30(6):632–9.
60. Armon MP, et al. Anatomical suitability of abdominal aortic aneurysms for endovascular repair. Br J Surg. 1997;84:178–80.
61. Becquemin JP, et al. A randomized controlled trial of endovascular aneurysm repair versus open surgery for abdominal aortic aneurysms in low- to moderate-risk patients. J Vasc Surg. 2011;53(5):1167–73. e1.
62. Carrafiello G, et al. Endovascular treatment of ruptured abdominal aortic aneurysms: aorto-uni-iliac or bifurcated endograft? In La Radiologia medica. 2012;117:410–25.
63. Chaudhuri A. Contralateral iliac occlusion can be successfully achieved using an amplatz vascular plug during aorto-uni-iliac endovascular aneurysm repair. EJVES Extra. 2012;23(2):365.
64. Chuter TA, et al. Aortomonoiliac endovascular grafting combined with femorofemoral bypass: an acceptable compromise or a preferred solution? Semin Vasc Surg. 1999;12(3): 176–81.
65. Grieve R, et al. Endovascular strategy or open repair for ruptured abdominal aortic aneurysm: one-year outcomes from the IMPROVE randomized trial. Eur Heart J. 2015.
66. Hinchliffe RJ, et al. A randomised trial of endovascular and open surgery for ruptured abdominal aortic aneurysm–results of a pilot study and lessons learned for future studies. Eur J Vasc Endovasc Surg. 2006;32(5):506–13; discussion 514–5.
67. Hinchliffe RJ, et al. Durability of femorofemoral bypass grafting after aortouniiliac endovascular aneurysm repair. J Vasc Surg. 2003;38(3):498–503.
68. Hinchliffe RJ, et al. Endovascular repair of ruptured abdominal aortic aneurysm–a challenge to open repair? results of a single centre experience in 20 patients. Eur J Vasc Endovasc Surg. 2001;22(6):528–34.
69. Hinchliffe RJ, Braithwaite BD, European BiFab Study Collaborators. A Modular aortouniiliac endovascular stent-graft is a useful device for the treatment of symptomatic and ruptured infrarenal abdominal aortic aneurysms: one-year results from a multicentre study. Eur J Vasc Endovasc Surg. 2007;34(3):291–8.
70. Hoornweg LL, et al. The amsterdam acute aneurysm trial: suitability and application rate for endovascular repair of ruptured abdominal aortic aneurysms. Eur J Vasc Endovasc Surg. 2007;33(6):679–83.
71. Ivancev K, et al. Abdominal aortic aneurysms: experience with the Ivancev-Malmö endovascular system for aortomonoiliac stent-grafts. J Endovasc Surg. 1997;4(3):242–51.
72. Nasim A, et al. Is endoluminal abdominal aortic aneurysm repair using an aortoaortic (tube) device a durable procedure? Ann Vasc Surg. 1998;12:522–8.
73. Parodi JC, Palmaz JC, Barone HD. Transfemoral intraluminal graft implantation for abdominal aortic aneurysms. Ann Vasc Surg. 1991;5(6):491–9.
74. Peppelenbosch N, et al. Endograft treatment of ruptured abdominal aortic aneurysms using the talent aortouniiliac system: an international multicenter study. J Vasc Surg. 2006;43(6):1111–24.
75. Reimerink J, et al. Endovascular repair versus open repair of ruptured abdominal aortic aneurysms: a multicenter randomized controlled trial. Ann Surg. 2013;258(2):248–56.
76. Rose DFG, et al. Anatomical suitability of ruptured abdominal aortic aneurysms for endovascular repair. J Endovasc Ther. 2003;10(3):453–7.
77. Smit JGM, Van Marle J. Repair of abdominal aortic aneurysms with aorto-uni-iliac stentgraft and femoro-femoral bypass. S Afr J Surg. 2012;50(2):33–6.
78. Tang T, et al. Comparison of the endurant bifurcated endograft vs. aorto-uni-iliac stent-grafting in patients with abdominal aortic aneurysms: experience from the ENGAGE registry. J Endovasc Ther. 2013;20(2):172–81.

79. Thompson MM, et al. Aortomonoiliac endovascular grafting: difficult solutions to difficult aneurysms. J Endovasc Surg. 1997;4(2):174–81.
80. Thompson MM, et al. Comparison of computed tomography and duplex imaging in assessing aortic morphology following endovascular aneurysm repair. Br J Surg. 1998;85(3):346–50.
81. Visser JJ, et al. Endovascular repair versus open surgery in patients with ruptured abdominal aortic aneurysms: clinical outcomes with 1-year follow-up. J Vasc Surg. 2006;44(6):1148–55.
82. Volodos', N.L. et al.. A case of distant transfemoral endoprosthesis of the thoracic artery using a self-fixing synthetic prosthesis in traumatic aneurysm. Grudnaia khirurgiia (Moscow, Russia);1988(6), pp.84–86.
83. Walker SR, et al. A study on the patency of the inferior mesenteric and lumbar arteries in the incidence of endoleak following endovascular repair of infra-renal aortic aneurysms. Clin Radiol. 1998;53(8):593–5.
84. Walker SR, et al. Early complications of femorofemoral crossover bypass grafts after aorta uni-iliac endovascular repair of abdominal aortic aneurysms. J Vasc Surg. 1998;28(4):647–50.
85. White GH, Yu W, May J. Endoleak–a proposed new terminology to describe incomplete aneurysm exclusion by an endoluminal graft. J Endovasc Surg. 1996;3(1):124–5.
86. Yusuf SW, et al. Early results of endovascular aortic aneurysm surgery with aortouniiliac graft, contralateral iliac occlusion, and femorofemoral bypass. J Vasc Surg. 1997;25(1):165–72.
87. Yusuf SW, et al. Emergency endovascular repair of leaking aortic aneurysm. Lancet. 1994;344(8937):1645.

Physician Modified Endovascular Grafts for Treating Ruptured Abdominal Aortic Aneurysms

88. Anderson JL, Berce M, Hartley DE. Endoluminal aortic grafting with renal and superior mesenteric artery incorporation by graft fenestration. J Endovasc Ther. 2001;8(1):3–15.
89. Starnes BW, Quiroga E, Hutter C, Tran NT, Hatsukami T, Meissner M, et al. Management of ruptured abdominal aortic aneurysm in the endovascular era. J Vasc Surg. 2010;51(1):9–17.
90. Starnes BW. Physician-modified endovascular grafts for the treatment of elective, symptomatic, or ruptured juxtarenal aortic aneurysms. J Vasc Surg. 2012;56(3):601–7.
91. Starnes BW, Tatum B. Early report from an investigator-initiated investigational device exemption clinical trial on physician-modified endovascular grafts. J Vasc Surg. 2013;58(2):311–7.

Endovascular Aneurysm Sealing for Ruptured Abdominal Aortic Aneurysm

92. Krievins DK, Holden A, Savlovskis J, Calderas C, Donayre CE, Moll FL, Katzen B, Zarins CK. EVAR using the Nellix Sac-anchoring endoprosthesis: treatment of favorable and adverse anatomy. Eur J Vasc Endovasc Surg. 2011;42:38–46.
93. Donayre CE, Zarins CK, Krievins DK, Holden A, Hill A, Calderas C, Velez J, White RA. Initial clinical experience with a sac-anchoring endoprosthesis for aortic aneurysm repair. J Vasc Surg. 2011;53:574–82.

94. Böckler D, Holden A, Thompson M, Hayes P, Krievins D, de Vries JP, Reijnen MM. Multicenter nellix EndoVascular aneurysm sealing system experience in aneurysm sac sealing. J Vasc Surg. 2015;62(2):290–8.
95. Egorova N, Giacovelli J, Greco G, Gelijns A, Kent CK, McKinsey JF. National outcomes for the treatment of ruptured abdominal aortic aneurysm: comparison of open versus endovascular repairs. J Vasc Surg. 2008;48:1092–100.
96. Hoornweg LL, Storm-Versloot MN, Ubbink DT, Koelemay MJ, Legemate DA, Balm R. Meta analysis on mortality of ruptured abdominal aortic aneurysms. Eur J Vasc Endovasc Surg. 2008;35:558–70.
97. Reimerink JJ, Hoornweg LL, Vahl AC, Wisselink W, van den Broek TA, Legemate DA, Reekers JA, Balm R, Amsterdam Acute Aneurysm Trial Collaborators. Endovascular repair versus open repair of ruptured abdominal aortic aneurysms: a multicenter randomized controlled trial. Ann Surg. 2013;258:248–56.
98. IMPROVE Trial Investigators, Powell JT, Sweeting MJ, Thompson MM, Ashleigh R, Bell R, Gomes M, Greenhalgh RM, Grieve R, Heatley F, Hinchliffe RJ, Thompson SG, Ulug P. Endovascular or open repair strategy for ruptured abdominal aortic aneurysm: 30 day outcomes from IMPROVE randomised trial. BMJ. 2014;348:f7661.
99. Sweeting MJ, Ulug P, Powell JT, Desgranges P, Balm R, Ruptured Aneurysm Trialists. Ruptured aneurysm trials: the importance of longer-term outcomes and meta-analysis for 1-year mortality. Eur J Vasc Endovasc Surg. 2015;50(3):297–302.
100. Grieve R, Gomes M, Sweeting MJ, Ulug P, Hinchliffe RJ, Thompson MM, Thompson SG, Ashleigh R, Greenhalgh RM, Powell JT, IMPROVE trial investigators. Endovascular strategy or open repair for ruptured abdominal aortic aneurysm: one-year outcomes from the IMPROVE randomized trial. Eur Heart J. 2015;36(31):2061–9.
101. Holden A. Endovascular sac sealing concept: will the Endologix Nellix solve the deficiencies? J Cardiovasc Surg. 2014;56(3):339–53.
102. Truijers M, van Sterkenburg SM, Lardenoije JW, Reijnen MM. Endovascular repair of a ruptured para-renal aortic aneurysm using the NellixTM endovascular system and parallel chimney grafts. J Endovasc Ther 2015;22(3):291–4. doi: 10.1177/1526602815579899. Epub 2015 Apr 22.
103. de Bruin JL, Brownrigg JR, Karthikesalingam A, Patterson BO, Holt PJ, Hinchliffe RJ, Morgan RA, Loftus IM, Thompson MM. Endovascular aneurysm sealing for the treatment of ruptured abdominal aortic aneurysms. J Endovasc Ther. 2015;22:283–7.
104. Coppi G, Saitta G, Lauricella A, Silingardi R. Treatment of a ruptured abdominal aortic aneurysm with an adverse anatomy using the nellix endovascular aneurysm sealing system. J Vasc Interv Radiol. 2015;26:606–8.
105. Malkawi A, de Bruin J, Loftus I, Thompson M. Treatment of a juxta-renal aneurysm with the Nellix endovascular aneurysm sealing system and chimney stent. J Endovasc Ther. 2014;21:541–7.
106. Dijkstra ML, Lardenoye JW, van Oostayen JA, Zeebregts CJ, Reijnen MM. Endovascular aneurysm sealing for juxtarenal aneurysm using the Nellix device and chimney covered stents. J Endovasc Ther. 2014;21:541–7.
107. Larzon T, Skoog P. One hundred percent of ruptured aortic abdominal aneurysms can be treated endovascularly if adjunct techniques are used such as chimneys, periscopes and embolization. J Cardiovasc Surg (Torino). 2014;55(2):169–78.
108. Karthikesalingam A, Cobb RJ, Khoury A, Choke EC, Sayers RD, Holt PJ, Thompson MM. The morphological applicability of a novel endovascular aneurysm sealing (EVAS) system (Nellix) in patients with abdominal aortic aneurysms. Eur J Vasc Endovasc Surg. 2013;46:440–5.
109. Maila M, Veith F, Ivancev K, Sonesson B. Balloon occlusion of the aorta during endovascular repair of ruptured abdominal aortic aneurysm. J Endovasc Ther. 2005;12(5):556–9.
110. Saito N, Matsumoto H, Yagi T, Hara Y, Hayashida K, Motomura T, Mashiko K, Iida H, Yokota H, Wagatsuma Y. Evaluation of the safety and feasibility of resuscitative endovascular balloon occlusion of the aorta. J Trauma Acute Care Surg. 2015;78(5):897–903.
111. Koike Y, Nishimura J, Hase S, Yamasaki M. Sac angiography and glue embolization in emergency endovascular aneurysm repair for ruptured abdominal aortic aneurysm. Cardiovasc Intervent Radiol. 2015;38(2):457–62.

Aortocaval Fistula

112. Alexander JJ, Imbembo AL. Aorto-vena cava fistula. Surgery. 1989;105:1–12.
113. Torigian DA, Carpenter JP, Roberts DA. Mycotic aortocaval fistula: efficient evaluation by bolus-chase MR angiography. J Magn Reson Imaging. 2002;15:195–8.
114. Kuint J, Bilik R, Heyman Z, et al. Congenital aortocaval fistula in the newborn: a case report. J Pediatr Surg. 1998;33:743–4.
115. de Andrade DR, Wood CA, Tedesco J. Aortocaval fistula due to remote gunshot wound. Am J Med. 2002;113:699–700.
116. Gorombey Z, Gomory A, Bekassy SM. Iatrogenic aortocaval fistula secondary to intervertebral disc surgery: a case report. Acta Chir Scand. 1984;150:585–7.
117. Dragas M, Davidovic L, Pejkic S, et al. Aorto-left renal vein fistula is a rare complication of abdominal aortic aneurysm with unique clinical presentation. J Vasc Surg. 2010;52:1658–61.
118. Maeda H, Umezawa H, Goshima M, et al. Surgery for ruptured abdominal aortic aneurysm with an aortocaval and iliac vein fistula. Surg Today. 2007;37:445–8.
119. Houben PF, Bollen EC, Nuyens CM. "Asymptomatic" ruptured aneurysm: a report of two cases of aortocaval fistula presenting with cardiac failure. Eur J Vasc Surg. 1993;7:352–4.
120. Lebon A, Agueznai M, Labombarda F. High-output heart failure resulting from chronic aortocaval fistula. Circulation. 2013;127:527–8.
121. Yancy DM, Guichard JL, Ahmed MI, et al. Cardiomyocyte mitochondrial oxidative stress and cytoskeletal breakdown in the heart with a primary volume overload. Am J Physiol Heart Circ Physiol. 2015;308:H651–3.
122. Steinke TM, Reber PU, Hakki H, Kniemeyer HW. Haematuria and an abdominal aneurysm – warning of an aortocaval fistula. Eur J Endovasc Surg. 1999;18:530–1.
123. Oda T, Yasunaga H, Hosokawa Y, et al. Preoperative computed tomographic diagnosis of an aortocaval fistula associated with aneurysm of the abdominal aorta. Ann Thorac Cardiovasc Surg. 2011;17:531–3.
124. Bhatia M, Platon A, Khabiri E, Becker C, Poletti PA. Contrast-enhanced ultrasonography versus MR angiography in aortocaval fistula: case report. Abdom Imaging. 2010;35:376–80.
125. Bolognesi R, Tsialtas D, Straneo U, Pexxola D, Manca C. The diagnosis by a Doppler color echocardiographic method of an aortocaval fistula following the rupture of an aortic aneurysm into the inferior vena cava. Cardiologia. 1991;36:147–52.
126. Egan DJ, Saul T, Herbert-Cohen D, Lewiss RE. Bedside ultrasound diagnosis of an aortocaval fistula in the emergency department. J Emerg Med. 2014;47:55–7.
127. Brightwell RE, Pegna V, Boyne N. Aortocaval fistula: current management strategies. ANZ J Surg. 2013;83:31–5.
128. Nakad G, AbiChedid G, Osman R. Endovascular treatment of major abdominal arteriovenous fistulas: a systematic review. Vasc Endovasc Surg. 2014;48:388–95.
129. Melas N, Saratzis A, Saratzis N, et al. Inferior vena cava stent-graft placement to treat endoleak associated with an aortocaval fistula. J Vasc Endovasc Surg. 2011;30:640–4.
130. Madani A, Leung S, Obrand D. Open repair of inflammatory abdominal aortic aneurysm and aortocaval fistula using retrograde balloon occlusion. Vasc Endovasc Surg. 2014;48:80–2.
131. Calligaro KD, Dougherty MJ. Surgical treatment of abdominal aortic aneurysm-inferior vena cava fistula. In: Stanley J, Veith F, Wakefield T, editors. Current therapy in vascular and endovascular surgery. 5th ed. Philadelphia: Elsevier; 2014.
132. Hecker BR, Lynch C. Intraoperative diagnosis and treatment of massive pulmonary embolism complicating surgery on the abdominal aorta. Br J Anaesth. 1983;55:689–91.
133. Brunkwall J, Lanne T, Bergentz SE. Acute renal impairment due to a primary aortocaval fistula is normalized after a successful operation. Eur J Vasc Endovasc Surg. 1999;17:191–6.

Dealing with Ruptured Common Iliac Artery Aneurysms

134. Santilli SM, Wernsing SE, Lee ES. Expansion rates and outcomes for iliac artery aneurysms. J Vasc Surg. 2000;31(1 Pt 1):114–21.
135. Huang Y, Gloviczki P, Duncan AA, Kalra M, Hoskin TL, Oderich GS, et al. Common iliac artery aneurysm: expansion rate and results of open surgical and endovascular repair. J Vasc Surg. 2008;47(6):1203–10; discussion 10–1.
136. Vammen S, Lindholt J, Henneberg EW, Fasting H. A comparative study of iliac and abdominal aortic aneurysms. Int Angiol. 2000;19(2):152–7.
137. Richardson JW, Greenfield LJ. Natural history and management of iliac aneurysms. J Vasc Surg. 1988;8(2):165–71.
138. Krupski WC, Selzman CH, Floridia R, Strecker PK, Nehler MR, Whitehill TA. Contemporary management of isolated iliac aneurysms. J Vasc Surg. 1998;28(1):1–11; discussion –3.
139. Patel NV, Long GW, Cheema ZF, Rimar K, Brown OW, Shanley CJ. Open vs. Endovascular repair of isolated iliac artery aneurysms: a 12-year experience. J Vasc Surg. 2009;49(5):1147–53.
140. Ijaz S, Geroulakos G. Ruptured internal iliac artery aneurysm mimicking a hip fracture. Int Angiol. 2001;20(2):187–9.
141. Appel N, Duncan JR, Schuerer DJ. Percutaneous stent-graft treatment of superior mesenteric and internal iliac artery pseudoaneurysms. J Vasc Interv Radiol. 2003;14(7):917–22.
142. Atsuta Y, Inaba M, Goh K, Azuma N, Akasaka N, Asada H, et al. Isolated iliac artery aneurysm caused by fibromuscular dysplasia: report of a case. Surg Today. 2003;33(8):639–41.
143. Dix FP, Titi M, Al-Khaffaf H. The isolated internal iliac artery aneurysm--a review. Eur J Vasc Endovasc Surg. 2005;30(2):119–29.
144. Boules TN, Selzer F, Stanziale SF, Chomic A, Marone LK, Dillavou ED, et al. Endovascular management of isolated iliac artery aneurysms. J Vasc Surg. 2006;44(1):29–37.
145. Loos MJ, Scheer M, van der Vliet JA, Warle MC. Ruptured iliac artery aneurysm presenting as acute right heart failure and cardiac arrest. Ann Vasc Surg. 2015;29(2):363 e5–7.
146. Atin HL. Rupture of an iliac-artery aneurysm into the sigmoid colon; report of a case. N Engl J Med. 1958;258(8):366–9.
147. Cardon JM, Cardon A, Joyeux A, Vidal V, Noblet D. Endovascular repair of iliac artery aneurysm with endoprosystem I: a multicentric French study. J Cardiovasc Surg (Torino). 1996;37(3 Suppl 1):45–50.
148. Ruebben A, Tettoni S, Muratore P, Rossato D, Savio D, Rabbia C. Percutaneous endoluminal bypass of iliac aneurysms with a covered stent. Cardiovasc Intervent Radiol. 1998;21(4):339–42.
149. Kirkwood ML, Saunders A, Jackson BM, Wang GJ, Fairman RM, Woo EY. Aneurysmal iliac arteries do not portend future iliac aneurysmal enlargement after endovascular aneurysm repair for abdominal aortic aneurysm. J Vasc Surg. 2011;53(2):269–73.
150. Parlani G, Zannetti S, Verzini F, De Rango P, Carlini G, Lenti M, et al. Does the presence of an iliac aneurysm affect outcome of endoluminal AAA repair? an analysis of 336 cases. Eur J Vasc Endovasc Surg. 2002;24(2):134–8.
151. Sandhu RS, Pipinos II. Isolated iliac artery aneurysms. Semin Vasc Surg. 2005;18(4):209–15.
152. Sakamoto I, Sueyoshi E, Hazama S, Makino K, Nishida A, Yamaguchi T, et al. Endovascular treatment of iliac artery aneurysms. Radiographics. 2005;25 Suppl 1:S213–27.
153. Marin ML, Veith FJ, Lyon RT, Cynamon J, Sanchez LA. Transfemoral endovascular repair of iliac artery aneurysms. Am J Surg. 1995;170(2):179–82.
154. Dorros G, Cohn JM, Jaff MR. Percutaneous endovascular stent-graft repair of iliac artery aneurysms. J Endovasc Surg. 1997;4(4):370–5.
155. Krajcer Z, Khoshnevis R, Leachman DR, Herman H. Endoluminal exclusion of an iliac artery aneurysm by Wallstent endoprosthesis and PTFE vascular graft. Tex Heart Inst J. 1997;24(1):11–4.
156. Kritpracha B, Pigott JP, Russell TE, Corbey MJ, Whalen RC, DiSalle RS, et al. Bell-bottom aortoiliac endografts: an alternative that preserves pelvic blood flow. J Vasc Surg. 2002;35(5):874–81.
157. Alvarez Marcos F, de la Torre A G, Alonso Perez M, Llaneza Coto JM, Camblor Santervas LA, Zanabili Al Sibbai AA, et al. Use of aortic extension cuffs for preserving hypogastric

blood flow in endovascular aneurysm repair with aneurysmal involvement of common iliac arteries. Ann Vasc Surg. 2013;27(2):139–45.
158. Yano OJ, Morrissey N, Eisen L, Faries PL, Soundararajan K, Wan S, et al. Intentional internal iliac artery occlusion to facilitate endovascular repair of aortoiliac aneurysms. J Vasc Surg. 2001;34(2):204–11.
159. Rayt HS, Bown MJ, Lambert KV, Fishwick NG, McCarthy MJ, London NJ, et al. Buttock claudication and erectile dysfunction after internal iliac artery embolization in patients prior to endovascular aortic aneurysm repair. Cardiovasc Intervent Radiol. 2008;31(4):728–34.
160. Parodi JC, Ferreira M. Relocation of the iliac artery bifurcation to facilitate endoluminal treatment of abdominal aortic aneurysms. J Endovasc Surg. 1999;6(4):342–7.
161. Faries PL, Morrissey N, Burks JA, Gravereaux E, Kerstein MD, Teodorescu VJ, et al. Internal iliac artery revascularization as an adjunct to endovascular repair of aortoiliac aneurysms. J Vasc Surg. 2001;34(5):892–9.
162. Rhee RY, Muluk SC, Tzeng E, Missig Carroll N, Makaroun MS. Can the internal iliac artery be safely covered during endovascular repair of abdominal aortic and iliac artery aneurysms? Ann Vasc Surg. 2002;16(1):29–36.
163. Lobato AC, Camacho-Lobato L. The sandwich technique to treat complex aortoiliac or isolated iliac aneurysms: results of midterm follow-up. J Vasc Surg. 2013;57(2 Suppl):26S–34.
164. Lepidi S, Piazza M, Scrivere P, Menegolo M, Antonello M, Grego F, et al. Parallel endografts in the treatment of distal aortic and common iliac aneurysms. Eur J Vasc Endovasc Surg. 2014;48(1):29–37.
165. Heckenkamp J, Brunkwall J, Luebke T, Aleksic M, Schondube F, Stojanovic T. Novel chimney-graft technique for preserving hypogastric flow in complex aortoiliac aneurysms. J Cardiovasc Surg (Torino). 2012;53(6):773–6.
166. DeRubertis BG, Quinones-Baldrich WJ, Greenberg JI, Jimenez JC, Lee JT. Results of a double-barrel technique with commercially available devices for hypogastric preservation during aortoilac endovascular abdominal aortic aneurysm repair. J Vasc Surg. 2012;56(5):1252–9.
167. Ricci C, Ceccherini C, Cini M, Vigni F, Leonini S, Tommasino G, et al. Single-center experience and 1-year follow-up results of "sandwich technique" in the management of common iliac artery aneurysms during EVAR. Cardiovasc Intervent Radiol. 2012;35(5):1195–200.
168. Karthikesalingam A, Hinchliffe RJ, Holt PJ, Boyle JR, Loftus IM, Thompson MM. Endovascular aneurysm repair with preservation of the internal iliac artery using the iliac branch graft device. Eur J Vasc Endovasc Surg. 2010;39(3):285–94.
169. Wong S, Greenberg RK, Brown CR, Mastracci TM, Bena J, Eagleton MJ. Endovascular repair of aortoiliac aneurysmal disease with the helical iliac bifurcation device and the bifurcated-bifurcated iliac bifurcation device. J Vasc Surg. 2013;58(4):861–9.
170. Wyers MC, Schermerhorn ML, Fillinger MF, Powell RJ, Rzucidlo EM, Walsh DB, et al. Internal iliac occlusion without coil embolization during endovascular abdominal aortic aneurysm repair. J Vasc Surg. 2002;36(6):1138–45.
171. Mehta M, Veith FJ, Ohki T, Cynamon J, Goldstein K, Suggs WD, et al. Unilateral and bilateral hypogastric artery interruption during aortoiliac aneurysm repair in 154 patients: a relatively innocuous procedure. J Vasc Surg. 2001;33(2 Suppl):S27–32.
172. Razavi MK, DeGroot M, Olcott 3rd C, Sze D, Kee S, Semba CP, et al. Internal iliac artery embolization in the stent-graft treatment of aortoiliac aneurysms: analysis of outcomes and complications. J Vasc Interv Radiol. 2000;11(5):561–6.
173. Lyden SP, Sternbach Y, Waldman DL, Green RM. Clinical implications of internal iliac artery embolization in endovascular repair of aortoiliac aneurysms. Ann Vasc Surg. 2001;15(5):539–43.
174. Ha CD, Calcagno D. Amplatzer Vascular Plug to occlude the internal iliac arteries in patients undergoing aortoiliac aneurysm repair. J Vasc Surg. 2005;42(6):1058–62.
175. Farahmand P, Becquemin JP, Desgranges P, Allaire E, Marzelle J, Roudot-Thoraval F. Is hypogastric artery embolization during endovascular aortoiliac aneurysm repair (EVAR) innocuous and useful? Eur J Vasc Endovasc Surg. 2008;35(4):429–35.
176. Schoder M, Zaunbauer L, Holzenbein T, Fleischmann D, Cejna M, Kretschmer G, et al. Internal iliac artery embolization before endovascular repair of abdominal aortic aneurysms: frequency, efficacy, and clinical results. AJR Am J Roentgenol. 2001;177(3):599–605.

177. Criado FJ, Wilson EP, Velazquez OC, Carpenter JP, Barker C, Wellons E, et al. Safety of coil embolization of the internal iliac artery in endovascular grafting of abdominal aortic aneurysms. J Vasc Surg. 2000;32(4):684–8.
178. Mehta M, Veith FJ, Darling RC, Roddy SP, Ohki T, Lipsitz EC, et al. Effects of bilateral hypogastric artery interruption during endovascular and open aortoiliac aneurysm repair. J Vasc Surg. 2004;40(4):698–702.
179. Lee CW, Kaufman JA, Fan CM, Geller SC, Brewster DC, Cambria RP, et al. Clinical outcome of internal iliac artery occlusions during endovascular treatment of aortoiliac aneurysmal diseases. J Vasc Interv Radiol. 2000;11(5):567–71.
180. Kritpracha B, Pigott JP, Price CI, Russell TE, Corbey MJ, Beebe HG. Distal internal iliac artery embolization: a procedure to avoid. J Vasc Surg. 2003;37(5):943–8.
181. Tefera G, Turnipseed WD, Carr SC, Pulfer KA, Hoch JR, Acher CW. Is coil embolization of hypogastric artery necessary during endovascular treatment of aortoiliac aneurysms? Ann Vasc Surg. 2004;18(2):143–6.
182. Wolpert LM, Dittrich KP, Hallisey MJ, Allmendinger PP, Gallagher JJ, Heydt K, et al. Hypogastric artery embolization in endovascular abdominal aortic aneurysm repair. J Vasc Surg. 2001;33(6):1193–8.
183. Jean-Baptiste E, Brizzi S, Bartoli MA, Sadaghianloo N, Baque J, Magnan PE, et al. Pelvic ischemia and quality of life scores after interventional occlusion of the hypogastric artery in patients undergoing endovascular aortic aneurysm repair. J Vasc Surg. 2014;60(1):40–9, 9 e1.
184. Lin PH, Bush RL, Chaikof EL, Chen C, Conklin B, Terramani TT, et al. A prospective evaluation of hypogastric artery embolization in endovascular aortoiliac aneurysm repair. J Vasc Surg. 2002;36(3):500–6.
185. Karch LA, Hodgson KJ, Mattos MA, Bohannon WT, Ramsey DE, McLafferty RB. Adverse consequences of internal iliac artery occlusion during endovascular repair of abdominal aortic aneurysms. J Vasc Surg. 2000;32(4):676–83.
186. Kritpracha B, Comerota AJ. Unilateral lower extremity paralysis after coil embolization of an internal iliac artery aneurysm. J Vasc Surg. 2004;40(4):819–21.
187. Lin TW, Kan CB. Endovascular repair of ruptured iliac artery aneurysm. Acta Cardiol Sin. 2010;26:198–200.
188. Shimabukuro K, Miyauchi T, Takemura H. Rupture of left common iliac artery aneurysm. J Vasc Surg. 2007;45(5):1083.
189. Plaza-Martinez A, Gomez-Palones F, Zaragoza-Garcia JM, Martinez-Parreno C, AlRaies-Bolanos B, Ortiz-Monzon E. Endovascular treatment of a ruptured iliac aneurysm previously excluded. Ann Vasc Surg. 2009;23(6):785 e13–6.
190. Buck DB, Bensley RP, Darling J, Curran T, McCallum JC, Moll FL, et al. The effect of endovascular treatment on isolated iliac artery aneurysm treatment and mortality. J Vasc Surg. 2015;62:331–5.
191. Chaer RA, Barbato JE, Lin SC, Zenati M, Kent KC, McKinsey JF. Isolated iliac artery aneurysms: a contemporary comparison of endovascular and open repair. J Vasc Surg. 2008;47(4):708–13.
192. Cynamon J, Lerer D, Veith FJ, Taragin BH, Wahl SI, Lautin JL, et al. Hypogastric artery coil embolization prior to endoluminal repair of aneurysms and fistulas: buttock claudication, a recognizable but possibly preventable complication. J Vasc Interv Radiol. 2000;11:573–7.
193. Iliopoulos JI, Howanitz PE, Pierce GE, Kueshkerian SM, Thomas JH, Hermreck AS. The critical hypogastric circulation. Am J Surg. 1987;154:671–5.

Management of Ruptured Abdominal Aortic Aneurysms in Association with Aortic Dissection

194. DiMusto PD, Williams DM, Patel HJ, Trimarchi S, Eliason JL, Upchurch GR. Endovascular management of type B aortic dissection. J Vasc Surg. 2010;52:26S–36.
195. Criado FJ. Aortic dissection: a 250-year perspective. Tex Heart Inst J. 2011;38:694–700.

196. Swee W, Dake MD. Endovascular management of thoracic dissections. Circulation. 2008;117:1460–73.
197. Umaña JP, Lai DT, Mitchell RS, Moore KA, Rodriguez F, Robbins RC, et al. Is medical therapy still the optimal treatment strategy for patients with acute type B aortic dissections? J Thorac Cardiovasc Surg. 2002;124:896–910.
198. IMPROVE trial investigators. Endovascular or open repair strategy for ruptured abdominal aortic aneurysm: 30 day outcomes from IMPROVE randomised trial. BMJ. 2014;348:f7661.
199. Dimusto PD, Upchurch GR. The pathogenesis of abdominal aortic aneurysms. https://www.vascularweb.org/research/Pages/the-pathogenesis-of-abdominal-aortic-aneurysms.aspx.
200. DeBakey ME, McCollun CH, Crawford ES, Morris Jr GC, Howell J, Noon GP, et al. Dissection and dissecting aneurysms of the aorta: twenty year follow-up of five hundred twenty-seven patients treated surgically. Surgery. 1982;92:1118–33.
201. Lee JJ, Dimick JB, Williams DM, Henke PK, Deeb GM, Eagle KA, et al. Existence of abdominal aortic aneurysms in patients with thoracic aortic dissections. J Vasc Surg. 2003;38:671–5.
202. van Bogerijen GH, Tolenaar JL, Rampoldi V, Moll FL, van Herwaarden JA, Jonker FH, Eagle KA, Trimarchi S. Predictors of aortic growth in uncomplicated type B aortic dissection. J Vasc Surg. 2014;59:1134–43.
203. Ali MM, Flahive J, Schanzer A, Simons JP, Aiello FA, Doucet DR, et al. In patients stratified by preoperative risk, endovascular repair of ruptured abdominal aortic aneurysms has a lower in-hospital mortality and morbidity than open repair. J Vasc Surg. 2015;61:1399–407.
204. Conrad MF, Cambria RP. Aortic dissection. In: Cronenwett J, Johnston W, editors. Rutherford's vascular surgery. 7th ed. Philadelphia: Elsevier Health Sciences; 2010. p. 2090–109.
205. Reimerink JJ, Hoornweg LL, Vahl AC, Wisselink W, Balm R. Controlled hypotension in patients suspected of a ruptured abdominal aortic aneurysm: feasibility during transport by ambulance services and possible. Eur J Vasc Endovasc Surg. 2010;40:54–9.
206. Sharafuddin MJ, Sun RC, Lysandrou AJ, Amin PB, Nicholson RM, Sharp WJ, Kresowik TF. Endovascular management of ruptured/leaking descending thoracic and visceral aortic aneurysms using branch snorkels technique. J Vasc Surg. 2012;56:1191.
207. Lee JT, Lee GK, Chandra V, Dalman RL. Comparison of fenestrated endografts and the snorkel/chimney technique. J Vasc Surg. 2014;60:849–56.
208. Tashiro J, Baqai A, Goldstein LJ, Salsamendi JT, Taubman M, Rey J. "Cheese wire" fenestration of a chronic aortic dissection flap for endovascular repair of a contained aneurysm rupture. J Vasc Surg. 2014;60:497–9.
209. Norberto EM, Gutiérrez VM, Taylor J, Vaquero C. Coil embolization of persistent false lumen after stent graft repair of type B aortic dissection. J Vasc Surg. 2011;54:201–4.
210. Idrees J, Roselli EE, Shafii S, Reside J, Lytle BW. Outcomes after false lumen embolization with covered stent devices in chronic dissection. J Vasc Surg. 2014;60:1507–13.
211. Roselli EE, Idrees J, Reside J, Susan Shafii S. Use of covered stent devices for false lumen embolization in chronic dissection: a novel approach. Ann Thorac Surg. 2014;98:737–9.

Surgical Conversion for Rupture After EVAR

212. Brewster DC, Jones JE, Chung TK, Lamuraglia GM, Kwolek CJ, Watkins MT, et al. Long-term outcomes after endovascular abdominal aortic aneurysm repair: the first decade. Ann Surg. 2006;244(3):426–38.
213. Stark M, Suresh A, Alexander J, Cragg A. An analysis of variables affecting aortic neck length with implications for fenestrated endovascular repair of abdominal aortic aneurysm. Ann Vasc Surg. 2014;28(4):808–15.
214. Lee JT, Ullery BW, Zarins CK, Olcott C, Harris Jr EJ, Dalman RL. EVAR deployment in anatomically challenging necks outside the IFU. Eur J Vasc Endovasc Surg. 2013;46(1):65–73.
215. Schanzer A, Greenberg RK, Hevelone N, Robinson WP, Eslami MH, Goldberg RJ, et al. Predictors of abdominal aortic aneurysm sac enlargement after endovascular repair. Circulation. 2011;123(24):2848–55.

216. Sternbergh 3rd WC, Carter G, York JW, Yoselevitz M, Money SR. Aortic neck angulation predicts adverse outcome with endovascular abdominal aortic aneurysm repair. J Vasc Surg. 2002;35(3):482–6.
217. Turney EJ, Steenberge SP, Lyden SP, Eagleton MJ, Srivastava SD, Sarac TP, et al. Late graft explants in endovascular aneurysm repair. J Vasc Surg. 2014;59(4):886–93.
218. Abbruzzese TA, Kwolek CJ, Brewster DC, Chung TK, Kang J, Conrad MF, et al. Outcomes following endovascular abdominal aortic aneurysm repair (EVAR): an anatomic and device-specific analysis. J Vasc Surg. 2008;48(1):19–28.
219. Vourliotakis G, Bos WT, Beck AW, Van Den Dungen JJ, Prins TR, Verhoeven EL. Fenestrated stent-grafting after previous endovascular abdominal aortic aneurysm repair. J Cardiovasc Surg (Torino). 2010;51(3):383–9.
220. Martin Z, Greenberg RK, Mastracci TM, Eagleton MJ, O'Callaghan A, Bena J. Late rescue of proximal endograft failure using fenestrated and branched devices. J Vasc Surg. 2014;59(6):1479–87.
221. Mehta M, Paty PS, Roddy SP, Taggert JB, Sternbach Y, Kreienberg PB, et al. Treatment options for delayed AAA rupture following endovascular repair. J Vasc Surg. 2011;53(1):14–20.
222. Chaar CI, Eid R, Park T, Rhee RY, Abu-Hamad G, Tzeng E, et al. Delayed open conversions after endovascular abdominal aortic aneurysm repair. J Vasc Surg. 2012;55(6):f1562–9 e1.
223. Kelso RL, Lyden SP, Butler B, Greenberg RK, Eagleton MJ, Clair DG. Late conversion of aortic stent grafts. J Vasc Surg. 2009;49(3):589–95.
224. Schermerhorn ML, Buck DB, O'Malley AJ, Curran T, McCallum JC, Darling J, et al. Long-term outcomes of abdominal aortic aneurysm in the Medicare population. N Engl J Med. 2015;373(4):328–38.
225. Lyden SP, McNamara JM, Sternbach Y, Illig KA, Waldman DL, Green RM. Technical considerations for late removal of aortic endografts. J Vasc Surg. 2002;36(4):674–8.
226. May J, White GH, Harris JP. Techniques for surgical conversion of aortic endoprosthesis. Eur J Vasc Endovasc Surg. 1999;18(4):284–9.
227. Koning OH, Hinnen JW, van Baalen JM. Technique for safe removal of an aortic endograft with suprarenal fixation. J Vasc Surg. 2006;43(4):855–7.
228. Popplewell MA, Garnham AW, Hobbs SD. A new technique to explant an infected aortic endograft. J Vasc Surg. 2015;62(2):512–4.
229. Candell L, Tucker LY, Goodney P, Walker J, Okuhn S, Hill B, et al. Early and delayed rupture after endovascular abdominal aortic aneurysm repair in a 10-year multicenter registry. J Vasc Surg. 2014;60(5):1146–52.
230. Antoniou GA, Georgiadis GS, Antoniou SA, Neequaye S, Brennan JA, Torella F, et al. Late rupture of abdominal aortic aneurysm after previous endovascular repair: a systematic review and meta-analysis. J Endovasc Ther. 2015;22(5):734–44.

Chapter 14
Randomized Trials: What is the Evidence?

**James Budge, Benjamin Patterson, Matt M. Thompson,
Frank J. Veith, and Caron B. Rockman**

Randomized Trials: What is the Evidence?

James Budge, Benjamin Patterson, Matt Thompson

Key Points
- Endovascular surgery for rAAA is clinically effective, cost-effective, and associated with shorter hospital stay.
- Endovascular repair should be offered to most patients that are anatomically suitable.
- Hospitals that perform rAAA repair should be able to perform both open and endovascular repair.

Introduction

Open surgical treatment of a ruptured aortic abdominal aneurysm (rAAA) has historically been the sole treatment modality available, and in many centers remains the only one offered despite the first endovascular repair being described in 1994

J. Budge • B. Patterson • M.M. Thompson, MD (✉)
St George's Vascular Institute, St George's Hospital,
Blackshaw Road Tooting, London SW17 0QT, UK
e-mail: matt.thompson@stgeorges.nhs.uk

F.J. Veith, MD
New York University, Langone Medical Center, New York, NY, USA

The Cleveland Clinic, Cleveland, OH, USA
e-mail: fjvmd@msn.com

C.B. Rockman, MD
New York University, Langone Medical Center, New York, NY, USA

B.W. Starnes et al. (eds.), *Ruptured Abdominal Aortic Aneurysm*,
DOI 10.1007/978-3-319-23844-9_14

[17]. Widespread uptake of the technique has been slow, but the development by early adopters has allowed for the improvement of protocols and identification of logistical issues that have required specific solutions [9–11].

Over time the need for larger datasets and randomized controlled trial (RCTs) has been increasingly debated, largely prompted by the results of a pilot RCT [5] and analysis of national databases [4,6,16]. The latter studies analyzed the Medicare dataset and the hospital episode statistics (HES) data in the USA and UK, respectively, demonstrating better 30-day mortality outcomes with endovascular repair of rAAA (between 21 and 30 %) when compared to open surgical repair. These results have been subject to some criticism due to a perception that there is an inherent patient selection bias and that these are mixed cohorts of symptomatic and ruptured aneurysms.

There are three main trials that will be discussed in this chapter, two trials in which patients were selected anatomically, AJAX [13] and ECAR [2], and one that represents a pragmatic clinical practice, IMPROVE [13]. The design and utility of these trials are discussed below.

RCT Trials: AJAX, ECAR, and IMPROVE (Design)

AJAX (Amsterdam Acute Aneurysm Trial)

The AJAX trial recruited patients between April 2004 and February 2011 in three centers in Amsterdam. Patients were mainly recruited from two academic medical centers and one teaching hospital but also recruited from seven regional hospitals where transfer was possible. Patients who were deemed fit and anatomically suitable for both EVAR and OSR were randomized. Those that could not undergo CTA, EVAR, or OSR were excluded.

A total of 520 patients with a clinical suspicion of rAAA were identified, and 466 were admitted to one of the three trial centers. rAAA was confirmed by CTA in 395 patients, and after exclusion due to anatomy and other factors, 116 patients were randomized. 59 were assigned to OSR and 57 assigned to EVAR (see Fig. 14.1).

The primary end point was the composite of death and severe complications at 30 days.

The main findings were that there was no difference in mortality at either 30 days (EVAR 21 % vs OSR 25 % $p=0.66$) or 6 months (EVAR 28 % vs OSR 31 % $p=0.84$) between open and endovascular repair. The AJAX trial also found no difference in severe complications (cardiac, bowel ischemia, reintervention, stroke, amputation, or cord ischemia) between the EVAR and OSR group at 30 days and at 6 months. Renal insufficiency was found to be significantly lower at 30 days and at 6 months in the EVAR when compared with OSR (11 % vs 31 %, respectively, at 30 days, $p=0.01$; 11 % vs 31 %, respectively, at 6 months). Encouragingly AJAX also found that mortality for OSR was lower than expected in comparison with a relatively contemporaneous meta-analysis (mortality of OSR = 48.5 %) [7].

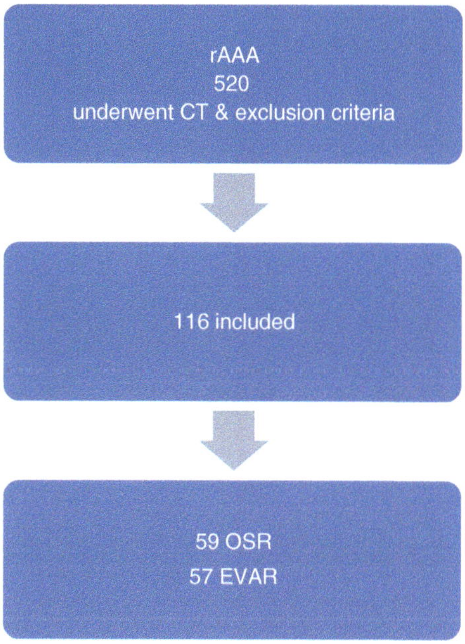

Fig. 14.1 Flowchart of AJAX recruitment

AJAX showed that mortality and severe morbidity were equal in EVAR and OSR at 30 days and at 6 months. The trial also presented lower than expected mortality, which was ascribed to the effect of performing surgery in centers with a high level of expertise, in patients with aortic anatomy suitable for endovascular repair (relatively long aortic neck). Limitations of the study include that only aorto-uni-iliac endoprosthesis was used with femoral to femoral crossover grafts in all patients, which is not representative of current practice. Secondly only 22 % of patients with rAAA in the trial region were included, most being excluded due to unsuitable anatomy (46 %). This is likely to mean that the overall mortality rate was underestimated as morphologically complex aneurysms were excluded. Due to the hypothesis of a higher mortality with OSR, the study may not have been sufficiently powered to discriminate a smaller difference of mortality between OSR and EVAR in this particular group of patients with relatively favorable anatomy.

ECAR (Ruptured Aortoiliac Aneurysm: Endo Versus Surgery)

The ECAR trial recruited from January 2008 to January 2013, and 107 patients were enrolled across 14 centers. 56 patients were assigned to the EVAR group and 51 to OSR (see Fig. 14.2) [3].

The primary end point of this study was 30-day mortality, with secondary end points of 30-day rates of cardiovascular, pulmonary, gastrointestinal, renal, and neurological morbidity. Time spent in ITU and volume of blood transfusion received were also end points.

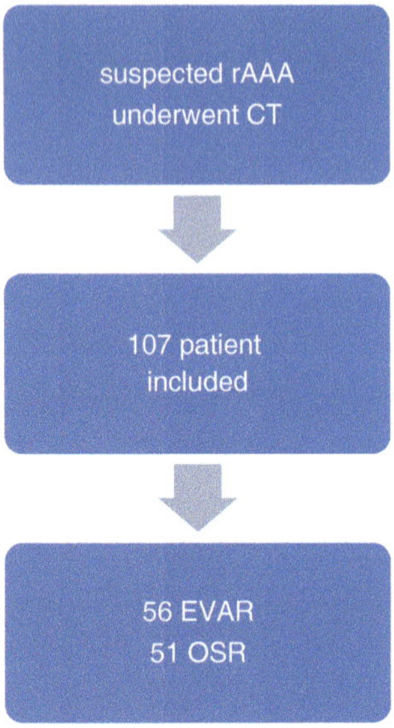

Fig. 14.2 Flowchart of ECAR recruitment

The main outcome of the ECAR trial was similar to that of the AJAX trial, demonstrating that 30-day (18 % EVAR vs 24 % OSR) and 1-year mortality (30 % EVAR vs 35 % OSR) was not statistically different between the OSR and EVAR groups. Analysis of secondary outcomes observed that EVAR was associated with less severe complications. There were reduced rates of pulmonary complications in the EVAR group (15.5 % vs 41.5 % in OSR $p=0.05$), reduced requirements for blood transfusion (6.8 units EVAR vs 10.9 OSR $p=0.02$), and less intensive use of hospital resources (significantly shorter ITU stay in EVAR vs OSR; 7 vs 11.9 days, $p=0.01$).

As with AJAX this study only addressed the question of EVAR vs OSR in a stable group of patients with particular anatomy that would allow EVAR to occur, and once again the trial may not have been sufficiently powered due to better than expected outcomes with OSR.

IMPROVE

The IMPROVE trial recruited from September 2009 to July 2013, recruiting patients from 29 British centers and one Canadian center. During this time 613 patients were randomized to OSR or EVAR (see Fig. 14.3), with randomization occurring at a clinical diagnosis of AAA and often before CTA to determine anatomical suitability for EVAR. These patients had varying levels of hemodynamic stability, but clearly moribund patients were excluded. The trial design meant that IMPROVE did include some patients without a diagnosis of ruptured aneurysm, but specified analyses defined that this was not a cause of bias in the trial.

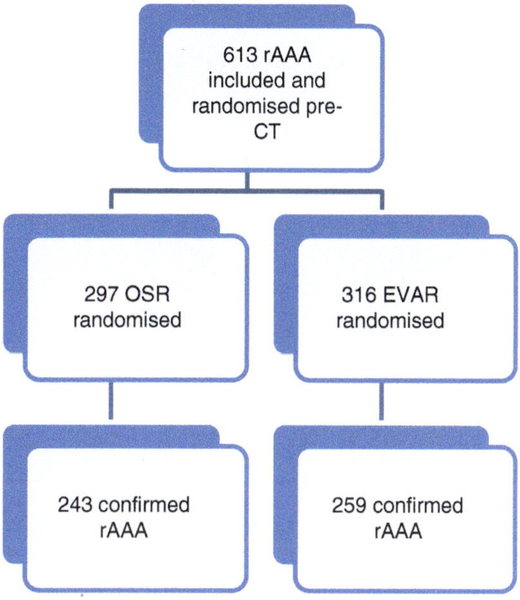

Fig. 14.3 Flowchart of IMPROVE recruitment

Due to the differences in study design, IMPROVE was better able to assess the efficacy of an endovascular first strategy and was more generalizable to the entire ruptured aneurysm patient population. In addition the heterogeneity of trial hospitals more accurately represented the variety of sites that a patient may present to as opposed to only selected expert centers.

Although the AJAX and ECAR trials may appear similar to the IMPROVE trial, they are in fact answering very different questions (see Table 14.1 for a comparison between the three studies). ECAR and AJAX as described above only address a small percentage of the target population, i.e., those that are hemodynamically stable and have undergone a CT which documents rupture and has favorable anatomy for EVAR.

Analysis of Findings from the IMPROVE Trial

30-Day Outcomes

The 30-day results from the IMPROVE trial demonstrated that the mortality for patients randomized to either EVAR or OSR was not statistically different. The trial observed that women benefit more from endovascular repair, and this was thought in part to be because women had a higher risk of mortality than men for OSR (57 % vs 32 %) when compared to EVAR in which they were more comparable (37 % vs 35 %).

Table 14.1 A comparison between AJAX, ECAR, and IMPROVE

	AJAX	ECAR	IMPROVE
Number of randomized	116	107	613
Number of study sites	3	14	30
Randomized before or after CT	After	After	Before (mostly)
Primary end point	30-day composite of death and severe complications	30-day mortality	30-day mortality
Secondary end points	Length of hospital and ITU stay, duration of intubation/ ventilation, use of blood products	30-day cardiovascular, pulmonary, gastrointestinal, renal, and neurological morbidity; time spent in ITU and volume of blood transfusion	Reintervention, hospital discharge, health-related quality of life, cost, quality-adjusted life years, cost-effectiveness
Mortality of EVAR vs OSR, 30 days	EVAR 21 % OSR 25 %	EVAR 18 % OSR 24 %	EVAR 35 % OSR 37 %
Mortality EVAR vs OSR, 1 year	(6 months) EVAR 28 (6 months) OSR 31	30 % EVAR 35 % OSR	41 % EVAR 45 % OSR

EVAR also demonstrated a trend toward better outcomes for the most seriously ill and older people, which was thought to be due to the minimally invasive nature of the surgery placing less of a physiological strain on these patients. Similarly local anesthesia was also shown to have better outcome than general anesthesia. Many have suggested that permissive hypotension may have a beneficial effect in patients with rAAA in the same way that it has been demonstrated in those with hypovolemic shock following trauma. Contrary to this, permissive hypotension with a systolic blood pressure of under 70 mmHg was associated with increased mortality (51 % if lowest recorded <70 vs 34 % >70) [12]. This finding should be interpreted with some caution as it is well known that patients who develop profound and refractory hypotension are less likely to survive than those in which this does not occur. Similarly, the finding that suggested a better outcome in patients treated under local anesthesia should be interpreted cautiously.

Hospital stay was reduced in the EVAR patients when compared to the OSR group (17 days vs 26 days), and significantly more patients were discharged home after their intervention in the EVAR group. This was part of the reason that IMPROVE also showed that an endovascular strategy was fiscally beneficial, with EVAR calculated to give an incremental net benefit of £3877 compared to OSR at 1 year, despite an allowance of £4000–10,000 per device used and the possible increase in operative theater staff and other additional intervention costs.

IMPROVE did attempt to also include the cost of readmission and reintervention associated with EVAR, but this was performed using a health services questionnaire.

The IMPROVE investigators identified time of presentation as a factor that affected mortality with out-of-hours presentation being higher (odds ratio 1.47 $p=0.048$). Efficacy of EVAR vs OSR was unchanged however when randomized to in or out of hours [12].

1-Year Follow-Up Data

The recently reported 1-year follow-up of the IMPROVE trial [14] has continued to reflect the 30-day data. There was no difference observed in all-cause mortality at 1 year (41.1 % EVAR vs 45.1 % OSR) and also no difference in aneurysm-related mortality (33.9 % in EVAR vs 39.3 % in OSR). Of note half of these deaths occurred within 24 h and the majority of the rest within 30 days.

In the longer follow-up, patients randomized to EVAR had an improved health-related quality of life and reduced costs and were more likely to be discharged home sooner. A cost-effectiveness analysis demonstrated benefit to the EVAR first strategy.

Morphology

Due to the randomization procedure in the IMPROVE study mostly occurring before CTA, the effect of morphology on mortality could be studied [8]. The effect of six morphological parameters (maximum aortic diameter, aneurysm neck diameter, length and conicality, proximal neck angle, and maximum common iliac diameter) was studied to see the effect on a 30-day mortality and reintervention. There were no significant correlations between the six morphological variables seen.

Analysis of these data demonstrated that by far the greatest predictor of mortality was aneurysm neck length and that each 15-mm increase in neck length equated to a reduction in 30-day mortality of approximately 20 %. This relationship could also be seen in the 24-h period, during which half deaths seen occurred. It was also the most likely factor to preclude EVAR.

The importance of neck length as a key factor may also go some way in explaining why randomization after CT makes EVAR look more favorable in terms of early mortality in contemporary cohort studies, as without a suitable neck length, EVAR would not be technically possible. It also explains why to some extent women are seen to benefit so greatly from EVAR, as they often have shorter aneurysm necks [8]. One benefit of EVAR in women is that the distal landing zone is often in common iliac instead of requiring extension into the external iliac which reduces potential morbidity. This is due to a lower incidence of aortoiliac aneurysms in women as well as the smaller average diameter of the distal common iliac [8].

Based on these findings it is clear that the relationship between neck length and mortality significantly confounds the influence of choice of repair strategy on early survival after rAAA.

Individual Patient Meta-analysis of the Randomized Controlled Trials

The three RCTs discussed have been incorporated into an individual patient meta-analysis [15]. Due to the difference in design between AJAX and ECAR when compared with IMPROVE, only the patients that were amenable to EVAR from IMPROVE were included in this analysis.

Part of the rationale of this study was that the three trials assumed higher rates of mortality in the OSR group than observed, meaning perhaps they were insufficiently powered to discriminate a smaller difference in mortality observed in comparison with EVAR. In addition it was felt that advances in perioperative care techniques could potentially have improved 30-day survival in comparison with earlier reports [1], and this was the reason the primary outcome of the meta-analysis was 90-day mortality.

The meta-analysis included 836 patients from the three trials and once again showed that there was no early mortality benefit to EVAR, although there was a weak trend toward EVAR at 90 days in those eligible for both OSR and EVAR (odds ratio = 0.74; 95 % CI 0.51–1.08). The meta-analysis also once again showed the benefit was particularly significant in women. The analysis also showed earlier hospital discharges were seen in the EVAR group when compared to those who underwent OSR (hazard ratio = 1.24 95 % CI 1.04–1.47), inferring that the incidence of serious morbidity was less.

Conclusion

According to a recent trial evidence, EVAR did not achieve a significant mortality benefit in comparison with OSR at 30 days or 1 year. Despite this many other benefits such as shorter hospital stay, better quality of life, possible increased benefit to women, and improved cost-effectiveness were observed. Based on these findings, all centers treating rAAA should be in a position to offer EVAR as the treatment of choice to anatomically suitable patients. This presents significant issues in terms of resources usage and staff training, but the reported increased mortality in patients presenting “out of hours” means that this would represent a useful investment of time and money. These factors reinforce the idea that the best way to reduce mortality following rAAA is to treat patients in specialist centers with sufficient resources, and this should be taken into account when planning services.

The Recent Randomized Trials of EVAR Versus Open Repair for Ruptured AAAs Are Misleading

Frank J. Veith and Caron B. Rockman

Many vascular surgeons are convinced that EVAR is superior to open repair for the treatment of ruptured abdominal aortic aneurysms (RAAAs) [18]. However, the issue of which form of repair is best remains controversial. Those who question the superiority of EVAR in this setting claim that much of the data showing superior outcomes for EVAR are flawed by patient selection [19]. This view is supported by reports of comparative series showing no improvement in operative mortality with EVAR compared to open repair [20]. Thus, the vascular community remains somewhat divided, and many have demanded level 1 evidence from randomized comparisons of the two procedures to settle the issue.

Three such randomized controlled trials (RCTs) have recently published or presented their results: the AJAX or Amsterdam (Dutch) trial [21], the ECAR or French trial [22], and the IMPROVE or UK trial [23]. All three trials concluded that 30-day mortality outcomes after EVAR for RAAA are no better than those after open repair. However, we are concerned that in all three trials these conclusions are rendered unjustified or misleading because of serious flaws or misinterpretation of the trial data. This communication addresses the specifics.

The AJAX trial enrolled 520 patients with ruptured AAA, of which only 116 (22 %) were randomized over a 7-year period. The ECAR trial had similar limitations in that it too randomized only 107 patients over a 5-year period. In addition to excluding many patients from randomization, both trials had the potentially serious flaw of excluding hypotensive or unstable RAAA patients who were treated by open repair or not treated at all. Such high risk patients are most likely to be the ones who would have better outcomes with EVAR than with open repair. In both trials, significant delays in EVAR patients favored outcomes in open repair patients; EVAR patients in AJAX had a mean extra delay of 30 min, and EVAR patients in ECAR had a mean extra delay of nearly 90 min. Thus, exclusion of these high risk patients, and delays in EVAR patients receiving treatment, may have precluded these trials from demonstrating any advantage EVAR might have had over open repair in the overall population of patients with RAAAs. Moreover, in both of these trials, three adjuncts generally believed to improve EVAR outcomes in RAAA cases were used in a suboptimal fashion. Improved utilization of preoperative fluid restriction (hypotensive hemostasis) [18], supra-aortic balloon control [24], and adjunctive open abdomen treatment of abdominal compartment syndrome [25] might have further improved the EVAR outcomes in both trials.

The larger UK IMPROVE trial was conducted in 30 high volume centers (including one from Canada). This trial was carefully planned and conducted [26], and much useful information was collected [27, 28]. However, its most important findings were detailed in the report of its 30-day outcomes [23]. In the IMPROVE trial, although 652 possible RAAA patients were excluded for various reasons, the trialists did randomize 613 patients with a diagnosis of RAAA to either an "*Endovascular Strategy*" group (316 patients) or an "*Open Repair*" group (297 patients). Patients were randomized before CT scans were performed. The 30-day mortality in the Endovascular Strategy group was 35 %; in the Open Repair group it was 37 % ($p=0.67$). Obviously there was no significant difference between these two groups based upon these percentages, and therefore a primary conclusion of the main IMPROVE trial article was "A strategy of endovascular repair was not associated with significant reduction in 30-day mortality" [23]. This was unfortunately paraphrased in various news report headlines as, "NO DIFFERENCE BETWEEN ENDOVASCULAR & OPEN REPAIR FOR RUPTURED *ANEURYSMS*" [29].

However, the detailed data from the IMPROVE trial must be examined closely to see why these conclusions may be misleading (Table 14.2) [23]. Of the patients initially randomized to the Endovascular Strategy group, only 154 (about half) were actually treated by EVAR; 112 had an open repair and 17 had no treatment. As patients were randomized to the Endovascular Strategy group before CT scans were performed, the most common reason for patients in this group to ultimately receive open repair was anatomic unsuitability for EVAR. The 30-day mortality for those patients ultimately treated by EVAR in this group was 27 % (42 of 154), while for those treated by open repair in this group it was 38 % (43 of 112) ($p=0.06$). Of the patients randomized to the Open Repair group, 36 actually had EVAR, 220 had open repair, and 19 had no treatment. The 30-day mortality in this Open Repair group was 22 % (8 of 36) for those undergoing EVAR and 37 % (81 of 220) for those undergoing open repair ($p=0.09$). Overall in the two randomized groups, taken together, the 30-day mortality for RAAA patients actually treated by EVAR was *25 %* (*46 of 186*), and for those actually treated by open repair, it was *38 %* (*128 of 336*) (*p < 0.002*).[1]

The superiority of EVAR over open repair within each of the two separate randomized groups approached statistical significance, and was highly statistically significant when data from the two groups were combined (when one takes into account the procedures that the patients actually had). Clearly the conclusion of the IMPROVE trial should have been, in patients with a RAAA, if they can be treated by EVAR, their 30-day survival will be superior to those patients who undergo open repair. If one adds that patients undergoing EVAR are less likely to receive expectant or no definitive treatment [30], the conclusion is inescapable: EVAR, if it can be performed, is superior to open repair for the treatment of patients with RAAAs.

[1]Four patients in the Endovascular Strategy group had an attempt at EVAR, but required conversion to open repair. All 4 died within 30 days. These 4 patients were included in the EVAR deaths but not in the open repair deaths in the Endovascular Strategy group calculations. However, in the calculations of the overall 30-day mortality rates for the two randomized groups taken together, these 4 patients were excluded from the EVAR deaths and included in the open repair deaths. If these 4 patients were included in the EVAR deaths and excluded from the open repair deaths in the calculations for the combined groups, the 30-day mortalities would have been 26.3 % (50/190) for EVAR and 37.3 % (124/332) for open repair ($p=0.01$).

Table 14.2 Detailed 30-day mortality data from the IMPROVE Trial [23]

Treatment	Number of patients treated	Number of deaths in 30 days	30-day mortality (%)
316 patients randomized to endovascular strategy[a]			
EVAR	150	38 (combined: 42)	25.3 (combined: 27.3)
EVAR attempted Converted to open repair	4	4	100
Open repair	112	43	38.4
No Repair	17	16	94.1
297 patients randomized to open repair[b]			
EVAR	36	8	22.2
Open repair	220	81	36.8
No repair	19	19	100
Actual treatment results in the two randomized groups combined			
EVAR	186	46	24.7
Open repair	336	128	38.1

[a]8 patients had a symptomatic unruptured AAA but were included in this treatment analysis; 33 patients had another non-aneurysmal diagnosis and were not included in this treatment analysis
[b]14 patients had a symptomatic unruptured AAA but were included in this treatment analysis; 22 patients had another non-aneurysmal diagnosis and were not included in this treatment analysis

A secondary conclusion is equally inescapable. Those treating RAAA patients must learn how to perform EVAR in the RAAA setting, including acquiring expertise in all the adjuncts and strategies that can improve EVAR outcomes in such patients. Further RCTs in this setting will be difficult to do and in our opinion are unnecessary.

References

Randomized Trials: What Is the Evidence?

1. Björck M. Surgery for ruptured abdominal aortic aneurysm. BMJ. 2014;348.
2. Desgranges P, Kobeiter H, Castier Y, Senechal M, Majewski M, Krimi A. The Endovascularie vs Chirurgie dans les Aneurysmes Rompus Protocol trial update. J Vasc Surg. 2010;51(267):70.
3. Desgranges P, Kobeiter H, Katsahian S, Bouffi M, Gouny P, Favre JP, Alsac JM, Sobocinski J, Julia P, Alimi Y, Steinmetz E, Haulon S, Alric P, Canaud L, Castier Y, Jean-Baptiste E, Hassen-Khodja R, Lermusiaux P, Feugier P, Destrieux-Garnier L, Charles-Nelson A, Marzelle J, Majewski M, Bourmaud A, Becquemin JP. Editor's Choice – ECAR (Endovasculaire ou Chirurgie dans les Anevrysmes aorto-iliaques Rompus): a french randomized controlled trial of endovascular versus open surgical repair of ruptured aorto-iliac aneurysms. Eur J Vasc Endovasc Surg. 2015;50(3):303–10.

4. Egorova N, Giacovelli J, Greco G, Gelijns A, Kent CK, McKinsey JF. National outcomes for the treatment of ruptured abdominal aortic aneurysm: comparison of open versus endovascular repairs. J Vasc Surg. 2008;48(1092):100.
5. Hinchliffe RJ, Bruijstens L, MacSweeney ST, Braithwaite BD. A randomised trial of endovascular and open surgery for ruptured abdominal aortic aneurysms—results of a pilot study. Eur J Vasc Endovasc Surg. 2006;5(506):13.
6. Holt PJ, Karthikesalingam A, Poloniecki JD, Hinchliffe RJ, Loftus IM, Thompson MM. Propensity scored analysis of outcomes after ruptured abdominal aortic aneurysm. Br J Surg. 2010;97(496):503.
7. Hoornweg LL, Storm-Versloot MN, Ubbink DT, Koelemay MJ, Legemate DA, Balm R.Meta analysis on mortality of ruptured abdominal aortic aneurysms. Eur J Vasc Endovasc Surg. 2008;35(5):558–70.
8. Investigators IMPROVE Trial. The effect of aortic morphology on perioperative mortality of ruptured abdominal aortic aneurysm. Eur Heart J. 2015;36(1328):1334.
9. Malina M, Veith F, Ivancev K, Sonesson B. Balloon occlusion of the aorta during endovascular repair of ruptured abdominal aortic aneurysm. J Endovasc Ther. 2005;12:556–9.
10. Mayer D, Pfammatter T, Rancic Z, Hechelhammer L, Wilhelm M, Veith FJ, Lachat M. et al.. 10 years of emergency endovascular aneurysm repair for ruptured aortoiliac aneurysms: lessons learned. Ann Surg. 2009;249(3):510–5.
11. Mayer D, Rancic Z, Meier C, Pfammatter T, Veith FJ, Lachat M. Open abdomen treatment following endovascular repair of ruptured abdominal aortic aneurysms. J Vasc Surg. 2009;50(1):7.
12. Powell JT, Hinchliffe RJ, Thompson MM, Sweeting MJ, Ashleigh R, Bell R, Gomes M, Greenhalgh RM, Grieve RJ, Heatley F, Thompson SG, Ulug P. Observations from the IMPROVE trial concerning the clinical care of patients with ruptured abdominal aortic aneurysm. Br J Surg. 2014;101(3):216–24; discussion 224.
13. Reimerink JJ, Hoornweg LL, Vahl AC, Wisselink W, van den Broek TA, Legemate DA, Reekers JA, Balm R. Endovascular repair versus open repair of ruptured abdominal aortic aneurysms: a multicenter randomized controlled trial. Ann Surg. 2013;258(2):248–56.
14. Richard Grieve MG, Sweeting MJ, Ulug P, Hinchliffe RJ, Thompson MM, Thompson SG, Ashleigh R, Greenhalgh RM, Powell JT. Endovascular strategy or open repair for ruptured abdominal aortic aneurysm: one-year outcomes from the IMPROVE randomized trial. Eur Heart J. 2015;36(31):2061–9.
15. Sweeting MJ, Balm R, Desgranges P, Ulug P, Powell JT, Ruptured Aneurysm T. Individual-patient meta-analysis of three randomized trials comparing endovascular versus open repair for ruptured abdominal aortic aneurysm. Br J Surg. 2015;102(10):1229–39.
16. Veith FJ, Powell JT, Hinchliffe RJ. Is a randomized trial necessary to determine whether endovascular repair is the preferred management strategy in patients with ruptured abdominal aortic aneurysms? J Vasc Surg. 2010;52(4):1087–93.
17. Yusuf SW, Whitaker SC, Chuter TA, Wenham PW, Hopkinson BR. Emergency endovascular repair of leaking aortic aneurysm. Lancet. 1994;344(8397):1645.

The Recent Randomized Trials of EVAR Versus Open Repair for Ruptured AAAs Are Misleading

18. Veith FJ, Lachat M, Mayer D, Malina M, Holst J, Mehta M, Verhoeven EL, Larzon T, Gennai S, Coppi G, Lipsitz EC, Gargiulo NJ, van der Vliet JA, Blankensteijn J, Buth J, Lee WA, Biasi G, Deleo G, Kasirajan K, Moore R, Soong CV, Cayne NS, Farber MA, Raithel D, Greenberg RK, van Sambeek MR, Brunkwall JS, Rockman CB, Hinchliffe RJ, RAAA Investigators. Collected world and single center experience with endovascular treatment of ruptured abdominal aortic aneurysms. Ann Surg. 2009;250:818–24.

19. Von Allman RS, Schmidli J, Dick F. Regarding endovascular vs open repair for ruptured abdominal aortic aneurysm. J Vasc Surg. 2013;57:897.
20. Saqib N, Park SC, Park T, Rhee RY, Chaer RA, Makaroun MS, Cho JS. Endovascular repair of ruptured abdominal aortic aneurysm does not confer survival benefits over open repair. J Vasc Surg. 2012;56:614–9.
21. Reimerink JJ, et al. Endovascular repair versus open repair of ruptured abdominal aortic aneurysms: a multicenter randomized controlled trial. Ann Surg. 2013;258:248–56.
22. Desgranges P, KobeiterH, Katsahian S, Bouffi M, Gouny P, Favre JP, Alsac JM, et al for the ECAR Investigators. A french randomized controlled trial of endovascular versus open surgical repair of ruptured aorto-iliac aneurysms. Eur J Vasc Endovasc Surg. 2015;50:303–10.
23. IMPROVE trial Investigtors, Powell JT, Sweeting MJ, Thompson MM, Ashleigh R, Bell R, Gomes M, Greenhalgh RM, Grieve R, Heatley F, Hinchliffe RJ, Thompson SG, Ulug P. Endovascular or open repair strategy for ruptured abdominal aortic aneurysm: 30 day outcomes from IMPROVE randomised trial. BMJ. 2014;348:f7661.
24. Berland TL, Veith FJ, Cayne NS, Mehta M, Mayer D, Lachat M. Technique of supraceliac balloon control of the aorta during endovascular repair of ruptured abdominal aortic aneurysms. J Vasc Surg. 2013;57:272–5.
25. Mayer D, Rancic Z, Meier C, Pfammatter T, Veith FJ, Lachat M. Open abdomen treatment following endovascular repair of ruptured abdominal aortic aneurysms. J Vasc Surg. 2009;50:1–7.
26. IMPROVE Trial Investigators, Powell JT, Thompson SG, Thompson MM, Grieve R, Nicholson AA, Ashleigh R, Hassan T, Moore F, Walker A, Braithwaite BD, Hinchliffe RJ, Greenhalgh RM, Cheshire NJ, Howell SJ, Soong CV. The immediate management of the patient with rupture: open versus endovascular repair (IMPROVE) aneurysm trial–ISRCTN 48334791 IMPROVE trialists. Acta Chir Belg. 2009;109:678–80.
27. IMPROVE trial investigators, Powell JT, Hinchliffe RJ, Thompson MM, Sweeting MJ, Ashleigh R, Bell R, Gomes M, Greenhalgh RM, Grieve RJ, Heatley F, Thompson SG, Ulug P. Observations from the IMPROVE trial concerning the clinical care of patients with ruptured abdominal aortic aneurysm. Br J Surg. 2014;101:216–24.
28. IMPROVE Trial Investigators. An endovascular strategy for suspected ruptured abdominal aortic aneurysm brings earlier home discharge but not early survival or cost benefits. Eur J Vasc Endovasc Surg. 2014;47:333–4.
29. IMPROVE Trial 30-day results: no difference between endovascular and open repair for ruptured aneurysms. Vascular News Issue 61, January 2014, Biba Medical, p. 1–2.
30. Mayer D, Aeschbacher S, Pfammatter T, Veith FJ, Norgren L, Magnuson A, Rancic Z, Lachat M, Hörer T, Skoog P, Larzon T. Complete replacement of open repair for ruptured abdominal aortic aneurysms by endovascular aneurysm repair: a two-center 14-year experience. Ann Surg. 2012;256:688–96.

Chapter 15
Postoperative Intensive Care Unit Management After Ruptured Abdominal Aortic Aneurysm

John Kuckelman, Alexander Niven, and Matthew J. Martin

Introduction

Among all vascular pathologies and emergencies, arguably the most dramatic and rapidly fatal is the rupture of an aortic aneurysm. Many of these patients do not survive long enough to be transported to an operating room or even to a hospital. Among those who do survive to a hospital, there is a wide spectrum of presentations ranging from relatively stable hemodynamics to impending cardiovascular collapse and arrest. Similar to stroke and myocardial infarction, the one factor that has consistently been shown to reduce morbidity and mortality is minimizing the time from arrival to operative intervention ("door to OR" time). Despite this, operative mortality after a ruptured abdominal aortic aneurysm (AAA) has been reported to be 40–60 % [1–3]. Among the approximately 50 % who do survive, there is an equally high incidence of major postoperative morbidity and long-term debility. The incidence of postoperative complications is severalfold higher among this cohort when compared to elective AAA repair, and intensive care unit (ICU) and total hospital stays are typically longer and protracted.

The goal of this chapter is to provide a practical, chronological approach to the ICU management practices and principles in the critically ill patient following emergent repair of a ruptured abdominal aortic aneurysm (rAAA). Although endovascular techniques have now been extended to many patients with rAAA and have been associated with significantly lower postoperative morbidity and mortality, a standard open approach is often necessary in these patients. This chapter will

J. Kuckelman, DO • M.J. Martin, MD, FACS (✉)
Department of Surgery, Madigan Army Medical Center, Tacoma, WA, USA
e-mail: matthew.j.martin16.mil@mail.mil

A. Niven, MD
Department of Internal Medicine, Madigan Army Medical Center, Tacoma, WA, USA

B.W. Starnes et al. (eds.), *Ruptured Abdominal Aortic Aneurysm*,
DOI 10.1007/978-3-319-23844-9_15

primarily focus on the ICU management following open emergent aortic procedures, but the same basic principles of resuscitation, stabilization, and optimization will apply to all patients with major physiologic disturbance regardless of the surgical approach. Anticipation, rapid recognition, and immediate appropriate management of these common postoperative complications are essential to optimize and maximize the chances of a successful patient recovery and to avoid potentially preventable deaths or complications.

From Operating Room to ICU

Patients are frequently unstable following emergent AAA repair, and safe transport to the ICU requires the presence of a physician, transportable continuous monitoring, resuscitation meds, a defibrillator, and either manual bag valve mask or battery-powered ventilator. On arrival to the ICU, a comprehensive handoff should be executed detailing the patient identification, pertinent general and cardiac history, and intraoperative events. Key intraoperative information includes the length of the case, hemodynamic stability during the case, amount and type of resuscitation used, as well as total blood product utilization and breakdown. Critical care management will be significantly impacted by type of rupture (contained vs uncontained) and type of repair (open vs EVAR), aortic cross clamp time and location (supraceliac, juxta-renal, iliac), and the type of aortic, renal, and mesenteric reconstructions.

Most patients on arrival to the ICU will have large-bore central venous access (cordis or similar trauma resuscitation catheter) which should be maintained until active bleeding is excluded and hemodynamic stability maintained. Arterial line monitoring and Foley catheter placement are common to provide continuous data to facilitate ongoing resuscitation efforts. The patient may often be receiving ongoing resuscitation, as well as on one or multiple continuous infusions of sedatives, analgesics, inotropes, and vasopressors. All of these should be detailed and reported to the receiving team, including the current doses and the trends (increasing or decreasing doses) prior to arrival. Respiratory therapy should be standing by to place the patient on the ventilator and appropriate levels of ventilator support as dictated by the clinical condition and the most recent settings from the operating room.

Initial Assessment and Stabilization

Patients immediately following emergent AAA repair are frequently tenuous and hemodynamically labile. Variables to consider in acute perioperative management include intravascular volume status, baseline cardiopulmonary status, and clinical and laboratory evidence of coagulopathy and ongoing bleeding. Low-grade distributive shock may also be present in patients with massive blood loss and resuscitation. Initial clinical assessment in addition to continuous hemodynamic monitoring should include a baseline cardiac, chest, and abdominal exam, careful assessment of lower extremity pulses and muscle compartments, electrocardiogram, and portable chest radiograph. Initial laboratory assessment should include CBC, PT/PTT, serum chemistry, and lactate at a minimum to assess for evidence of ongoing bleeding, coagulopathy, and end-organ perfusion.

Intravascular Volume Assessment

Preoperative and intraoperative blood loss and intraoperative resuscitation volumes provide only a rough estimate of intravascular volume status, and urine output is frequently an insensitive marker of end-organ perfusion following prolonged hypotension or suprarenal clamping. Accurate measurement of central venous pressure will require placement of a triple-lumen catheter through large-bore access devices, and other common available assessment tools include continuous assessment of stroke volume variation, ultrasound assessment of inferior vena cava diameter and collapsibility, or bedside echocardiography to assess baseline cardiac function and filling.

Bleeding and Resuscitation

The immediate postoperative period is frequently marked by significant fluid shifts, and thrombocytopenia and coagulopathy are common. The incidence of clinically significant postoperative bleeding in the ruptured AAA patient ranges from 3 to 25 %, with approximately 3 % of patients requiring reoperation. Massive transfusion is defined as the administration of ten or more units of packed red blood cells (PRBCs) in less than a 24-h period. Many ruptured AAA patients will meet these criteria, and the accompanying risk of both consumptive and dilutional coagulopathy – especially in the presence of hypothermia and acidosis – must be aggressively managed in subsequent critical care management. Blood products should be the initial resuscitation fluids of choice in patients who meet these criteria, and generalization of trauma data that had demonstrated reductions in mortality, organ failure, and blood product consumption with the implementation of a predefined massive transfusion protocol that rapidly provides specified types and numbers of blood products early in resuscitation in this setting is appropriate [4]. The appropriate ratio of PRBCs, fresh frozen plasma (FFP), platelets, and cryoprecipitate remains controversial. The PROPPR trial demonstrated that initial empiric resuscitation with a ratio of 1:1:2 (three units FFP, 0 doses platelets, and six units PRBCs followed by alternating two units PRBCs and one unit plasma, with one unit of platelets with the second and subsequent even numbered containers) was not inferior to a 1:1:1 ratio (six units plasma, six units of pooled platelets, and six units of PRBCs) previously published in military trauma literature, although the latter group achieved hemostasis more frequently and had less deaths from exsanguination in the first 24 h [5]. The PROMITT trial also demonstrated that initial empiric resuscitation with a ratio of two units of packed red blood cells (PRBCs) to one unit of fresh frozen plasma was not inferior to traditional 1:1 resuscitation strategies described in the military trauma literature, and early platelet transfusions given after four–six units of PRBCs and FFP have been shown to reduce transfusion requirements and mortality in trauma patients following massive hemorrhage. Although there has been long-standing concern that the use of blood that has been stored for an extended period may be harmful in critical illness, a recent prospective randomized control trial has shown that there is no difference in the multiple organ dysfunction score for patients who received blood stored up to 21 days [6]. Aggressive correction of hypothermia and hypocalcemia is essential in these patients, and cryoprecipitate may be used in patients with fibrinogen levels (<100 mg/dl) [7].

Thromboelastography (TEG, ROTEM) can provide valuable information to augment information provided by traditional INR, PTT, hematocrit, platelet counts, and fibrinogen and help direct transfusion therapy [8]. TEG measures fibrinolytic index (a measure of fibrinolysis), r value (a reflection of the intrinsic clotting cascade), and the alpha angle and K values (measures of the speed of solid clot formation) using a pin hanging from a torsion wire that is inserted into a standardized volume of patient blood held in a continuously rotating container. Animal studies have shown that 30 min of aortic cross clamping does not result in thrombolysis, but does increase clotting activity and decrease speed of clot formation and fibrinogen levels especially after unclamping from a supraceliac location [9]. A number of studies in both cardiovascular surgery and mixed surgical critical care populations have demonstrated reductions in intraoperative blood loss and transfusion requirements with the use of TEG to drive targeted transfusion therapy with blood components, fibrinogen concentrate, four-factor prothrombin complex, and factor XIII concentrate. Algorithms employing targeted transfusion management using thromboelastography and whole blood impedance aggregometry (Multiplate) have been proposed, but remain labor intensive with limited availability and still require validation in randomized controlled trials [10]. TEG has also been shown to effectively monitor adequate heparinization intraoperatively during vascular surgery and therefore may have a role in the critical care management of these issues in the postoperative setting as well [11]. Limited data are available on the use of antifibrinolytic therapy in this setting, with concerns of thrombotic complications, acute kidney injury, and seizures limiting indications for use without further study on appropriate patient selection and dosing [12–15]. Targeted transfusion therapies therefore show promise to reduce transfusion requirements and reduce the risk of transfusion-related acute lung injury (TRALI), transfusion acute circulatory overload (TACO), and subsequent negative immunomodulatory effects (TRIM) that may increase nosocomial infectious complications, but more work is needed in this area. Intraoperative autotransfusion is also an important consideration to mitigate these potential transfusion-related complications.

Anticoagulation can also be a compounding issue in the bleeding postoperative patient. Patients with elevated PTT from intraoperative heparin use may be reversed with protamine sulfate, although the short half-life of unfractionated heparin (30–60 min) may obviate this need. Low-molecular-weight heparin compounds may also be reversed by protamine. Current guidelines advocate the use of four-factor prothrombin complex concentrate (PCC) with or without FFP for major bleeding associated with vitamin K antagonists and would be the preferred management in addition to vitamin K administration for patients on therapeutic anticoagulation presenting with aortic rupture [16]. PCC is administered in stratified weight-based dosing of 25, 35, or 50 IU/kg dosing based on initial INR. Currently there are no FDA-approved agents to reverse the factor Xa (apixaban, rivaroxiban) and IIa (bivalirudin) inhibitors. However, activated prothrombin complex concentrates (PCC), factor eight inhibitor bypassing activity (FEIBA), and recombinant activated factor VII have been used successfully in these patients with severe bleeding or trauma. Arapazine and Andexanet alpha have been developed as possible antidotes for the Xa inhibitors and Idarucizamab for IIa inhibitors. Modified thrombin has been suggested for reversal of the anticoagulant effects of dabigatran, a direct thrombin inhibitor [17].

In the absence of significant bleeding, judicious crystalloid administration remains the resuscitation fluid of choice to maintain adequate intravascular volume and renal perfusion. Lactated Ringers are typically the crystalloid of choice as its composition does not contain large amounts of chloride that may lead to hyperchloremic acidosis and acute kidney injury [7]. Judicious administration of fluids is key in these patients and should be guided using a combination of the assessments listed above to guide intravascular volume status, as fluid overload contributes directly to length of stay, transfusion requirements, and complications such as pulmonary edema, post-op ileus, and cardiac complications [18].

Evaluation and Management of Ongoing Hemodynamic Instability

The differential diagnosis of continued hemodynamic lability after bleeding has been excluded, and intravascular volume depletion has been treated with either blood products or crystalloids that include either cardiogenic or distributive shock. The release of pro-inflammatory cytokines following a massive surgical insult is well described and can frequently be best managed with low-dose norepinephrine to counter the predominantly vasodilatory effects that follow. Table 15.1 provides a comprehensive review of the different vasoactive medications. Vasopressin, a hormonal agent with strong vasoconstriction effects, should be avoided in the early resuscitation of ruptured AAA patient due to its effects on splanchnic circulation. As bowel ischemia is a major risk after emergent rAAA repair, strong unopposed vasoconstrictors such as vasopressin or phenylephrine should be avoided particularly while the volume status has not yet been optimized [7, 19]. The most recent randomized trial of dopamine and norepinephrine in a mixed population of patients in shock showed no difference in outcomes but an increased incidence of

Table 15.1 Inotropic, vasopressor, and vasodilatory agents commonly used after cardiac surgery

Agent	Class	Effect(s)	Indications
Epinephrine	Catecholamine	Inotrope	Low CO
		Vasopressor (higher doses)	Hypotension
Norepinepherine	Catecholamine	Vasopressor	Hypotension
			Excessive vasodilatation
		Some inotrope	Vasoplegia
			Low CO
Dopamine	Catecholamine	Inotrope	Low CO
		Some vasopressor	Hypotension
Dobutamine	Catecholamine	Inotrope	Low CO
		Systemic vasodilator	Decrease LV afterload
Milrinone (Amrinone; enoximone)			
Milrinone (Amrinone; enoximone)	Phosphodiesterase inhibitor	Inotrope	
		Systemic vasodilator	Decrease right ventricular afterload
		Lusitrope	Decrease LV afterload
		Pulmonary vasodilator	
Vasopressin	Hormone	Vasopressor	Hypotension
			Excessive vasodilatation
			Vasoplegia
Levosimendan	Calcium sensitizer	Inotrope	Low CO
		Lusitrope	
Sodium nitroprusside NO donor	cGMP stimulator	Arterial vasodilator	Low CO with high BP
			Decreased LV afterload
			Decreased BP
Nicardipine	Calcium channel blocker	Arterial vasodilator	Low CO with high BP
			Decreased LV afterload
			Decreased BP
Nitroglycerin NO Donor	cGMP stimulator	Venous vasodilator	Decreased LV preload
			Decreased BP
			Treat or prevent coronary vasospasm

Reprinted with permission from Stephens et al. [7]
See text for discussion
CO cardiac output, *LV* left ventricle, *NO* nitric oxide, *cGMP* cyclic guanosine monophosphate, *BP* blood pressure

arrhythmias in patients receiving dopamine, making the latter agent less desirable in this setting [20].

Cardiovascular disease is common in patients with abdominal aortic aneurysms, and cardiac complications are common in the postoperative setting. Ongoing hemodynamic instability should prompt a review of recent cardiovascular history and available data, and an echocardiogram can be helpful in the absence of this information to identify evidence of heart failure with reduced ejection fraction and the presence of focal wall motion abnormalities that may suggest an underlying significant ischemic burden. After careful assessment to exclude an underlying acute coronary syndrome or arrhythmia, inotropic therapy with dobutamine or milrinone may be necessary to maintain adequate cardiac output and end-organ perfusion.

Myocardial Infarction

The most common cause of death after successful repair of a ruptured AAA is postoperative myocardial infarction. A large retrospective study of 1135 patients who underwent elective open AAA repair at the Cleveland Clinic identified active myocardial ischemia on preoperative imaging in 16 % of this population and severe but correctable CAD in 29 % of patients who underwent coronary angiography. Despite this aggressive risk stratification, cardiac events still accounted for 23 % of late deaths following surgery [21]. The cumulative incidence of a late cardiac event after open AAA has been reported to be 14.9 % at 5 years and interestingly does not substantially differ between patients undergoing open or endovascular aneurysm repair (EVAR) (3.2 and 2.6 events per 100 person-years, respectively) [22, 23]. Although controversial, data continue to be published supporting reductions in long-term cardiovascular risk with preoperative cardiovascular intervention [24].

Myocardial infarction can occur in AAA patients from acute plaque rupture (ST elevation MI or non-ST elevation MI type 1) or due to reduced myocardial oxygen supply and/or increased myocardial oxygen demand in the absence of a direct coronary artery process (type II) [25]. Acute cardiac decompensation related to physiologic stress (Takotsubo's or stress-induced cardiomyopathy) or embolic events from vascular manipulation are less common but also seen and can have a similar presentation.

Recognition of MI in these patients can be challenging, as postoperative pain, the use of sedation and analgesics, and other critical care interventions may distract from or obscure typical angina symptoms. The Vascular Surgery Group Cardiac Risk Index, a simple scoring system that recently was shown to outperform the Revised Cardiac Risk Index, is one method to help proactively identify patients at high risk for cardiac events (Table 15.2) [26]. In addition to age, aortic cross clamp duration, volume of blood transfusion, emergency operation, and use of vasopressors during aortic cross clamp have also been identified as independent risk factors for postoperative complications [27].

Table 15.2 The Vascular Surgery Group Cardiac Risk Index (VSG-CRI) scoring system

Risk factor	# points
Age ≥80 years	4
Age 70–79	3
Age 60–69	2
CAD	2
CHF	2
COPD	2
Creatinine >1.8	2
Insulin-dependent diabetes	1
Long-term beta-blockade	−1

Risk of adverse cardiac events

VSG-CRI score	Risk of adverse cardiac outcome (%)
0–3	2.6
4	3.5
5	6
6	6.6
7	8.9
8 or more	14.3

All patients following emergent AAA surgery should receive a baseline and serial daily ECGs on ICU arrival, recognizing that the greatest risk of myocardial ischemia is in the first 5 days. ST segment changes on ECG are sensitive but not specific for the diagnosis of a MI and will be present without active cardiac ischemia in approximately one third of patients undergoing major vascular surgery. Cardiac enzyme evaluation using a troponin I assay should be performed whenever cardiac symptoms and new ECG changes are present, and some have argued that this should be done routinely in the postoperative period. This is because troponin I elevations are very specific for MI and have been associated with increased risk of mortality over the next 18 months and may benefit from more intensive management of their coronary artery disease [28]. Bedside transthoracic echocardiogram can also be helpful to identify focal wall motion abnormalities with or without a depressed ejection fraction that may increase clinical suspicion for clinically significant ischemia.

Rapid recognition and management is the key to the treatment of an acute myocardial infarction. Supplemental oxygen should be administered immediately, along with sublingual nitroglycerin with an additional intravenous infusion, if signs and symptoms of ischemia persist. Oral or intravenous beta-blocker therapy should be strongly considered provided there is no evidence of heart failure or shock or high-grade conduction abnormalities on ECG. High-intensity statin therapy should be initiated and continued in all patients, and antiplatelet therapy with aspirin is typically safe. Anticoagulation with unfractionated heparin is also generally acceptable should there be concern for acute plaque rupture and still provides the option of reversal should bleeding occur. An ACE inhibitor should be started and continued indefinitely in all patients with a left ventricular ejection fraction of <40 %. As the risk of thrombolytics is generally not acceptable in the setting of recent aortic surgery, patients with STEMI or refractory ischemia despite aggressive medical intervention will require urgent revascularization with either PCI using a radial artery approach or coronary bypass. The use of intra-aortic balloon pump counterpulsation for patients in cardiogenic shock in this setting is contraindicated [7, 25, 29].

Atrial Fibrillation

Atrial fibrillation is reported to occur in approximately 10 % of open abdominal aortic aneurysm surgery postoperatively. Risk factors include a history of cerebrovascular disease, myocardial ischemia, fluid shifts, electrolyte abnormalities, and withdrawal from home meds such as beta-blockers, occult thyroid disease, and untreated sleep apnea. Patients who develop atrial fibrillation are more likely to develop congestive heart failure and have a longer length of stay [30]. Rate control is the most important intervention in this setting to preserve adequate left ventricular filling and reduce the risk of progressive myocardial ischemia and can generally be accomplished with beta-blockers in patients with a preserved left ventricular ejection fraction. Calcium channel blockers or digoxin may be used as added therapy in cases that are difficult to control. Amiodarone can also be effective in refractory cases and should be considered first-line therapy in patients with a severely reduced ejection fraction. Hemodynamically unstable patients should undergo timely electrical cardioversion, but success rates with this intervention can be reduced even with coadministration of an antiarrhythmic due to the high sympathetic tone frequently present in these cases.

Ventilator Management

The majority of patients following emergent AAA repair will remain intubated and sedated upon ICU transfer until they can demonstrate stable hemodynamics and no evidence of clinically significant bleeding that requires aggressive management. Extubation within the first 6 h of ICU arrival correlates with less nosocomial complications and shorter ICU stay and should be strongly considered if no contraindications exist [7]. Endovascular techniques are associated with less time on the ventilator due to less overall physiological insult as well as decreased requirement of sedation for pain control [29].

An ICU admission portable chest radiograph is helpful to both confirm placement and exclude complications from central lines placed emergently in the operating room and to identify potential barriers to early extubation. Most AAA patients have a history of tobacco abuse and are at risk for chronic obstructive pulmonary disease. Patients with clinically significant COPD may have evidence of hyperinflation (more than nine posterior ribs completely visible) or hyperlucency in the upper lung fields due to air trapping and upper lobe predominant emphysema most common in smoking-related lung disease. Chest radiograph can also identify pulmonary infiltrates that may suggest TRALI, TACO, or underlying left ventricular dysfunction and when present should prompt early and aggressive assessment of intravascular volume and examination for myocardial ischemia.

Assist-control ventilation is generally preferred initially to minimize patient work of breathing until hemodynamics stabilize. Typical starting tidal volume and respiratory rate are 6–8 ml/kg and 12–15, respectively, which should be adjusted based on initial pH and initial peak and plateau pressures measured on the ventilator. The vast majority of these patients will have a metabolic acidosis on initial ICU presentation, and management of this finding should focus on continued resuscitation with mechanical ventilation simply serving as an adjunct to stabilize pH and reduce the risk of arrhythmia [31, 32]. Elevated peak pressures with a low plateau pressure should prompt suctioning to clear the endotracheal tube and central airways of mucus plugging, followed by bronchodilator administration if persistent for likely underlying obstructive lung disease. Severe COPD patients may benefit from slower respiratory rates and low tidal volumes to reduce the risk of dynamic air trapping and barotrauma. Elevated peak and plateau pressures combined with diffuse infiltrates on chest radiograph are concerning for problems with lung compliance and should prompt a lung-protective ventilator strategy (tidal volumes of <6 cc/kg ideal body weight, titrated to keep the plateau pressure less than 30 cmH_2O, and consideration of higher levels of PEEP). FiO_2 should initially be set at 100 % and then weaned to a PaO_2 of 70 mmHg or greater, with an initial PEEP of 5 cmH_2O.

Attempts at ventilator liberation should begin as rapidly as possible once hemodynamics have stabilized and pain, bleeding, acidosis, and myocardial ischemia have been addressed. Patients who are alert enough to protect their airway and demonstrate an appropriate rapid shallow breathing index (RSBI, frequency/tidal volume in L) of <105 should be considered for a spontaneous breathing trial using either CPAP or T piece and extubated in 30 min if doing well. Multiple studies have shown that the prophylactic use of noninvasive positive pressure ventilation immediately post-extubation, especially in patients with COPD, can reduce the risk of reintubation [33].

The Early Postoperative ICU Course

The first 24–48 h of ICU care in the critically ill patient generally focus on initial resuscitation, support, correction of immediately life-threatening physiologic or metabolic abnormalities, and stabilization. This period will set the stage for the next phase of care and will play out over the first 3–5 days of the ICU stay, and the ultimate outcome will largely depend on the amount and degree of end-organ dysfunction that results from both the initial insult (rAAA with shock) and the initial resuscitation (reperfusion syndromes). It is important to note that the resuscitation can play an equal (or even greater) part in many of the complications and organ failure syndromes that are seen after rAAA. As described above, a balanced and judicious resuscitation using reliable and meaningful end points and avoiding massive over-resuscitation (particularly with standard crystalloid solutions) has been shown to result in significantly lower morbidity and potentially even lower mortality. Following this initial period of intensive care and resuscitation, patients will generally sort into one of three possible categories: (1) rapid stabilization and immediate recovery of end-organ function, (2) continued and progressive deterioration despite maximal efforts, or (3) stabilization but evidence of developing or ongoing single or multi-organ dysfunction syndromes (MODS). It is this third population where most of the gains with attentive and evidence-based ICU care can be realized.

Abdominal Compartment Syndrome

Abdominal compartment syndrome (ACS) is one of the most feared complications among all surgical patients and particularly after emergent abdominal aortic surgery. All rAAA patients regardless of the method of repair should be considered to be at high risk for developing ACS, and we recommend routine focused monitoring postoperatively in this patient population. Although ACS is primarily thought of as a complication after open abdominal surgery, there is a significant risk of ACS even among patients who undergo endovascular repair. Epidemiologic studies have demonstrated an incidence of ACS in 30–50 % of patients after open rAAA repair and in up to 30 % of emergent endovascular repairs [34–36]. The etiology and causes of ACS after rAAA repair are multifactorial and have been related to the amount of fluid resuscitation, the presence and depth of presenting shock, the volume of retroperitoneal hematoma, the duration of ischemia, and the development of postoperative abdominal complications such as ischemic bowel [37]. Understanding these factors and the common causes of ACS allows the ICU physician to anticipate and potentially even prevent the development of ACS. Diagnostic clues to developing or frank ACS can range from subtle physiologic changes to complete cardiorespiratory collapse, and the key to avoiding unnecessary morbidity or death is always earlier recognition and intervention.

The most important diagnostic strategy is to appreciate the potential risk for developing ACS in an individual patient by identifying the presence and number of risk factors as described above. These patients should then be closely monitored for the early physiologic indicators of developing ACS combined with routine serial monitoring of intra-abdominal pressure. Early clues to developing intra-abdominal hypertension include progressive tachycardia, tachypnea (if spontaneously ventilating), decreasing urine output, and decreasing mean arterial pressures. Unfortunately these are all relatively nonspecific signs of ACS, but should prompt at least consideration of the diagnosis. More specific indicators of ACS include worsening abdominal distension and firmness on exam, steadily decreasing pulmonary compliance, decreasing mean arterial pressures (MAP), and sudden oliguria or anuria that is not responsive to volume expansion. It is important to also understand that the signs of decreasing pulmonary compliance will depend on the mode of ventilation, with rising peak or mean airway pressures on a volume-controlled mode or decreasing tidal volumes on a pressure-controlled mode. Early changes in pulmonary compliance may be less obvious in the patient on ventilator modes that automatically compensate for compliance changes (such as pressure release volume-controlled ventilation). Similarly, decreases in blood pressure may be less appreciated in the patient on vasopressor agents that are being titrated to a certain MAP, so the dose of vasopressor should also be followed closely. Systemic markers of perfusion or metabolic acidosis (lactate, base deficit) may be elevated late in the course of ACS, but they are not reliable early indicators. The best indicators of ACS include rising peak airway pressures, decreasing MAP and/or increased vasopressor requirement, and decreased urine output in the setting of increasing abdominal distension and abdominal pressures.

There are now published international consensus guidelines on ACS that have standardized the diagnostic criteria and provide evidence-based recommendations for interventions and therapeutic options [38, 39]. The preferred method of assessment of intra-abdominal pressure (IAP) is via bladder pressures obtained with the patient supine, relaxed, and measured at the midaxillary line. Intra-abdominal hypertension is defined as a sustained intra-abdominal pressure (IAP) ≥12 mmHg, while ACS is characterized by a sustained IAP ≥20 mmHg. Some have proposed that calculating an actual abdominal perfusion pressure (defined as MAP-IAP) is superior to the above definition, with a perfusion pressure <60 mmHg indicating ACS [39]. We recommend routine serial assessments of IAP via the bladder catheter in all patients after emergent repair of a rAAA and that these be continued until the patient is out of the early high-risk period (initial 2–3 days) and has no clinical signs of elevated IAP. If the patient develops elevated IAP, then initial interventions to present progression to ACS include diuresis or dialysis/hemofiltration for volume overload, a trial of intravenous paralytic agents, and assessment for any abdominal complications (such as hemorrhage, bowel ischemia) [38, 40]. There is also a select subgroup of patients that will develop ACS due to massive ascites, and these patients can often be treated successfully by large-volume paracentesis and either repeat paracentesis as needed or placement of a temporary drainage catheter for continuous evacuation of fluid.

Although some of these temporizing maneuvers can delay or even prevent progression to ACS, the majority of patients that develop true ACS will require an emergent decompressive laparotomy. The key technical steps to successful decompression are to widely open the skin and abdominal fascia, to perform a thorough exploration to identify any pathologic process underlying the ACS (such as bleeding, ischemic bowel, bowel obstruction with massive dilation), and to perform a temporary abdominal closure with enough laxity to avoid recurrent ACS. However open abdomen and temporary closure techniques are not without complications. There is a higher risk of infection, fistula formation, skin necrosis, and abdominal wall retraction with loss of domain following decompressive laparotomy. Mortality is also significantly higher among patients who develop ACS after ruptured AAA repair. In one recent series, mortality with ACS was 62 % among patients who had undergone open repair and

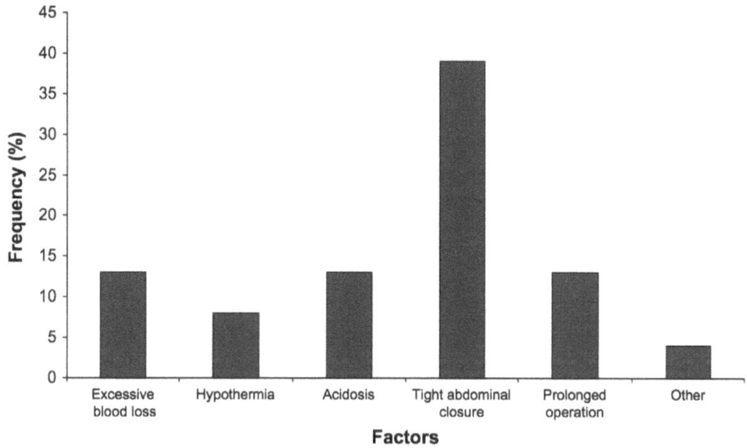

Fig. 15.1 Choi et al. evaluated factors influencing a surgeon's decision of prophylactic laparotomy for suspected ACS in rAAA for abdominal compartment syndrome (Reprinted with permission from Choi et al. [40])

was a strikingly high 83 % among the endovascular group [34]. The high rates of postoperative ACS and the associated morbidity/mortality have prompted some to propose prophylactically leaving the abdomen open at the time of initial open repair, with delayed closure performed once the patient is out of the high-risk time window. We would recommend strong consideration of this approach in any patient undergoing open repair who is requiring ongoing fluid and vasopressor resuscitation, with significant bowel distension/edema or with undue fascial tension or elevated airway pressures during fascial closure [37, 40, 41]. In the patient with elevated IAP that progresses after an endovascular repair, decompressive laparotomy should be considered before the development of ACS. The results of a study by Choi et al. are shown in Fig. 15.1 and display what factors most commonly weighed into a surgeon deciding to progress to decompressive laparotomy [40]. As the ACS in this patient population is often attributed to the large retroperitoneal hematoma that would otherwise be evacuated with an open approach, an alternative-described treatment modality is the placement of a percutaneous image-guided catheter into the hematoma and infusing thrombolytics to break up and evacuate the clot [42]. Finally, the decision to perform a decompressive laparotomy must also be made with consideration of the patient's overall status and likelihood of survival, aligned with any known advanced directives and the wishes of the patient or their surrogate decision-makers.

Acute Kidney Injury

The incidence of acute kidney injury (AKI) in all patients undergoing elective and ruptured AAA surgery has been reported to be 15–22 % and likely underestimates the risk in the latter population [43–45]. Another recent retrospective review of 140 patients undergoing emergent AAA repair identified an incidence of acute kidney injury of 75.7 %, for example, with 78.3 % of which occurring in the first 24 h in the ICU [46]. Postoperative AKI has been associated with a higher risk of death and prolonged hospitalization in this population, with only 63.4 % of survivors at 1 year demonstrating complete kidney recovery.

Risk factors for AKI in emergent AAA procedures include baseline chronic kidney disease, greater intraoperative blood loss and transfusion requirements, need for mechanical ventilation and vasoactive therapy, higher illness severity scores, and detectable postoperative troponin I values [46]. Other associated factors identified from elective AAA repair include diabetes, procedural duration, kidney ischemic time during aortic cross clamping of >100 min, rhabdomyolysis, low cardiac output, intravenous contrast administration, rhabdomyolysis from lower extremity reperfusion, and athero-embolization during aortic manipulation [43, 44, 47]. In some circumstances it is acceptable to intraoperatively sacrifice the left renal vein for exposure during these emergent repairs. If the gonadal vein is not preserved, then renal failure is more likely to develop from venous congestion; acute renal failure is associated with 60–80 % mortality after repair of ruptured AAA [48].

Oliguria and anuria with a rise in creatinine despite appropriate resuscitation are the first markers of AKI in this setting and should be evaluated with urine studies to exclude prerenal etiologies using the factional excretion of sodium and urea (FENa, FEUrea) and urine microscopy. A FENa of >1 % and the presence of muddy brown casts in the urine sediment are highly suggestive of acute tubular necrosis from an ischemic renal injury.

Prevention and management strategies for AKI are limited. Efforts should be taken in all patients to maintain adequate intravascular volume to ensure appropriate renal perfusion and minimize vasopressors and other nephrotoxic medications when possible. Daily review and appropriate dosing adjustments of all medications with renal metabolism and excretion are important in the setting of a reduced creatinine clearance. Forced diuresis using loop diuretics or mannitol is not encouraged, as these interventions increase the risk of volume depletion and further renal injury. In patients with preexisting kidney disease, the use of renal vasodilators such as fenoldopam may decrease risk of concomitant AKI postoperatively [7, 49]. Renal replacement therapy should be initiated early in the setting of acidosis, electrolyte disorders, volume overload, or uremia symptoms that are refractory to medical management, and more severe AKI is associated with a lower incidence of renal recovery (OR 5.01, 95 % CI 2.34–19.7, $p<0.001$) [50].

Acute Limb Ischemia

High mortality is also associated with the development of critical limb ischemia following ruptured AAA repair. Development of acute limb ischemia can potentially be caused by multiple different etiologies including postoperative thromboembolic disease, prolonged preoperative and intraoperative ischemia, extremity compartment syndrome from reperfusion, or distal embolization of plaque or clot from aortic clamping and intraoperative manipulation. In addition, aortic manipulation can put the patient at risk for dislodgement of cholesterol particles with resultant cholesterol emboli. These differ from atherothrombotic emboli in that they are typically smaller and cause ischemia more distally in smaller vessels. Virtually any end organ may be affected by cholesterol emboli, and the true incidence is unknown. Physical signs of this phenomenon can go well beyond limb ischemia and may include fever, skin petechiae, and signs of end-organ damage such as renal azotemia, worsening respiratory distress, or even neurologic changes. The presence of livedo reticularis in this setting is strongly associated with cholesterol emboli syndrome. Blue toe syndrome or ischemia to distal extremities following both elective and emergent aortic surgery has also been associated with cholesterol emboli [51]. The importance of rapid identification and intervention for postoperative limb ischemia is well described in the available literature. In one series of 46 emergent ruptured AAA repairs (all done open), there was a 17 % incidence of postoperative critical limb ischemia [52]. These required a variety of interventions including attempts at operative repair, thrombolysis, or catheter embolectomy. Ultimately, 63 % of the patients who developed limb ischemia progressed to frank limb necrosis. The overall mortality due to critical limb ischemia for the entire cohort was 11 %, and among those who developed limb ischemia, the mortality rate was 83 % [52].

As with abdominal compartment syndrome, all patients who undergo emergent repair for a ruptured AAA should have routine postoperative monitoring done to identify any signs of impending or current limb ischemia. This can be complicated by the multiple factors in these patients that can compromise the reliability and accuracy of the physical exam of the extremities. These can include hypotension, vasopressors, preexisting vascular disease, edema, venous stasis changes, and obesity. It is critical for the operative team to assure that there is adequate distal flow to the extremities following the rAAA repair and to establish a new baseline extremity vascular exam that can be reliably compared to subsequent examinations for any significant change. The other key component is to then accurately communicate (and preferably demonstrate) the key parts of that exam to the ICU team who will be involved in the patient's postoperative care. This should include documentation of both the pulse and Doppler exam for the femoral, popliteal, and all three pedal vessels to characterize which have a palpable pulse, which have only a Doppler signal, and which have neither. Subsequent vascular checks should be done on these patients hourly during the initial resuscitation and stabilization period and should preferably be done by the same person during each shift. There should be clear instructions to notify the ICU and operative team immediately for any significant change in the exam indicating worsening perfusion. This includes the loss of any palpable pulse, the change from palpable to Doppler signal only, and of most concern the complete loss of pulse and Doppler signals in any vessel. It is important to recognize developing limb ischemia as early as possible in order to initiate prompt interventions to improve or restore flow. As the development of limb ischemia is associated with a high mortality in addition to a high rate of limb loss, this monitoring and early intervention process can be lifesaving in addition to limbsaving.

Interventions for the development of limb ischemia can include any of the following alone or in combination: chemical anticoagulation, thrombolysis, catheter-based lysis or thrombectomy, infusion of vasodilators, endovascular angioplasty and/or stenting, operative thrombectomy/embolectomy, revision or repair of anastomoses, and operative revascularization of the affected extremity. A full description of all of these options is beyond the scope of this chapter, but meticulous attention to proper ICU care and management may minimize the time to identification and intervention of this postoperative complication or may even prevent it from developing. Avoidance of both over- and under-resuscitation can help reestablish steady perfusion and avoid repeat periods of relative low-flow or no-flow ischemia. Although correction of coagulopathy is often emphasized in the critically ill postoperative patient, there is a growing appreciation of the multiple phenotypes of coagulation abnormalities during and after shock, including a predisposition to thrombotic complications rather than hemorrhagic complications. Complete normalization of all coagulation parameters should not be used as a target in the non-bleeding patient after a major vascular reconstruction. The increasing use of thromboelastography (TEG) may allow for better appreciation of the current dynamic clotting and clot lysis function in an individual patient and avoid over- or undertreating coagulopathy based off of standard coagulation parameters such as the prothrombin time and partial thromboplastin time. If acute postoperative limb ischemia or threatened limb ischemia develops, then therapeutic anticoagulation with heparin should usually be started immediately for suspected thromboembolism. This may be effective alone in improving perfusion and effecting resolution of any partially obstructing thrombus, but if gross loss of tissue is impending or occurring, then immediate endovascular or operative intervention is typically necessary. In the event that tissue loss is too advanced or extremity revascularization is not possible or will not be tolerated due to the severity of illness, then an amputation should be considered. In rare cases with extremity necrosis in patients who are too unstable to tolerate any operative intervention, a temporizing "medical amputation" can be performed by placement of a proximal extremity tourniquet to occlude both inflow and outflow or by placing the extremity in dry ice until they are stable enough to tolerate a formal surgical amputation [53–55].

Extremity compartment syndrome deserves special mention in any discussion of the ICU and care and monitoring in this patient population. All post-op ruptured AAA patients are at risk for development of compartment syndrome of the lower extremities, and in addition to the limb concerns, it can impact multiple areas of their ICU care including the cardiovascular and renal systems. Patients at particularly high risk include those with prolonged shock, longer durations of preoperative and/or intraoperative limb ischemia (>4–6 h), lack of palpable pedal pulses after surgery, and those with concurrent venous thrombosis and decreased venous return. Regardless of the individual risk factors, all patients should be closely monitored for compartment syndrome following an emergent rAAA repair. The classic early signs of compartment syndrome including severe pain, sensory deficits, loss of toe/foot extension are frequently not reliable in this patient population as the exam is compromised by narcotics, sedation, and often mechanical ventilation. Serial examination of the calf compartments, preferably by the same person or groups of people, should be performed to detect increased swelling and tenseness. Soft compartments with an intact distal vascular exam do not require any further evaluation. If there is increasing concern for a compartment syndrome based on the physical exam, then either compartment pressures should be measured at the bedside or operative fasciotomies should be performed. Similar to abdominal compartment syndrome, compartment pressures above 15 mmHg should raise concern, and those above 20–25 mmHg should prompt intervention. Although several authors have proposed using a perfusion pressure (MAP-compartment pressure) to diagnose compartment syndrome, this has primarily been validated in isolated orthopedic trauma and not in the vascular or ICU patient population. Several others have examined the use of a cutaneous near-infrared spectroscopy monitor to monitor for compartment syndrome and have reported increased sensitivity and specificity when compared to standard clinical criteria and physical examination [56–58]. In addition to providing earlier warnings of impending compartment syndrome, this technology has the advantage of being noninvasive, portable, and continuous. The risk of postoperative extremity compartment syndrome is almost exclusively limited to the calf, although rarely thigh and gluteal compartment syndromes have been reported and should be considered for the patient with evidence of rhabdomyolysis and an unconcerning calf exam. For the patient with failed attempts at restoration of perfusion or irreversible major tissue loss, emergent amputation may be necessary and lifesaving. This is crucial in the setting of a post-op ruptured AAA patient as any increased metabolic demand such as tissue necrosis may be the inciting cause of additional cardiopulmonary stress with resultant major morbidity or mortality [52].

In addition to evaluation of the extremity, any suspected or proven compartment syndrome should prompt immediate assessment for rhabdomyolysis, myoglobinuria, and acute kidney injury with serial laboratory studies (serum CPK, urine myoglobin, and BUN/creatinine). Fluids should be titrated to maintain UOP of at least 30–50 cc/h, and if the CPK is greater than 5000, then we recommend increasing the goal UOP to 80–100 cc/h. Although mannitol and bicarbonate administration are commonly advocated adjuncts for rhabdomyolysis, there is no high-quality evidence demonstrating any benefit to these therapies above standard fluid resuscitation. We reserve these therapies for the patient with a CPK >10,000 and that is rising despite standard fluid resuscitation and positive urine myoglobin. The most common error we see in this area is underestimation of the amount of bicarbonate required to truly alkalinize the urine. We will typically give an immediate bolus of 1–2 ampules (50–100 meq) of sodium bicarbonate (NaHCO3), followed by a continuous infusion of D5W with 100–150 meq NaHCO3/l running at 100–150 cc/h. Confirmation of urine alkalization can be obtained with a simple bedside urine dipstick for pH. Intermittent mannitol boluses may also be given if the patient is failing to adequately respond to the measures above, but should not be given to the anuric patient.

Adrenal Insufficiency

The physiologic stress and relative hemodynamic instability that often accompanies the presentation of a ruptured AAA create a decidedly vulnerable environment for the adrenal gland. The incidence of adrenal insufficiency (AI) is approximately 30 % overall after ruptured AAA repair, and it is reported that up to 67 % of patients with unexplained postoperative hypotension have underlying AI. Table 15.3 highlights the systemic physiologic impact of AI on overall outcomes between those who have AI during recovery after rAAA and those who do not [59]. The stress of the vascular event and major surgery can increase cortisol production tenfold and cease the typical diurnal cycling of cortisol production. The robust blood supply to the adrenal gland is protective from supraceliac clamping; however, the combination of blood loss, mechanical interruption, and microvascular thrombosis or emboli make adrenal ischemia and AI a real possibility that should be considered in all patients [59]. Additional important factors that are critical to elucidate are any history of prior AI, current or recent use of steroid medications, prior adrenal surgery or radiation, and whether any medications have been administered that can interfere with adrenal glucocorticoid and/or mineralocorticoid production. One of the more commonly used medications that can suppress adrenocortical function is etomidate, a commonly used induction agent for rapid sequence intubation. Among patients with septic shock, the incidence of AI was found to be 76 % after etomidate administration versus 51 % with no etomidate [60]. Several other series in shock states (including hemorrhagic shock) have confirmed these findings and also suggest a possible adverse impact on survival [60–62]. However, others have challenged these findings, particularly with a single dose of etomidate [63, 64]. We prefer to avoid etomidate if possible in this patient population and also assume that some degree of adrenal insufficiency is likely in the post-op patient with hypotension despite adequate volume replacement and who received etomidate for intubation or during surgery.

Table 15.3 Effect of adrenal insufficiency on outcomes

	AI group		Non-AI group		
	N	%	*N*	%	*P* value
Bowel ischemia	1	17	3	21	1
Respiratory failure	3	50	8	57	0.63
Myocardial infarction	1	17	3	21	1
Acute renal failure	2	33	5	35	1
Wound problems	1	17	3	21	1
Sepsis	3	50	8	57	0.2
Death	1	17	2	14	0.21
Discharge status					
Home	0	0	4	29	0.04
Extended care	5	83	8	57	

Reprinted with permission from Parikshak et al. [59]
AI adrenal insufficiency, *N* number

It is well understood that cortisol production is intimately involved in the production and activation of catecholamines that regulate not only vascular tone but cardiac function as well. The classic clinical picture of AI is profound hypotension that is not responsive to intravenous volume expansion and pressor medications. Individuals with unidentified AI are therefore at risk of requiring a larger amount of fluid resuscitation, higher doses of vasopressor medications, and the expected resultant increase in complications, organ failures, and mortality [59]. However, these factors can be difficult to isolate and attribute to AI in the complicated post-op rAAA patient who is hypotensive and requiring large-volume resuscitation. The criteria for diagnosis of AI and for initiation of supplemental low-dose (or "stress dose") steroids have undergone a number of changes and modifications over the past decade as new high-quality controlled data has become available [65–67]. Previous recommendations for diagnosing AI in critically ill patients focused on laboratory testing to evaluate serum cortisol levels, cortisol response to a corticotropin stimulation test, or both. Although these results have been shown to be predictive of outcomes, they have not been shown to be reliable for guiding initiation or continuation of therapy [67–69]. The most widely accepted current guidelines in critically ill patients come from the Surviving Sepsis Campaign (www.survivingsepsis.org), and although they focus on septic shock, their algorithms have been widely adopted among diverse ICU populations with shock from varying etiologies [70, 71]. For suspected AI, therapy should be initiated with low-dose hydrocortisone (200–300 mg/day intravenously) based on clinical assessment alone and should not rely on or be delayed for the results of laboratory testing of cortisol levels or a corticotropin (ACTH) stimulation test. Adrenal insufficiency should be suspected in all patients with hypotension despite adequate or ongoing volume expansion and requiring high dose or increasing doses of vasopressor medications and in the absence of another identified cause of the refractory shock. Empiric steroid therapy should be immediately initiated in these patients using hydrocortisone (or equivalent agent) at a dose of 50–100 mg every 8 h. Specific additional mineralocorticoid supplementation (typically with fludrocortisone) is not recommended unless there is some etiology or concern for severe mineralocorticoid deficiency that is being inadequately supplemented by the hydrocortisone. Exogenous steroid treatment should be implemented for the improved outcomes for these patients when hypotension remains unexplained after the first 24 h. Boluses of hydrocortisone are typically used initially with 100 mg immediately followed by 50–100 mg IV every 8 h. Hydrocortisone is typically preferred over dexamethasone or other formulations because of its added benefit of mineralocorticoid activity, although some intensivists advocate adding a specific mineralocorticoid agent (such as fludrocortisone).

Ischemic Colitis

Ischemic colitis is one of the most feared and morbid conditions or complications after abdominal aortic surgery and is particularly well described after both elective and emergent AAA repair. Although the etiology is often assumed to be simple interruption of the colon blood supply, typically in the inferior mesenteric artery distribution, the actual cause is frequently multifactorial. It can include preexisting atherosclerotic or thrombotic disease of the mesenteric vessels, anatomic variation or absence of collateral vessels to the colon, ligation or exclusion of the hypogastric arteries, hypotension with low-flow states, medications, vasopressor use, and infection. The risk of ischemic colitis is substantially higher in ruptured AAA patients in comparison to those undergoing elective repair and will also vary highly depending on the aggressiveness of screening. Clinically significant ischemic colitis is demonstrated in approximately 5 % of elective open AAA repairs, with an increase to 35 % in emergent ruptured AAA repairs [72, 73]. When routine or aggressive endoscopic surveillance is employed, up to 65 % of patients will have some evidence of ischemic colitis after open repair of a ruptured AAA [72, 74]. Much less data is available on ischemic colitis after endovascular repair, but several series have described an incidence of 1.4–1.7 % for all endovascular AAA repairs [75, 76]. The incidence in EVAR for rAAA is undoubtedly higher, but has not been well characterized. Of interest, the presence of atheroemboli as the primary source of colonic ischemia is much more common following endovascular repair and carries an overall poor prognosis. The presentation and clinical significance of postoperative ischemic colitis exists along a broad spectrum, from relatively asymptomatic disease limited to the mucosa and identified on endoscopy to full-thickness colon necrosis with perforation. However, there is a clear and significant increase in overall mortality among patients with clinically evident ischemic colitis to 40–60 % and up to 90 % in the presence of necrosis with perforation [77, 78].

A detailed discussion of the identification and management of this complication is comprehensively discussed separately in this book. Of specific importance to the ICU physician caring for these patients is to maintain a high index of suspicion for ischemic colitis, as a delay in diagnosis is one of the strongest factors associated with poor outcomes. The diagnosis should be considered in any patient who is failing to respond to resuscitation or who demonstrates rapid decompensation after an initial 24–72-h period of stability. More specific signs such as worsening abdominal distension, abdominal pain and fevers, bloody and/or frequent bowel movements, and leukocytosis should prompt a focused evaluation, typically with flexible endoscopy to assess the colonic mucosa. Because this entity almost universally involves the left colon in the inferior mesenteric artery territory, a bedside flexible sigmoidoscopy is sufficient to evaluate the primary areas at risk (Fig. 15.2). Medical management is the preferred treatment for mild to moderate ischemia without evidence of full-thickness involvement, colon necrosis, perforation, or peritonitis. This consists of bowel rest, intravenous volume expansion, intravenous antibiotics, and close monitoring for progression versus resolution. Any patient who develops evidence of an acute abdomen or abdominal compartment syndrome should be presumed to have ischemic colon with necrosis until proven otherwise and should undergo immediate laparotomy and segmental versus total abdominal colectomy. Other interventions that may have benefit are avoiding the use of vasopressor agents with strong or unopposed vasoconstrictive effects that preferentially affect mesenteric flow and withholding full-dose enteral feeding to allow bowel rest and mucosal recovery and healing.

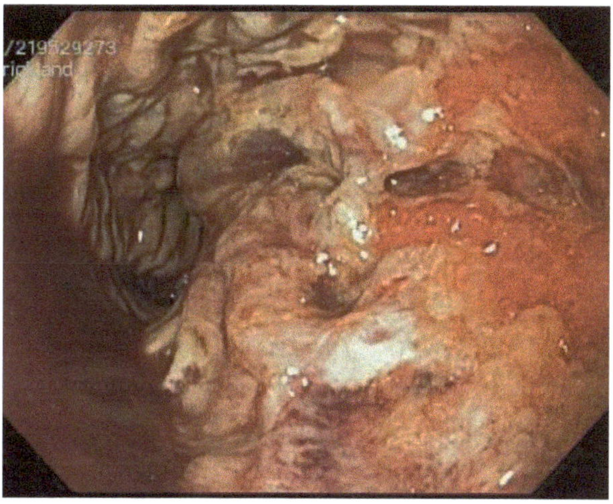

Fig. 15.2 Examination of the sigmoid colon via flexible endoscopy 3 days after open repair of a ruptured abdominal aortic aneurysm reveals pale mucosa, vascular congestion, and large ulcerations consistent with ischemic colitis

Standard Daily Critical Care Principles and Practice

The acute care issues and complications of a ruptured AAA have been addressed as they will appear during a typical postoperative ICU stay. More generalized standard ICU "best practices" still very much apply to the post-op ruptured AAA patient and should briefly be reviewed. One of the most important factors in providing consistently high-quality ICU care is to have a standard and systematic approach to the initial evaluation and all subsequent daily evaluations of the ICU patient. This is even more important in the complicated vascular patient who often has multiple preexisting comorbidities, medications, several consulting services, and more than one active ICU issue or problem. Methods to simplify, protocolize, and automate the care of these patients, and particularly the aspects of care with strong evidence-based support, have been consistently found to result in improved outcomes and decreased errors or "near misses." The use of standardized data collection systems, preformatted rounding sheets, ICU care protocols or "bundles," and daily care checklists are key components to enhance care and to ensure that important things aren't overlooked or forgotten (i.e., DVT prophylaxis, nutrition, oral care, positioning, etc.). Finally, the ultimate impact of this process will be significantly lessened or even nullified if the information is restricted to only the physicians on either the ICU or the surgical team. Daily rounds should also include the key nonphysician personnel who will be involved in the care of the patient, including the ICU nurse and any nursing assistants, respiratory therapy, etc. Additional benefit will be derived through having larger multidisciplinary rounds at least weekly, with involvement of key personnel including nutrition, physical and occupational therapy, speech pathology, an ICU pharmacologist, social work, and case management.

Daily ICU rounds can often be characterized as a large "data dump" followed by discussion and planning and then execution. Although actions and interventions are often emphasized, it is important to be able to distinguish between doing things to "optimize" the patient versus doing things to try and "normalize" them. The history of critical care is littered with abandoned practices that attempted to intervene to make some parameter in the ICU patient look like it does in a healthy patient. Table 15.4 contains several key examples of these, such as tight glucose control (targeted to glucose level of 90–110 mg/dl), that in the end turned out to be more harmful than helpful. This section will be presented in a system-based fashion, which has become the preferred organizational framework for standard ICU rounds at most major medical centers.

Neurologic/Pain Management

Neurologic management and care can be broken down to analgesia, sedation, and delirium prevention or management. Patients should be monitored closely to ensure adequate pain control, and a validated system of pain measurement should be utilized. Specifically, it is recommended that post-op ruptured AAA patients have a thoracic epidural in place if at all possible, which can provide superior pain control with lower doses of narcotics and/or local anesthetic infusion. Opioid analgesia is the first line for intravenous or oral analgesia, but must be balanced against the known side-effect profiles including respiratory depression, worsening of delirium, urinary retention, and constipation. This should be supplemented with nonnarcotic medications such as nonsteroidal anti-inflammatory drugs and acetaminophen whenever possible. The combination of scheduled intravenous ketorolac and acetaminophen can work wonders in reducing musculoskeletal pain and decreasing the total narcotic requirement, particularly among elderly patients. If there is concomitant neuropathic pain, then gabapentin or similar agents can be added [79]. For patients with refractory pain despite all of the above, or with significant side effects or intolerance to narcotics, a low-dose ketamine infusion (2 ug/kg/min) will almost always be effective and is well tolerated without the hemodynamic effects or respiratory depression seen with higher doses of narcotics [80, 81].

Sedation of the ICU patient remains one of the more challenging and frequently misunderstood aspects of ICU care. There is a common assumption that all intubated patients need to be heavily sedated and that sedation must be delivered as a continuous intravenous infusion. This approach has now been clearly shown to result in avoidable morbidity and even mortality and should be abandoned. The first question that must be asked for every patient is whether they require sedation at all, and if so, whether it can be achieved with intermittent dosing of short-acting agents. In many cases, patients felt to be "difficult to sedate" due to agitation actually will respond to improved pain control and do not require heavier sedation. All ICU sedation should be managed via a protocolized approach that includes options for continuous versus intermittent dosing, contains a validated and objective sedation scoring system that is used to titrate the sedation, and provides for daily "sedation holidays" to better assess the patient's neurologic status and whether they require continued sedation at all. There are multiple readily available and validated sedation

Table 15.4 Abandoned ICU paradigms based on "normalization" of key parameters

Variable	Rationale for intervention	Suggested intervention	Actual impacts	Current approach
O_2 delivery	Low O_2 delivery creates an oxygen "deficit," end-organ hypoxia, and injury	Drive O_2 delivery to "supranormal" levels to make up for the oxygen deficit	Increased complications including pulmonary edema, abdominal compartment syndrome	Optimize oxygen delivery to minimally acceptable level, no supranormal goals
Glucose control	Hyperglycemia leading to increased infections and organ injury	Tight glycemic control to keep glucose 90–110 mg/dl	Increased need for insulin drips, longer ICU stays, increased hypoglycemia, no benefit	Maintain moderate euglycemia with acceptable glucose levels of up to 150–180 mg/dl
Arterial carbon dioxide (pCO_2) and pH	Hypercapnia causing metabolic acidosis, loss of enzyme function, and coagulopathy	Titrate minute ventilation to keep pCO_2 in normal range (35–40)	Increased tidal volumes and respiratory rates with increased exposure to ventilator-induced lung injury	Allow permissive hypercapnia as long as pH >7.2, added benefit of increased O_2 delivery with acidosis
Hematocrit	Anemia resulting in decreased O_2 delivery, increased cardiac work	Liberal transfusion of packed red blood cells to keep Hgb >10 g/dl	Increased blood transfusions, increased infectious complications and exposures to blood-borne pathogens	Restrictive transfusion only for Hgb <7 g/dl in most patients or for symptomatic anemia
Tidal volumes	Low tidal volumes leading to atelectasis, respiratory acidosis, hypoxia	Deliver "normal" tidal volumes of 10–15 cc/kg/breath	Increased airway pressures, increased barotrauma and volutrauma, worse outcomes in ARDS	Low tidal volume ventilation of 4–6 cc/kg, avoidance of elevated peak airway pressures
Estimated protein/calorie needs, albumin/prealbumin levels	Critical illness associated with protein wasting and prolonged negative nitrogen balance, low albumin/prealbumin despite nutritional supplementation	Calculate protein/calorie requirements and multiply by some "stress factor" to deliver supranormal levels of protein and nonprotein calories, early and liberal use of TPN	Overfeeding syndromes, increased CO_2 production, increased nitrogenous waste production, increased fat mass with no muscle/protein-sparing effect	Early initiation of enteral nutrition with initial low caloric dose slowly titrated to meet resting energy expenditure; delayed initiation of TPN if enteral not possible; avoidance of excess protein/calories

scoring systems, such as the Ramsay sedation score (RSS) and the Richmond Agitation-Sedation Score (RASS), and sedation orders should be written to titrate to a specific score and not to meaningless categories such as "titrate to moderate sedation" [82, 83]. In select cases where deeper sedation is required or sedation assessment is compromised by either medications (such as paralytic agents) or organic brain disorders, advanced neuromonitors such as the bispectral index system (BIS) can provide continuous and objective data on depth of sedation [84, 85].

There is significant debate in the literature regarding the optimal choice of sedating agents, and each class of medications has its own pros and cons in this patient population. The choice of agent should depend on the level of sedation that is required, the anticipated duration of sedation, the patient's age and renal/liver function, the desired dosing schedule (continuous versus intermittent), and the individual sedation and side-effect profile of the medication. Benzodiazepines are common first-line agents for ICU sedation and can produce effective and sustained sedation as well as amnestic effects. Side effects can include decreased blood pressure, paradoxical increased agitation (particularly in elderly patients), and significant depression of respiratory drive. Midazolam and lorazepam are the two most commonly utilized agents for ICU sedation, and both are effective agents with relatively short durations of onset and action when given intermittently. However, there is a widespread misperception that midazolam is a superior agent for continuous infusion due to the short duration of action and ability to quickly awaken the patient after stopping the infusion. After 24–48 h of continuous infusion, midazolam has similar long-term effects as the other long-acting benzodiazepines due to the systemic accumulation of the drug and its active metabolites. We recommend intermittent dosing of benzodiazepines when possible, with repeated additional small doses as needed for inadequate sedation or intermittent agitation. These agents should be minimized or altogether avoided in the patient at high risk for delirium or with established delirium [79].

Alternative agents such as propofol and dexmedetomidine (Precedex) have gained widespread use and acceptance in all ICU populations, primarily due to their advantages over benzodiazepines in terms of rapid onset and clearance (propofol) and less hemodynamic and respiratory effects (dexmedetomidine). Propofol infusion has particularly gained favor as the preferred agent when a short duration of sedation is anticipated (typically less than 72 h). It has a rapid onset when initiated and similarly rapid clearance when held, even after continuous infusion for >24 h. However, its use may be limited in the post-op ruptured AAA patient with hypotension or with labile hemodynamics. Continuous infusion should not be continued beyond 3–4 days, and patients should be monitored for the rare but frequently fatal "propofol infusion syndrome," characterized by lactic acidosis, heart failure, rhabdomyolysis, hyperkalemia, and renal failure [86]. Dexmedetomidine is a newer agent that induces sedation as well as analgesia via central alpha-2 adrenergic agonism and has no respiratory depressant effects. Patients are typically easy to arouse from sedation on this agent, and its use has been associated with significantly shorter times to extubation versus standard agents such as benzodiazepines [87, 88]. Similar to propofol, this agent does have negative cardiovascular effects such as hypotension and bradycardia and should not be used during periods of hemodynamic instability or lability [89].

Delirium is one of the more morbid but simultaneously preventable complications of prolonged ICU care. The first principle of delirium is that it should be a diagnosis of exclusion, and alternative metabolic or physiologic causes for confusion/agitation (such as hypoxia, hypercarbia, uremia, etc.) should be sought out and treated. Daily implementation of early mobilization, consistent schedules of care and activity, and day-night cycling is paramount in the prevention of ICU delirium. Delirium should be monitored with scoring tools such as the Confusion Assessment Method for the ICU (CAM-ICU) or the Intensive Care Delirium Screening Checklist (ICDSC) [79]. Ruptured AAA patients are at significant risk for developing postoperative delirium due to multiple factors including their typically advanced age, multiple comorbidities, polypharmacy, requirement for frequent pain medication, and their overall severity of illness. Furthermore patients with preexisting dementia or history of smoking or alcoholism will be at a compounded risk for ICU delirium and should be closely monitored for early signs. Treatment of delirium is largely based on the above measures as well as the minimization of narcotics, avoidance of benzodiazepines (unless alcohol withdrawal related) or other sedating medications, and avoidance of other central nervous system medications. Implementation of rivastigmine is not advised. The use of select atypical antipsychotics and dexmedetomidine are preferred and may reduce the duration and length of ICU delirium. All regularly administered home medications should be restarted as soon as is appropriate [79]. Finally, acute mental status changes or encephalopathy related to thromboembolic or ischemic events throughout the initial treatment and repair of a ruptured AAA should stay high on your differential. New ischemia, intracranial hemorrhage, or cerebral vascular disease may be detected with computed tomography or magnetic resonance imaging and should be considered to rule out an anatomic lesion before attributing abnormalities to simple delirium. Treatment for the majority of these postoperative CNS events is largely supportive; however, certain circumstances (such as a focal embolism) may benefit from neurovascular intervention.

Cardiac

The majority of cardiac concerns and management have been addressed in the first parts of this chapter. Daily rounding and routine ICU cardiovascular care should focus on optimization of postoperative cardiac performance, judicious resuscitation and hemodynamic support, identification of cardiovascular complications (such as myocardial infarction), and prevention of additional complications. Two of the most common cardiovascular concerns in the post-op rAAA patient are myocardial infarction (described in detail above) and congestive heart failure or volume overload syndromes. Obtaining a formal bedside echocardiogram in the postoperative period can be very helpful to assess the volume status and cardiac performance after the stress of the aneurysm rupture and surgical repair and to establish a new baseline for future comparisons. Many surgeons and intensivists are becoming facile at simplified bedside echocardiography which can provide reliable estimates of cardiac performance and volume status, which can help to guide resuscitation and avoid the need for invasive monitoring [90]. Although the priority during the initial resuscitation and stabilization period is supporting organ perfusion and avoiding hypotension, patients on preoperative beta-blockers should have these continued or resumed (usually in intravenous form) as soon as possible. After the initial resuscitation and stabilization period, home medications such as oral beta-blockers and statins should be restarted as soon as possible and have been associated with a decreased incidence of adverse cardiac events during not only the hospital admission but over the initial months to year after surgery. Although invasive hemodynamic monitoring with a pulmonary artery catheter was routinely used in the past to guide postoperative resuscitation, they have largely been abandoned in favor of simpler and more reliable measures or "end points," such as lactate, central venous O_2 saturation, and bedside echocardiography. It should again be highlighted that myocardial infarction and cardiac arrhythmias are the most common causes of death in these patients, and we routinely assess rAAA patients with serum troponin measurements as well as electrocardiograms following surgery. In patients with suspected volume overload, serial measurements of serum BNP can be helpful to confirm the diagnosis and to guide the initiation and response to diuresis or to dialysis/hemofiltration for volume removal.

Pulmonary

The key aspects of postoperative pulmonary evaluation and management have been described above in the section on ventilator management. Following emergent surgical intervention for ruptured AAA, patients are at significantly increased risk of major pulmonary complications. Two of the most common in the ICU population are acute respiratory distress syndrome (ARDS) and ventilator-associated pneumonia (VAP). Although pulmonary support with mechanical ventilation is almost universally required for at least 24 h after emergent surgery for rAAA, the overriding principle in minimizing the risk of additional pulmonary morbidity should be separation of the patient from mechanical ventilation at the earliest opportunity. This does not mean premature extubation, which itself carries a risk of additional morbidity, but means early and aggressive attempts at ventilator weaning and extubation as soon as reasonable criteria are met. If it appears that prolonged mechanical ventilation will be required or if the patient fails one or more attempts at extubation, then consideration of a tracheostomy should be entertained.

ARDS is characterized as a diffuse and heterogeneous alveolar and interstitial lung injury characterized by vascular permeability leading to pulmonary edema, loss of pulmonary compliance, and refractory hypoxemia. The previously utilized consensus conference definitions distinguished the milder acute lung injury from the more severe ARDS based primarily on the PaO_2/FiO_2 ratio. The newer and now widely adopted Berlin criteria for ARDS has eliminated the diagnosis of ALI and instead provides clear criteria for diagnosing ARDS and then subcategorizing the severity. The Berlin criteria for ARDS includes the following: hypoxia occurring within 1 week of a clear inciting event or new onset of respiratory distress, characteristic chest x-ray findings of diffuse bilateral interstitial infiltrates that is not caused by cardiogenic fluid overload, and a decrease in the PaO_2/FiO_2 ratio to less than 300. The severity of ARDS is further subcategorized by the PaO_2/FiO_2 ratio into mild (200–300), moderate (100–200), or severe (less than 100) with a normal PEEP level of 5 mmHg [91].

Lung-protective strategies are key in the management of ARDS and include low tidal volumes (4–6 ml/kg), low plateau pressures (<30 mmHg), permissive hypercapnia, and appropriate PEEP. PEEP should be started at a lower level [5–10] and then titrated up only as needed to accomplish appropriate oxygenation (PaO_2 55–80 mmHg or SpO_2 of 88–95 %) (Table 15.5) [92]. A meta-analysis by Gu et al. has shown that these lung-protective strategies should be employed from the time of initial intubation and mechanical ventilation to improve outcomes in surgical patients [31]. Permissive hypercapnia to a pH of 7.2 is safe and well tolerated and helps to achieve low plateau pressure and low tidal volumes. Sodium bicarbonate or THAM may be utilized for patients whose pH decreases below 7.2, or a different ventilator mode may be attempted. Early prone positioning of patients with severe ARDS was recently found to significantly decrease 28- and 90-day mortality and should be utilized if there is difficulty achieving minimal levels of oxygenation with supine positioning [93].

Rescue or salvage mechanical ventilation may be required in severe ARDS. High-frequency oscillatory ventilation (HFOV) has been used in attempts to improve oxygenation in these patients. This type of strategy employs constant inflation with oxygen with minute exchanges of CO_2 with 2–5 Hz oscillation. Although recent studies have shown no mortality benefit with HFOV, it will almost always improve oxygenation and should be used selectively for patient's failing standard modes [94]. Venovenous extracorporeal membrane oxygenation (ECMO) is the use of machine-directed blood oxygenation and carbon dioxide extraction, while the lungs are bypassed to promote ventilation-free time to heal. Indication for ECMO includes one of the following: severe refractory hypoxemia, severe hypercapnia, or continue

Table 15.5 A simplified conservative fluid management protocol in ARDS

CVP (recommended)	PAOP (optional)	MAP ≥60 mmHg and off vasopressors ≥12 h	
		UOP <0.5 ml/kg/h	UOP >0.5 mL/kg/h
>8	>12	Furosemide; reassess in 1 h	Furosemide; reassess in 4 h
4–8	8–12	Fluid bolus; reassess in 1 h	Furosemide; reassess in 4 h
<4	<8	Fluid bolus; reassess in 1 h	No intervention; reassess in 4 h

Recommended furosemide dosing = begin with 20 mg bolus or 3 mg/ml infusion or last known effective dose high plateau pressure despite optimal standard management. Anticoagulation is required and any contraindication to this is an absolute contraindication to ECMO. Recent evidence taken from the H1N1 pandemic and other randomized control trials has displayed a survival benefit in severe refractory ARDS [95, 96].

Ventilator-associated pneumonia (VAP) and hospital-acquired pneumonias (HAP) are the second most common nosocomial infections and are associated with the highest mortality. VAP should be expected in all patients that have had at least two episodes of fever, leukocytosis/leukopenia, purulent sputum, or hypoxia. Empiric antibiotic therapy should be initiated within the first 24 h of diagnosis, which should be based on clinical findings as well as results of bronchoalveolar lavage quantitative cultures. The most common bacteria include *Streptococcus* species, MRSA, *Enterococcus*, *Pseudomonas*, *Haemophilus*, *Enterobacter*, *Proteus* species, *E. coli* and *Klebsiella.* Antibiotic treatment should be tailored as specific microbial agents are identified through cultures, and the majority of VAP can be treated with an 8-day course of antibiotics [97, 98]. It is important to note that antibiotic-resistant organisms are more common with VAP/HAP. Risk factors that should be minimized in the ICU patient include colonization of the oropharynx, nasogastric or endotracheal tubes, and use of acid-suppressing medications [99, 100]. Additional preventive efforts include elevation of the head of the bed (particularly with enteral feeding), weekly circuit changes, closed suction drainage of secretions, and the use of oral chlorhexidine [101].

Renal and Genitourinary

Aside from the previously discussed recognition and treatment of acute kidney injury – daily electrolyte, acid base, and Foley catheter management should be closely monitored throughout the initial period of critical illness. However, after stabilization there is little role for routine daily labs unless there is some clinical concern or ongoing process such as diuresis, electrolyte imbalance or active replacement, bleeding or hemodynamic change, or for adjustment of parenteral nutrition formulas or additives. Automatic electrolyte replacement protocols should be used to promptly manage deficiencies rather than relying on daily review and recognition, unless there is some critical range deficiency or worsening imbalance despite protocolized replacement. Electrolyte homeostasis is important for cardiac myocardial stabilization, acid-base regulation, and will promote faster return and maintenance of GI motility. Foley catheters should be removed as soon as possible to prevent urinary tract infections (UTI) and should not be left in simply for convenience or for "monitoring" outside of ongoing resuscitation or large-volume diuresis. If urinary tract infections do occur, they should be considered a complicated UTI, urine should be cultured and appropriate antibiotic therapy should be initiated and later tailored. A repeat urinalysis should be obtained after completion of treatment to confirm resolution.

Gastrointestinal/Nutrition

Post-op ileus will always occur after open repair of a ruptured AAA, especially those repairs done through an open transabdominal approach. However, a major ileus can be seen with any type of critical illness and can certainly occur even with an endovascular rAAA repair. In addition, the presence of a large retroperitoneal hematoma can cause significant abdominal pain, distension, ileus, and even obstructive symptoms for up to 1–2 weeks after repair. This does not mean that prolonged periods of NPO are required, but full early enteral nutrition within the first 24–48 h will rarely be tolerated in this patient cohort. A prolonged ileus may present with a significantly delayed return of bowel function, persistent nausea with or without vomiting, and recurrent bouts of abdominal distension. Dilated bowel with air fluid levels and gas distally may be seen on acute abdominal series and can be difficult to distinguish from an early postoperative small bowel obstruction. This should be managed with bowel decompression with placement of a nasogastric tube, correction of electrolyte abnormalities, and patient observation. Nearly all post-op ileus will resolve, and even most early post-op small bowel obstructions are successfully managed nonoperatively. However, this can have significant impact on the delivery of adequate postoperative nutritional support.

A full discussion of the complex issues around ICU nutrition is beyond the scope of this chapter, and two excellent sources for evidence-based guidelines are the Canadian Critical Care Nutrition Guidelines and the Society of Critical Care Medicine Nutrition Guidelines [102–104]. One of the common misconceptions in ICU care is that patients require and will benefit from aggressive delivery of supranormal levels of calories and protein, based on the fact that they are severely "stressed" and the well-recognized syndrome of critical illness protein wasting. During the acute phases of severe critical illness, there is a systemic inability to properly process large amounts of nutrients, so overfeeding with protein and carbohydrates will generally lead to increased nitrogenous waste product production, hyperglycemia, increased fat mass, and little impact on protein accumulation. This has been confirmed by multiple controlled trials that have demonstrated little to no benefit to providing higher levels of protein or caloric intake [102, 105]. A second area of debate centers around the route of administration: enteral versus parenteral (TPN). It has become generally accepted that enteral feeding is preferred over TPN, but this appears to primarily be due to its ability to enhance gut barrier function rather than any nutritional superiority. Current evidence-based guidelines support the early initiation of enteral feeds within 24–48 h of ICU admission if possible and that these should be started at a slow rate (20 cc/HR) and not rapidly advanced until tolerance has been demonstrated for 24–48 h. A reasonable early caloric goal for the critically ill patient is 10–20 kcal/kg/day and protein of 1–1.5 g/kg/day, and this can then be advanced based on tolerance and as the acute illness is improving. In the patient who cannot tolerate enteral feeds, there is no benefit to starting early TPN unless there is moderate to severe preexisting malnutrition. For all others, current guidelines are to start TPN at day 5–7 if enteral is not possible or not tolerated after several trials [102, 106]. If TPN is initiated, there should be strict attention paid to electrolyte balance and contents, aseptic line placement and care techniques, and resumption of oral or enteral nutrition at the earliest possible time [107].

Endocrine

Euthyroid sick syndrome or low T3 syndrome is a relatively newly discovered and researched area for critically ill patients. This can be characterized as abnormal thyroid lab values to include low T3, high rT3, with normal or low levels of T4 and TSH. Euthyroid sick syndrome has associated with increased mortality in critically ill patients; however no good evidence currently exists as to why and the effect of thyroid supplementation. Thus thyroid levels should not be evaluated in an ICU patient unless there is a specific concern related to the patient's thyroid. Moreover, TSH alone is not sufficient in the evaluation of the thyroid in the critically ill patient and T3, rT3, and T4 should also be measured [108].

Glycemic control in the critically ill patient has been well studied. Hyperglycemia is associated with increased risk for infection, impaired wound healing, and sepsis, although the directionality and causality of this relationship are still unclear. It can be difficult to control blood sugar in the setting of elevated physiologic stress, pre-existing diabetes, administration of enteral or parental nutrition, and catecholamine use, and this will typically require either an aggressive intermittent regimen of insulin or a continuous infusion with frequent titration. Very tight glucose control (goal of 90–110 mg/dl) using continuous infusions and frequent adjustments became widely accepted after initial studies demonstrated a potential benefit in reduction of infections and improved mortality [109]. Subsequent larger randomized studies such as the NICE-SUGAR trial demonstrated the superiority of less strict maintenance of blood glucose with a target of less than 180 mg/dl. This resulted in decreased complications and improved survival in comparison to tight control and with significantly fewer episodes of severe hypoglycemia [110].

Prophylaxis

Patient who have undergone repair of a ruptured AAA are categorized by the ACCP as high risk for development of deep venous thrombosis. However, they are also at increased risk of major bleeding or significant complication from a major bleed. Therefore, until major risk of bleeding has subsided, mechanical prophylaxis with sequential compression devices should be used. Once there is no longer considered to be a high risk of major bleeding, then it is prudent to start chemical prophylaxis with either low-molecular-weight heparin or unfractionated heparin. In almost all cases of rAAA repair, this can safely be initiated within 24–48 h of surgery unless there are signs of ongoing bleeding or a clinically significant coagulopathy. This should be continued throughout their hospital stay and continued in select patients after discharge based on their individual risk factors, mobility level, and comorbid conditions [111].

GI prophylaxis with acid-suppressing medications has been showed to prevent the development of stress-induced ulcers in patients with coagulopathy, burns, or respiratory failure requiring >48 h of mechanical ventilation. The majority of patients who undergo repair of a rAAA will fall into this patient population (typically due to the mechanical ventilation criteria) and should receive stress ulcer prophylaxis from the time of ICU admission. Arguably the most effective stress ulcer prophylaxis is the administration of enteral feeding, and there is debate about whether these medications need to be continued once enteral feeding is initiated. Although there is ample evidence that proton pump inhibitors are more effective at acid suppression than older histaminc receptor blockers, there is no difference in survival or other outcome measures among the different acid-suppressing medications. The choice can be based upon local formularies, cost analysis, and ease of administration. These medications should not be routinely continued beyond the ICU stay, and stress ulcer prophylaxis is safe to discontinue once the previously mentioned independent risk factors have resolved [112].

Daily Checklist

A daily rounding checklist should be routinely completed every day for patients recovering from ruptured AAA repair. This should include an account of all tubes, lines, and drains and consideration of removal. Nutrition status should be addressed daily as well as a plan for implementation. Quality skin care and checks need to be done daily to identify any areas of skin breakdown. Early mobilization should be reviewed daily and the use of physical therapy involved early. Coordination of care among the multiple services that are likely involved is crucial to the successful multidisciplinary management of these complex patients. Given the significant morbidity associated with ruptured AAA, a comprehensive and honest discussion should be done with the patient and patient's family to decide goals of care, code status, and potential for transition to a more comfort or palliative-based care.

References

1. Bown MJ, Sutton AJ, Bell PR, Sayers RD. A meta-analysis of 50 years of ruptured abdominal aortic aneurysm repair. Br J Surg. 2002;89:714–30. doi:10.1046/j.1365-2168.2002.02122.x; published online EpubJun.
2. Kantonen I, Lepantalo M, Brommels M, Luther M, Salenius JP, Ylonen K. Mortality in ruptured abdominal aortic aneurysms. The Finnvasc Study Group. Eur J Vasc Endovasc Surg Off J Eur Soc Vasc Surg. 1999;17:208–12; published online EpubMar.
3. Katz DJ, Stanley JC, Zelenock GB. Operative mortality rates for intact and ruptured abdominal aortic aneurysms in Michigan: an eleven-year statewide experience. J Vasc Surg. 1994;19:804–15; discussion 816–7; published online EpubMay.

4. Cotton BA, Au BK, Nunez TC, Gunter OL, Robertson AM, Young PP. Predefined massive transfusion protocols are associated with a reduction in organ failure and postinjury complications. J Trauma. 2009;66:41–8. doi:10.1097/TA.0b013e31819313bb; discussion 48–9; published online EpubJan.
5. Holcomb JB, Tilley BC, Baraniuk S, Fox EE, Wade CE, Podbielski JM, del Junco DJ, Brasel KJ, Bulger EM, Callcut RA, Cohen MJ, Cotton BA, Fabian TC, Inaba K, Kerby JD, Muskat P, O'Keeffe T, Rizoli S, Robinson BR, Scalea TM, Schreiber MA, Stein DM, Weinberg JA, Callum JL, Hess JR, Matijevic N, Miller CN, Pittet JF, Hoyt DB, Pearson GD, Leroux B, van Belle G, PROPPR Study Group. Transfusion of plasma, platelets, and red blood cells in a 1:1:1 vs a 1:1:2 ratio and mortality in patients with severe trauma: the PROPPR randomized clinical trial. JAMA. 2015;313:471–82. doi:10.1001/jama.2015.12; published online EpubFeb 3.
6. Steiner ME, Assmann SF, Levy JH, Marshall J, Pulkrabek S, Sloan SR, Triulzi D, Stowell CP. Addressing the question of the effect of RBC storage on clinical outcomes: the Red Cell Storage Duration Study (RECESS) (Section 7). Transfus Apher Sci Off J World Apher Assoc Off J Eur Soc Haemapheresis. 2010;43:107–16. doi:10.1016/j.transci.2010.05.014; published online EpubAug.
7. Stephens RS, Whitman GJ. Postoperative critical care of the adult cardiac surgical patient. Part I: routine postoperative care. Crit Care Med. 2015;43:1477–97. doi:10.1097/CCM.0000000000001059; published online EpubJul.
8. Da Luz LT, Nascimento B, Shankarakutty AK, Rizoli S, Adhikari NK. Effect of thromboelastography (TEG(R)) and rotational thromboelastometry (ROTEM(R)) on diagnosis of coagulopathy, transfusion guidance and mortality in trauma: descriptive systematic review. Crit Care. 2014;18:518. doi:10.1186/s13054-014-0518-9).
9. Anagnostopoulos PV, Shepard AD, Pipinos II, Raman SB, Chaudhry PA, Mishima T, Morita H, Suzuki G. Analysis of coagulation changes associated with supraceliac aortic crossclamping using thromboelastography. J Surg Res. 2001;98:52–8. doi:10.1006/jsre.2001.6162; published online EpubJun 1.
10. Gorlinger K, Dirkmann D, Hanke AA. Potential value of transfusion protocols in cardiac surgery. Curr Opin Anaesthesiol. 2013;26:230–43. doi:10.1097/ACO.0b013e32835ddca6; published online EpubApr.
11. Martin P, Greenstein D, Gupta NK, Walker DR, Kester RC. Systemic heparinization during peripheral vascular surgery: thromboelastographic, activated coagulation time, and heparin titration monitoring. J Cardiothorac Vasc Anesth. 1994;8:150–2; published online EpubApr.
12. Henry DA, Carless PA, Moxey AJ, O'Connell D, Stokes BJ, Fergusson DA, KerK. Antifibrinolytic use for minimising perioperative allogeneic blood transfusion. Cochrane Database Syst Rev. 2011;16(3):CD001886. doi:10.1002/14651858.CD001886.pub4).
13. Hutton B, Joseph L, Fergusson D, Mazer CD, Shapiro S, Tinmouth A. Risks of harms using antifibrinolytics in cardiac surgery: systematic review and network meta-analysis of randomised and observational studies. BMJ. 2012;345:e5798. doi:10.1136/bmj.e5798).
14. Koster A, Schirmer U. Re-evaluation of the role of antifibrinolytic therapy with lysine analogs during cardiac surgery in the post aprotinin era. Curr Opin Anaesthesiol. 2011;24:92–7. doi:10.1097/ACO.0b013e32833ff3eb; published online EpubFeb.
15. Makhija N, Sarupria A, Kumar Choudhary S, Das S, Lakshmy R, Kiran U. Comparison of epsilon aminocaproic acid and tranexamic Acid in thoracic aortic surgery: clinical efficacy and safety. J Cardiothorac Vasc Anesth. 2013;27:1201–7. doi:10.1053/j.jvca.2013.04.003; published online EpubDec.
16. Holbrook A, Schulman S, Witt DM, Vandvik PO, Fish J, Kovacs MJ, Svensson PJ, Veenstra DL, Crowther M, Guyatt GH, American College of Chest Physicians. Evidence-based management of anticoagulant therapy: antithrombotic therapy and prevention of thrombosis, 9th ed: American College of Chest Physicians evidence-based clinical practice guidelines. Chest. 2012;141:e152S–84. doi:10.1378/chest.11-2295; published online EpubFeb.
17. Greinacher A, Thiele T, Selleng K. Reversal of anticoagulants: an overview of current developments. Thromb Haemost. 2015;113:931–42. doi:10.1160/TH14-11-0982; published online EpubMay.

18. Piljic D, Petricevic M, Piljic D, Ksela J, Robic B, Klokocovnik T. Restrictive versus standard fluid regimen in elective minilaparotomy abdominal aortic repair-prospective randomized controlled trial. Thorac Cardiovasc Surg. 2015. doi:10.1055/s-0035-1548736; published online EpubMar 31
19. Stephens S, Whitman GJ. Postoperative critical care of the adult cardiac surgical patient: part II: procedure-specific considerations, management of complications, and quality improvement. Crit Care Med. 2015;43(9):1995–2014. doi:10.1097/CCM.0000000000001171; published online EpubJul 1.
20. De Backer D, Biston P, Devriendt J, Madl C, Chochrad D, Aldecoa C, Brasseur A, Defrance P, Gottignies P, Vincent JL, Investigators SI. Comparison of dopamine and norepinephrine in the treatment of shock. N Engl J Med. 2010;362:779–89. doi:10.1056/NEJMoa0907118; published online EpubMar 4.
21. Hertzer NR, Mascha EJ, Karafa MT, O'Hara PJ, Krajewski LP, Beven EG. Open infrarenal abdominal aortic aneurysm repair: the Cleveland Clinic experience from 1989 to 1998. J Vasc Surg. 2002;35:1145–54; published online EpubJun.
22. Onohara T, Komori K, Kume M, Ishida M, Ohta S, Takeuchi K, Matsumoto T, Sugimachi K. Increased plasma fibrinogen level and future risk of coronary artery disease after repair of abdominal aortic aneurysm. J Am Coll Surg. 2000;191:619–25; published online EpubDec.
23. Brown LC, Thompson SG, Greenhalgh RM, Powell JT, Endovascular Aneurysm Repair Trial Participants. Incidence of cardiovascular events and death after open or endovascular repair of abdominal aortic aneurysm in the randomized EVAR trial 1. Br J Surg. 2011;98:935–42. doi:10.1002/bjs.7485; published online EpubJul.
24. Onohara T, Inoue K, Furuyama T, Ohno T. Preoperative cardiovascular assessment and late cardiovascular events after elective abdominal aortic aneurysm repair. Ann Vasc Surg. 2015;29(8):1533–42. doi:10.1016/j.avsg.2015.05.026; published online EpubJul 16.
25. Amsterdam EA, Wenger NK, Brindis RG, Casey Jr DE, Ganiats TG, Holmes Jr DR, Jaffe AS, Jneid H, Kelly RF, Kontos MC, Levine GN, Liebson PR, Mukherjee D, Peterson ED, Sabatine MS, Smalling RW, Zieman SJ, American College of Cardiology, American Heart Association Task Force on Practice Guidelines, Society for Cardiovascular Angiography, Interventions, Society of Thoracic Surgeons, American Association for Clinical Chemistry. 2014 AHA/ACC guideline for the management of patients with non-ST-elevation acute coronary syndromes: a report of the American College of Cardiology/American Heart Association Task Force on Practice Guidelines. J Am Coll Cardiol. 2014;64:e139–228. doi:10.1016/j.jacc.2014.09.017; published online EpubDec 23.
26. Bertges DJ, Goodney PP, Zhao Y, Schanzer A, Nolan BW, Likosky DS, Eldrup-Jorgensen J, Cronenwett JL, Vascular Study Group of New England. The Vascular Study Group of New England Cardiac Risk Index (VSG-CRI) predicts cardiac complications more accurately than the Revised Cardiac Risk Index in vascular surgery patients. J Vasc Surg. 2010;52:674–683, 683.e671–683.e673. doi:10.1016/j.jvs.2010.03.031; published online EpubSep.
27. Kim GS, Ahn HJ, Kim WH, Kim MJ, Lee SH. Risk factors for postoperative complications after open infrarenal abdominal aortic aneurysm repair in Koreans. Yonsei Med J. 2011;52:339–46. doi:10.3349/ymj.2011.52.2.333; published online EpubMar.
28. Ali ZA, Callaghan CJ, Ali AA, Sheikh AY, Akhtar A, Pavlovic A, Nouraei SA, Dutka DP, Gaunt ME. Perioperative myocardial injury after elective open abdominal aortic aneurysm repair predicts outcome. Eur J Vasc Endovasc Surg Off J Eur Soc Vasc Surg. 2008;35:413–9. doi:10.1016/j.ejvs.2007.10.007; published online EpubApr.
29. Qin C, Chen L, Xiao YB. Emergent endovascular vs. open surgery repair for ruptured abdominal aortic aneurysms: a meta-analysis. PLoS One. 2014;9:e87465. doi:10.1371/journal.pone.0087465).
30. Noorani A, Walsh SR, Tang TY, Sadat U, Cooper DG, Callaghan CJ, Varty K, Gaunt ME. Atrial fibrillation following elective open abdominal aortic aneurysm repair. Int J Surg. 2009;7:24–7. doi:10.1016/j.ijsu.2008.09.002; published online EpubFeb.
31. Gu WJ, Wang F, Liu JC. Effect of lung-protective ventilation with lower tidal volumes on clinical outcomes among patients undergoing surgery: a meta-analysis of randomized

controlled trials. CMAJ Can Med Assoc J J Assoc Med Can. 2015;187:E101–9. doi:10.1503/cmaj.141005; published online EpubFeb 17.
32. Oba Y, Salzman GA. Ventilation with lower tidal volumes as compared with traditional tidal volumes for acute lung injury. N Engl J Med. 2000;343:813; author reply 813–4; published online EpubSep 14.
33. McCurdy BR. Noninvasive positive pressure ventilation for acute respiratory failure patients with chronic obstructive pulmonary disease (COPD): an evidence-based analysis. Ont Health Technol Assess Ser. 2012;12:1–102.
34. Rubenstein C, Bietz G, Davenport DL, Winkler M, Endean ED. Abdominal compartment syndrome associated with endovascular and open repair of ruptured abdominal aortic aneurysms. J Vasc Surg. 2015;61:648–54. doi:10.1016/j.jvs.2014.10.011; published online EpubMar.
35. Karkos CD, Menexes GC, Patelis N, Kalogirou TE, Giagtzidis IT, Harkin DW. A systematic review and meta-analysis of abdominal compartment syndrome after endovascular repair of ruptured abdominal aortic aneurysms. J Vasc Surg. 2014;59:829–42. doi:10.1016/j.jvs.2013.11.085; published online EpubMar.
36. Mehta M, Darling 3rd RC, Roddy SP, Fecteau S, Ozsvath KJ, Kreienberg PB, Paty PS, Chang BB, Shah DM. Factors associated with abdominal compartment syndrome complicating endovascular repair of ruptured abdominal aortic aneurysms. J Vasc Surg. 2005;42:1047–51. doi:10.1016/j.jvs.2005.08.033; published online EpubDec.
37. Mayer D, Rancic Z, Veith FJ, Pecoraro F, Pfammatter T, Lachat M. How to diagnose and treat abdominal compartment syndrome after endovascular and open repair of ruptured abdominal aortic aneurysms. J Cardiovasc Surg (Torino). 2014;55:179–92; published online EpubApr.
38. Cheatham ML, Malbrain ML, Kirkpatrick A, Sugrue M, Parr M, De Waele J, Balogh Z, Leppaniemi A, Olvera C, Ivatury R, D'Amours S, Wendon J, Hillman K, Wilmer A. Results from the international conference of experts on intra-abdominal hypertension and abdominal compartment syndrome. II. Recommendations. Intensive Care Med. 2007;33:951–62. doi:10.1007/s00134-007-0592-4; published online EpubJun.
39. Malbrain ML, Cheatham ML, Kirkpatrick A, Sugrue M, Parr M, De Waele J, Balogh Z, Leppaniemi A, Olvera C, Ivatury R, D'Amours S, Wendon J, Hillman K, Johansson K, Kolkman K, Wilmer A. Results from the international conference of experts on intra-abdominal hypertension and abdominal compartment syndrome. I. Definitions. Intensive Care Med. 2006;32:1722–32. doi:10.1007/s00134-006-0349-5; published online EpubNov.
40. Choi JY, Burton P, Walker S, Ghane-Asle S. Abdominal compartment syndrome after ruptured abdominal aortic aneurysm. ANZ J Surg. 2008;78:648–53. doi:10.1111/j.1445-2197.2008.04466.x; published online EpubAug.
41. Bozeman MC, Ross CB. Intra-abdominal hypertension and abdominal compartment syndrome in association with ruptured abdominal aortic aneurysm in the endovascular era: vigilance remains critical. Crit Care Res Pract. 2012;2012:151650. doi:10.1155/2012/151650.
42. Horer T, Skoog P, Pirouzram A, Larzon T. Tissue plasminogen activator-assisted hematoma evacuation to relieve abdominal compartment syndrome after endovascular repair of ruptured abdominal aortic aneurysm. J Endovasc Ther Off J Int Soc Endovasc Spec. 2012;19:144–8. doi:10.1583/11-3699.1; published online EpubApr.
43. Ellenberger C, Schweizer A, Diaper J, Kalangos A, Murith N, Katchatourian G, Panos A, Licker M. Incidence, risk factors and prognosis of changes in serum creatinine early after aortic abdominal surgery. Intensive Care Med. 2006;32:1808–16. doi:10.1007/s00134-006-0308-1; published online EpubNov.
44. Tallgren M, Niemi T, Poyhia R, Raininko E, Railo M, Salmenpera M, Lepantalo M, Hynninen M. Acute renal injury and dysfunction following elective abdominal aortic surgery. Eur J Vasc Endovasc Surg Off J Eur Soc Vasc Surg. 2007;33:550–5. doi:10.1016/j.ejvs.2006.12.005; published online EpubMay.
45. West CA, Noel AA, Bower TC, Cherry Jr KJ, Gloviczki P, Sullivan TM, Kalra M, Hoskin TL, Harrington JR. Factors affecting outcomes of open surgical repair of pararenal aortic aneurysms: a 10-year experience. J Vasc Surg. 2006;43:921–7. doi:10.1016/j.jvs.2006.01.018; discussion 927–8; published online EpubMay.

46. Kopolovic I, Simmonds K, Duggan S, Ewanchuk M, Stollery DE, Bagshaw SM. Risk factors and outcomes associated with acute kidney injury following ruptured abdominal aortic aneurysm. BMC Nephrol. 2013;14:99. doi:10.1186/1471-2369-14-99).
47. Macedo E, Castro I, Yu L, Abdulkader RR, Vieira Jr JM. Impact of mild acute kidney injury (AKI) on outcome after open repair of aortic aneurysms. Ren Fail. 2008;30:287–96. doi:10.1080/08860220701857522).
48. Grant SW, Grayson AD, Grant MJ, Purkayastha D, McCollum CN. What are the risk factors for renal failure following open elective abdominal aortic aneurysm repair? Eur J Vasc Endovasc Surg Off J Eur Soc Vasc Surg. 2012;43:182–7. doi:10.1016/j.ejvs.2011.11.018; published online EpubFeb.
49. Taylor PR, Reidy J, Scoble JE. Endovascular abdominal aortic aneurysm repair and renal function. Nephrol Dial Transplant Off Publ Eur Dial Transplant Assoc Eur Ren Assoc. 2006;21:2362–5. doi:10.1093/ndt/gfl264; published online EpubSep.
50. Kopolovic I, Simmonds K, Duggan S, et al. Risk factors and outcomes associated with acute kidney injury following ruptured abdominal aortic aneurysm. BMC Nephrol. 2013;14:99.
51. Saric M, Kronzon I. Cholesterol embolization syndrome. Curr Opin Cardiol. 2011;26:472–9. doi:10.1097/HCO.0b013e32834b7fdd; published online EpubNov.
52. Wang L, Xin SJ, Liu K, Zhang J, Hu HD, Yang D, Li GX, Duan ZQ. Critical limb ischemia during perioperative period of open surgery for rupture abdominal aortic aneurysm: treatment and prognosis. Zhonghua Yi Xue Za Zhi. 2013;93:653–5; published online EpubMar 5.
53. Nuzzo RM. Dry ice freezing as a prelude to surgical amputation. Orthopedics. 1982;5:169–75. doi:10.3928/0147-7447-19820201-05; published online EpubFeb 1.
54. Still Jr JM, Wray CH, Moretz WH. Selective physiologic amputation: a valuable adjunct in preparation for surgical operation. Ann Surg. 1970;171:143–51; published online EpubJan.
55. Gibbel MI, Atkins RA, Burns A. The use of dry ice refrigeration when delaying an inevitable amputation. Am J Surg. 1960;99:326–9; published online EpubMar.
56. Bariteau JT, Beutel BG, Kamal R, Hayda R, Born C. The use of near-infrared spectrometry for the diagnosis of lower-extremity compartment syndrome. Orthopedics. 2011;34:178. doi:10.3928/01477447-20110124-12; published online EpubMar.
57. Gentilello LM, Sanzone A, Wang L, Liu PY, Robinson L. Near-infrared spectroscopy versus compartment pressure for the diagnosis of lower extremity compartmental syndrome using electromyography-determined measurements of neuromuscular function. J Trauma. 2001;51:1–8; discussion 8–9; published online EpubJul.
58. Giannotti G, Cohn SM, Brown M, Varela JE, McKenney MG, Wiseberg JA. Utility of near-infrared spectroscopy in the diagnosis of lower extremity compartment syndrome. J Trauma. 2000;48:396–9; discussion 399–401; published online EpubMar.
59. Parikshak M, Shepard AD, Reddy DJ, Nypaver TJ. Adrenal insufficiency in patients with ruptured abdominal aortic aneurysms. J Vasc Surg. 2004;39:944–50. doi:10.1016/j.jvs.2004.01.020; published online EpubMay.
60. Mohammad Z, Afessa B, Finkielman JD. The incidence of relative adrenal insufficiency in patients with septic shock after the administration of etomidate. Crit Care. 2006;10:R105. doi:10.1186/cc4979.
61. Chan CM, Mitchell AL, Shorr AF. Etomidate is associated with mortality and adrenal insufficiency in sepsis: a meta-analysis*. Crit Care Med. 2012;40:2945–53. doi:10.1097/CCM.0b013e31825fec26; published online EpubNov.
62. Cotton BA, Guillamondegui OD, Fleming SB, Carpenter RO, Patel SH, Morris Jr JA, Arbogast PG. Increased risk of adrenal insufficiency following etomidate exposure in critically injured patients. Arch Surg. 2008;143:62–7. doi:10.1001/archsurg.143.1.62; discussion 67; published online EpubJan.
63. Majesko A, Darby JM. Etomidate and adrenal insufficiency: the controversy continues. Crit Care. 2010;14:338. doi:10.1186/cc9338).
64. Mullins ME, Theodoro DL. Lack of evidence for adrenal insufficiency after single-dose etomidate. Arch Surg. 2008;143:808–9. doi:10.1001/archsurg.143.8.808-c; author reply 809; published online EpubAug.

65. Stein DM, Jessie EM, Crane S, Kufera JA, Timmons T, Rodriguez CJ, Menaker J, Scalea TM. Hyperacute adrenal insufficiency after hemorrhagic shock exists and is associated with pooroutcomes. J Trauma Acute Care Surg. 2013;74:363–70. doi:10.1097/TA.0b013e31827e2aaf; discussion 370; published online EpubFeb.
66. Maxime V, Lesur O, Annane D. Adrenal insufficiency in septic shock. Clin Chest Med. 2009;30:17–27, vii. doi:10.1016/j.ccm.2008.10.003; published online EpubMar.
67. Sprung CL, Annane D, Keh D, Moreno R, Singer M, Freivogel K, Weiss YG, Benbenishty J, Kalenka A, Forst H, Laterre PF, Reinhart K, Cuthbertson BH, Payen D, Briegel J, Group CS. Hydrocortisone therapy for patients with septic shock. N Engl J Med. 2008;358:111–24. doi:10.1056/NEJMoa071366; published online EpubJan 10.
68. Beigel J, Eichacker P. Hydrocortisone and fludrocortisone improved 28-day survival in septic shock and adrenal insufficiency. ACP J Club. 2003;138:44; published online EpubMar-Apr.
69. Spurzem JR. On the diagnosis of adrenal insufficiency in severe sepsis and septic shock. Am J Respir Crit Care Med. 2007;175:1095. doi:10.1164/ajrccm.175.10.1095; author reply 1095; published online EpubMay 15.
70. Miller J. Surviving sepsis: a review of the latest guidelines. Nursing. 2014;44:24–30. doi:10.1097/01.NURSE.0000444530.66327.de; quiz 30–21; published online EpubApr.
71. Vassalos A, Rooney K. Surviving sepsis guidelines 2012. Crit Care Med. 2013;41:e485–6. doi:10.1097/CCM.0b013e31829644e8; published online EpubDec.
72. Assadian A, Senekowitsch C, Assadian O, Hartleb H, Hagmuller GW. Diagnostic accuracy of sigmoidoscopy compared with histology for ischemic colitis after aortic aneurysm repair. Vascular. 2008;16:243–7; published online EpubSep-Oct.
73. Hagihara PF, Ernst CB, Griffen Jr WO. Incidence of ischemic colitis following abdominal aortic reconstruction. Surg Gynecol Obstet. 1979;149:571–3; published online EpubOct.
74. Forde KA, Lebwohl O, Wolff M, Voorhees AB. The endoscopy corner: reversible ischemic colitis – correlation of colonoscopic and pathologic changes. Am J Gastroenterol. 1979;72:182–5; published online EpubAug.
75. Geraghty PJ, Sanchez LA, Rubin BG, Choi ET, Flye MW, Curci JA, Thompson RW, Sicard GA. Overt ischemic colitis after endovascular repair of aortoiliac aneurysms. J Vasc Surg. 2004;40:413–8. doi:10.1016/j.jvs.2004.05.022; published online EpubSep.
76. Miller A, Marotta M, Scordi-Bello I, Tammaro Y, Marin M, Divino C. Ischemic colitis after endovascular aortoiliac aneurysm repair: a 10-year retrospective study. Arch Surg. 2009;144:900–3. doi:10.1001/archsurg.2009.70; published online EpubOct.
77. Bjorck M. Intestinal ischaemia after aortoiliac surgery – a case-control study within the Swedvasc registry. Eur J Surg Suppl Acta Chir Suppl. 1998;(581):37–9.
78. Bjorck M, Bergqvist D, Troeng T. Incidence and clinical presentation of bowel ischaemia after aortoiliac surgery – 2930 operations from a population-based registry in Sweden. Eur J Vasc Endovasc Surg Off J Eur Soc Vasc Surg. 1996;12:139–44; published online EpubAug.
79. Barr J, Fraser GL, Puntillo K, Ely EW, Gelinas C, Dasta JF, Davidson JE, Devlin JW, Kress JP, Joffe AM, Coursin DB, Herr DL, Tung A, Robinson BR, Fontaine DK, Ramsay MA, Riker RR, Sessler CN, Pun B, Skrobik Y, Jaeschke R, American M. College of Critical Care, Clinical practice guidelines for the management of pain, agitation, and delirium in adult patients in the intensive care unit. Crit Care Med. 2013;41:263–306. doi:10.1097/CCM.0b013e3182783b72; published online EpubJan.
80. Imani F, Faiz HR, Sedaghat M, Hajiashrafi M. Effects of adding ketamine to fentanyl plus acetaminophen on postoperative pain by patient controlled analgesia in abdominal surgery. Anesthesiol Pain Med. 2014;4:e12162. doi:10.5812/aapm.12162; published online EpubFeb.
81. Unlugenc H, Gunduz M, Ozalevli M, Akman H. A comparative study on the analgesic effect of tramadol, tramadol plus magnesium, and tramadol plus ketamine for postoperative pain management after major abdominal surgery. Acta Anaesthesiol Scand. 2002;46:1025–30; published online EpubSep.
82. Dawson R, von Fintel N, Nairn S. Sedation assessment using the Ramsay scale. Emerg Nurs J RCN Accid Emerg Nurs Assoc. 2010;18:18–20. doi:10.7748/en2010.06.18.3.18.c7825; published online EpubJun.

83. Mendes CL, Vasconcelos LC, Tavares JS, Fontan SB, Ferreira DC, Diniz LA, Alves ES, Villar EJ, Albuquerque CD, Silva SL. Ramsay and Richmond's scores are equivalent to assessment sedation level on critical patients. Rev Bras Ter Intensiva. 2008;20:344–8; published online EpubDec.
84. Mason KP, Michna E, Zurakowski D, Burrows PE, Pirich MA, Carrier M, Fontaine PJ, Sethna NF. Value of bispectral index monitor in differentiating between moderate and deep Ramsay Sedation Scores in children. Paediatr Anaesth. 2006;16:1226–31. doi:10.1111/j.1460-9592.2006.01975.x; published online EpubDec.
85. Mondello E, Siliotti R, Noto G, Cuzzocrea E, Scollo G, Trimarchi G, Venuti FS. Bispectral index in ICU: correlation with Ramsay score on assessment of sedation level. J Clin Monit Comput. 2002;17:271–7; published online EpubJul.
86. Papaioannou V, Dragoumanis C, Theodorou V, Pneumatikos I. The propofol infusion 'syndrome' in intensive care unit: from pathophysiology to prophylaxis and treatment. Acta Anaesthesiol Belg. 2008;59:79–86.
87. MacLaren R, Preslaski CR, Mueller SW, Kiser TH, Fish DN, Lavelle JC, Malkoski SP. A randomized, double-blind pilot study of dexmedetomidine versus midazolam for intensive care unit sedation: patient recall of their experiences and short-term psychological outcomes. J Intensive Care Med. 2015;30:167–75. doi:10.1177/0885066613510874; published online EpubMar.
88. Reardon DP, Anger KE, Adams CD, Szumita PM. Role of dexmedetomidine in adults in the intensive care unit: an update. Am J Health Syst Pharm AJHP Off J Am Soc Health Syst Pharm. 2013;70:767–77. doi:10.2146/ajhp120211; published online EpubMay 1.
89. Szumita PM, Baroletti SA, Anger KE, Wechsler ME. Sedation and analgesia in the intensive care unit: evaluating the role of dexmedetomidine. Am J health Syst Pharm AJHP Off J Am Soc Health Syst Pharm. 2007;64:37–44. doi:10.2146/ajhp050508; published online EpubJan 1.
90. Jensen MB, Sloth E. Echocardiography for cardiopulmonary optimization in the intensive care unit: should we expand its use? Acta Anaesthesiol Scand. 2004;48:1069–70. doi:10.1111/j.1399-6576.2004.00465.x; published online EpubOct.
91. Force ADT, Ranieri VM, Rubenfeld GD, Thompson BT, Ferguson ND, Caldwell E, Fan E, Camporota L, Slutsky AS. Acute respiratory distress syndrome: the Berlin Definition. JAMA. 2012;307:2526–33. doi:10.1001/jama.2012.5669; published online EpubJun 20.
92. Ventilation with lower tidal volumes as compared with traditional tidal volumes for acute lung injury and the acute respiratory distress syndrome. The Acute Respiratory Distress Syndrome Network. N Engl J Med. 2000;342:1301–8. doi:10.1056/NEJM200005043421801, published online EpubMay 4.
93. Guerin C. Prone ventilation in acute respiratory distress syndrome. Eur Respir Rev Off J Eur Respir Soc. 2014;23:249–57. doi:10.1183/09059180.00001114; published online EpubJun.
94. Young D, Lamb SE, Shah S, MacKenzie I, Tunnicliffe W, Lall R, Rowan K, Cuthbertson BH, Group OS. High-frequency oscillation for acute respiratory distress syndrome. N Engl J Med. 2013;368:806–13. doi:10.1056/NEJMoa1215716; published online EpubFeb 28.
95. Brodie D, Bacchetta M. Extracorporeal membrane oxygenation for ARDS in adults. N Engl J Med. 2011;365:1905–14. doi:10.1056/NEJMct1103720; published online EpubNov 17.
96. Agerstrand CL, Bacchetta MD, Brodie D. ECMO for adult respiratory failure: current use and evolving applications. ASAIO J. 2014;60:255–62. doi:10.1097/MAT.0000000000000062; published online EpubMay–Jun.
97. Stoeppel CM, Eriksson EA, Diaz-Flores R, Coffie P, Koshy J, Kacir C, Hawkins K, Minei J, Minshall C. Guiding the management of intubated patients with pneumonia and ventilator-associated events using serial catheter-directed bronchoalveolar lavage. J Trauma Acare Surg. 2014;76:1264–9. doi:10.1097/TA.0000000000000219; published online EpubMay.
98. Chastre J, Wolff M, Fagon JY, Chevret S, Thomas F, Wermert D, Clementi E, Gonzalez J, Jusserand D, Asfar P, Perrin D, Fieux F, Aubas S, Pneum ATG. Comparison of 8 vs 15 days of antibiotic therapy for ventilator-associated pneumonia in adults: a randomized trial. JAMA. 2003;290:2588–98. doi:10.1001/jama.290.19.2588; published online EpubNov 19.

99. Bonten MJ, Weinstein RA. Infection control in intensive care units and prevention of ventilator-associated pneumonia. Semin Respir Infect. 2000;15:327–35; published online EpubDec.
100. Chastre J. Ventilator-associated pneumonia: what is new? Surg Infect (Larchmt). 2006;7 Suppl 2:S81–5. doi:10.1089/sur.2006.7.s2-81).
101. Rotstein C, Evans G, Born A, Grossman R, Light RB, Magder S, McTaggart B, Weiss K, Zhanel GG. Clinical practice guidelines for hospital-acquired pneumonia and ventilator-associated pneumonia in adults. Can J Infect Dis Med Microbiol J Can Mal Infect Microbiol Med AMMI Can. 2008;19:19–53; published online EpubJan.
102. Dhaliwal R, Cahill N, Lemieux M, Heyland DK. The Canadian critical care nutrition guidelines in 2013: an update on current recommendations and implementation strategies. Nutr Clin Pract Off Publ Am Soc Parenter Enteral Nutr. 2014;29:29–43. doi:10.1177/0884533613510948; published online EpubFeb.
103. Heyland DK, Dhaliwal R, Day A, Jain M, Drover J. Validation of the Canadian clinical practice guidelines for nutrition support in mechanically ventilated, critically ill adult patients: results of a prospective observational study. Crit Care Med. 2004;32:2260–6; published online EpubNov.
104. McClave SA, Martindale RG, Vanek VW, McCarthy M, Roberts P, Taylor B, Ochoa JB, Napolitano L, Cresci G, A. S. P. E. N. Board of Directors, American College of Critical Care, M. Society of Critical Care Medicine. Guidelines for the provision and assessment of nutrition support therapy in the adult critically Ill patient: Society of Critical Care Medicine (SCCM) and American Society for Parenteral and Enteral Nutrition (A.S.P.E.N.). JPEN J Parenter Enteral Nutr. 2009;33:277–316. doi:10.1177/0148607109335234; published online EpubMay-Jun.
105. Cahill NE, Dhaliwal R, Heyland DK. Response to "The Canadian Critical Care Nutrition Guidelines in 2013: importance of nasojejunal enteral feeding tube design in improving rates of small bowel enteral feeding in patients with high gastric residual volumes". Nutr Clin Pract Off Publ Am Soc Parenter Enteral Nutr. 2014;29:561. doi:10.1177/0884533614538287; published online EpubJul 16.
106. Silk DB. The Canadian Critical Care Nutrition guidelines in 2013: importance of nasojejunal enteral feeding tube design in improving rates of small bowel enteral feeding in patients with high gastric residual volumes. Nutr Clin Pract Off Publ Am Soc Parenter Enteral Nutr. 2014;29:559–60. doi:10.1177/0884533614538286; published online EpubJul 16.
107. Casaer MP, Van den Berghe G. Nutrition in the acute phase of critical illness. N Engl J Med. 2014;370:2450–1. doi:10.1056/NEJMc1404896; published online EpubJun 19.
108. Economidou F, Douka E, Tzanela M, Nanas S, Kotanidou A. Thyroid function during critical illness. Hormones. 2011;10:117–24; published online EpubApr–Jun.
109. van den Berghe G, Wouters P, Weekers F, Verwaest C, Bruyninckx F, Schetz M, Vlasselaers D, Ferdinande P, Lauwers P, Bouillon R. Intensive insulin therapy in critically ill patients. N Engl J Med. 2001;345:1359–67. doi:10.1056/NEJMoa011300; published online EpubNov 8.
110. NICE-SUGAR Study Investigators for the Australian Group, New Zealand Intensive Care Society Clinical Trials Group, the Canadian Critical Care Trials Group. Intensive versus conventional glucose control in critically ill patients with traumatic brain injury: long-term follow-up of a subgroup of patients from the NICE-SUGAR study. Intensive Care Med. 2015;41:1037–47. doi:10.1007/s00134-015-3757-6; published online EpubJun.
111. Guyatt GH, Akl EA, Crowther M, Gutterman DD, Schuunemann HJ, American College of Chest Physicians Antithrombotic Therapy, Prevention of Thrombosis Panel. Executive summary: antithrombotic therapy and prevention of thrombosis, 9th ed: American College of Chest Physicians evidence-based clinical practice guidelines. Chest. 2012;141:7S–47. doi:10.1378/chest.1412S3; published online EpubFeb.
112. Mohebbi L, Hesch K. Stress ulcer prophylaxis in the intensive care unit. Proceedings (Bayl Univ Med Cent). 2009;22:373–6; published online EpubOct.

Chapter 16
Postoperative Complications

Kevin Kniery, Scott R. Steele, Martin Björck, Anders Wanhainen, Anthony M. Roche, Hernando Olivar, Koichiro Nandate, Shahram Aarabi, Surbhi Mathur, Joseph Cuschieri, Khanjan H. Nagarsheth, and Saum A. Rahimi

K. Kniery, MD
Department of Surgery, Division of Colorectal Surgery,
Madigan Army Medical Center, Tacoma/Fort Lewis, WA, USA

S.R. Steele, MD (✉)
Vice Chairman for Clinical Affairs, Department of Surgery, Chief,
Division of Colorectal Surgery,
University Hospitals Case Medical Center,
11100 Euclid Avenue, Cleveland,
OH 44106, USA

Professor of Surgery, Case Western Reserve University,
11100 Euclid Avenue, Cleveland, OH 44106, USA
e-mail: scott.steele@UHhospitals.org, harkersteele@mac.com

M. Björck (✉) • A. Wanhainen
Department of Surgical Sciences, Section of Vascular Surgery,
Uppsala University, Uppsala, Sweden
e-mail: martin@bjorck.pp.se

A.M. Roche • H. Olivar • K. Nandate
Department of Anesthesiology and Pain Medicine,
University of Washington, Seattle, WA, USA

S. Aarabi, MD
Fellow Division of Vascular Surgery, Department of Surgery,
University of Washington, Seattle, WA, USA

S. Mathur, MD • J. Cuschieri
Department of Surgery, University of Washington,
Seattle, WA, USA

K.H. Nagarsheth, MD, MBA • S.A. Rahimi, MD, FACS
Division of Vascular Surgery, Rutgers – Robert Wood Johnson Medical School,
New Brunswick, NJ, USA

B.W. Starnes et al. (eds.), *Ruptured Abdominal Aortic Aneurysm*,
DOI 10.1007/978-3-319-23844-9_16

Key Points

- Endovascular repair has dramatically decreased the incidence of ischemic colitis following elective and even ruptured abdominal aortic aneurysm repair.
- Ischemic colitis remains a wide-ranging disease process with variable presentation and severity.
- The key to good outcomes remains a high index of suspicion, early diagnosis, and initial supportive care (NPO, intravenous fluids, intravenous antibiotics).
- Surgery is reserved for those patients with perforation, gangrene, sepsis, (chronically) smoldering disease, and/or stricture.

Ischemic Colitis After Ruptured Abdominal Aortic Aneurysm Repair

Kevin Kniery and Scott R. Steele

Introduction

Ischemic colitis is one of the most feared complications following an abdominal aortic aneurysm (AAA) repair. At a very basic level, it occurs when blood flow to the colon is interrupted or diminished and supply does not equal colonic demand (Fig. 16.1). Although Shaw and Green [1] were the first to report a case of ischemic colitis in 1953 following ligation of the inferior mesenteric artery during an abdominal aortic aneurysm repair, alterations to the colon secondary to a lack of adequate blood supply have been recognized for over a century. The evolution in understanding this disease process continued over the next few decades, with Boley in 1963 [2] being first to report that colonic ischemia was a reversible process secondary to

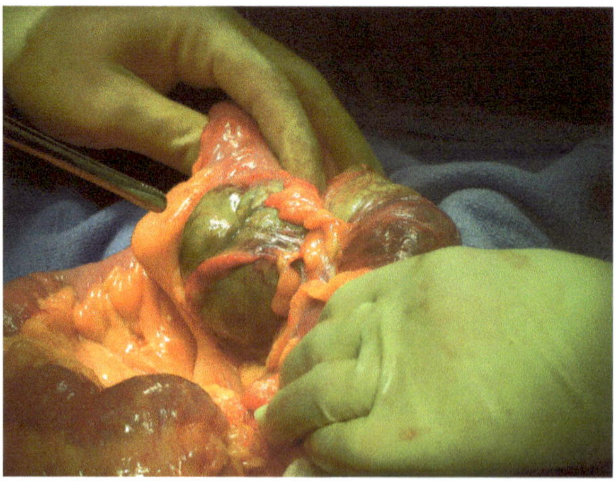

Fig. 16.1 Intraoperative photo demonstrating full-thickness serosal changes in ischemic colitis

vascular occlusion and Marston and associates coining the term "ischemic colitis" 3 years later after depicting its three stages of evolution (transient ischemia, late ischemic stricture, and gangrene) along with the natural history of the disease [3].

The causes of ischemic colitis are numerous, though the exact etiology of the initial insult is often difficult to pinpoint—especially in elderly, debilitated patients with multiple contributing comorbidities. In addition, the differential diagnosis remains vast, with inflammatory and infectious colitis heading the list and often with similar presentations. Regardless of its etiology, patient outcome depends markedly on the severity and extent of the ischemic insult and is largely influenced by the clinician's ability to make a prompt diagnosis and initiate appropriate management.

Historically, ischemic colitis following vascular surgery was associated with mortality rates approaching 45–67 % [4]. Unfortunately, even more recent reports have demonstrated only modest improvements. Currently, ischemic colitis is the most common form of gastrointestinal ischemia, accounting for 50–60 % of all cases, translating to ~1 in 2000 hospital admissions [5]. The incidence of colonic ischemia specifically following repair of a ruptured AAA (rAAA) is 4–5 times higher than an elective repair, increasing from ~1–6 % to ~17–35 % [6]. Not surprisingly, the outcomes are significantly worse in patients that have a delayed diagnosis or present with a more advanced state of ischemic colitis, such as those patients with a concomitant perforation. In these cases, mortality rates have been reported to be >90 % [7]. In one retrospective study of 222 patients after a rAAA repair, ischemic colitis was the most common cause of death, even above multi-organ system failure and myocardial infarction [8]. It is easy to then understand why early diagnosis is of chief importance. Unfortunately, clinical parameters to identify patients with colonic ischemia lack specificity, which is even more limited in the rAAA population. In this chapter, we will review the pathophysiology, risk factors, diagnostics, and treatment options for patients who suffer ischemic colitis after a rAAA.

Pathophysiology

Regardless of the underlying etiology, the pathophysiology of ischemic colitis revolves around an inadequate blood supply to the colon. In patients suffering from a rAAA, there are numerous potential etiologies of this decreased blood flow including perioperative hemorrhage resulting in a loss of overall blood volume, prolonged hypotension, splanchnic vasoconstriction due to shock and vasopressors, and cross clamping or balloon occlusion of the aorta. The surgical repair itself, for both the open and endovascular (EVAR) approaches, occludes blood flow (at least temporarily) through the inferior mesenteric artery (IMA), which directly supplies the left colon. In addition, embolization of debris (thrombus and plaque) may occur from opening the aneurysmal sac or manipulation of the graft and wires inside the sac. These embolic phenomena can cause a less predictable variation of ischemic colitis, with numerous reports of right-sided colonic and even small bowel ischemia [9].

However, there is an intrinsic protective mechanism already in place. Although the colon derives its blood supply from branches of the major vessels [i.e., superior mesenteric artery (SMA) and inferior mesenteric artery (IMA)], it is the extensive collateral circulation that allows this ischemic process to be avoided in many cases. The two main collateral routes are via the marginal artery of Drummond that parallels the colon and gives rise to the vasa recta, and the meandering mesenteric artery (or arc of Riolan) which, while not always present, can represent another potential connection between the SMA and IMA systems. In addition, the IMA and internal iliac arteries communicate via the superior and middle hemorrhoidal arteries, while the left colic branch of the IMA contributes to overlap of the transverse colon that is supplied mostly by branches of the SMA. In an otherwise healthy patient, the vast vascular network would prevent any significant degree of colonic ischemia after ligation of the IMA. Yet, patients who suffer a rAAA generally have severe vascular comorbidities and are often in physiologic extremis, which explains why there is such a higher rate of colonic ischemia despite this collateral circulation. Certain parts of the colon are more prone to fluctuations in blood flow, leading to the all-too-common "rounds" question with answers consisting of the splenic flexure (i.e., Sudeck's) and rectosigmoid junction (i.e., Griffiths). It is felt that these are the most vulnerable segments given that there is incomplete anastomosis of the marginal artery in these two locations. The next most common area affected is the cecum, likely secondary to low blood flow in the terminal branches of the ileocolic artery combined with varying presence and competency of the right colic artery [10–12].

Ischemic colitis is not an all or nothing process. The earliest manifestations are witnessed at the mucosal level, those furthest away from the vasa recta [10, 13] (Fig. 16.2). As such, there is a progression in the stages of ischemic colitis: (a) Grade I, transient mucosal ischemia; (b) Grade II, mucosal and muscularis involvement that may result in healing with fibrosis and stricture formation; and (c) Grade III, transmural ischemia and infarction which results in gangrene and perforation [14] (Fig. 16.3). Importantly, sepsis can occur in the absence of transmural ischemia, as an ischemic mucosa loses its barrier function and allows bacterial translocation to occur, which may result in sepsis.

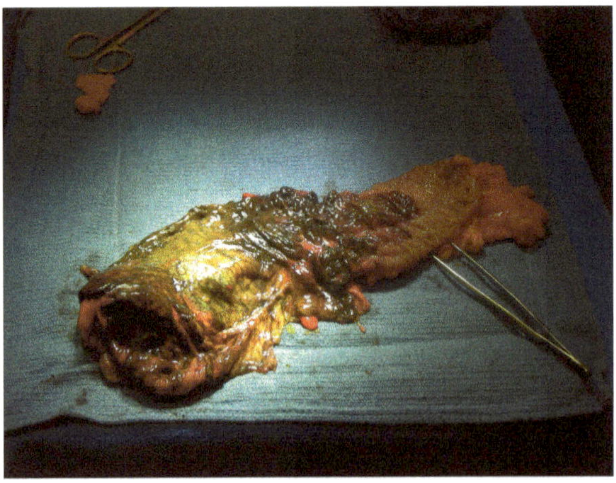

Fig. 16.2 Mucosal changes with ischemic colitis

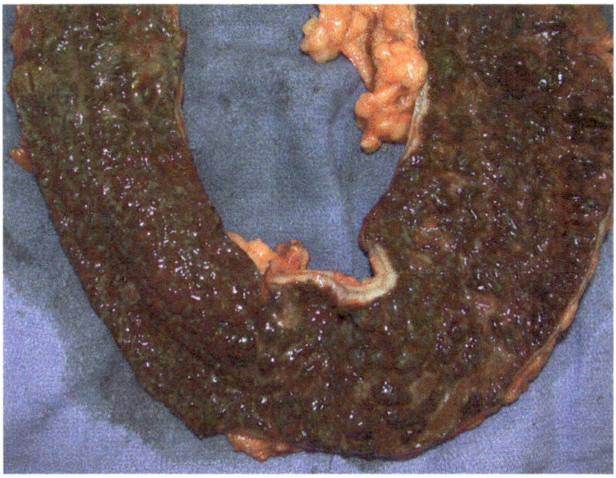

Fig. 16.3 Full-thickness changes with gangrenous ischemic colitis

Risk Factors for the Development of Ischemic Colitis

There are certain risk factors that clearly put a patient with an AAA at higher risk of suffering ischemic colitis. The greatest risk factor is the focus of this chapter; a patient with a rAAA has a two- to fourfold increased risk for ischemic colitis. Interestingly, those underdoing surgery with a symptomatic aneurysm (even in the absence of rupture) have higher rates of ischemic colitis than elective repair based on size criteria alone in the absence of symptoms. Other independent risk factors for colonic ischemia include renal insufficiency, open versus endovascular repair, operative time >4 h, prolonged cross clamp, preoperative hypotension, aorto-bifemoral graft placement, and postoperative acidosis [15, 16].

Many of these make intuitive sense. Others have second- or third-order ramifications that promote the onset of ischemic colitis. For example, renal insufficiency itself results in a decreased ability to handle changes in volume, clear toxins, and recovery from any physiological insult. Yet, in addition, it is thought to be a marker of systemic atherosclerotic disease, which would be reflected in the mesenteric vessels that directly supply the colon, therefore decreasing the colon's tolerance to hypotension. Worsening of renal insufficiency following repair may also represent a reflection of the severity of hypotension the patient endured perioperatively.

While the exact operative time that correlates with the onset of ischemic colitis is likely more variable, when the length of surgery is over 4 h, studies have shown a four- to sixfold increase in incidence [16]. This is likely related both to the technical difficulty of the surgery and associated hypotension and blood requirement needed during the operation. Open repair is another independent risk factor for colonic ischemia, as demonstrated in one large national database review that showed that open elective AAA repair had a rate of 2.2 % versus 0.5 % with elective EVAR repair [4]. A small randomized trial comparing open and endovascular repair in patients with rAAA found half the rate of colonic ischemia (8 % vs. 4 %) when using EVAR, but it was underpowered to reach significance [17]. However, it is remarkable to witness the drastic drop in onset with the use of endovascular approaches, even in the setting of rupture.

Some surgeons have recommended reimplanting the IMA to allow restoration of direct "forward flow" from the aorta to the left colon. While controversial, IMA reimplantation with an open repair has multiple studies, including a randomized controlled trial, that have failed to show a decreased rate of colonic ischemia with IMA reimplantation when compared with ligation of the IMA and maintenance of normothermia and normal blood pressures. On the other hand, common vascular surgery dogma is to do whatever possible to prevent pelvic ischemia because once it occurs, it is likely not reversible and is associated with high morbidity rates [18]. With this in mind, many surgeons will reimplant based on intraoperative findings such as poor backflow from the IMA (<40 mmHg) or decreased antimesenteric vasculature Doppler signals [16, 19]. An additional tool used in the past was laser Doppler flowmetry, which measures the erythrocyte flux to bowel segments and has been specifically shown to be a successful tool to determine the necessity of reimplanting the IMA [20]. More recent advances, such as the intraoperative availability of indocyanine green [21, 22] that can demonstrate real-time perfusion, may soon find its way into this intraoperative algorithm for evaluating colonic ischemia—even though it still not applicable to EVAR cases. Other more traditional operative tools such as Doppler or Wood's lamp with fluorescent dyes can only be used in open surgery to help determine bowel viability. In contrast, there is a device available that can be used in open and endovascular aneurysm repairs that utilizes a probe placed in the rectum and measures tissue oxygen saturation. It has been shown to be sensitive in predicting colonic ischemia if the saturation drops below fifty percent of baseline. This tool can provide objective evidence to allow the opportunity to revascularize the IMA or the hypogastrics [23]. While promising, the current data is limited, and ultimately only longer-term data with a wider experience will determine its role in the evaluation and treatment of ischemic colitis.

The importance of hypogastric preservation also appears to be predicated highly on the method of repair—endovascular versus open. In open surgery, there are higher rates of colonic ischemia when hypogastric aneurysms are present or if both hypogastrics are ligated [24]. With endovascular repair, there is literature that states there are only minimal complications associated with embolization of the hypogastrics [25–27] and other series reporting increased risk of colonic ischemia if they are not preserved [28, 29]. In the setting of rAAA, there is only anecdotal evidence when discussing preserving hypogastrics, but given the extremis that patients are often in, it is likely prudent to preserve any potential collaterals to the colon, if possible. Yet, the surgeon must take into account the stability of the patient and weigh any downside that may occur with the additional operative time that another procedure would require.

Additional risk factors for the development of ischemic colitis that have no randomized data, but have been reported in small retrospective studies, include previous colonic surgery and pelvic irradiation. This should also make sense, as patients who have had previous colonic surgery have likely had the collaterals between the SMA and IMA disrupted. While there was a substantial rate of colonic ischemia in this subset of patients, these reports have been largely underpowered [16]. Yet, even a patent meandering marginal artery (arc of Riolan) has been shown to have some protective effects against ischemic colitis [30].

Finally, pelvic irradiation leads to obliteration of the microvasculature to the sigmoid and rectum, creating conditions ripe for small vessel ischemic changes. Furthermore, these radiation effects are cumulative and progressive, a fact often overlooked. Although it has not been widely studied, this appears to be a real association with patients at a higher risk of developing ischemic colitis [31]. Furthermore, this may be a precipitating factor not only in early disease but helps to explain the underlying disorder that leads to chronic changes such as colonic stricture.

Diagnosis

The key to diagnosing ischemic colitis first and foremost involves a high degree of suspicion by the treating provider, especially given the drastic improvements in outcomes for patients that are recognized and treated promptly. Unfortunately, the signs and symptoms vary drastically and are remarkably inconsistent from patient to patient. Occasionally, ischemic colitis is recognized intraoperatively; however, that tends to be way too late. Despite a somewhat "textbook" presentation for more severe forms, the mean time to diagnosis remains ~5.5 days [14].

This delay is secondary to the wide-ranging spectrum of disease—from mild mucosal sloughing to severe (perforation and sepsis). In some cases, the majority of symptoms are often self-limited and nonspecific. The most common symptoms encountered are left lower quadrant pain, bloating, and diarrhea. The diarrhea is a consequence of mucosal sloughing which causes colonic peristalsis. Depending on the extent and severity of the ischemia, patients can present with melena, hematochezia, watery diarrhea, or even no diarrhea at all. The abdominal pain may be limited to the hypogastrium or left lower quadrant or in more severe cases present with frank peritonitis and diffuse pain. Similar to the symptomology, the imaging and laboratory studies are generally nonspecific. Plain films may show colonic dilatation and/or fluid levels. More advanced cases may have pneumatosis, portal venous gas, or pneumoperitoneum.

Historically, barium enemas were used, often showing mucosal edema suggested by thumbprinting or colonic strictures with more chronic disease. In general, barium should be avoided in this setting. Water-soluble enemas may demonstrate similar findings but are much less commonly used. The workhorse of radiology tests remains the CT scan. Although they are not initially as sensitive, later in the course, they can be more helpful showing colonic wall thickening and an inflamed edematous mesentery/fat stranding. CT also provides the ability to evaluate the bowel as well as the surrounding tissue. In this light, mucosal enhancement, intramural air, bowel dilatation, or even more ominous signs such as portal venous gas can be visualized. It can also be a very useful test in ruling out other diagnoses [32]. In general, angiography does not help in patients with acute ischemic changes and is rarely used for vessel patency (embolic/thrombotic) or to rule out other sources.

Laboratory examinations are similarly nonspecific for ischemic colitis, and no marker exists to date that is specific in identifying colonic ischemia. For more advanced cases, a leukocytosis and metabolic acidosis may be present. Occasionally, electrolyte and renal abnormalities (i.e., hypokalemia, rising BUN/Cr) may be present due to severe diarrhea combined with a lack of oral intake. Serum lactate levels may be elevated, though generalized systemic hypoperfusion or tissue hypoxia may also cause this, and is therefore not a specific marker. Unfortunately, many of these concerning lab values such as lactate, creatinine, acidosis, or leukocytosis are all commonly seen postoperatively after a rAAA. A small prospective study of 12 patients who underwent open AAA repair reported an elevated d-lactate (uncommon isomer of more common L-lactate) could be detected within 2 h postoperatively in patients with ischemic colitis compared to patients without ischemic colitis [13]. Yet, this has yet to achieve widespread clinical use.

Colonoscopy remains the most sensitive and specific study available for diagnosis of ischemic colitis (Fig. 16.4). Some suggest that any concern for colonic ischemia warrants an endoscopic evaluation and even argue routine endoscopy after rAAA using a flexible sigmoidoscopy should be performed within 24 h of the surgery. Endoscopy has a diagnostic accuracy of 78–98 % for ischemic colitis [33], in part due to the wide extent of changes and characteristics ischemia has when viewed endoscopically. In the acute phase, the bowel will demonstrate hyperemia, edema, friable mucosa, ulcerations, and petechial hemorrhages. As the ischemia progresses, evidence of submucosal edema and hemorrhage may appear as bluish-black blebs or nodules protruding into the lumen of the bowel [34]. When full-thickness transmural ischemia occurs, the mucosa typically appears gray or black, indicating gangrene. If the ischemia is more chronic, changes such as strictures and fibrosis would be endoscopy also allows the examiner to sample the colonic mucosa for pathologic assessment to help differentiate inflammatory, infectious (e.g., *C. difficile*), and ischemic etiologies. In reality, biopsy (Fig. 16.5) is rarely useful and is more likely to demonstrate either nonspecific ischemic or inflammatory changes

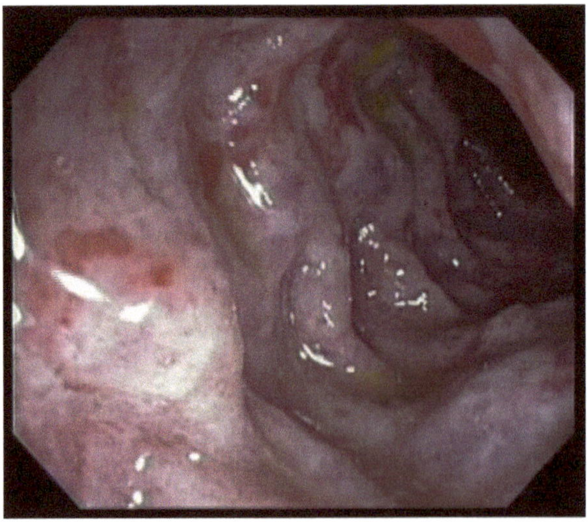

Fig. 16.4 Ischemic colitis seen on colonoscopy

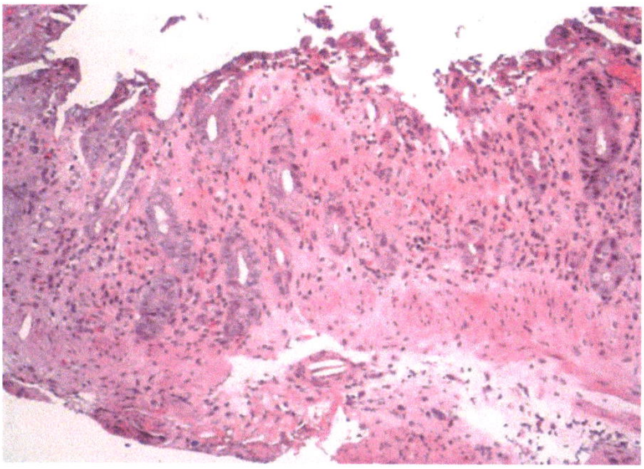

Fig. 16.5 Histology of ischemic colitis demonstrating sloughing of the mucosa and inflammatory cells

and rarely shows the ghost cells that are classic for ischemia [11]. It is important to recognize that endoscopy is not without its own potential hazards. Air insufflation may result in distention of the bowel, diminishing colonic blood flow and may actually worsen the colonic ischemia [9]. In addition, the ischemic wall of the colon is fragile and at an increased risk of perforation. Chronically, endoscopy will demonstrate a smooth stricture without an associated mass, consisted with the fibrotic process that occurs over time [35].

Endoscopic Surveillance Following rAAA

There have been two prospective studies that have evaluated the effectiveness of routine colonoscopic screening in all patients who survive after the initial repair of a rAAA (Figs. 16.6 and 16.7). The first study by Megalopoulas et al. [36] identified preoperative risk factors (hypotension, temperature, pH, > 6 units PRBCs, fluid sequestration >5 L) that correlated with the presence of ischemic colitis. The authors concluded that when less than four were present, they were unlikely to develop colonic ischemia and therefore did not need routine endoscopic screening. One criticism of this study was that it is difficult to extrapolate to outside hospitals, as many of the parameters depend on the overall management of the patient apart from the use of endoscopy. To address this deficiency, Tottrup and colleagues prospectively screened 41 patients who survived a rAAA with colonoscopy in the first 24 h following surgery. Only nine of their patients developed colonic ischemia, and there were no perioperative or intraoperative clinical or biochemical parameters that were sufficiently reliable to distinguish patients with colonic ischemia versus those without [6]. Their conclusion was that the worse outcomes associated with a delayed diagnosis of colonic ischemia after rAAA warrant all patients to undergo routine endoscopic surveillance [37].

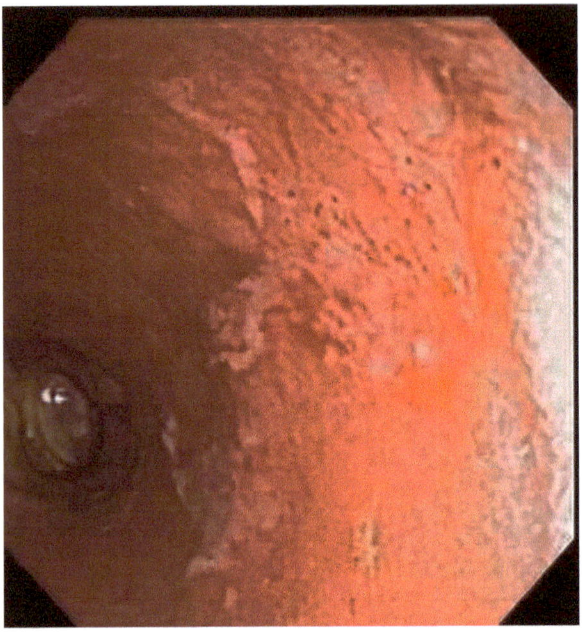

Fig. 16.6 Mild changes seen on colonoscopy with early ischemic colitis

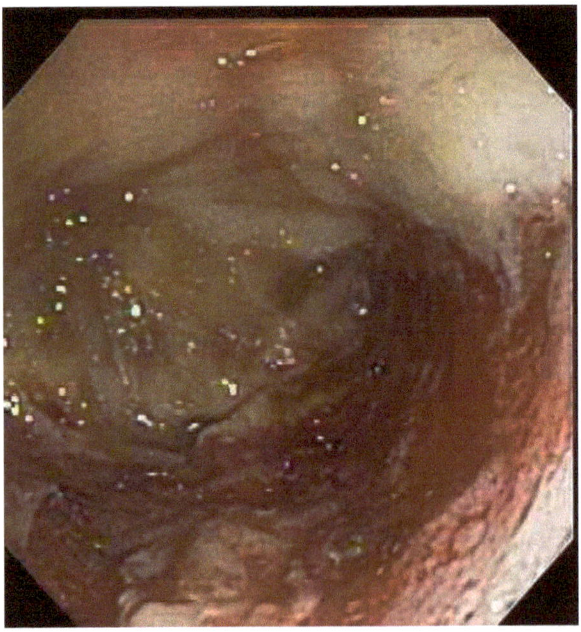

Fig. 16.7 Gangrenous changes seen on colonoscopy

Conversely, routine surveillance has been questioned by those who feel colonoscopy does not necessarily change the management of patients and can even exacerbate the problem by placing a scope in a friable segment of bowel and filling it with pressurized air. They argue that if a patient has suggestive symptoms along with radiologic and examination findings concerning for severe ischemic colitis, they should undergo an exploration. On the other hand, if a patient has clinical signs of ischemic colitis but lacks peritoneal signs or sepsis, they should undergo supportive therapy alone. This argument is supported by a study that showed that clinicians are unable to differentiate mucosal versus transmural necrosis reliably with colonoscopic evaluation [38].

Treatment Options

Once ischemic colitis is identified, treatment falls into two categories depending on the degree of injury: supportive therapy and colectomy. As most patients present with only mucosal ischemia, their clinical course is often relatively benign and warrant supportive therapy alone. Supportive therapy consists primarily of fluid resuscitation, blood pressure support, bowel rest, and antibiotics. Broad-spectrum antibiotics should typically be started due to risk for bacterial and endotoxin translocation following disruption of the mucosal membrane. Vasopressors should be used cautiously and only in septic patients. Alpha agonists are likely to worsen colonic ischemia by further reducing splanchnic blood flow. Beta-adrenergics can be considered as a first-line option if fluid therapy is inadequate to maintain blood pressure. However, pressor requirement should prompt the physician to consider if an abdominal exploration is warranted. The majority of these patients have a poor nutritional status at baseline and a high metabolic demand and will likely have a prolonged time that they will be NPO; therefore, early parenteral nutrition is often required.

Serial abdominal exams, laboratory testing, and plain film labs should be performed to monitor for worsening in their condition. Approximately 10 % of patients will fail supportive therapy and ultimately require a colectomy. Failure of supportive therapy can be obvious with signs of peritonitis, or it can be more insidious. There are patients that will continue to have persistent pain, leukocytosis, low-grade fevers, tachycardia, tender abdominal exam, but not frank peritonitis. After ruling out other sources of sepsis, abdominal exploration with colectomy is often undertaken, as the devitalized colon serves as the source for persistent problems. Decisions on when to repeat flexible endoscopy vary, but likely should be repeated if there are no resolution in symptoms, an acute change in symptoms, or prior to beginning an oral diet.

When Grade III or transmural/gangrene is identified, emergent colectomy is almost always indicated. This subset of patients, even with colectomy, have mortality rates >50 %. Patients who suffer a rAAA, compared to an elective AAA repair, and develop colonic ischemia are more likely to undergo a colectomy [4]. This is due to the larger physiologic insult that occurs with rupture. Interestingly, one study found patients undergoing colectomy for ischemic colitis after elective EVAR had significantly higher mortality than patients undergoing colectomy for rAAA or open AAA repair. This should not be misinterpreted; however, as EVAR is generally much safer and associated with lower rates of ischemic colitis. More likely, this finding reflects the delay in diagnosis, as suspicion is generally lower after elective EVAR, or the differing mechanism of the ischemic insult (i.e., cardiac) [4].

With rare exceptions, all patients with evidence of bowel infarction or perforation require surgical exploration. The greatest challenge associated with abdominal exploration is determining which portion of bowel is salvageable and which is non-viable. When evaluating the bowel intra-abdominally, it is important to remember that the serosa may appear healthy, even when there is actually full-thickness mucosal and muscularis necrosis. It is often helpful to combine an endoscopic evaluation to help determine the level of bowel viability (even despite its relative lack of accuracy). Laser Doppler flowmetry and spectrophotometry are all techniques that can assist clinical judgment in deciding bowel viability and what requires resection and what can be salvaged. Furthermore, palpation of mesenteric pulses, detecting Doppler signals on the antimesenteric portion of the bowel wall, and Wood's lamp evaluation of the bowel wall following administration of fluorescein dye intravenously are all described techniques to help separate perfused from non-perfused bowel. Some surgeons will routinely perform a second look operation in 24–48 h, whereas others will perform it selectively when there is higher concern for intestinal viability (see Algorithm).

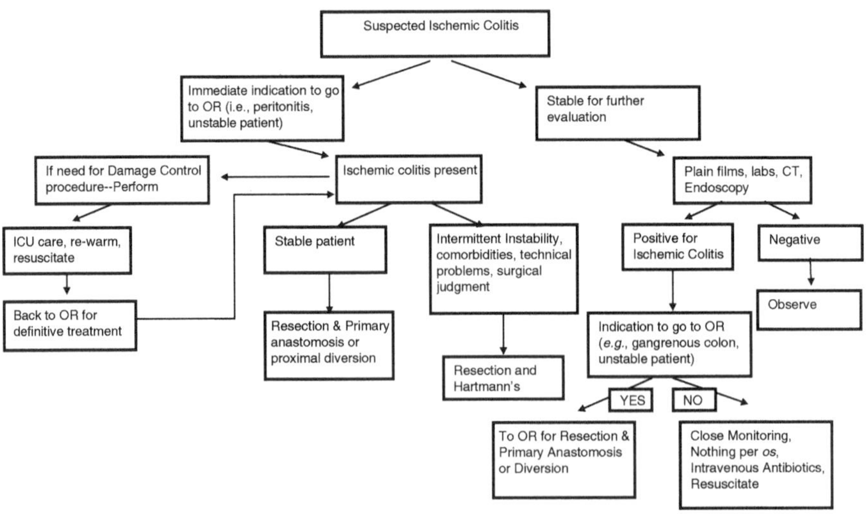

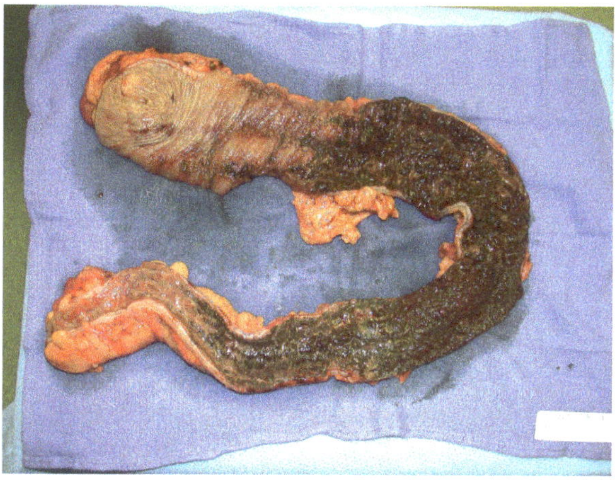

Fig. 16.8 Total abdominal colectomy for colonic ischemia

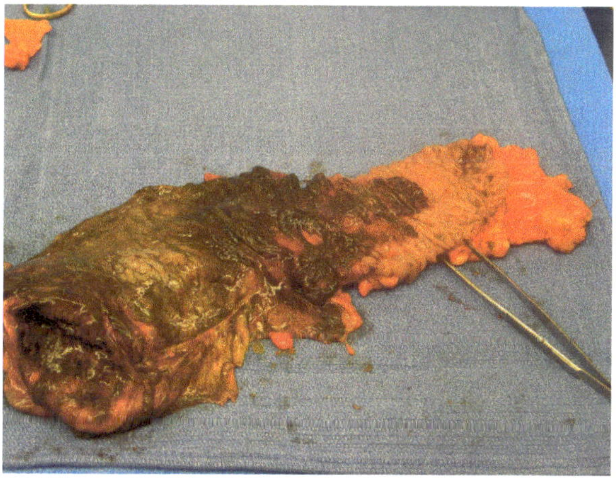

Fig. 16.9 Segmental resection for demonstrating colonic ischemia

Operative therapy must consider both the need for bowel resection and vascular reconstruction. The surgeon must balance the need to avoid leaving behind necrotic bowel with the potential morbidity of overzealous resection leading to short bowel syndrome, although the intraoperative judgment of the well-trained surgeon remains one of the most important factors. In most cases, surgical resection involves a total abdominal colectomy with end ileostomy (Fig. 16.8). Although primary anastomosis after a subtotal or partial colectomy (Fig. 16.9) with a proximal diversion may be considered in isolated hemodynamically stable patients with healthy bowel margins, this is often a poor choice [34]. Regardless of the approach, the need for an exploration and bowel resection in the acute setting has been associated with mortality rates as high as 40 %, particularly when the patients has multiple underlying comorbidities [39].

Finally, vascular repair involves first determining the patency of the vessel supplying the at risk portion of the colon. In addition, determining whether there is antegrade flow to the iliac vessels that may provide potential pelvic collaterals is crucial. While the technical aspects of vascular reconstruction are beyond the scope of this chapter, options for dealing with the inferior mesenteric artery or other major visceral vessels include resection of the base of the vessel along with a small cuff of aortic wall (Carrel patch) and reimplanting it in the aorta or graft, patch angioplasty of the stenotic opening, bypass grafting, or endarterectomy of the atherosclerotic plaque [40–42]. In either light, embarking on a complex vascular reconstruction should not be undertaken lightly and again needs to be weighed against the potential downside of prolonged operative time, excess blood loss, and failure of the repair.

Conclusion

Ischemic colitis is the leading cause of death after repair of a rAAA. With few operative or clinical parameters that are sensitive or specific for colonic ischemia, suspicion must remain high in the postoperative period. Early identification and treatment of this feared complication is the only clear way to help reduce morbidity and mortality.

Abdominal Compartment Syndrome Following Ruptured Abdominal Aortic Aneurysm

Martin Björck and Anders Wanhainen
Martin Björck is a member of the Executive Committee of the World Society of Abdominal Compartment Syndrome (website: wsacs.org)

Introduction

The knowledge that a tense abdomen is a life-threatening condition is very old, with observations from ancient Greece and during the Middle Ages. The twentieth century was a golden age of understanding human physiology, including the importance of intra-abdominal hypertension (IAH) and the abdominal compartment syndrome (ACS). It is often a consequence of aggressive resuscitation after major bleeding, thus partly an iatrogenic condition [43, 44]. In the first paper naming the condition, the vascular surgeon Irving Kron described it following ruptured abdominal aortic aneurysm (rAAA) [45]. The association between IAH/ACS and colonic ischemia following rAAA repair was demonstrated in multiple investigations [46–51]. Survival can be improved if the hypoperfusion of the abdominal organs created by IAH/ACS is prevented or reversed timely [46, 50, 51]. The purpose of this chapter is to offer guidance how that can be accomplished.

Definition of IAH/ACS

"IAH is defined by a sustained or repeated pathological elevation in intra-abdominal pressure (IAP) >12 mmHg." This is the definition of IAH, as first stated in the 2005 Consensus document [43], and unaltered in the 2013 Updated Consensus Definitions and Clinical Practice Guidelines [52]. It was shown in basic research, and in clinical studies, that an IAP above 12 mmHg affects organ function negatively. In particular renal function is affected at this relatively low pressure. Please note the words "sustained or repeated." A single elevated value, maybe the result of the patient being in pain, is not sufficient. This threshold for negative effects on organ function is important to consider in patients operated on for rAAA, since multiple prospective clinical studies have shown that it is uncommon that the IAP is less than 12 mmHg in the early postoperative period after open surgery [49, 50, 53, 54]. The situation after EVAR for rAAA is less well studied [55], but if hemodynamically instable patients are treated with EVAR, there is no reason to believe the situation to be different [51]. Although the evidence-based approach used in the revision of the guidelines did not find support for a subdefinition of low abdominal perfusion pressure (APP = MAP-IAP <60 mmHg), it is a clinical observation that hypotensive patients are more sensitive to IAH.

ACS is defined as a sustained IAP >20 mmHg (with or without an APP <60 mmHg) that is associated with new organ dysfunction/failure [52]. Again, the exact wording is important: "a sustained IAP >20 mmHg" means that the measurement has to be repeated at least once, and it needs to be associated with a "new organ dysfunction/failure," with a timely deterioration of vital organ function. ACS is never defined as a mere measurement of IAP but the combination of this high IAP and its effect on vital organ function!

There are many ways to measure IAP. Almost everyone measures IAP in the bladder, intermittently or continuously. For details, please consult the guidelines [44, 52]. Our preferred method is the Foley manometer method, with the advantage that it can easily be applied outside of the ICU, which is a great advantage after EVAR for rAAA, since those patients seldom need to stay in the ICU after surgery.

How Common Is IAH/ACS After rAAA Repair?

One of the problems in answering this question is the fact that prior to 2005 [43], there was not a consensus definition of ACS, and even after 2005, some investigators have continued to use "homemade" definitions of ACS. The incidence will depend on several factors. The routines for resuscitation are of paramount importance. Balogh et al. showed that the administration of crystalloids is an independent risk factor for ACS in abdominal trauma patients [56]. We have reasons to believe that this is true in any bleeding patient. A policy of preoperative permissive hypotension may decrease the risk of IAH/ACS.

Mell et al. showed that patients who received less than one unit of plasma for every two units of red blood cells during rAAA repair had a four times higher mortality than those given more plasma [57], highlighting the importance of a massive transfusion protocol. Massive transfusion protocols, which are discussed in another chapter of this book, do not only reduce mortality, they also reduce the risk of fluid overload and risk of ACS.

The introduction of endovascular aneurysm repair (EVAR) [58, 59] by Volodos in 1985 transformed aortic surgery. The application of EVAR on patients with rAAA was first described by Veith in 2000 [60]. Although it has not been possible to show an advantage in survival of this technique in randomized trials, it is natural that the surgical technique used for elective surgery that surgeons feel comfortable with will also be used in emergencies. How the use of EVAR on patients with rAAA affects the incidence of IAH/ACS is controversial, however.

If measured consistently, IAP >20 mmHg occurs in about half of the patients after open repair (OR) of a rAAA, and 20 % develop ACS [53, 54]. In many series on patients operated on for rAAA with EVAR, a selection of more circulatory stable patients took place, however, resulting in a lower incidence of IAH/ACS [55]. The Zürich group that treats virtually all ruptured patients with EVAR and monitors IAP on a regular basis reported a higher incidence of ACS, however: 20 % (20/102) [51], similar to the results after OR. In a prospective cohort study in four Swedish hospitals, the risk to require treatment with open abdomen (OA) was similar after EVAR (3/86, 3.4 %) and OR (14/115, 2.5 %) [61].

In a nationwide, population-based study during 2008–2013 in Sweden, 6612 aortic repairs were studied, 1341 (20.3 %) of them for rupture and 28 % of them with EVAR. [62] ACS was registered prospectively in the national vascular registry (Swedvasc) and developed in 6.8 % after OR and in 6.9 % after EVAR, $p = 1.0$. Among those with ACS, decompression laparotomy (DL) was performed in 77.3 % after OR and in 84.6 % after EVAR, $p = 0.433$. Interestingly, the abdomen was not closed at OR in 10.7 %. Adding these figures approximately 15 % were treated with OA, one in seven patients. In conclusion, IAH/ACS is a common problem after rAAA repair, irrespective of which surgical technique used.

Risk Factors for ACS After rAAA Repair

Although most patients develop IAH after surgery for rAAA, the risk to develop the ACS increases when one or multiple of the risk factors given in Table 16.1 are present. These factors were either identified as general risk factors for ACS, described in the Guidelines from the World Society of the Abdominal Compartment Syndrome [44, 52] (www.wsacs.org), or they were identified in the already mentioned nationwide, population-based study [62].

Can ACS Be Prevented? Medical Management?

Being aware of the risk factors (Table 16.1), and if possible avoiding them, is an obvious preventive strategy. It is also possible to treat IAH in a proactive way, preventing further deterioration of the patient and development of ACS. This treatment is sometimes referred to as "medical management," or "conservative management," which is not an appropriate label since it can be quite aggressive.

The therapeutic alternatives are described in Table 16.2. There are two mechanisms through which the IAP can be reduced. One mechanism is volume reduction of the intra-abdominal cavity. Evacuation of the retroperitoneal hematoma after EVAR for rAAA has been attempted using surgical approach through the lateral/dorsal part of the abdominal wall. Another alternative was described by Hörer et al. who inserted tissue plasminogen activator (tPA) through a 20 F catheter placed in the hematoma with CT guidance, in 13 patients [63]. None of these techniques are truly minimally invasive, and major bleeding was reported. Although we lack personal experience of these techniques, decompression laparotomy seems both safer and more effective.

Table 16.1 Risk factors for ACS after rAAA repair

Preoperative risk factors	Intraoperative risk factors	Postoperative risk factors
Hypotension Unconsciousness Massive fluid resuscitation (>5 L) No permissive hypotension Preoperative intubation Morbid obesity (BMI > 35)	Massive transfusion (>10U/24 h) Coagulopathy No massive transfusion protocol Hypothermia (<33° C) Acidosis (pH < 7.2) Intraoperative bleeding >5 L Prolonged operation Prolonged cross clamping Need of occlusion balloon (EVAR)	Continued need of transfusions Continued bleeding (e.g. through endoleakage after EVAR) Fluid overload (capillary leakage) Renal failure Respiratory failure (especially if elevated intrathoracic pressure) Intestinal failure/Ileus Liver failure/ascites

These risk factors were identified in the references [44] (general risk factors for ACS) and [62] (a large population-based cohort study)

Table 16.2 Nonsurgical treatment of intra-abdominal hypertension

Reducing intra-abdominal volume	Improving compliance of the abdominal wall
Evacuating the retroperitoneal hematoma: (a) Lumbectomy (b) tPA-assisted hematoma evacuation Drainage of free intra-abdominal fluid Drainage of intragastric contents Enema, drainage of fecal contents Reducing fluid overload	Pain relief (a) Avoid opioids, if possible (b) Epidural analgesia Neuromuscular blockade Reducing fluid overload

Drainage of gastric content is important, but early enteral nutrition should not be halted [64], since bowel movements are of strategic importance. We initiate enteral feeding the first postoperative day, even in the presence of IAH, but the gastric contents are drained twice daily to avoid accumulation. Enemas and other activities to stimulate the fecal flow are seldom effective after rAAA repair. Early enteral nutrition and avoiding opioids are more effective. It is common that the IAP increases hours before the first bowel emptying, when bowel movements start, after which the IAP drops substantially. Free drainable fluid in the abdominal cavity is uncommon, but may occur if there is hepatic or pancreatic pathology.

Abdominal compliance (AC) measures the ease of abdominal expansion, expressed as a change (delta = Δ) in intra-abdominal volume (IAV) per change in intra-abdominal pressure (IAP): $AC = \Delta IAV/\Delta IAP$. This is a dynamic variable dependent on baseline IAV and IAP, as well as on reshaping and stretching capacity of the abdominal wall. The first phenomenon is that the abdomen transforms from an oval into a circular shape (reshaping, see Fig. 16.10), followed by stretching and finally followed by a rapid increase in IAP. In a recent review of AC the most important conclusion was that patients with high IAP have a reduced AC, making the IAP very sensitive to small changes in IAV. [65] A critically ill patient with IAH may have a reshaped and quite rigid abdominal wall, where a small increase of IAV results in ACS. Inversely, a small decrease in IAV may result in a substantial decrease of IAP.

One of the most effective ways of decreasing the IAP is pain relief, but it is also strategically important to avoid opioids. During rAAA repair, there is seldom time to apply an epidural catheter prior to surgery, and after surgery, the patient often has coagulopathy. We routinely discuss with the anesthesiologists, postpone LMWH medication, give thrombocytes if necessary, and then apply epidural analgesia whenever possible.

Neuromuscular blockade (NMB) is an effective way of immediately reducing IAP when the patient is on the ventilator, which is often the case after rAAA repair with massive bleeding and transfusion, even if EVAR was used. It reduces IAP by 30–50 %, which is often sufficient to improve renal function, reduce fluid overload, and reverse the situation of increasing IAP before ACS develops. In a study on 191 trauma patients undergoing damage control laparotomy, 92 who were on NMB the first 24 h had higher primary fascial closure rate [66]. A large randomized French trial showed that NMB during 48 h was safe and improved survival in patients with acute respiratory failure, in 340 mixed ICU patients [67]. There are no published specific data on rAAA patients, but in our experience, it works well.

Reducing the fluid overload acts through both mechanisms, reducing intra-abdominal volume and making the abdominal wall more compliant, as the edema decreases. How this shall be best achieved is probably worth a special chapter, written by an intensivist. This issue is highly controversial, however. Many argue that colloids are beneficial in this situation, others that they only leak into the extracellular space, adding further to the fluid overload and affecting renal function negatively. We tend to use plasma in the first postoperative phase, when the patient often is coagulopathic, and hypertonic 20 % albumin combined with furosemide or renal replacement therapy later. If the patient is on the ventilator, an increased PEEP may help to recruit fluid from the lungs.

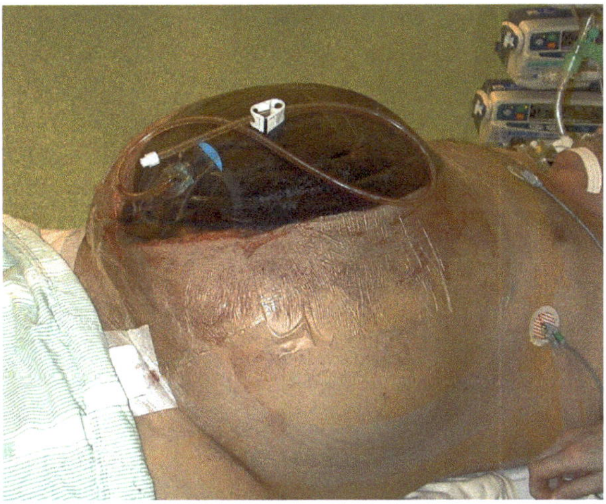

Fig. 16.10 A 70-year-old man was treated with EVAR electively despite an unfavorable anatomy because of obesity (110 kg) and chronic obstructive pulmonary disease. There was an acute rupture of the aneurysm, secondary to a distal type I endoleak. There was a long transport with helicopter to Uppsala. The patient was treated with an extension of the endograft covering the internal iliac artery, with a good result, but had increased his body weight to 125 kg. He had a MAP of 70 and an IAP of 18 and developed anuria. Despite not fulfilling the criteria of ACS, a DL was performed, resulting in improved renal function, with urinary outputs of 300 ml/h, the first hours post DL. This picture was taken during the first redressing, when a VACM was applied. Despite unfavorable conditions, the patient survived and the abdomen was closed with delayed primary fascial closure after 30 days. No incisional hernia developed

The fluid overload is often more iatrogenic than what is recognized. The Uppsala protocol is very restrictive with the administration of crystalloids from early resuscitation. Not all are aware of the fact that when we give fractionated blood products (erythrocytes, plasma, and thrombocytes, 1:1:1), to compensate for one liter of blood loss, 4–500 ml of saline solution is also added. Thus, even if only blood products are given, the transfusion to compensate for 10 l of blood loss will automatically result in a fluid overload of 4–5 l, making further administration of crystalloids dangerous.

Decompression Laparotomy (DL)

When ACS is incipient, or even manifest, the only effective treatment is DL. It should preferably be performed in the midline, from the costal arch to the symphysis pubis. If the primary laparotomy was a transverse incision, which fortunately is very rare after rAAA repair, that may need to be used again, but it will be less effective. To not open the entire abdomen is a classical beginner's mistake, less effective, and more difficult to close.

The timing of DL is important but a difficult subject to discuss. Ideally, the two strategies of early or delayed DL should be compared in a randomized design. It does not make sense to await severe organ dysfunction/failure before DL, but OA treatment is a morbid procedure associated with both morbidity and mortality.

When a decision to perform DL has been taken, often in the middle of the night, there may be a waiting list for OR. Other patients may have high priorities, in which case NMB can reduce the ischemic injury to the abdominal organs during waiting. It is important to inform the anesthesiologist that the patient needs to have an extra bolus of fluids prior to DL, to avoid hypotension, which is common during DL.

The effect of DL is often dramatic, reducing IAP, and improving oxygenation and urinary output. Effects on multiple organ failure scores (SOFA, APACHE) are not as quick, however, since multiple organ failure is not reversed quickly. In a recent multicentre study on 33 patients undergoing DL for overt ACS, with different pathologies including rAAA, the IAP decreased from 23 mmHg (range 21–27) to 12 mmHg (9–15) after 2 h [68].

Prophylactic Open Abdomen Treatment

Is it best to leave all patients open as a routine after OR of a rAAA, or is it better to close most patients (who do not have a very tense abdomen) and follow them closely in the postoperative period? This issue should ideally be investigated in a randomized study, but that has not taken place. The Mayo Clinic reported having left 19 % open after AAA repair (43/223) [69], and a similar experience was reported from Zürich [51].

Based on a systematic EBM review of the literature, the updated consensus document favors primary closure and IAP measuring [52]. They recommend "measuring IAP when any known risk factor for IAH/ACS is present in a critically ill or injured patient" and "use of protocolized monitoring and management of IAP versus not." Furthermore, "we could make no recommendation regarding the prophylactic use of the open abdomen".

The policy in Uppsala is to leave the patient open primarily after OR of a rAAA only if the abdomen is tense and difficult to close, in approximately 5–10 %. Most patients with rAAA are treated with EVAR. We monitor IAP every 4 h in all patients, more frequently the first hours and when IAH, early medical treatment and DL on demand. An algorithm was published [70]. In the largest study ever on ACS after rAAA repair, 1341 operations were studied. Among the 72 % operated on with OR, 10.7 % were left open [63].

Management of the Patient with Open Abdomen (OA)

Managing a patient with OA after rAAA repair is a vast topic; many review articles have been written on this subject [70–72]. The first issue is how to optimize the management of the open abdomen itself. It is important to maintain a sterile environment, to keep the intestines moist and protected from injury, and to protect the abdominal wall. A classification system of the open abdomen was developed, in order to facilitate training and research [73]. Preventing and controlling contamination, as well as lateralization of the abdominal wall, are key elements to enable to close the abdomen as soon as possible [52, 73, 74].

The importance of closing the abdomen as soon as possible was illustrated by the results of a recent publication from Helsinki, Finland [75]. They used a temporary abdominal closure (TAC) device including continuous negative pressure (the VACM method, see below), yet the open abdomen of their patients was progressively colonized so that 80 % of the patients had positive bacterial cultures after 2 weeks of OA treatment.

The choice of TAC has attracted much attention, and multiple solutions were developed [76]. The first to treat patients with OA were the pediatric surgeons, who started to repair omphalocele in the 1940s, using silastic coverage of the intestines. A similar system was later popularized in trauma surgery by the Colombian invention of the Bogotá bag, using the plastic bag from a drip that is sutured to the skin or the fascia. This system works well for a few days, but during a more prolonged treatment (which is necessary after rAAA repair), three major problems develop. Two of those were solved by the later development of the vacuum pack technique, developed in 1995 by Barker in Philadelphia, USA [77]: the active suction prevented leakage of fluids from the OA, and the surgical towels covered with plastic prevented adhesions to form between the intestines and the abdominal wall. This system was further refined by a commercially available ready-made system (V.A.C.® Abdominal Dressing System; KCI, San Antonio, Texas, USA).

A third problem, the lateralization of the abdominal wall, remained however, making it difficult to close patients who had been treated with OA >5 days. This was the reason why we developed a novel combination in Uppsala and Malmö, Sweden, the vacuum-assisted wound closure and mesh-mediated fascial traction (VACM) method, published in 2007 [78]. This is a combination of the commercially available VAC system with a prolene mesh that is sutured to the fascial edges to permit an active traction toward the midline. A multicenter study with this technique (including only patients with a need of OA during >4 days) showed an 89 % primary delayed fascial closure rate after a median time of 15 days with OA [79], and in a subgroup analysis of those treated for aortic disease, this figure was 100 % [61]. These results have been repeated independently at other major centers [80, 81] and is now the preferred TAC method in many centers worldwide.

The problem of lateralization was defined in the updated consensus document [52]: "Lateralization of the abdominal wall is the phenomenon where the musculature and fascia of the abdominal wall, most exemplified by the rectus abdominis muscles and their enveloping fascia, move laterally away from the midline with time." It is also included in the classification system of OA [73].

The Uppsala algorithm summarizing the management of patients after rAAA repair, regarding preventing and treating ACS, is summarized in Fig. 16.11.

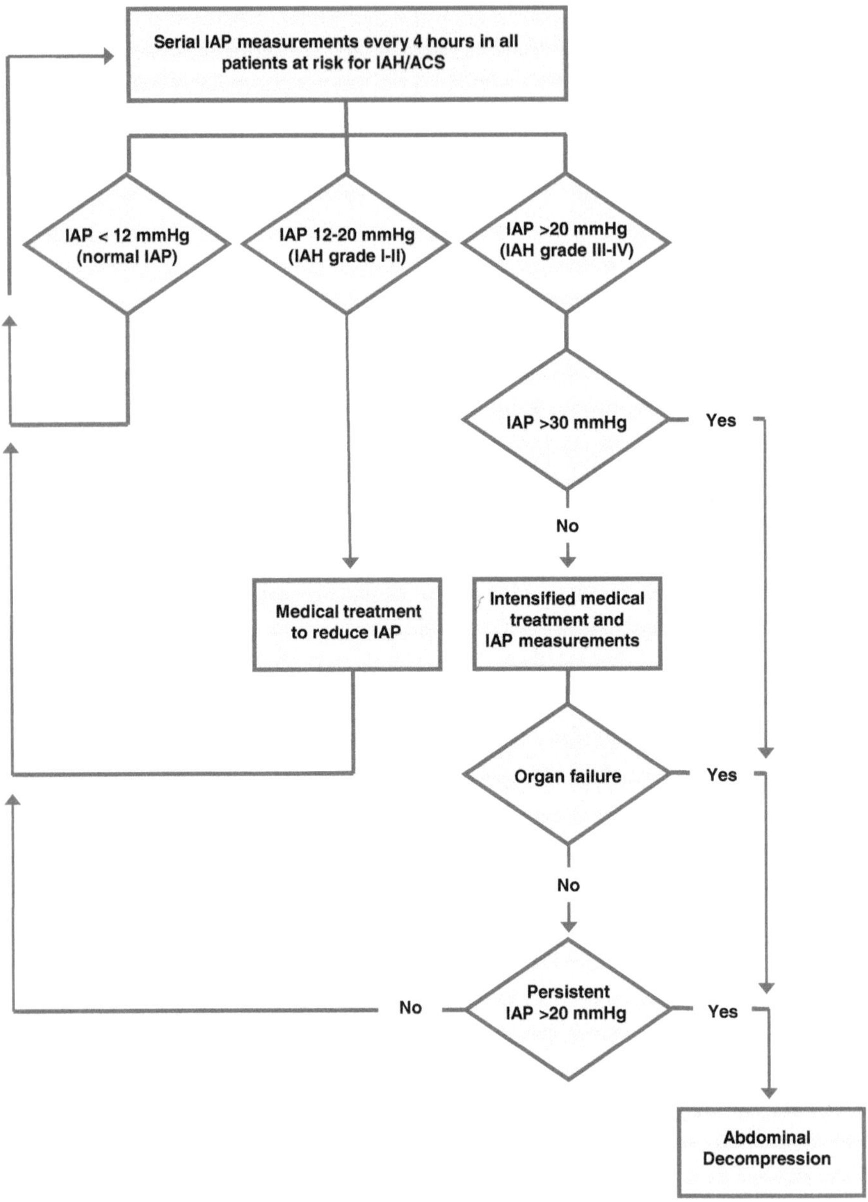

Fig. 16.11 The Uppsala algorithm to prevent and treat ACS

Prognosis

The overall mortality in the aforementioned international multicenter study on decompression laparotomy for ACS (including but not exclusively rAAA patients) was 28 % at 28 days and 55 % at 1 year; non-survivors were older (63 vs. 53 years)

[69]. The large population-based cohort study from Sweden, including 1341 rAAA repairs, showed the great impact that ACS has on the prognosis after rAAA [62]. Thirty-day mortality rate was 42.4 % with ACS versus 23.5 % without ACS, $p<0.001$, at 1 year 50.7 % versus 31.8 %, $p<0.001$. Furthermore, all registered complications, such as myocardial infarction, renal failure, multiple organ failure, ICU care >5 days, intestinal ischemia, bowel resection, and reoperation for bleeding, were all four to six times more common among the 94 patients who developed ACS after rAAA repair. Those results are actually rather encouraging, since untreated ACS has a mortality approaching 100 %, and maybe the fact that ACS has been recognized and treated for many years in Sweden is one of the explanations why survival after rAAA has increased over time [82].

Spinal Cord Protection in Emergency Aortic Surgery

Anthony M. Roche, Hernando Olivar, and Koichiro Nandate

Introduction

Spinal cord ischemia during endovascular repair of aortic aneurysms can lead to devastating neurological deficits including complete paraplegia. Depending on the type of aortic surgery, it has a quoted incidence of 2.5–13 % [83]. This variation differs based on extent of surgery, elective or emergency surgery, open versus endovascular techniques, as well as perioperative management. The available literature implicates an overall spinal cord injury (SCI) rate of 6–13 % [83] for open procedures, with thoracic endovascular aneurysm repairs (TEVAR) having an associated rate of 3–4 %. In a systematic review of SCI associated with TEVAR and cerebrospinal fluid drainage, Wong et al. found 46 eligible studies totaling 4936 patients. They discovered an overall SCI rate of 3.89 % [84]. There is a paucity of literature on SCI in emergency aortic surgery, and no studies specifically relating to SCI in emergency EVAR surgery. Since there is such a paucity of literature specifically on SCI in emergency endovascular aortic repairs, we present our institutional approach to spinal cord protection based on current literature with emphasis on overall patient safety.

Pathogenesis and Risk Factors

The pathogenesis of SCI is multifactorial; however, most injuries are the result of ischemia or ischemia–reperfusion injury. Spinal cord perfusion is a dynamic process, which is dependent on major segmental arteries and vast networks of collateral blood flow. In most circumstances of open or endovascular abdominal aortic aneurysm surgery, there is usually limited to no occlusion of major segmental arteries. The picture changes somewhat when a thoracic repair is indicated. In such scenarios, segmental arteries are usually implicated, especially with longer grafts or previous aortic procedures. This results in the spinal cord perfusion being increasingly dependent on the vulnerable and often inadequate collateral circulation. Hemodynamic disturbances and fluctuations inevitably lead to a reduction in collateral circulation flow.

Part of patient preparation for surgery, be it elective or emergency, should include some form of risk stratification for adverse perioperative outcomes. As is the case for adverse cardiac outcome risk assessment and subsequent stratified management bundles, it is prudent to assess the risk for SCI in aortic surgery. This enables the surgical team to better quantify the risk of SCI, improve patient counseling, and plan stepwise spinal cord protection strategies [85, 86].

Known risk factors for SCI in TEVAR include the following: previous aortic interventions; long aortic coverage, especially if the left subclavian and/or hypogastric arteries are covered; renal insufficiency (with creatinine levels greater than 1.5 mg/dL); and prolonged periods of hypotension (mean arterial pressures less than 65–70 mmHg) [87]. Furthermore, age, comorbidities (e.g., hypertension, hyperlipidemia, diabetes mellitus), and increasing number of aortic stents may also increase risk of SCI [83, 85, 88, 89]. Symptomatic disease or rupture has also been implicated, especially in open thoracic aortic surgery.

Spinal Cord Protection

As described above, an important first step is recognizing the risk of SCI. Based on that risk assessment, a stepwise approach can be employed to reducing the risk of spinal cord ischemia.

It is recommended as a minimum that hypotension be avoided during aortic surgery [87]. The basis of spinal cord perfusion rests with the simple equation:SPP = MAP – ITPLegend: SPP is spinal perfusion pressure, MAP is mean arterial pressure, and ITP is intrathecal pressure.

The goal of spinal cord perfusion pressure management is to remain as close to each patient's baseline as possible [83, 90]. This is less of a problem in mostly abdominal aortic surgery, regardless of open or endovascular technique, where it is less likely that segmental branches to the spinal cord will be covered or ligated. Fastidious control of SPP is especially important in circumstances of longer stents/grafts and in patients determined to be at higher risk of SCI. The underlying principle is to maintain spinal blood flow and oxygenation, thereby reducing the risk of ischemia or ischemia–reperfusion injury.

The avoidance of hypotension, although self-explanatory, can be described especially as reducing duration thereof. Sustained hypotensive periods, with MAPs below 65–70 mmHg for longer than 5–15 min, are associated with higher incidence of SCI. Strict BP management is therefore a crucial first step in reducing SCI [91]. This is a difficult goal to achieve, especially in compromised patients undergoing emergency procedures. One of the most effective measures that we perform at our institution during the initial surgical approach of patients with aortic emergencies is to achieve endovascular control of the aorta. Once the balloon is in place, intravascular accesses and invasive blood pressure monitoring as well as fluid resuscitation are initiated. If the patient does not tolerate light sedation, general anesthesia is induced. Permissive hypertension is described as a potential management strategy for patients with symptomatic SCI [91].

Our center uses the following algorithm for blood pressure management:

- Maintain intraoperative MAP >80 mmHg.
- Increase MAP to greater than 80–90 mmHg at the moment of graft deployment.
- Maintain the MAP greater than 80–90 mmHg postoperatively for 24–48 h.
- If neurologic symptoms are present at any time point, increase MAP to greater than 100 mmHg using vasopressors and/or inotropes.
- Lumbar CSF drainage (description to follow)

Although controversial, lumbar CSF drainage has been shown to be effective in the prevention and management of SCI during TEVAR and open thoracoabdominal aneurysm repair [90, 92–95]. As a result, it has been recommended as part of spinal cord protection algorithms. The rationale is, like MAP management, to improve spinal cord blood flow and oxygenation. In addition to increasing MAP, reducing CSF pressure (ITP) increases SPP. Lumbar CSF drains should be placed preoperatively, following existing national guidelines for neuraxial block placement and anticoagulants/patient coagulation status (see Table 16.3). Reasonable ITP pressure goals are be as follows:

- Less than 15 mmHg prior to graft deployment.
- Reduce ITP to less than 10 mmHg after graft deployment.
- Reduce ITP to less than 8 mmHg if neurologic symptoms develop.
- Allow rates of CSF drainage of 10–20 ml per hour.
- Discontinue lumbar CSF drains 24–72 h postoperatively (also following national guidelines regarding anticoagulants/patient coagulation status) (see Table 16.3).

Significant variation exists among centers regarding lumbar CSF drainage. Also, there is paucity of literature about the use of lumbar drains in emergency endovascular treatment of aortic pathology. Our center recommends placement in all TEVAR patients identified as high risk for SCI, and as a rescue measure when blood pressure management alone does not reverse SCI symptoms, and that have cardiovascular stability, which is sufficient enough to tolerate drain placement [83, 94, 96]. One important exception to this is patients with traumatic thoracic aortic injury to be treated with shorter thoracic endografts (less risk of SCI).

It is worth noting that lumbar CSF drains are not without risk; there are numerous complications described [97]. Potential risks include catheter breakage and retention of fragments in the intrathecal space, postdural puncture headache, epidural and subdural hematomas with or without cauda equina syndrome, meningitis, intracranial hemorrhage, and traumatic puncture [97]. In the setting of traumatic preoperative puncture (significant bleeding from the needle or catheter), elective TEVAR or open aortic surgery should be delayed. Although the incidence of these complications is low, they lead to high morbidity rates and potential independent mortality risk.

Table 16.3 University of Washington neuraxial access and anticoagulation protocol

Class	MOA	Drug	Catheter placement	While catheter in place	Catheter removal	Reinitiation of anticoagulation
Fibrinolytics	Activate plasminogen	Alteplase, Urokinase, Streptokinase	Contraindicated Avoid lumbar puncture/catheter placement	Contraindicated	Contraindicated	If fibrinolytics are required, check if neuraxial technique/catheter was placed within 10 days. If yes, medication is contraindicated
Anticoagulants	Direct thrombin (IIa) inhibition	Bivalirudin (Angiomax), desirudin (Iprivask), argatroban (no trade name), dabigatran (Pradaxa)	Contraindicated Insufficient data; avoid lumbar puncture/catheter placement	Contraindicated	Contraindicated	Not addressed, insufficient data
	Indirect thrombin (IIa) inhibition via AT III	Unfractioned heparin (UFH)	5 K U SQ BID—no restrictions on placement >10 K. Catheter placement 4 h after last dose. Check PTT and platelet before puncture *Check Plts if on heparin >4d	Ok if dose less than 10 K units (QD, BiD) TID doses or >10 K units. Contraindicated	Remove after 4 h of discontinuation	Reinitiate 4 h after catheter removal
	Indirect Xa inhibition via AT III	LMWH: dalteparin (Fragmin), enoxaparin (Lovenox) Fondaparinux	Dalteparin, enoxaparin. Catheter placement after 12 h of QD doses. 24 h for higher doses. *Fondaparinux:* contraindicated	LMWH QD doses ok. Avoid BID doses *Fondaparinux is contraindicated*	Remove after 12 h of discontinuation	Reinitiate after 6 h of catheter removal

	Direct Xa inhibition	Apixaban (Eliquis), rivaroxaban (Xarelto)	No specific recommendations. Weigh risks. Recommend to stop 48 h before puncture	No specific recommendations. Weigh risks. Not recommended	No specific recommendations. Weigh risks. Not recommended	No specific recommendations. Weigh risks. Xarelto manufacturer recommends reinitiate after 6 h of removal
	Vit K epoxide reductase inhibition (II, VII, IX, X)	Warfarin (coumadin)	Stop 5 days before, bridge to UFH or LMWH and follow recommendations. INR <1.4	Contraindicated	INR <1.5: remove + monitor x 24 h INR 1.5–3.0: remove w/caution; monitor until INR is normal INR >3.0: reduce dose or hold; no definitive removal recs.	Timing according to patient's risk of thromboembolic events and risk of surgical bleeding
Antiplatelets	COX inhibition (inhibits aggregation)	ASA, NSAIDs	No contraindication if solo agent	No contraindication if solo agent	No contraindication if solo agent	No contraindication if solo agent
	Gp IIb/IIA receptor inhibition (inhibits aggregation)	Eptifibatide (Integrilin), abciximab (ReoPro), tirofiban (Aggrastat)	Not recommended with ongoing therapy	Contraindicated	Contraindicated	
	PAR antagonist (inhibits aggregation)	Vorapaxar (Zontivity)	Not addressed given new FDA approval.			

(continued)

Table 16.3 (continued)

Class	MOA	Drug	Catheter placement	While catheter in place	Catheter removal	Reinitiation of anticoagulation
	ADP receptor blocker (inhibits activation)	Thienopyridine derivatives: clopidogrel (Plavix), ticlopidine (Ticlid), prasugrel (Effient)	Not recommended with ongoing therapy. Ok if discontinued for 5 days	Contraindicated	Contraindicated	Timing according to patient's risk of thromboembolic events and risk of surgical bleeding.
	PDE inhibition (inhibits activation)	Dipyridamole (Persantine), cilostazol (Pletal)	Not addressed. For Pletal, manufacturer recommends to discontinue 5 days before block placement	Not addressed	Not addressed	Not addressed
Herbals	Inhibit platelets	Garlic, ginkgo, ginseng	Not addressed presumed no restrictions	Not addressed presumed no restrictions	Not addressed presumed no restrictions	Not addressed presumed no restrictions

Modified from the American Society of Regional Anesthesia guidelines

Carotid to left subclavian artery transposition/bypass (CSCT) is a recognized and extremely useful technique for patients identified preoperatively as high risk for development of SCI [98]. It is especially of use in those undergoing TEVAR with long or multiple endografts, as well as those potentially requiring left subclavian artery occlusion by the endograft. In such patients, there are a number of preoperative imaging techniques to evaluate the left-sided vertebral arterial system. The main evaluation techniques are computed tomography (CT), magnetic resonance imaging (MRI), or angiography. If the left vertebral artery arises from the left subclavian artery, and the anterior spinal artery is left vertebral artery dominant, it is recommended to perform a pre-TEVAR CSCT. It is important to note that the anterior spinal artery arises superiorly from the vertebral arteries, other segmental arteries, as well as the hypogastric arteries, yet its most important anatomic/physiologic function is to supply two-thirds of spinal cord blood flow.

An intervention of potential benefit is distal aortic perfusion/bypass, through venoarterial cardiopulmonary bypass, with distal access to the femoral arterial system. This lessens the effect of the cross clamp on the hypogastric to spinal artery circulation, as bypass maintains a blood pressure in the hypogastric circulation. Some authors have advocated the use of axillo-femoral artery bypass to achieve similar effects in the femoral/hypogastric circulation.

Managed intentional hypothermia is described as a protection strategy in central nervous system (CNS) protection; however, there are little data to guide TEVAR or emergency EVAR surgery [99]. It is important to consider the potential benefit of hypothermia on CNS protection versus the potential adverse effects on the coagulation system, especially in the setting of aortic leak/rupture undergoing emergency EVAR. Some authors have recommended local hypothermia of the spinal cord, by circulating cold 0.9 % saline in the subarachnoid space. This has been reported to be of benefit; however, it is markedly invasive, extremely difficult to perform, and a technique which could have catastrophic complications if not performed well. As such, it is not something we would recommend unless a developing body of evidence suggests otherwise.

Multiple pharmacologic approaches have been studied for decades, among others steroids, naloxone, barbiturates, and papaverine. Although some of these interventions have shown some promise, none have been shown to be reliably effective in preventing or managing SCI.

Staged procedures have been reported to increase the development of the collateral circulation in circumstances of patients with combined thoracic and abdominal aortic disease. This development of the hypogastric and lumbar arteries allows improved aortic blood flow less dependent on the segmental artery of Adamkiewicz (arteria radicularis magna), present in over 80 % of the population. This artery usually arises from segmental vessels from T9 to T11.

Spinal cord monitoring is a modality which is showing significant promise. Neurophysiologic monitoring involves two main types of evoked potentials, somatosensory and motor. Somatosensory evoked potentials (SSEP) monitor and assess the function of the ascending sensory pathways from arms and legs to cranial scalp leads. Transcranial motor evoked potentials (tcMEP) are induced by the cranial scalp leads to assess function and signal conduction of the descending motor pathways. These modalities provide sensitive assessment of spinal cord function and can provide an early sign of developing SCI, especially intraoperatively when a patient may be under general anesthesia and unable to report changes in sensation or motor function [99]. Such early signs from SSEP and/or tcMEP enable clinicians to make early intraoperative precise interventions aimed at reducing or managing SCI, for example, blood pressure and ITP management.

Conclusion

SCI is a devastating complication of aortic surgery, most commonly in TEVAR surgery. Its incidence greater than 1 % necessitates centers to (a) preoperatively proactively assess risk of SCI, (b) have distinct protocols and guidelines in place for spinal cord protection by avoidance of perioperative hypotension, consider other management strategies in higher risk patients, (c) develop guidelines for emergent management of patients developing or with suspected SCI, and (d) consider newer monitoring strategies, e.g., SSEP and/or tcMEP [100].

Fastidious attention to detail, strict management guidelines, or early intervention in patients with developing or suspected SCI increases the risk of either avoiding SCI or improving partial or full recovery. These all require a system which is attentive to the risks, provides seamless communication and skillset in aiding early intervention, and one which follows current evidence of best practice.

Multisystem Organ Failure After Ruptured Abdominal Aortic Aneurysm

Shahram Aarabi, Surbhi Mathur, and Joseph Cuschieri

Introduction

Ruptured abdominal aortic aneurysm (rAAA) is the most lethal vascular surgical emergency. Without repair, rAAA is almost uniformly fatal [101]. With modern techniques of resuscitation and surgical management, the majority of patients presenting with rAAA survive [102]. This is in contrast to just 20 years ago where upwards of 50–70 % of patients with rAAA died despite arriving at a tertiary referral center alive [103]. Given the hemodynamic and circulatory factors of the disease and the associated ischemia–reperfusion injury, it is not surprising that rAAA has a high incidence of multisystem organ failure (MSOF) [104]. As a result of this improvement in overall initially mortality, an increased risk of MSOF and the subsequent challenges due to organ dysfunction continue to plague subsequent morbidity and recovery. Once MSOF develops, complications due to organ dysfunction and need for increased resource utilization occur leading to prolonged ICU stays, high resource consumption for organ failure support, and increased mortality, all at considerable financial and human cost [105].

Pathogenesis

rAAA is associated with a systemic inflammatory response syndrome (SIRS), characterized by increased microvascular permeability, neutrophil sequestration, and innate and adaptive immune dysfunction that leads to direct and indirect organ injury. Central to the development of this constellation of conditions is ischemia–reperfusion injury that characterizes rAAA. The initial control and subsequent resuscitation with both crystalloid and high-volume blood products further exacerbate immune dysregulation and dysfunction associated with rAAA. Ischemia–reperfusion injury following aortic hemorrhage, subsequent cross clamping, and resuscitation leads to activation of inflammatory pathways and their eventual dysregulation resulting in inflammatory-mediated injury to both local and distant organs. The two major organ systems most profoundly affected are the lungs, demonstrated by development of acute respiratory distress syndrome (ARDS), and the kidneys, demonstrated by development of acute kidney injury (AKI). In addition to the development of ARDS and AKI, all other organs are at risk due to this dysregulated immune state [104].

Clinically, ischemia–reperfusion injury is identified through the progressive development of coagulopathy, acidosis, and hypothermia. The development of this triad of clinical symptoms known as the "lethal triad" is a sequential and progressive clinical state leading to further disruption of the inflammatory response. Subsequent stressors (e.g., reintervention or infection) lead to a so-called "second-hit" phenomenon that causes further activation of inflammatory pathways. This second-hit hypothesis, however, has been recently challenged by a series of investigations evaluating severe hemorrhagic shock following injury similar in magnitude to that seen in rAAA [106–109]. This data would argue that the initial dysregulation in both innate and adaptive immunity occurs early following ischemia–reperfusion and these secondary hits are merely manifestations of altered immunity and established organ dysfunction [106–109]. Several inflammatory mediators liberated by this dysregulated immune state play an important role in this process (Fig. 16.12) and may serve as prognostic markers for the extent of injury. Further, there has been basic research that demonstrates modulating this immune response may be beneficial after rAAA repair. Among these studies, Harkin and colleagues have shown that C5a receptor antagonism can reduce local intestinal and remote lung injury in a model of rAAA [110]. However, clinically individual blockade of C5a or other inflammatory mediators has not been demonstrated to be beneficial in ischemia–reperfusion injury due to the remarkable redundancy of the immune system.

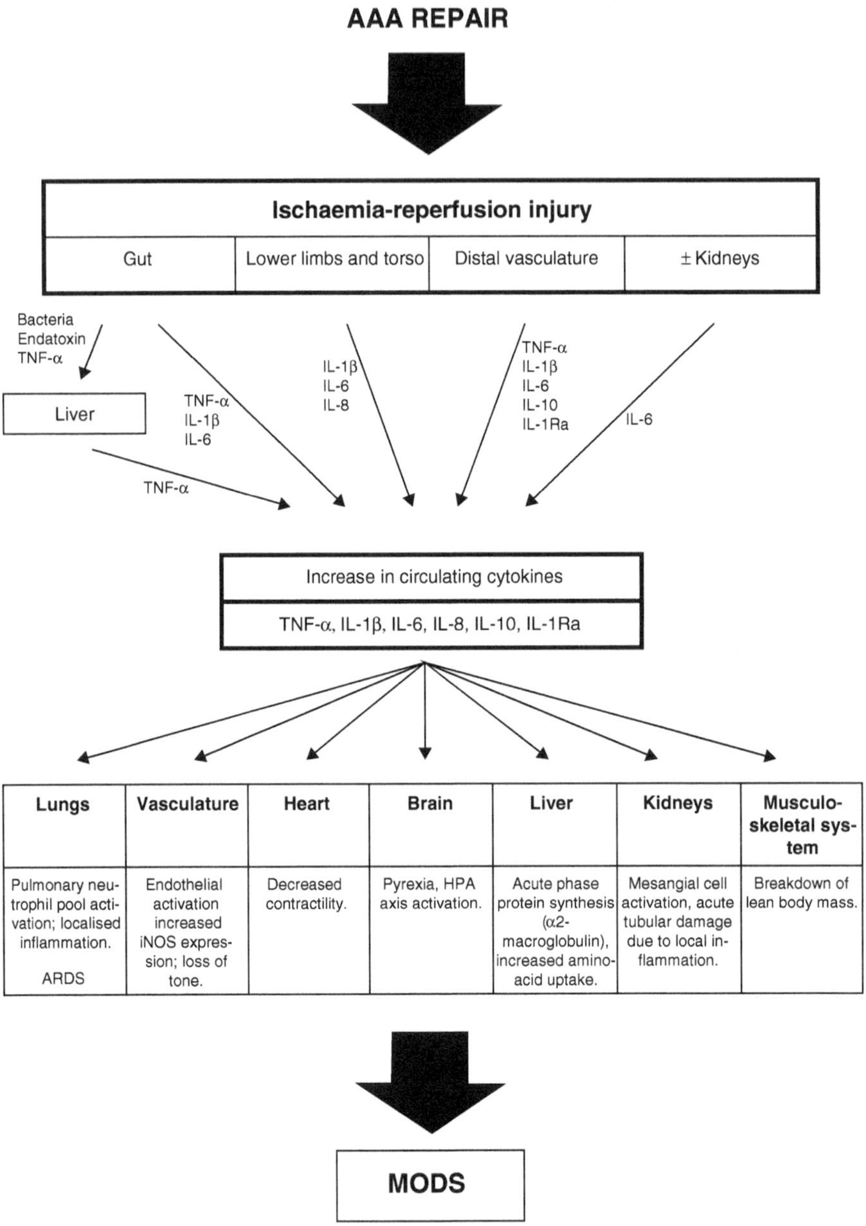

Fig. 16.12 Cytokine response to AAA repair and the pathogenesis of multiple organ dysfunction syndrome (MODS) [104]

Table 16.4 Cause of death among 29 patients who died within 30 days of endovascular aneurysm repair (*EVAR*) for ruptured abdominal aortic aneurysm (r-AAA)

Cause of death	EVAR	OSR
Intraoperative myocardial infarction/on table	5	12
Bleeding/coagulopathy	7[b]	29
Multisystem organ failure	5	16
Abdominal compartment syndrome	9	1
Colon ischemia	2	5
Acute respiratory distress syndrome[a]	1	6
Gastrointestinal hemorrhage	0	1
Pulmonary embolism	0	1
Acute hepatic failure	0	1

OSR open surgical repair

[a] Acute respiratory distress syndrome and 72 who died after OSR

[b] One patient with EVAR died on the table from bleeding

Incidence

MSOF among rAAA patients has been defined in various ways. Most of these require two or more of the following organ systems to meet criteria for severe dysfunction within a 24 h period: cardiovascular, respiratory, renal, hematologic, and neurologic. Historically, that is, in the pre-endovascular era, causes of death after rAAA repair included MSOF (37 %), cardiac or cardiorespiratory failure (26 %), transmural colon infarction (18 %), renal failure (10 %), and other unspecified causes (9 %) [103]. In a large contemporary series by Mehta and colleagues, causes of death among patients who died within 30 days of endovascular or open repair of rAAA were described [111]. These included myocardial infarction, bleeding, coagulopathy, MSOF, abdominal compartment syndrome (ACS), colon ischemia, acute respiratory distress syndrome (ARDS), gastrointestinal hemorrhage, pulmonary embolism, and acute hepatic failure [111]. Following either open or endovascular repair, the development of MSOF Once MSOF develops after rAAA repair is associated with a 50–70 % increased mortality rate [105]. Among survivors of endovascular repair for rAAA, complications included ACS (6.6 %), colon ischemia (5.5 %), acute respiratory failure (5.5 %), small bowel obstruction (1.1 %), lower extremity thrombosis (1.1 %), AKI requiring dialysis (1.1 %), MSOF (1.1 %), prolonged ileus (1.1 %), and pulmonary embolism (1.1 %) [111]. Among survivors after open surgical repair, complications included colon ischemia (16.5 %), acute respiratory failure (12.1 %), AKI (8.7 %), myocardial infarction (7.6 %), wound infection (7.6 %), acute cholecystitis (5.5 %), MSOF (3.3 %), ACS (3.3 %), gastrointestinal hemorrhage (1.1 %), acute hepatic failure (1.1 %), and sepsis (1.1 %) (Table 16.4) [111].

Risk Assessment

Various scoring systems have been used as predictors of survival in patients undergoing open surgical repair for rAAA. The Sequential Organ Failure Assessment score (SOFA) is based on six different organ systems: PaO2/FiO2 for respiratory failure, creatinine level or urine output for renal failure, bilirubin for liver failure, Glasgow Coma Scale for neurological impairment, platelet count for coagulopathy, and mean arterial pressure or administration of vasopressors for cardiovascular failure [112]. The Simplified Acute Physiology Score (SAPS II) (0–163) includes seventeen variables composed of twelve physiological variables, age, type of admission, and three different underlying disease variables [113]. The Simplified Therapeutic Intervention Scoring System-28 (TISS-28) score (1–78) is derived from 28 therapeutic activities performed in the ICU which are subdivided into seven groups: basic activities, ventilator support, cardiovascular support, renal support, neurological support, metabolic support, and specific interventions [114]. SOFA and SAPS II scoring systems have been applied to rAAA patients with validation of their utility in early prediction of in-hospital mortality [115]. However, overall prediction of the development of MSOF remains problematic. Interestingly, in hemorrhagic shock following trauma, it has been demonstrated that there is delayed clinical recovery due to MSOF using both clinical and genomic data [116]. This research may prove to be beneficial in treatment of other conditions incited by hemorrhagic shock, such as rAAA.

Procedural Factors Associated with Development of MSOF After rAAA Repair

The most contemporary series by Mehta et al. has shown that 30-day mortality for patients undergoing open surgical repair has been shown to be significantly higher than endovascular repair for rAAA (44.2 % vs. 24.2 %, $p<0.001$) [111]. Our experience has similarly shown that implementation of contemporary endovascular-first protocol for the treatment of a rAAA is associated with decreased perioperative morbidity and mortality, with higher likelihood of discharge to home and improved long-term survival [117, 118]. Most surgeons now believe that patients presenting with rAAA and appropriate anatomy should be offered endovascular repair as first-line treatment at experienced vascular centers [119–123]. The IMPROVE Trial has suggested that patients randomized to an endovascular strategy had reduced stay in the ICU and were discharged home earlier than were patients randomized to open repair [101]. Despite the clear trend toward endovascular repair of rAAA among vascular surgeons [124], some controversies still exist as to benefit of endovascular repair. The IMPROVE trial as well as various retrospective data show equivalent mortality rates in patients undergoing endovascular aneurysm repair (EVAR) for rAAA compared with those undergoing open repair [101, 125]. For further information in the controversial outcomes of IMPROVE trial, refer to Veith Chapter…

Prolonged aortic cross-clamp time during open rAAA repair is associated with MSOF, most notably increasing the rates of AKI and ARDS [126]. Suprarenal and supraceliac aortic clamping during the repair of rAAA are also positive predictors of mortality and have high rates of renal, hepatic, and intestinal injury [127]. With regard to endovascular repair, in our experience we have found that in patients in whom EVAR is attempted for rAAA despite not meeting accepted anatomic criteria for endovascular intervention, the mortality rate is 100 %. Other centers have confirmed this high mortality associated with conversion from endovascular repair to open repair for rAAA [128]. Taken together this data suggests that the overall incidence of MSOF following successful endovascular repair may be lower that open repair with a more rapid return to normal organ function. However, this has not been validated in a randomized clinical trial to date.

Reoperation and Reintervention

The reintervention rate for repair of rAAA, whether open or endovascular, remains high at approximately 20 % [101]. Reintervention after open rAAA repair occurs most commonly due to bleeding, bowel ischemia, or bowel obstruction [101]. Reintervention after endovascular rAAA repair occurs most commonly due to endoleak, graft migration, extremity complications, and limb ischemia [111]. Given that the rate of systemic complications is higher after open rAAA repair, there appears to be an overall reduction in the risk of MSOF overall following endovascular repair compared to open repair.

Abdominal Compartment Syndrome

ACS is characterized by progressive intra-abdominal dysfunction resulting from elevated intra-abdominal pressure (IAP). The term abdominal compartment syndrome was coined by Kron et al. in 1984, when they described the process following rAAA. The classic description of ACS includes a tense distended abdomen, increased IAP, decreased renal function, elevated peak airway pressure, hypoxia, and inadequate ventilation [129]. Although ACS was originally described after open rAAA repair, it is also a known complication after endovascular rAAA repair [130]. The pathophysiology of ACS after rAAA repair is multifactorial; obviously, free intraperitoneal or contained retroperitoneal aneurysm rupture can lead directly to increased intra-abdominal volume. Massive fluid resuscitation, massive transfusion, prolonged cross-clamp or intra-aortic occlusion balloon inflation times, and emergent conversion of modular bifurcated stent graft to unibodied device also contribute to elevated IAP via worsening of ischemia–reperfusion injury. The end result of intra-abdominal hypertension is impaired end-organ perfusion resulting in MSOF. The incidence of ACS after rAAA repair has fallen dramatically from 18 to 25 % in the pre-endovascular era to 1–6 % in contemporary series [101]. While some recent experience (including the IMPROVE trial) has shown equivalent incidence of ACS after endovascular versus open rAAA repair, several other series have shown a significantly higher incidence of ACS after open rAAA repair compared with EVAR. [101, 102, 131] In a study published by Starnes et al. in 2010, ACS was documented in 32 patients over the study period [102]. In the pre-protocol period, 24 patients developed ACS (all open repairs) and nine survived (62.5 % mortality). In the post-protocol period, eight patients had ACS: six open repairs with one survivor (83 % mortality) and two EVARs with one survivor (50 % mortality) [102].

A high index of suspicion is required to diagnose ACS, and patients should be monitored with serial abdominal examinations, bladder pressures, evidence of visceral malperfusion, and difficulty with ventilation. The treatment for ACS is emergent decompressive laparotomy which, depending on the stability of the patient, can be performed either in the ICU or in the operating room.

Colon Ischemia

Colon ischemia remains a serious complication after rAAA repair. In a contemporary series, colon ischemia was observed at a higher rate following open surgery (4 %) compared to EVAR (1.4 %) in treatment of rAAA [132]. Eighteen patients (52 %) died within the first postoperative month; however, the mortality rate due to colon ischemia was not statistically different between open surgery 14/27 (52 %) and EVAR 4/7 (50 %) [132]. Presumed causes of colon ischemia are nonocclusive mesenteric ischemia due to shock or vasopressor drugs, interruption of inferior mesenteric artery or internal iliac artery blood flow, and atheroembolization during repair. Again, a high index of suspicion—particularly among patients who arrive in the ICU after a difficult intraoperative course and requiring ongoing administration of vasoactive agents—is required for diagnosis. Abdominal pain, distension, evidence of ileus, bloody bowel movements, or unexplained clinical deterioration should lead to further workup with laboratory studies and sigmoidoscopy. First-line treatment includes bowel rest, resuscitation, and avoiding vasopressor use, with the majority of cases resolving with expectant management. Once the diagnosis is made, worsening clinical status may herald transmural necrosis or perforation, and laparotomy with colectomy is required for emergent treatment. The development of colon ischemia following rAAA repair is a predicator and potential causative factor in the development of MSOF following rAAA repair.

Cardiac Dysfunction

Various cardiac complications including myocardial infarction, arrhythmias, cardiac arrest, and congestive heart failure are associated with increased mortality after rAAA repair [111]. Patients with rAAA are at higher risk of ischemic heart disease than general population by virtue of similar risk factors and pathogenic mechanisms underlying both diseases [104]. As such, the rate of these complications remains high with myocardial infarction (8–17 %) and arrhythmias (20 %) occurring in a large proportion of patients undergoing rAAA repair [101, 133, 134]. A study done in 2001 has shown that patients with preoperative cardiac arrest following rAAA had an increased overall mortality (85 %) compared with those without cardiac arrest (36 %); of the 80 patients with preoperative cardiac arrest, 53 underwent surgical repair, and 12 of those patients survived (23 %) [135]. Myocardial infarction was observed in 18 % of patients in the postoperative period [135].

The application and removal of an aortic cross clamp also contribute to complex series of hemodynamic perturbations and create increased demand on the heart. Communication with the anesthesiologist while application and removal of aortic cross clamp, continuation of perioperative beta blockers and statins, appropriate resuscitation, and close monitoring in ICU are key to early diagnosis and management of these issues. However, as a result of the marked dysregulation of immune system following rAAA repair, cardiac dysfunction due to a number of secretory chemokines and cytokines that are likely cardiac depressants results in direct cardiac dysfunction. The onset and duration of this dysfunction have not been clearly identified.

Renal Dysfunction

One of the most frequent complications after rAAA repair is AKI with an incidence approaching 50 % in some series [136]. In this series, patients undergoing open rAAA repair had significantly higher rates of AKI compared with those undergoing EVAR (43 % vs. 26 %), despite the iodinated contrast loads and older average age the EVAR patients [137]. Severe AKI is also associated with higher mortality once it develops after rAAA repair [137]. These mortality rates at 30 days are 28 % (open) versus 5 % (endovascular) and at 12 months is 44 % (open) versus 13 % (endovascular) [137]. Factors associated with AKI after rAAA repair include perioperative hemorrhagic shock, intraoperative suprarenal aortic clamping, secondary ischemic injuries, and SIRS [136]. Monitoring of diuresis in the ICU is crucial to management in these patients, and early institution of renal replacement therapy should also be considered. It should be noted, however, that once patients progress to the point of anuric renal failure and dialysis, it is a harbinger of in-hospital mortality.

Respiratory Failure

Studies have shown that open surgical repair of rAAA is associated with higher pulmonary complications compared to endovascular repair (32.4 % vs. 21.7 %) [133]. Administration of large volume of fluids, blood products, prolonged cross-clamp duration, and preexisting pulmonary disease are some of the contributing factors for respiratory failure after rAAA. Management includes monitoring of patient in the ICU, continuation of ventilator support until patient is stabilized, as well as goal-directed fluid and blood product administration. Adjuncts to mechanical ventilation may be required in order to optimize oxygenation following the development of ARDS. In theory these include but are not limited to the use of inhaled nitric oxide, inhaled or systemic administered Flolan, prone positioning, and ECMO. In reality, patients with MSOF after rAAA repair will likely not tolerate many of these more aggressive interventions from a cardiovascular standpoint.

Limb Ischemia

Limb ischemia is a significant complication after the repair of rAAA which is usually diagnosed prior to leaving the operating room by doing mandatory Doppler and pulse examinations. If found, this should be further investigated with aortography and run-off, with access being obtained via the contralateral common femoral artery as that suspected with pathology. The most common causes of limb ischemia after open rAAA repair are problems associated with the distal anastomosis, distal embolus, and occasionally with iliac artery dissection. In our experience, attempting to deal with these issues via endovascular approach first is preferable, reserving reopening of the laparotomy and revising the original anastomosis for cases where endovascular intervention fails. The IMPROVE trial revealed the rate of reintervention due to limb ischemia after open repair following rAAA is 7 % and after endovascular repair is 8 % [101]. Crossover femoral artery to femoral artery bypass can be a valuable "bail-out" procedure when a patient with rAAA has the complication of unilateral limb ischemia and an absent femoral pulse on the side of the ischemic limb. Following endovascular repair, the most common causes of limb ischemia are occlusive issues with the iliac limb extension or distal embolus [138]. Again, these issues should be dealt with via endovascular methods when possible. If this is not possible, then femoral artery to femoral artery bypass or open embolectomy may be required.

Spinal Ischemia

Spinal cord ischemia is a rare complication after open rAAA repair, with an incidence varying from 1 to 2.8 % [139]. This manifests as paraplegia and paresis which can be difficult to diagnose early in patients who are intubated and sedated. Factors associated with spinal cord ischemia include interruption of pelvic blood supply, prolonged cross clamping, preoperative and intraoperative hypotension, and embolization. Unfortunately, there is little to do to prevent or treat this issue other than good surgical technique and appropriate perioperative hemodynamic management and resuscitation.

Strategies to Reduce Multisystem Organ Failure After rAAA

A dedicated ICU team is crucial to providing appropriate resuscitation, close hemodynamic monitoring, and the identification of early complications that are key to ensuring good outcomes in patients after rAAA repair. Appropriate fluid and vasoactive agent management postoperatively plays an important role in the prevention of multisystem organ failure after rAAA. Patients need to be closely monitored in the ICU after rAAA repair with an arterial line, central venous line, Foley catheter, continuous telemetry, serial laboratory tests (ABG, lactate, CBC, BMP, coagulation profile), and serial abdominal, peripheral vascular, and compartment checks. There should be judicious use of crystalloids and blood products to balance adequate resuscitation and prevention of coagulopathy on the one hand with avoidance of pulmonary complications and abdominal compartment syndrome on the other. A combination of central venous pressure, pulse pressure variation, point of care inferior vena cava, and cardiac sonography can be very useful in determining fluid status in these complex patients. Other monitors such as a pulmonary artery catheter (i.e., Swan–Ganz catheter), FloTrac, CardioQ, PiCCO, and LiDCO may also be helpful given particular institutional and provider expertise.

Although attempts to minimize the development of MSOF should be the first-line strategy in managing rAAA patients, there are patients in whom MSOF development is unavoidable. In these patients, it is imperative that the appropriate support measures be in place to minimize progression of organ failure and allow for optimal organ recovery. Often this becomes a game of balance with treatment of one organ system necessarily compromising another (e.g., fluid resuscitation in renal compromise which may worsen pulmonary function). However, the ultimate restoration of overall homeostasis will decrease the systemic inflammatory response and eventually be optimal for all organ systems. Additionally, consistent attempts to minimize the development of additional organ failure by rapidly correcting and identifying complications such as ACS, colon ischemia, limb ischemia, and infection must occur, and this is best accomplished through a high intensity ICU care model.

Dedicated ICU teams and regionalized care with high-volume aortic centers have shown promise in improving outcomes in patients with rAAA [140]. Specifically, regionalization of care has shown improved mortality and decreased length of stay and cost for rAAA patients [121, 141]. However, although currently merely supportive, future therapies will be directed at mitigating and controlling the dysregulated immunity associated with ischemia–reperfusion. But these therapies, contrary to previous trials will need to be patient specific dealing with individual differences in their immune dysregulation with the hope of inhibiting the development of MSOF.

Management of Endoleaks After rEVAR

Khanjan H. Nagarsheth and Saum A. Rahimi

Background

Since Parodi introduced the concept of endovascular aortic aneurysm repair (EVAR) in 1990 [142], endovascular techniques and technology have gained much acceptance in managing not only elective but also ruptured AAA. Today dozens of large single center and multicenter studies have documented the feasibility and safety of rEVAR, and many have gone on to show short- and long-term survival advantage of rEVAR when compared to open surgical repair [143–148]. The debate however continues as controversial conclusions from the most recent randomized trial have failed to indicate rEVAR survival advantage when compared to ruptured open surgical repair [145] (*more on this discussed in later chapter by Veith*). With ongoing technological advancements in imaging, devices, and techniques, it is reasonable to believe that outcomes will continue to improve for rEVAR and may one day become the gold standard for repair of ruptured abdominal aortic aneurysms (rAAA).

Endovascular aortic aneurysm repair for rAAA has complications that are unique to this surgical technique such as graft migration, contrast-induced nephropathy, and, in particular, endoleaks. Endoleaks are defined as persistence of blood flow into the aneurysm sac, following deployment of an endoluminal stent graft. This particular adverse event can prove to be worrisome as persistent blood flow can continue to pressurize the aneurysm sac and can lead to both sac expansion and rupture. The ideal method of detection and management of endoleaks following rEVAR remains a source of controversy. Although there are five major types of endoleaks discussed in the literature, there are only three that are clinically relevant at the time of rEVAR. In this chapter, we will review the classification of endoleaks and relevance and management options of these endoleaks following rEVAR.

Classification

Endoleaks were first described in 1997 and five major types were identified [149]. They coined the term "endoleak" to describe the inability to obtain or maintain a secure seal between a vessel wall and a transluminally implanted intra-aneurysmal graft. Following this, the Society for Vascular Surgery and the American Association for Vascular Surgery (SVS/AAVS) further standardized the classification of endoleaks [150]. The classification of endoleaks was based on either time of occurrence relative to the EVAR procedure or the site of origin [151].

Endoleaks occurring within 30 days of the EVAR procedure were deemed a primary endoleak, and those that occurred following this 30-day window were called secondary endoleaks [152]. Those endoleaks that appeared after resolution, be it spontaneous or following intervention, were termed recurrent endoleaks. This system of classification had helped in terms of standardizing terminology based on the temporal relationship between time of procedure and identification of endoleak but did not help in management decision.

Another classification system based on origin of blood flow into the aneurysm was devised to aid in determining management. The anatomic classification of endoleaks is based on how blood is flowing into the aneurysm sac. The Ad Hoc Committee for Standardized Reporting Practices in Vascular Surgery created four major types of endoleaks and a fifth group that was an endoleak of unidentified origin.

Type I endoleaks are due to continued blood flow into the aneurysm sac through a channel between the arterial surface and the endoluminal stent graft at either the proximal or distal ends of the graft. This type I endoleak is further subclassified into type Ia for leaks occurring at the proximal extent of the graft and type Ib for those occurring at the distal extent of the graft. In the case of an aorto-uni-iliac (AUI) device, persistent blood flow around the contralateral iliac occlusion device is termed a type Ic endoleak. A type II endoleak occurs when there is blood flow into the aneurysm sac from collateral vessels, the inferior mesenteric artery, or lumbar artery branches. Since there is a robust system of collateral vessels in this region, it is important to identify both the inflow and outflow vessels contributing to the type II endoleak. Type III endoleaks are caused by either a tear in the fabric of the graft, disruption of the graft, modular disconnection, or even graft disintegration over time. Type III endoleaks are further subclassified into type IIIa if the leak is due to modular disconnection and type IIIb if there is a tear in the fabric covering of the stent graft. The type IIIb endoleak is again further stratified into minor or major if the tear is less than 2 mm or greater than or equal to 2 mm in size, respectively.

Management Options

Type I Endoleaks

Type I endoleaks must be dealt with expeditiously when they are encountered. This is because blood is entering the aneurysm sac directly with systemic arterial pressure. Dias and colleagues found that up to 93 % of systemic pressure was transmitted into the sac from type I endoleaks [153]. This can result in the sac being highly pressurized and increases the risk of aneurysm expansion and rupture. As many as 10 % of patients will have a type I endoleak within the first 30 days and require reintervention [154].

Historically, certain criteria were used to describe proximal aortic neck anatomy that was suitable for an endovascular repair. These anatomic features included an infra-renal section of healthy aorta: measuring 10–15 mm in length, at most 32 mm in diameter, angulation of less than 60°, minimal thrombus or calcification in the neck, and no evidence of tapered or reversed taped anatomy [155, 156]. Advancements in the technology of endoluminal aortic stent grafts have helped to reduce type Ia endoleaks and facilitate performing EVAR in even more challenging neck anatomy. If a type Ia endoleak occurs, there are several endovascular treatment options available. The first step should involve gently inflating a compliant balloon at the proximal or distal extent of the stent graft to obtain better wall apposition. If the endoleak persists after ballooning, and there is still healthy infrarenal aortic length available, placing a proximal or distal extension cuff may be an option as well [157]. If there is still an endoleak, placing a bare metal stent—such as a balloon mounted, stainless steel Palmaz stent (Cordis Endovascular, Fremont, CA)—can aid in providing increased radial force and pushing the aortic endoluminal stent against the arterial wall.

For patients who survive beyond the rEVAR and have a persistent type Ia endoleak, embolization procedures may be attempted using a variety of thrombogenic coils, embolic devices, and n-butyl 2-cyanoacrylate adhesive and fibrin glue embolization [156–160]. With the addition of these adjunctive measures, previous authors have reported resolution of type Ia endoleaks in up to 92.3 % of cases [158]. Injection of fibrin glue has also been shown in animal models to reduce systemic pressure transmitted to the aortic wall, thereby reducing wall stress. Therefore, the use of fibrin glue may serve to eliminate type Ia endoleaks and reduce wall stress [161]. It should be noted that employing these endovascular procedures to treat a type Ia endoleak could significantly increase the operative time in rEVAR that can be detrimental to an unstable patient. There is a paucity of evidence showing the utility of these techniques in the treatment of a rAAA, but nevertheless, these are options available to the surgeon or interventionalist.

More recently, the introduction of chimneys, snorkels, and fenestrated aortic endoluminal stent grafts has shown even further reduction in the rates of type Ia endoleaks. In the case of treating rAAA with rEVAR, if the patient still has a large type Ia endoleak, the decision must be made whether or not to employ these techniques. These procedures increase the operative time and morbidity for patients and therefore should be used sparingly with the current generation of devices available, when treating an unstable patient [162].

Endoleaks occurring at the distal extent of an endoluminal stent graft, type Ib, are most commonly due to hostile iliac artery anatomy. This hostile anatomy can include aneurysmal degeneration or a very tortuous course causing imprecise deployment of the stent graft. Additionally, if there is significant calcific disease of the iliac arteries, this can interfere with good wall apposition of the stent graft. In most cases, type Ib endoleaks are treatable with distal extension of the stent graft. Often times this will require coverage of the hypogastric artery and extension into the external iliac artery. In the case of a rAAA, if the patient is unstable, we advocate the use of this technique without coil embolization of the hypogastric artery. This will often times result in a type II endoleak but may allow for stabilization of the patient so this can be addressed at a later time. In their recent work, Quinn and colleagues found a lower incidence of type II endoleaks in rEVAR patients but hypothesized that this may be due to a selection bias, as the rEVAR patients may have died before a type II endoleak developed [163].

If the hypogastric artery needs to be covered to achieve seal, it should first be coil embolized to prevent occurrence of a type II endoleak. In cases where the hypogastric artery needs to be preserved or there is aneurysmal degeneration of the common iliac artery, one may employ use of the "sandwich" technique or iliac branched device [164]. Currently iliac branched devices are still in investigational trials and not available for general use. The "sandwich" technique is an alternative that requires placing two parallel endoluminal stents into an iliac artery limb graft to recreate the iliac bifurcation. The authors recommend oversizing the cross-sectional area of the combined grafts to 30 % greater than the cross section of the iliac limb. This is done to reduce the chance of a type III endoleak. The purpose of this technique is to prevent the relatively high incidence of buttock claudication with unilateral hypogastric artery coverage or pelvic ischemia when the hypogastric artery is covered bilaterally [165].

Though these techniques are well tolerated in the elective setting, they do increase operative time and complexity. Therefore, these results may not be translated the same way when performed in conjunction with rEVAR. Current evidence would suggest that under elective circumstances, nearly 1/3 of type I endoleaks might resolve in select patients with conservative management. However, with paucity of data, it is unlikely that rEVAR patients with untreated type I endoleaks would have favorable outcomes.

Type II Endoleaks

Type II endoleaks complicate almost 30 % of EVAR performed for AAA [166]. These are the most commonly encountered endoleaks and, as mentioned previously, are the results of retrograde flow from lumber arteries, the inferior mesenteric artery, or collateral vessels. The classification for type II endoleaks is based upon the number of vessels contributing to the leak. Type IIa endoleaks occur due to a single vessel, whereas type IIb endoleaks are due to multiple vessels flowing into the aneurysm sac. Up to 80 % of type II endoleaks will spontaneously resolve and require no further intervention within 6 months of the initial aneurysm repair. For those type II endoleaks that persist beyond 6 months, there is an increased risk of aneurysm sac enlargement and increased rupture risk [167]. Quinn and colleagues found a higher rate of type II endoleaks in elective EVAR compared to rEVAR (20.1 % vs. 9 %, $p<0.001$) [163]. As mentioned earlier, this may be a result of elective EVAR surviving longer and have a type II endoleak detected. In the setting of rEVAR, there is never an indication to urgently repair a type II endoleak, but if there is expansion of the sac at follow up, then intervention may be warranted.

There are different recommendations found throughout the literature in regard to when to intervene on type II endoleaks, but a consensus appears to exist that if the aneurysm sac is growing, it should be repaired [168]. The mere presence of a type II endoleak is not an indication for repair, and this was shown in the EUROSTAR data. The EUROSTAR study identified nine delayed ruptures following EVAR in 421 patients with a type II endoleak. Eight of these nine patients had a simultaneously occurring type I endoleak, and following multivariate regression analysis, the presence of a type II endoleak was not found to be a statistically significant risk factor for AAA rupture [169]. However, the EUROSTAR trial did identified patients with type II endoleaks to have a higher need for secondary interventions and open conversions, but not aneurysm rupture. This data was also corroborated by others that have shown the persistence of type II endoleaks to have an association with increased risks for secondary interventions and a small yet persistent risk for aneurysm rupture when associated with aneurysm sac growth [167].

If the decision is made to intervene upon a type II endoleak, there are several options available to treat this entity. These options are divided into three categories: transarterial, direct puncture of the aneurysm sac, and surgical ligation. Transarterial methods are typically employed first once an intervention is deemed necessary. Aortography is performed initially to help exclude a type I endoleak. Then selective angiography of the superior mesenteric and hypogastric arteries should be performed to identify late filling of the inferior mesenteric artery (IMA) and contrast blush in the aneurysm sac. If blush is seen, a microcatheter can be advanced into the IMA for either coil or polymer embolization. An important caveat to this technique is that embolization should not be performed if the origin of the IMA cannot be reached. The risk of distal IMA embolization is colonic ischemia, and this risk is mitigated by selectively embolization of the IMA at its origin [170]. With this technique, there is risk of recanalization of the feeding vessel or new collateral vessels forming to feed the aneurysm sac, thereby requiring reintervention [171].

The next approach to treat type II endoleaks is via direct puncture of the aneurysm sac. This procedure is performed in conjunction with computed tomography (CT), fluoroscopy, or ultrasound guidance. Access must be obtained into the endoleak cavity, and once this is confirmed with injection of contrast, the cavity can be closed using a variety of coils, glues, and hemostatic agents. Success for this technique is reported in the literature as over 80 % at 1 year [172].

If this technique is not successful, percutaneous translumbar access can be attempted. This procedure requires the patient to be in prone position and the left lumbar arteries are preferred for access to avoid the vena cava. Most interventionalists and surgeons will approach this with either ultrasound or fluoroscopic guidance, and once access is obtained, the best results are with selective embolization into the aneurysm sac [173, 174].

Surgical options for treatment of type II endoleaks should be reserved for patients with identified expansion of the aneurysm sac after attempts have been made transarterially or via direct sac puncture. Clipping of feeding vessels can be performed laparoscopically and has shown good results [175]. Care should be taken to clip these vessels close to the aneurysm sac, to avoid ischemic complications. It is often difficult to identify the exact feeding vessel during open exploration from outside the aneurysm sac. The aneurysm sac should be opened and the thrombus evacuated, and the intra-sac ligation of the feeding vessels needs to be performed to control all possible branches feeding the aneurysm sac. Following this, the sac should close over the endoluminal stent graft with imbricating sutures to reduce any possible dead space.

Type III Endoleaks

As mentioned previously, type III endoleaks are subdivided into two major categories, type IIIa, due to modular disconnections in the endoluminal graft, and type IIIb, which occur secondary to tears in the fabric covering the graft. With current generations of endoluminal aortic stent grafts, type III endoleaks are very rare, and the reported incidence is anywhere from 0 to 4 % in the literature [176].

Type IIIa endoleaks occur when there is separation of modular components of the stent graft. The reason for this separation is due to the arterial pressure and flow entering the graft. This pressure causes the graft to slowly take on the outer curvature of the aneurysm sac, and if there is insufficient stent graft overlap, separation will occur. Erosion of the fabric component of an endoluminal stent graft represents a type IIIb endoleak. One proposed mechanism for this occurring includes a primary stent suture break that allows the stent to become mobile and move as blood flows through the graft. Over time this movement can cause erosions in the fabric [177]. All type III endoleaks should be repaired as soon as they are identified, as they result in a direct communication between the arterial system and the aneurysm sac [178].

Treatment of type III endoleaks aims at restoring the integrity of the graft-aneurysm interface. Relining the damaged graft or bridging the section of separation with an additional component stent graft can usually repair this. If the gap or tear is too large, the rEVAR can be converted to an AUI with contralateral iliac limb occlusion, and then a femoral to femoral artery crossover bypass is constructed.

Conclusions

In cases of rAAA with hostile anatomy, rEVAR can be performed and, even if an endoleak is present, serve as a bridge until the patient stabilizes. After the patient is stable, the endoleak can be addressed, depending on the type encountered. Some endoleaks are of very low clinical significance and self-limited but those that provide a direct connection between the systemic arterial pressure and aneurysm sac require urgent attention and repair. Emerging technologies in the field of aortic repair are pushing the boundaries in terms of what anatomy can be approached endovascularly, and many are aimed at reducing the occurrence of endoleaks. Surveillance should continue lifelong following rEVAR to help detect clinically significant endoleaks that may require reintervention.

References

Ischemic Colitis After Ruptured Abdominal Aortic Aneurysm Repair

1. Shaw RS, Green TH. Massive mesenteric infarction following inferior mesenteric artery ligation in resection of the colon for carcinoma. N Engl J Med. 1953;248:890.
2. Boley SJ, Schwartz S, Lash J, Sternhill V. Reversible vascular occlusion of the colon. Surg Gynecol Obstet. 1963;116:53–60.
3. Marston A, Pheils MT, Thomas ML, Morson BC. Ischemic colitis. Gut. 1966;7(1):1–15.
4. Perry RJ, Martin MJ, Eckert MJ, Sohn VY, Steele SR. Colonic ischemia complicating open vs endovascular abdominal aortic aneurysm repair. J Vasc Surg. 2008;48(2):272–7.
5. Brandt LJ, Boley SJ. Colonic ischemia. Surg Clin N Am. 1992;72:203–29.
6. Tottrup M, Fedder AM, Jensen RH, Tottrup A, Laustsen J. The value of routine flexible sigmoidoscopy within 48 hours after surgical repair of ruptured abdominal aortic aneurysms. Ann Vasc Surg. 2013;27(6):714–8.
7. Bjorck M, Bergqvist D, Troeng T. Incidence and clinical presentation of bowel ischaemia after aortoiliac surgery – 2930 operations from a population-based registry in Sweden. Eur J Vasc Endovasc Surg Off J Eur Soc Vasc Surg. 1996;12(2):139–44.
8. Sandison AJ, Panayiotopoulos Y, Edmondson RC, Tyrrell MR, Taylor PR. A 4-year prospective audit of the cause of death after infrarenal aortic aneurysm surgery. Br J Surg. 1996;83(10):1386–9.
9. Longo WE, Ballantyne GH, Gusberg RJ. Ischemic colitis: patterns and prognosis. Dis Colon Rectum. 1992;35(8):726–30.

10. Longo WE, Lee TC, Barnett MG, et al. Ischemic colitis complicating abdominal aortic aneurysm surgery in the U.S. veteran. J Surg Res. 1996;60(2):351–4.
11. Gandhi SK, Hanson MM, Vernava AM, Kaminski DL, Longo WE. Ischemic colitis. Dis Colon Rectum. 1996;39(1):88–100.
12. Yamazaki T, Shirai Y, Tada T, Sasaki M, Sakai Y, Hatakeyama K. Ischemic colitis arising in watershed areas of the colonic blood supply: a report of two cases. Surg Today. 1997;27(5):460–2.
13. Assadian A, Assadian O, Senekowitsch C, et al. Plasma D-lactate as a potential early marker for colon ischaemia after open aortic reconstruction. Eur J Vasc Endovasc Surg. 2006;31(5):470–4.
14. Neary P. Gastrointestinal complications of abdominal aortic aneurysms, diagnosis, screening and treatment of abdominal, thoracoabdominal and thoracic aortic aneurysms, Prof Reinhart Grundmann, editors. 2011(Chapter 2.3):245–68.
15. Neary P, Hurson C, Briain DO, Brabazon A, Mehigan D, Keaveny TV, et al. Abdominal aortic aneurysm repair and colonic infarction: a risk factor appraisal. Colorectal Dis Off J Assoc Coloproctol Great Britain Ireland. 2007;9(2):166–72.
16. Becquemin JP, Majewski M, Fermani N, Marzelle J, Desgrandes P, Allaire E, et al. Colon ischemia following abdominal aortic aneurysm repair in the era of endovascular abdominal aortic repair. J Vasc Surg. 2008;47(2):258–63; discussion 63.
17. Reimerink JJ, Hoornweg LL, Vahl AC, Wisselink W, van den Broek TA, Legemate DA, et al. Endovascular repair versus open repair of ruptured abdominal aortic aneurysms: a multicenter randomized controlled trial. Ann Surg. 2013;258(2):248–56.
18. Welborn 3rd MB, Seeger JM. Prevention and management of sigmoid and pelvic ischemia associated with aortic surgery. Semin Vasc Surg. 2001;14(4):255–65.
19. Senekowitsch C, Assadian A, Assadian O, Hartleb H, Ptakovsky H, Hagmuller GW. Replanting the inferior mesentery artery during infrarenal aortic aneurysm repair: influence on postoperative colon ischemia. J Vasc Surg. 2006;43(4):689–94.
20. Redaelli CA, Schilling MK, Carrel TP. Intraoperative assessment of intestinal viability by laser Doppler flowmetry for surgery of ruptured abdominal aortic aneurysms. World J Surg. 1998;22(3):283–9.
21. Yamamoto M, Sasaguri S, Sato T. Assessing intraoperative blood flow in cardiovascular surgery. Surg Today. 2011;41(11):1467–74.
22. Boni L, David G, Mangano A, Dionigi G, Rausei S, Spampatti S, Cassinotti E, Fingerhut A. Clinical applications of indocyanine green (ICG) enhanced fluorescence in laparoscopic surgery. Surg Endosc. 2014;29:2046–55. [Epub ahead of print].
23. Lee ES, Bass A, Arko FR, Heikkinen M, Harris EJ, Zarins CK, et al. Intraoperative colon mucosal oxygen saturation during aortic surgery. J Surg Res. 2006;136(1):19–24.
24. Bjorck M, Troeng T, Bergqvist D. Risk factors for intestinal ischaemia after aortoiliac surgery: a combined cohort and case–control study of 2824 operations. Eur J Vasc Endovasc Surg Off J Eur Soc Vasc Surg. 1997;13(6):531–9.
25. Dadian N, Ohki T, Veith FJ, Edelman M, Mehta M, Lipsitz EC, et al. Overt colon ischemia after endovascular aneurysm repair: the importance of microembolization as an etiology. J Vasc Surg. 2001;34(6):986–96.
26. Mehta M, Veith FJ, Ohki T, Cynamon J, Goldstein K, Suggs WD, et al. Unilateral and bilateral hypogastric artery interruption during aortoiliac aneurysm repair in 154 patients: a relatively innocuous procedure. J Vasc Surg. 2001;33(2 Suppl):S27–32.
27. Wolpert LM, Dittrich KP, Hallisey MJ, Allmendinger PP, Gallagher JJ, Heydt K, et al. Hypogastric artery embolization in endovascular abdominal aortic aneurysm repair. J Vasc Surg. 2001;33(6):1193–8.
28. Arko FR, Lee WA, Hill BB, Fogarty TJ, Zarins CK. Hypogastric artery bypass to preserve pelvic circulation: improved outcome after endovascular abdominal aortic aneurysm repair. J Vasc Surg. 2004;39(2):404–8.
29. Karch LA, Hodgson KJ, Mattos MA, Bohannon WT, Ramsey DE, McLafferty RB. Adverse consequences of internal iliac artery occlusion during endovascular repair of abdominal aortic aneurysms. J Vasc Surg. 2000;32(4):676–83.

30. Ernst CB, Hagihara PF, Daughtery ME, Sachatello CR, Griffen Jr WO. Ischemic colitis incidence following abdominal aortic reconstruction: a prospective study. Surgery. 1976;80(4):417–21.
31. Israeli D, Dardik H, Wolodiger F, Silvestri F, Scherl B, Chessler R. Pelvic radiation therapy as a risk factor for ischemic colitis complicating abdominal aortic reconstruction. J Vasc Surg. 1996;23(4):706–9.
32. Balthazar EJ, Yen BC, Gordon RB. Ischemic colitis: CT evaluation of 54 cases. Radiology. 1999;211:381–8.
33. Brandt CP, Piotrowski JJ, Alexander JJ. Flexible sigmoidoscopy. A reliable determinant of colonic ischemia following ruptured abdominal aortic aneurysm. Surg Endosc. 1997;11(2):113–5.
34. Macdonald PH. Ischaemic colitis. Best Pract Res Clin Gastroenterol. 2002;16:51–61.
35. Steele SR. Ischemic colitis complicating major vascular surgery. Surg Clin North Am. 2007;87(5):1099–114, ix.
36. Megalopoulos A, Vasiliadis K, Tsalis K, Kapetanos D, Bitzani M, Tsachalis T, et al. Reliability of selective surveillance colonoscopy in the early diagnosis of colonic ischemia after successful ruptured abdominal aortic aneurysm repair. Vasc Endovascular Surg. 2007;41(6):509–15.
37. Champagne BJ, Darling 3rd RC, Daneshmand M, Kreienberg PB, Lee EC, Mehta M, et al. Outcome of aggressive surveillance colonoscopy in ruptured abdominal aortic aneurysm. J Vasc Surg. 2004;39(4):792–6.
38. Houe T, Thorboll JE, Sigild U, Liisberg-Larsen O, Schroeder TV. Can colonoscopy diagnose transmural ischaemic colitis after abdominal aortic surgery? An evidence-based approach. Eur J Vasc Endovasc Surg Off J Eur Soc Vasc Surg. 2000;19(3):304–7.
39. Scharff JR, Longo WE, Vartanian SM, et al. Ischemic colitis: spectrum of disease and outcome. Surgery. 2003;134:624–30.
40. Schneider DB, Nelken NA, Messina LM, Ehrenfeld WK. Isolated inferior mesenteric artery revascularization for chronic visceral ischemia. J Vasc Surg. 1999;30(1):51–8.
41. Rapp JH, Reilly LM, Qvarfordt PG, Goldstone J, Ehrenfeld WK, Stoney RJ. Durability of endarterectomy and antegrade grafts in the treatment of chronic visceral ischemia. J Vasc Surg. 1986;3(5):799–806.
42. Bailey JA, Jacobs DL, Bahadursingh A, Longo WE. Endovascular treatment of segmental ischemic colitis. Dig Dis Sci. 2005;50(4):774–9.

Abdominal compartment syndrome following ruptured abdominal aortic aneurysm

43. Malbrain ML, Cheatham ML, Kirkpatrick A, Sugrue M, Parr M, de Waele J, et al. Results from the International Conference Experts on Intra-abdominal Hypertension and Abdominal Compartment Syndrome. I Definitions. Intensive Care Med. 2006;32:1722–32.
44. Cheatham ML, Malbrain ML, Kirkpatrick A, Sugrue M, Parr M, de Waele J, et al. Results from the International Conference Experts on Intra-abdominal Hypertension and Abdominal Compartment Syndrome. II Recommendations. Intensive Care Med. 2007;33:951–62.
45. Kron IL, Harmon PK, Nolan SP. The measurement of intra-abdominal pressure as a criterion for abdominal re-exploration. Ann Surg. 1984;199:28–30.
46. Björck M, Hedberg B. Early detection of major complications after abdominal aortic surgery: predictive value of sigmoid colon and gastric intramucosal pH monitoring. Br J Surg. 1994;81:25–30.
47. Björck M, Troëng T, Bergqvist D. Risk factors for intestinal ischaemia after aortoiliac surgery. A combined cohort and case–control study of 2824 operations. Eur J Vasc Endovasc Surg. 1997;13:531–9.

48. Björck M, Broman G, Lindberg F, Bergqvist D. pHi-monitoring of the sigmoid colon after aortoiliac surgery. A five-year prospective study. Eur J Vasc Endovasc Surg. 2000;20:273–80.
49. Makar RR, Badger SA, O'Donell ME, Loan W, Lau LL, Soong CV. The effects of abdominal compartment hypertension after open and endovascular repair of a ruptured abdominal aortic aneurysm. J Vasc Surg. 2009;49:866–72.
50. Djavani K, Wanhainen A, Valtysson J, Björck M. Colonic ischaemia and intra-abdominal hypertension following open repair of ruptured abdominal aortic aneurysm. Br J Surg. 2009;96:621–7.
51. Mayer D, Rancic Z, Meier C, Pfammatter T, Veith FJ, Lachat M. Open abdomen treatment following endovascular repair of ruptured abdominal aortic aneurysms. J Vasc Surg. 2009;50(1):1–7.
52. Kirkpatrick A, Roberts DJ, De Waele J, Jaeschke R, Malbrain ML, De Kuelenaer B, Duchesne J, Björck M, et al. Intra-abdominal hypertension and the abdominal compartment syndrome: updated consensus definitions and clinical practice guidelines from the world society of the abdominal compartment syndrome. Intensive Care Med. 2013;39:1190–206.
53. Platell CF, Hall J, Clarke G, Lawrence-Brown M. Intra-abdominal pressure and renal function after surgery to the abdominal aorta. Aust N Z J Surg. 1990;60:213–6.
54. Djavani K, Wanhainen A, Björck M. Intra-abdominal hypertension and abdominal compartment syndrome following surgery for ruptured abdominal aortic aneurysm. Eur J Vasc Endovasc Surg. 2006;31:581–4.
55. Djavani-Gidlund K, Wanhainen A, Björck M. Intraabdominal hypertension and abdominal compartment syndrome after endovascular repair of ruptured abdominal aortic aneurysm. Eur J Vasc Endovasc Surg. 2011;41:742–7.
56. Balogh Z, McKinley BA, Cocanour CS, Kozar RA, Valdivia A, Sailors RM, et al. Supranormal trauma resuscitation causes more cases of abdominal compartment syndrome. Arch Surg. 2003;138:637–43.
57. Mell MW, O'Neil AS, Callcut RA, Acher CW, Hoch JR, Tefera G, Turnipseed WD. Effect of early plasma transfusion on mortality in patients with ruptured abdominal aortic aneurysm. Surgery. 2010;148:955–62.
58. Volodos NL, Shekhanin VE, Karpovich IP, Troian VI, Gur'ev IA. [A self-fixing synthetic blood vessel endoprosthesis]. Vestn Khir Im I I Grek. 1986;137:123–5.
59. Volodos NL. The 30th anniversary of the first clinical application of endovascular stentgrafting. Eur J Vasc Endovasc Surg. 2015;49:495–7.
60. Ohki T, Veith FJ. Endovascular grafts and other image-guided catheter-based adjuncts to improve the treatment of ruptured aortoiliac aneurysms. Ann Surg. 2000;232:466–79.
61. Sörelius K, Wanhainen A, Acosta S, Svensson M, Djavani-Gidlund K, Björck M. Open abdomen treatment after aortic aneurysm repair with vacuum-assisted wound closure and mesh-mediated fascial traction. Eur J Vasc Endovasc Surg. 2013;45:588–94.
62. Ersryd S, Djavani-Gidlund K, Wanhainen A, Björck M. Editor's choice: Abdominal compartment syndrome after surgery for abdominal aortic aneurysm: a nationwide population-based study. Eur J Vasc Endovasc Surg. 2016; 52:158–165.
63. Hörer T, Skoog P, Pirouzram A, Larzon T. Tissue plasminogen activator–assisted hematoma evacuation to relieve abdominal compartment syndrome after endovascular repair of ruptured abdominal aortic aneurysm. J Endovasc Ther. 2012;19:144–8.
64. Reintam Blaser A, Starkopf J. Should we use early enteral nutrition in all intensive care patients? Int J Abdom Res. 2013;1:59–63.
65. Reintam Blaser A, Björck M, De Keulenaer B, Regli A. Abdominal compliance: a bench-to-bedside review. J Trauma Acute Care Surg. 2015;78:1044–53.
66. Abouassaly CT, Dutton WD, Zaydfudim V, Dossett LA, Nunez TC, Fleming SB, Cotton BA. Postoperative neuromuscular blocker use is associated with higher primary fascial closure rates after damage control laparotomy. J Trauma. 2010;69:557–61.
67. Papazian L, Forel J-M, Gacouin A, et al. Neuromuscular blockers in early respiratory distress syndrome. N Engl J Med. 2010;363:1107–16.

68. DeWaele JJ, Kimball E, Malbrain M, Nesbitt, Cohen J, Kaloiani V, Ivantury R, Mone M, Debergh D, Bjorck. Laparotomy for Abdominal Compartment Syndrome. Br J Surg. 2016;103:709–15.
69. Oelschlager BK, Boyle EM, Johansen K, Meissner MH. Delayed abdominal closure in the management of ruptured abdominal aortic aneurysms. Am J Surg. 1997;172:411–5.
70. Björck M, Wanhainen A. Management of abdominal compartment syndrome and the open abdomen. Eur J Vasc Endovasc Surg. 2014;47:279–87.
71. Björck M, Wanhainen A, Djavani K, Acosta S. The clinical importance of monitoring intra-abdominal pressure after ruptured abdominal aortic aneurysm repair. Scand J Surg. 2008;97:183–90.
72. Björck M. Management of the tense abdomen or difficult abdominal closure following operation for ruptured AAA. Semin Vasc Surg. 2012;25:35–8.
73. Björck M, Bruhin A, Cheatham M, Hinck D, Kaplan M, Manca G, Wild T, Windsor A. Classification, an important step to improve the management of patients with an open abdomen. World J Surg. 2009;33:1154–7.
74. Björck M, D'Amours SK, Hamilton AER. Closure of the open abdomen. Am Surg. 2011;77:S58–61.
75. Rasilainen SK, Mentula PJ, Leppäniemi AK. Microbial colonization of open abdomen in critically ill surgical patients. World J Emerg Surg. 2015;10:25.
76. Boele van Hensbroek P, Wind J, Dijkgraaf MG, Busch OR, Goslings JC. Temporary closure of the abdomen: a systematic review on delayed primary fascial closure in patients with an open abdomen. World J Surg. 2009;33:199–207.
77. Brock WB, Barker DE, Burns RP. Temporary closure of open abdominal wounds: the vacuum pack. Am Surg. 1995;61:30–5.
78. Petersson U, Acosta S, Björck M. Vacuum-assisted wound closure and mesh-mediated fascial traction – a novel technique for late closure of the open abdomen. World J Surg. 2007;31:2133–7.
79. Acosta S, Bjarnason T, Pettersson U, Pålsson B, Wanhainen A, Svensson M, Djavani K, Björck M. Multicentre prospective study of fascial closure rate after open abdomen with vacuum and mesh-mediated fascial traction. Br J Surg. 2011;98:735–43.
80. Seternes A, Myhre HO, Dahl T. Early results after treatment of open abdomen after aortic surgery with mesh traction and vacuum-assisted wound closure. Eur J Vasc Endovasc Surg. 2010;40:60–4.
81. Rasilainen SK, Mentula PJ, Leppäniemi AK. Vacuum and mesh-mediated fascial traction for primary closure of the open abdomen in critically ill surgical patients. Br J Surg. 2012;99:1725–32.
82. Mani K, Björck M, Wanhainen A. Changes in the management of infrarenal abdominal aortic aneurysm disease in Sweden. Br J Surg. 2013;100:638–44.

Spinal Cord Protection in Emergency Aortic Surgery

83. Ullery BW, Cheung AT, Fairman RM, et al. Risk factors, outcomes, and clinical manifestations of spinal cord ischemia following thoracic endovascular aortic repair. J Vasc Surg. 2011;54(3):677–84.
84. Wong CS, Healy D, Canning C, Coffey JC, Boyle JR, Walsh SR. A systematic review of spinal cord injury and cerebrospinal fluid drainage after thoracic aortic endografting. J Vasc Surg. 2012;56(5):1438–47.
85. Amabile P, Grisoli D, Giorgi R, Bartoli JM, Piquet P. Incidence and determinants of spinal cord ischaemia in stent-graft repair of the thoracic aorta. Eur J Vasc Endovasc Surg. 2008;35(4):455–61.

86. Estrera AL, Miller 3rd CC, Huynh TT, et al. Preoperative and operative predictors of delayed neurologic deficit following repair of thoracoabdominal aortic aneurysm. J Thorac Cardiovasc Surg. 2003;126(5):1288–94.
87. Buth J, Harris PL, Hobo R, et al. Neurologic complications associated with endovascular repair of thoracic aortic pathology: Incidence and risk factors. a study from the European Collaborators on Stent/Graft Techniques for Aortic Aneurysm Repair (EUROSTAR) registry. J Vasc Surg. 2007;46(6):1103–10; discussion 1110–1101.
88. Czerny M, Eggebrecht H, Sodeck G, et al. Mechanisms of symptomatic spinal cord ischemia after TEVAR: insights from the European Registry of Endovascular Aortic Repair Complications (EuREC). J Endovasc Ther. 2012;19(1):37–43.
89. Desai ND, Pochettino A, Szeto WY, et al. Thoracic endovascular aortic repair: evolution of therapy, patterns of use, and results in a 10-year experience. J Thorac Cardiovasc Surg. 2011;142(3):587–94.
90. Augoustides JG, Stone ME, Drenger B. Novel approaches to spinal cord protection during thoracoabdominal aortic interventions. Curr Opin Anaesthesiol. 2014;27(1):98–105.
91. Cheung AT, Pochettino A, McGarvey ML, et al. Strategies to manage paraplegia risk after endovascular stent repair of descending thoracic aortic aneurysms. Ann Thorac Surg. 2005;80(4):1280–8; discussion 1288–1289.
92. Feezor RJ, Lee WA. Strategies for detection and prevention of spinal cord ischemia during TEVAR. Semin Vasc Surg. 2009;22(3):187–92.
93. Hnath JC, Mehta M, Taggert JB, et al. Strategies to improve spinal cord ischemia in endovascular thoracic aortic repair: outcomes of a prospective cerebrospinal fluid drainage protocol. J Vasc Surg. 2008;48(4):836–40.
94. Keith Jr CJ, Passman MA, Carignan MJ, et al. Protocol implementation of selective postoperative lumbar spinal drainage after thoracic aortic endograft. J Vasc Surg. 2012;55(1):1–8; discussion 8.
95. Uchida N. How to prevent spinal cord injury during endovascular repair of thoracic aortic disease. Gen Thorac Cardiovasc Surg. 2014;62(7):391–7.
96. Bobadilla JL, Wynn M, Tefera G, Acher CW. Low incidence of paraplegia after thoracic endovascular aneurysm repair with proactive spinal cord protective protocols. J Vasc Surg. 2013;57(6):1537–42.
97. Riambau V, Capoccia L, Mestres G, Matute P. Spinal cord protection and related complications in endovascular management of B dissection: LSA revascularization and CSF drainage. Ann Cardiothorac Surg. 2014;3(3):336–8.
98. Matsumura JS, Lee WA, Mitchell RS, et al. The Society for Vascular Surgery Practice Guidelines: management of the left subclavian artery with thoracic endovascular aortic repair. J Vasc Surg. 2009;50(5):1155–8.
99. Weigang E, Hartert M, Siegenthaler MP, et al. Perioperative management to improve neurologic outcome in thoracic or thoracoabdominal aortic stent-grafting. Ann Thorac Surg. 2006;82(5):1679–87.
100. Etz CD, Weigang E, Hartert M, et al. Contemporary spinal cord protection during thoracic and thoracoabdominal aortic surgery and endovascular aortic repair: a position paper of the vascular domain of the European Association for Cardio-Thoracic Surgerydagger. Eur J Cardiothorac Surg. 2015;47(6):943–57.

Multisystem Organ Failure After Ruptured Abdominal Aortic Aneurysm

101. Investigators IT, et al. Endovascular or open repair strategy for ruptured abdominal aortic aneurysm: 30 day outcomes from IMPROVE randomised trial. BMJ. 2014;348:f7661.
102. Starnes BW, et al. Management of ruptured abdominal aortic aneurysm in the endovascular era. J Vasc Surg. 2010;51(1):9–17; discussion 17–8.

103. Johansen K, et al. Ruptured abdominal aortic aneurysm: the Harborview experience. J Vasc Surg. 1991;13(2):240–5; discussion 245–7.
104. Bown MJ, et al. Cytokines and inflammatory pathways in the pathogenesis of multiple organ failure following abdominal aortic aneurysm repair. Eur J Vasc Endovasc Surg. 2001;22(6):485–95.
105. Bown MJ, et al. The systemic inflammatory response syndrome, organ failure, and mortality after abdominal aortic aneurysm repair. J Vasc Surg. 2003;37(3):600–6.
106. Hietbrink F, et al. Kinetics of the innate immune response after trauma: implications for the development of late onset sepsis. Shock. 2013;40(1):21–7.
107. Asehnoune K, Roquilly A, Abraham E. Innate immune dysfunction in trauma patients: from pathophysiology to treatment. Anesthesiology. 2012;117(2):411–6.
108. Kasten KR, et al. Divergent adaptive and innate immunological responses are observed in humans following blunt trauma. BMC Immunol. 2010;11:4.
109. Adams JM, et al. Early trauma polymorphonuclear neutrophil responses to chemokines are associated with development of sepsis, pneumonia, and organ failure. J Trauma. 2001;51(3):452–6; discussion 456–7.
110. Harkin DW, et al. Complement C5a receptor antagonist attenuates multiple organ injury in a model of ruptured abdominal aortic aneurysm. J Vasc Surg. 2004;39:196–206.
111. Mehta M, et al. Endovascular repair of ruptured infrarenal abdominal aortic aneurysm is associated with lower 30-day mortality and better 5-year survival rates than open surgical repair. J Vasc Surg. 2013;57(2):368–75.
112. Vincent JL, et al. The SOFA (Sepsis-related Organ Failure Assessment) score to describe organ dysfunction/failure. On behalf of the Working Group on Sepsis-Related Problems of the European Society of Intensive Care Medicine. Intensive Care Med. 1996;22(7):707–10.
113. Le Gall JR, Lemeshow S, Saulnier F. A new Simplified Acute Physiology Score (SAPS II) based on a European/North American multicenter study. JAMA. 1993;270(24):2957–63.
114. Miranda DR, de Rijk A, Schaufeli W. Simplified therapeutic intervention scoring system: the TISS-28 items – results from a multicenter study. Crit Care Med. 1996;24(1):64–73.
115. Krenzien F, et al. Early prediction of survival after open surgical repair of ruptured abdominal aortic aneurysms. BMC Surg. 2014;14:92.
116. Xiao W, et al. A genomic storm in critically injured humans. J Exp Med. 2011;208(13):2581–90.
117. Mastracci TM, et al. Endovascular repair of ruptured abdominal aortic aneurysms: a systematic review and meta-analysis. J Vasc Surg. 2008;47(1):214–21.
118. Lesperance K, et al. Expanding use of emergency endovascular repair for ruptured abdominal aortic aneurysms: disparities in outcomes from a nationwide perspective. J Vasc Surg. 2008;47(6):1165–70; discussion 1170–1.
119. Ullery BW, et al. Association of an endovascular-first protocol for ruptured abdominal aortic aneurysms with survival and discharge disposition. JAMA Surg. 2015;150:1058–65.
120. Wallace GA, et al. Favorable discharge disposition and survival after successful endovascular repair of ruptured abdominal aortic aneurysm. J Vasc Surg. 2013;57(6):1495–502.
121. McPhee J, et al. Endovascular treatment of ruptured abdominal aortic aneurysms in the United States (2001–2006): a significant survival benefit over open repair is independently associated with increased institutional volume. J Vasc Surg. 2009;49(4):817–26.
122. Giles KA, et al. Decrease in total aneurysm-related deaths in the era of endovascular aneurysm repair. J Vasc Surg. 2009;49(3):543–50; discussion 550–1.
123. Mureebe L, et al. National trends in the repair of ruptured abdominal aortic aneurysms. J Vasc Surg. 2008;48(5):1101–7.
124. Mani K, Bjorck M, Wanhainen A. Changes in the management of infrarenal abdominal aortic aneurysm disease in Sweden. Br J Surg. 2013;100(5):638–44.
125. McHugh SM, et al. Endovascular versus open repair of ruptured abdominal aortic aneurysm. Surgeon. 2015.
126. Sayers R. Aortic Aneurysms, inflammatory pathways and Nitric Oxide. Ann R Coll Surg Engl. 2002;2002(84):239–46.
127. El-Sabrout RA, Reul GJ. Suprarenal or supraceliac aortic clamping during repair of infrarenal abdominal aortic aneurysms. Tex Heart Inst J. 2001;28(4):254–64.

128. Visser JJ, et al. Endovascular repair versus open surgery in patients with ruptured abdominal aortic aneurysms: clinical outcomes with 1-year follow-up. J Vasc Surg. 2006;44(6):1148–55.
129. An G, West MA. Abdominal compartment syndrome: a concise clinical review. Crit Care Med. 2008;36(4):1304–10.
130. Oelschlager BK, et al. Delayed abdominal closure in the management of ruptured abdominal aortic aneurysms. Am J Surg. 1997;173(5):411–5.
131. Mehta M, et al. Factors associated with abdominal compartment syndrome complicating endovascular repair of ruptured abdominal aortic aneurysms. J Vasc Surg. 2005;42(6): 1047–51.
132. Becquemin JP, et al. Colon ischemia following abdominal aortic aneurysm repair in the era of endovascular abdominal aortic repair. J Vasc Surg. 2008;47(2):258–63; discussion 263.
133. Greco G, et al. Outcomes of endovascular treatment of ruptured abdominal aortic aneurysms. J Vasc Surg. 2006;43(3):453–9.
134. Johnston KW. Ruptured abdominal aortic aneurysm: six-year follow-up results of a multicenter prospective study. Canadian Society for Vascular Surgery Aneurysm Study Group. J Vasc Surg. 1994;19(5):888–900.
135. Noel AA, et al. Ruptured abdominal aortic aneurysms: the excessive mortality rate of conventional repair. J Vasc Surg. 2001;34(1):41–6.
136. Gierek D, et al. Perioperative prognostic factors in patients with ruptured abdominal aortic aneurysms treated in the intensive care unit. Anaesth Intensive Care. 2013;45(1):25–9.
137. Ambler GK, et al. Incidence and outcomes of severe renal impairment following ruptured abdominal aortic aneurysm repair. Eur J Vasc Endovasc Surg. 2015;50:443–9.
138. Maldonado TS, et al. Ischemic complications after endovascular abdominal aortic aneurysm repair. J Vasc Surg. 2004;40(4):703–9; discussion 709–10.
139. Peppelenbosch N, et al. Emergency endovascular treatment for ruptured abdominal aortic aneurysm and the risk of spinal cord ischemia. J Vasc Surg. 2005;42(4):608–14.
140. Nathens AB, Brunet FP, Maier RV. Development of trauma systems and effect on outcomes after injury. Lancet. 2004;363(9423):1794–801.
141. van Beek SC, et al. Effect of regional cooperation on outcomes from ruptured abdominal aortic aneurysm. Br J Surg. 2014;101(7):794–801.

Management of Endoleaks After rEVAR

142. Parodi JC, Palmaz JC, Barone HD. Transfemoral intraluminal graft implantation for abdominal aortic aneurysms. Ann Vasc Surg. 1991;5:491–9.
143. Hinchliffe RJ, Bruijstens L, MacSweeney ST, Braithwaite BD. A randomised trial of endovascular and open surgery for ruptured abdominal aortic aneurysm—results of a pilot study and lessons learned for future studies. Eur J Vasc Endovasc Surg. 2006;32:506–13.
144. Reimerink JJ, Hoornweg LL, Vahl AC, Wisselink W, van den Broek TA, Legemate., DA, et al., Amsterdam Acute AneurysmTrial Collaborators. Endovascular repair versus open repair of ruptured abdominal aortic aneurysm: a multicenter randomized controlled trial. Ann Surg. 2013;258:248–56.
145. Powell JT, Sweeting MJ, Thompson MM, Ashleigh R, Bell R, Gomes M, et al., IMPROVE Trial Investigators. Endovascular or open repair strategy for ruptured abdominal aortic aneurysm: 30 day outcomes from IMPROVE randomised trial. Br Med J. 2014; 348:f7661.
146. Veith FJ, Lachat M, Mayer D, Malina M, Holst J, Mehta M. Collected world and single center experience with endovascular treatment of ruptured abdominal aortic aneurysms. Ann Surg. 2009;250(5):818–24.
147. Starnes BW, Quiroga E, Hutter C, Tran NT, Hatsukami T, Meissner M, et al. Management of ruptured abdominal aortic aneurysm in the endovascular era. J Vasc Surg. 2010;51:9–18.

148. Mehta M, Byrne J, Darling III RC, Paty PSK, Roddy SP, Kreienberg PB, et al. Endovascular repair of ruptured infrarenal abdominal aortic aneurysm is associated with lower 30-day mortality and better 5-year survival rates than open surgical repair. J Vasc Surg. 2013;57:368–75.
149. White GH, Yu W, May J. "Endoleak": a proposed new terminology to describe incomplete aneurysm exclusion by an endoluminal graft. J Endovasc Surg. 1996;3:124–5.
150. Chaikof EL, Blankensteijn JD, Harris PL, et al. Reporting standards for endovascular aortic aneurysm repair. J Vasc Surg. 2002;35:1048–60.
151. White GH, May J, Petrasek P, Waugh RC, Yu W. Type III and type IV endoleak: toward a complete definition of blood flow in the sac after endoluminal repair of AAA. J Endovasc Surg. 1998;5:305–9.
152. White GH, Yu W, May J, et al. Endoleak as a complication of endoluminal grafting of abdominal aortic aneurysms: classification, incidence, diagnosis, and management. J Endovasc Surg. 1997;4:152–68.
153. Dias NV, Ivancev K, Resch TA, et al. Endoleaks after endovascular aneurysm repair lead to nonuniform intra-aneurysm sac pressure. J Vasc Surg. 2007;46:197–203.
154. White SB, Stavropoulos SW. Management of endoleaks following endovascular aneurysm repair. Semin Interv Radiol. 2009;26(1):33–8.
155. Lee JT, Ullery BW, Zarins CK, Olcott IV C, et al. EVAR deployment in anatomically challenging necks outside the IFU. Eur J Vasc Endovasc Surg. 2013;46(1):65–73.
156. Rosen RJ, Green RM. Endoleak management following endovascular aneurysm repair. J Vasc Interv Radiol. 2008;19:37–43.
157. Kim JK, Noll RE, Tonnessen BH, Sternbergh WC. A technique for increased accuracy in the placement of the "giant" Palmaz stent for treatment of type IA endoleak after endovascular abdominal aneurysm repair. J Vasc Surg. 2008;48:755–7.
158. Maldonado TS, Rosen RJ, Rockman CB, et al. Initial successful management of type I endoleak after endovascular aortic aneurysm repair with n-butyl cyanoacrylate adhesive. J Vasc Surg. 2003;38:664–70.
159. Zanchetta M, Faresin F, Pedon L, et al. Fibrin glue aneurysm sac embolization at the time of endografting. J Endovasc Ther. 2005;12:579–82.
160. Grisafi JL, Boiteau G, Detschelt E, et al. Endoluminal treatment of type IA endoleak with Onyx. J Vasc Surg. 2010;52:1346–9.
161. Pacanowski JP, Stevens SL, Freeman MB, et al. Endotension distribution and the role of thrombus following endovascular AAA exclusion. J Endovasc Ther. 2002;9:639–51.
162. Glebova NO, Selvarajah S, Orion KC, Black 3rd JH, et al. Fenestrated endovascular repair of abdominal aortic aneurysms is associated with increased morbidity but comparable mortality with infrarenal endovascular aneurysm repair. J Vasc Surg. 2015;61(3):604–10.
163. Quinn AA, Mehta M, Teymouri MT, et al. The incidence and fate of endoleaks varies between ruptured and elective endovascular abdominal aortic aneurysm repair. JVS (in press).
164. Smith MT, Gupta R, Jazaeri O, Rochon PJ, et al. Preservation of interal iliac arterial flow during endovascular aortic aneurysm repair using the "Sandwich" technique. Semin Intervent Radiol. 2013;30:82–6.
165. Mehta M, Veith FJ, Darling RC, et al. Effects of bilateral hypogastric artery interruption during endovascular and open aortoiliac aneurysm repair. J Vasc Surg. 2004;40(4):698–702.
166. El Batti S, Cochennec F, Roudot-Thoraval F, Becquemin JP. Type II endoleaks after endovascular repair of abdominal aortic aneurysm are not always a benign condition. J Vasc Surg. 2013;57(5):1291–7.
167. Jones JE, Atkins MD, Brewster DC, et al. Persistent type 2 endoleak after endovascular repair of abdominal aortic aneurysm is associated with adverse late outcomes. J Vasc Surg. 2007;46(1):1–8.
168. Bernhard VM, Mitchell RS, Matsumura JS, et al. Ruptured abdominal aortic aneurysm after endovascular repair. J Vasc Surg. 2002;35:1155–62.
169. Van Marrewijk C, Buth J, Harris PL, et al. Significance of endoleaks after endovas- cular repair of abdominal aortic aneurysm: the EUROSTAR experience. J Vasc Surg. 2002;35:461–73.

170. Martin ML, Dolmatch BL, Fry PD, Machan LS. Treatment of type II endoleaks with Onyx. J Vasc Interv Radiol. 2001;12:629–32.
171. Baum RA, Carpenter JP, Golden MA, et al. Treatment of type 2 endoleaks after endovascular repair of abdominal aortic aneurysms: comparison of transarterial and translumbar techniques. J Vasc Surg. 2002;35(1):23–9.
172. Mansueto G, Cenzi D, Scuro A, et al. Treatment of type II endoleak with a transcatheter transcaval approach: results at 1-year follow-up. J Vasc Surg. 2007;45:1120–7.
173. Baum RA, Cope C, Fairman RM, Carpenter JP. Translumbar embolization of type 2 endoleaks after endovascular repair of abdominal aortic aneurysms. J Vasc Interv Radiol. 2001;12(1):111–6.
174. Stavropoulos SW, Park J, Fairman R, Carpenter J. Type 2 endoleak embolization comparison: translumbar embolization versus modified transarterial embolization. J Vasc Interv Radiol. 2009;20(10):1299–302.
175. Zhou W, Lumsden AB, Li J. IMA clipping for a type II endoleak: combined laparoscopic and endovascular approach. Surg Laparosc Endosc Percutan Tech. 2006;16:272–5.
176. Wilt TJ, Lederle FA, Macdonald R, et al. Comparison of endovascular and open surgical repairs for abdominal aortic aneurysm. Evid Rep Technol Assess. 2006;144:1–113.
177. Wanhainen A, Nyman R, Mats-Ola E, Bjorck M. First report of a late type III endoleak from fabric tears of a Zenith stent graft. J Vasc Surg. 2008;48(3):723–6.
178. Stavropoulos SW, Charagundla SR. Imaging techniques for detection and management of endoleaks after endovascular aortic aneurysm repair. Radiology. 2007;243:641–55.

Martin Björck Martin Björck is a member of the Executive Committee of the World Society of Abdominal Compartment Syndrome (website: wsacs.org)

Chapter 17
Outcomes of Ruptured Aortic Aneurysm: Early and Late

Jessica P. Simons and Andres Schanzer

Overview of Outcomes

Abdominal aortic aneurysm (AAA) disease is the 13th leading cause of death in the United States, resulting in 16,000 deaths annually. It is the tenth leading cause of death in men over the age of 55 and the third leading cause of sudden death in elderly men. [Dartmouth Atlas of Vascular Health Care, http://www.dartmouthatlas.org/downloads/atlases/Vascular_Atlas.pdf, *accessed 4.5.15*] Ruptured AAA (rAAA), if untreated, is considered uniformly fatal. In a study of 56 patients with confirmed rAAA, median in-hospital survival was 2.2 h; however, 13 patients were still alive at 24 h, demonstrating that the time course can be quite variable [1].

Traditionally, it has been widely believed that approximately half of patients with rAAA will die before reaching a hospital; of those who do undergo repair, the perioperative mortality is reported to be greater than 50 % for an overall survival of rAAA of less than 25 % [2]. A systematic review and meta-analysis was published in 2013 that rigorously evaluated population-based mortality for rAAA [3]. Among nearly 15,000 patients in Finland, Sweden, Denmark, the United Kingdom, Australia, and New Zealand, the total mortality was estimated at 81 % (95 % confidence interval (CI), 78–83). The pre-hospital mortality was 32 % (range 27–37 %). When the studies were analyzed as a function of year of publication, categorizing studies published before 1990 as the "early period" and categorizing studies published after 1990 as the "recent period," a significant decline in overall mortality was noted in the recent period compared to the early period (74 % versus 86 %, $p = .002$). This reduction in mortality was attributed to declines

J.P. Simons, MD, MPH • A. Schanzer, MD (✉)
University of Massachusetts Medical School, Worcester, MA, USA
e-mail: Andres.Schanzer@umassmemorial.org

B.W. Starnes et al. (eds.), *Ruptured Abdominal Aortic Aneurysm*,
DOI 10.1007/978-3-319-23844-9_17

in pre-hospital mortality, nonintervention rate, and perioperative mortality. While the early mortality following rAAA has been well studied, there is a dearth of data on long-term outcomes following rAAA repair.

Permissive Hypotension

A policy of permissive hypotension for patients with rAAA prior to surgical hemorrhage control has been advocated for improving mortality. While hemorrhagic shock has traditionally been treated with aggressive fluid resuscitation prior to control of bleeding, this approach may exacerbate blood loss due to dilutional and hypothermic coagulopathy and secondary clot disruption by increased blood flow, perfusion pressure, and decreased viscosity [4]. In a systematic review of permissive hypotension, Roberts and colleagues found substantial evidence for benefits in survival, tissue perfusion, and total blood loss in animal studies [4]. However, high-quality studies of permissive hypotension in humans with rAAA were lacking, so evidence-based conclusions could not be drawn. In 2009, Reimerink and colleagues reported the safety and feasibility of this approach in patients suspected of having rAAA by first responders, using their experience in Amsterdam between 2006 and 2007 [5]. Their protocol entailed maintenance of systolic blood pressures between 80 and 100 mmHg, with restriction of fluids for patients with systolic pressures above 100 mmHg. Fluid boluses were only given for unresponsiveness or systolic pressure less than 80 mmHg. They concluded that this approach could safely be employed for patients suspected of having rAAA, despite a relatively low diagnostic accuracy by ambulance personnel.

Regionalization of Care

Another key component of pre-hospital strategies aimed at increasing survival for rAAA includes transport to centers that perform a high volume of aneurysm surgery [6]. Using the national data from Canada, Dueck and colleagues demonstrated a significantly increased hazard of death for patients with rAAA treated by surgeons with low annual volume of rAAA repair and surgeons without subspecialty training in vascular or cardiothoracic surgery [7]. Holt and colleagues examined the relationship of hospital volume and outcomes following repair of both intact AAA and rAAA. In their meta-analysis of nearly 46,000 procedures for rAAA, they reported a significant survival benefit (weighted odds ratio, 0.78; 95 % CI, 0.73–0.82) conferred at a threshold of 15 repairs per year [8]. The authors concluded that repair of both intact AAA and rAAA should be preferentially performed at high-volume centers in order to improve survival. Hafez and colleagues investigated referral and management patterns for rAAA in the United Kingdom and determined there was significant survival benefit associated with initial referral to a hospital with full, on-site vascular capabilities, even if it required a further distance of transport [9]. They found both a significant improvement in likelihood of intervention and in subsequent survival, leading them to conclude that care should be regionalized whenever possible in order to improve outcomes.

Standardized Protocols for Diagnosis and Management

One potential aspect of high-volume centers that may contribute to improved outcomes is the use of clearly defined protocols for diagnosis and management. As the use of endovascular aneurysm repair (EVAR) gained widespread acceptance, its application to the management of rAAA triggered many centers to develop specific protocols to facilitate this. In 2006, Mehta and colleagues published a description of their triage protocol for managing rAAA. This triage protocol enabled this large group of vascular surgeons servicing several different hospitals to convert in 2002 from an exclusively open repair strategy to a primarily endovascular treatment algorithm [10] Fig. 17.1.

Starnes and colleagues published a comparative experience, before and after implementation of a standardized protocol for management of rAAA [11]. In the era prior to implementation of a standardized protocol that incorporated preferential treatment with endovascular repair, the 30-day mortality was 57.8 %, compared with 35.3 % (p = .008) in the protocol era. After implementation of the standardized protocol, 48 % of patients underwent EVAR for rAAA, in contrast to <1 % (1 of 131) prior to implementation of the standardized protocol. The authors conclude that the survival benefit was due to both the adoption of a standardized protocol, as well as to the use of EVAR.

The benefits of a structured protocol for the diagnosis and management of rAAA are now so well recognized that it has been cited by some as a potential confounder in the assessment of the benefit of EVAR compared with open repair [12, 13]. In reviewing the literature, it can be difficult to separate the benefit from having a structured protocol in place from the potential benefit of EVAR compared to open surgery. The use of such protocols should be widely adopted [14].

Outcomes from Retrospective Studies

The majority of data on rAAA outcomes is derived from a variety of retrospective studies (case series, registries, large databases), which is common for emergent diagnoses such as this. Several authors have made efforts to correct for bias and confounding by using multivariable regression, propensity score matching, and subgroup analyses. Despite the retrospective nature of these data, the large body of published work has allowed for the performance of carefully structured meta-analyses and systematic reviews.

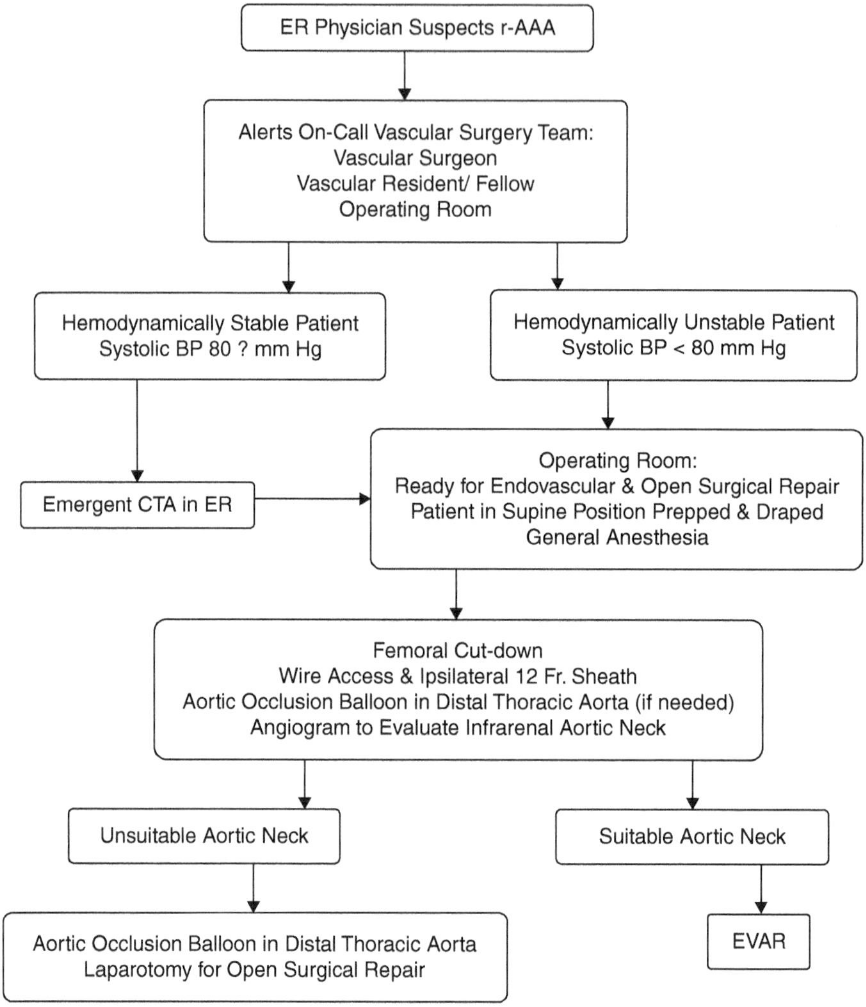

Fig. 17.1 A uniform triage protocol was established for endovascular repair of ruptured abdominal aortic aneurysms (rAAA). *ER* emergency room, *CTA* computed tomography angiography, *BP* blood pressure, *EVAR* endovascular aneurysm repair

Open Repair

In 2008, Hoornweg and colleagues published a systematic review and meta-analysis of 116 studies from 1991 to 2006 on open repair of rAAA [15]. They sought to evaluate trends in mortality over time, as well as the effect of hospital volume on outcomes. Among approximately 60,000 patients, the weighted mean overall perioperative mortality was 48.5 % (95 % CI, 48.1–48.9 %). The intraoperative mortality was reported in 37 studies, and the weighted mean was 13.3 % (95 % CI, 12.3–14.3 %). Over the 33 years of study, there was no significant change in overall

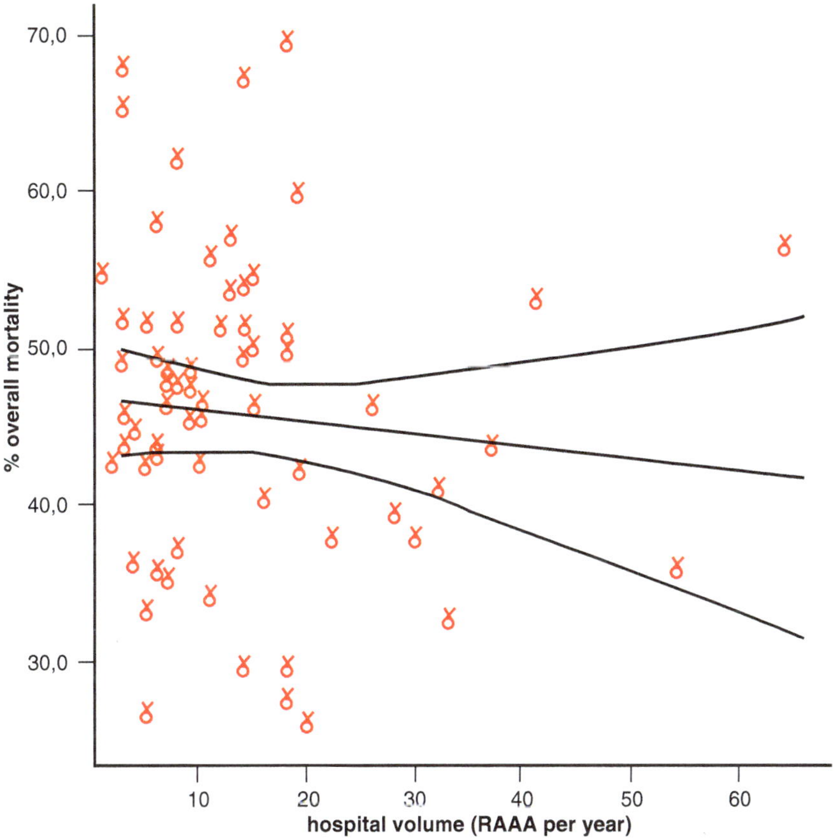

Fig. 17.2 Meta-regression of 69 studies reporting on % overall mortality (Y axis) against hospital volume (X axis) with 95 % CI

mortality as a function of time (1.6 % reduction, p = NS). Analysis of the 58 studies that included hospital volume revealed a significant positive association between annual hospital volume of rAAA repairs and overall mortality (p = .04). Unfortunately, the authors were unable to determine a threshold of rAAA hospital volume that is associated with improved mortality. Despite the limitations inherent to this study, the inclusion of over 60,000 patients provides valuable data on outcomes following open repair of rAAA (Fig. 17.2).

Endovascular Repair

In 2008, Mastracci and colleagues published a systematic review and meta-analysis of 18 studies between 1994 and 2006 on endovascular repair (EVAR) of rAAA [13]. The pooled mortality was 21 % (95 % CI, 13–29), with a broad range of reported outcomes across studies (0–45 % mortality). In fact, the authors conclude that in the presence of such substantial heterogeneity, the aggregated calculated point estimate cannot be considered reliable. Subgroup analyses that included only series where >30 cases were reported demonstrated a reduction in heterogeneity and a mortality of 19 % (95 % CI, 10–28). While EVAR for rAAA is widely practiced, rigorous analysis and interpretation of its results have been difficult.

Comparison of Open and Endovascular Repair

Several advantages of EVAR for rAAA repair compared to open surgery have been published, but the retrospective and other non-randomized study designs have been criticized for the potential selection bias that may be inherent to these studies. The primary concern has been that patients selected for EVAR may be more stable at their time of presentation, and this increased stability may be responsible for improved outcomes. In 2009, Hinchliffe and colleagues published a systematic review of the literature on EVAR for rAAA, specifically noting those that contained a "control" open repair group [12]. Despite having adopted EVAR for treatment of many patients with rAAA at the authors' center, they conclude that the evidence for its benefit is lacking. Conflicting results have been reported, and questions regarding the comparability of the two patient groups remain (Table 17.1).

Veith and colleagues published an account of the international experience with EVAR for rAAA in 2009 to assess its value and to explain the conflicting results that had been published to date [16]. They surveyed a number of centers throughout the world that were known to use EVAR to treat rAAA and collected data on the center as well as on the patients treated. They also included a single-center experience to detail one system that has been established to transition to a "EVAR-first" strategy for repair of all anatomically suitable rAAA; this included a protocol for diagnosis, the use of hypotensive hemostasis, the use of a hybrid operating suite, percutaneous technique with local anesthesia only until aortic control is achieved, supraceliac balloon occlusion, adequate device inventory, and close observation for abdominal compartment syndrome. The survey-based results showed a 30-day mortality of 21.1 % for EVAR for rAAA. While they note that this is clearly lower than results reported for open repair, they acknowledge that a bias may have been imparted with only the more hemodynamically stable patients being offered EVAR. To address this bias, they surveyed 13 centers that routinely perform EVAR even in unstable rAAA patients; these centers had established protocols, imaging technology, and providers experienced in the management of rAAA with EVAR. Among this group, the 30-day mortality was 19.7 % which was significantly less than the 36.3 % 30-day mortality for open repair at these centers ($p<.0001$). The authors concluded that EVAR, combined with a standardized approach to rAAA management, is the superior strategy for all anatomically suitable patients, and further study via randomized controlled trials is not needed.

Table 17.1 Data from published series from 1994 to 2009 where outcomes of endovascular repair for ruptured abdominal aortic aneurysms were compared with a control group undergoing open surgery

First author	Year	Study type	Patients treated by EVAR, No.	30-day mortality, %		P
				EVAR	Open repair	
Acosta	2007	Retrospective review	56	34	45	.16
Alsac	2005	Case series	17	23.5	50	.09
Anain	2007	Retrospective review	30	17	40	.19
Arya	2006	Prospective intent-to-treat	17	24	47	.14
Brandt	2005	Retrospective review	11	0	15	NS
Castelli	2005	Retrospective review	25	20	25	NS
Coppi	2006	Retrospective review	33	30	46	NS
Franks	2006	Retrospective study	21	11	54	NS
Hechelhammer	2005	Retrospective study	35	10.8	35	NS
Hinchliffe	2006	Prospective randomized	15	53	53	NS
Kapma	2005	Retrospective study	40	13	30	NS
Lee	2004	Retrospective study	13	4.69	25	NS
Mehta	2006	Prospective observation	40	18	51	…
Moore	2007	Prospective observation	20	5	25	NS
Najjer	2007	Retrospective review	15	6.7	13.6	NS
Ohki	2000	Retrospective study	18	10	0	NS
Ockert	2007	Retrospective review	29	31	31	<.99
Peppelenbosch	2003	Prospective study	26	31	50	NS
Scharrer-Pamler	2003	Retrospective review	24	20.8	40	NS
Vaddenini	2005	Retrospective study	9	22	26	NS
Visser	2006	Retrospective review	26	31	31	NS
Wibmer[a]	2008	Retrospective review	16	25[a]	29[a]	NS
Yilmaz	2002	Retrospective review	24	17	34	NS
Peppelenbosch	2006	Prospective study	49	35	39	NS
Verhoeven	2009	Prospective observation	36	28.1	13.9	.092
Sadat	2009	Prospective observation	17	6	17	…

EVAR endovascular aneurysm repair, *NS* not significant

[a]90-day mortality figures quoted

Randomized Controlled Trials

Randomized controlled trials have been suggested as the best means for addressing concerns of selection bias associated with retrospective and observational studies comparing EVAR and open repair of rAAA. In 2006, results of a single-center pilot randomized controlled trial, conducted in Nottingham, England, were reported [17]. This study was terminated after recruitment of only 32 patients. The overall mortality was 50 %, with no difference between open repair and EVAR. The French ECAR (Endovasculaire vs Chirurgie dans les Anévrysmes Rompus) trial, which began in

2008, is ongoing at the present time [18]. Two randomized controlled trials evaluating EVAR and open repair of rAAA have been performed to date: the Amsterdam Acute Aneurysm Trial [19] and the Immediate Management of Patients with Rupture: Open versus Endovascular Repair trial [20].

Amsterdam Acute Aneurysm Trial

The Amsterdam Acute Aneurysm Trial was a multicenter randomized controlled trial of patients suitable for both EVAR and open repair of rAAA from 2004 to 2011 [19]. Patients were treated at experienced centers, with 24-h on call staff capable of performing emergent EVAR repair. In cases where transfer was required to a designated center, an established protocol including the use of permissive hypotension was utilized. In accordance with the Dutch law, informed consent was not strictly required from the patient preoperatively. Anatomic suitability was strictly defined and confirmed both by the vascular surgeon and by a radiologist. A notable exclusion was those patients too unstable to obtain computed tomography angiography (71 exclusions of 520 screened). Aortic occlusion balloons prior to endograft placement were used at the discretion of the surgeon. Endovascular repair entailed aorto-uni-iliac endograft, contralateral iliac occlusion device, and femoral-femoral bypass. Sample size was set at 56 patients per group, based on an expected 30-day death and severe complications rate of 65 % for open repair and 40 % with EVAR. Analyses were performed according to an intention-to-treat principle. No significant difference was found (death and severe complications, 42 % in the EVAR group versus 47 % in the open group; 95 % CI, −13 to +23 %). The individual end point, 30-day mortality, was also not significantly different between the two groups (21 % for EVAR versus 25 % for open, absolute risk reduction = 4.4 %; 95 % CI, −11 to +20 %). Over the course of long-term follow-up (median, 1533 days), the survival curves did not separate demonstrating no significant difference in mortality between groups. The authors conclude that there was no significant benefit seen with EVAR for rAAA and postulate that the lack of benefit may be attributable to the low mortality rate achieved in the open repair group. An alternative explanation may be that the standardization of management and centralization of care at experienced trial centers resulted in excellent outcomes in both groups, and the study may have been underpowered to demonstrate a difference between groups.

Immediate Management of Patients with Rupture: Open Versus Endovascular Repair (IMPROVE) Trial

The IMPROVE Trial was a multicenter randomized controlled trial of EVAR and open repair for patients with rAAA from 2009 to 2013 [20]. In an effort to simulate the "real world," patients were randomized prior to obtaining CTA, with an expected estimate that 45 % of those initially randomized to EVAR would not have suitable anatomy, and would therefore undergo open repair instead. Patients were treated at experienced centers, with a designated team of providers available at least 2/3 of the week. They sought to enroll 600 patients based on an estimated 30-day mortality of 44.7 % in the open repair group and 30.4 % in the EVAR group. Analyses were performed according to an intention-to-treat principle with 316 patients randomized to EVAR and 297 patients randomized to open. No significant difference was found in 30-day mortality between the EVAR and open groups (35.4 % versus 37.4 %, respectively). Adjusted analyses also failed to identify a significant difference between treatment strategies. Secondary analyses demonstrated a significant difference in average lengths of stay and percentage of discharges to home, with these results favoring EVAR. Potential limitations of this study include the impact of randomizing patients prior to performing imaging; for patients with anatomy not suitable for EVAR, the intention-to-treat analyses would include those outcomes after open surgery in the EVAR group to which they had been randomized. This would potentially dilute any difference between the two strategies.

Much debate has occurred over the validity of the existing randomized trials. They have been criticized for the high rates of exclusion (>50 %), the use of intention-to-treat analyses, and other factors that would diminish the ability to detect a benefit with EVAR [21–23]. However, in aggregate, the three published randomized controlled trials comparing EVAR to open repair of rAAA are consistent (Table 17.2). They demonstrate no statistically significant benefit on 30-day mortality of EVAR compared with open repair for rAAA.

Predicting Outcomes After Repair of Ruptured Abdominal Aortic Aneurysm

Patient selection remains one of the most influential factors on outcomes after rAAA repair. However, this decision-making process remains challenging and complex. Several scoring systems have been developed to aid in prognostication for

Table 17.2 Results of randomized controlled trials

Study	Number randomized	30-day mortality: Endovascular repair	30-day mortality: Open repair	Significance
Nottingham pilot study [17]	15 randomized to EVAR; 17 randomized to open (terminated early)	53 %	53 %	N/A
Amsterdam Acute Aneurysm Trial [19]	57 randomized to EVAR; 59 randomized to open	21 %	25 %	NS
Immediate Management of Patients with Rupture: Open versus Endovascular Repair [20]	316 randomized to EVAR; 297 randomized to open	35.4%	37.4%	NS

Table 17.3 Preoperative factors incorporated in selected prediction models for 30-day mortality after repair of ruptured abdominal aortic aneurysm

Prediction model	Factors incorporated
Glasgow aneurysm score	Age, shock, myocardial disease, cerebrovascular disease, renal disease
Hardman index	Age >76 years, elevated creatinine, hemoglobin <9 mg/dL, myocardial ischemia, loss of consciousness
Edinburgh Ruptured Aneurysm Score	Hemoglobin <9 mg/dL, systolic blood pressure <90 mmHg, Glasgow Coma Score <15
Vascular Study Group of New England	Age >76 years, cardiac arrest, loss of consciousness, suprarenal clamp

patients undergoing rAAA repair. Some scoring systems have been limited to endovascular or open approaches, while others have factored type of repair into the model. Many of the AAA-specific prediction models have focused mainly on variables that are available preoperatively in order to inform preoperative decision-making. Other published models have included operative and postoperative variables to predict mortality postoperatively [24, 25]. An exhaustive review of all rAAA risk prediction models is beyond the scope of this chapter; some of the more commonly referenced scores are described below. Table 17.3 demonstrates the commonality of various predictors across these risk prediction models.

Glasgow Aneurysm Score

In 1994, Samy and colleagues reported a scoring system (the Glasgow aneurysm score, GAS) to predict mortality following open repair of AAA [26]. The score was additive, with higher values corresponding to higher mortality: (age in years) + (17 for shock) + (7 for myocardial disease) + (10 for cerebrovascular disease) + (14 for renal disease). The GAS has been studied extensively in the literature, with some recent modifications reported. In 2009, Visser and colleagues updated the score to include endovascular repair, with testing of the score in a more contemporary population of patients with rAAA [27]. This updated GAS added seven points for open repair; 30-day mortality estimates in this cohort ranged from approximately 10 to 60 %.

Hardman Index

In 1996, Hardman and colleagues described factors associated with 30-day mortality following open repair of rAAA [28]. The Hardman index was additive, based on the presence of various factors: age >76 years, serum creatinine level >190 mmol/L, hemoglobin level <9 g/dL, myocardial ischemia on electrocardiograph, and a history of loss of consciousness after hospital arrival. Mortality for those with no variables was 16 %, while those with three or more variables had 100 % mortality.

Edinburgh Ruptured Aneurysm Score

In 2007, Tambyraja and colleagues described a prediction model for in-hospital and/or 30-day mortality following open repair of rAAA [29]. Similar to the Hardman index, this score was additive, based on the number of factors present. However, it only incorporated three readily available preoperative factors: hemoglobin <9 g/dL, systolic blood pressure <90 mmHg, and Glasgow Coma Score <15. Mortality across risk strata ranged from 29 to 80 %.

Vascular Study Group of New England Score

In 2013, Robinson and colleagues derived and validated a risk score for predicting 30-day mortality after open repair of rAAA [30]. This score was derived from the prospectively collected Vascular Study Group of New England (VSGNE) database. This simple additive score assigned two points for age >76 years, two points for cardiac arrest, one point for loss of consciousness, and one point for the use of suprarenal clamp. Mortality across risk strata varied from 8 to 87 %.

Summary of Evidence

In summary, many lessons have been learned in the several decades of management of rAAA. The majority of data on outcomes were derived from retrospective and observational studies. Prior to the last decade, overall mortality from population-based studies was estimated to be >80 %, with nearly 1/3 dying before reaching a hospital. However, there is evidence that mortality has improved over time, likely due to a combination of factors. Notably, several best practices have been described including regionalization of care at experienced centers whenever possible, the use of permissive hypotension until bleeding is controlled, development of well-defined, multidisciplinary protocols for rapid diagnosis and treatment, and advances in perioperative critical care practices. While the use of EVAR, whenever anatomically feasible, has several theoretical advantages over open repair, studies have been plagued with bias and contradictory results, limiting the ability to make strong evidence-based recommendations. Several risk scoring systems have been developed to assist with prognostication and patient selection for repair of this life-threatening emergency.

References

1. van Beek SC, Vahl AC, Wisselink W, Balm R. Amsterdam acute aneurysm trial C. Fate of patients unwilling or unsuitable to undergo surgical intervention for a ruptured abdominal aortic aneurysm. Eur J Vasc Endovasc Surg. 2015;49(2):163–5.
2. Zarins CKHM, Hill BB. Aneurysmal vascular disease. In: Townsend CM, Jr BR, Evers BM, Mattox KL, editors. Sabiston textbook of surgery. Philadelphia: Elsevier; 2004.
3. Reimerink JJ, van der Laan MJ, Koelemay MJ, Balm R, Legemate DA. Systematic review and meta-analysis of population-based mortality from ruptured abdominal aortic aneurysm. Br J Surg. 2013;100(11):1405–13.
4. Roberts K, Revell M, Youssef H, Bradbury AW, Adam DJ. Hypotensive resuscitation in patients with ruptured abdominal aortic aneurysm. Eur J Vasc Endovasc Surg. 2006;31(4):339–44.
5. Reimerink JJ, Hoornweg LL, Vahl AC, Wisselink W, Balm R. Controlled hypotension in patients suspected of a ruptured abdominal aortic aneurysm: feasibility during transport by ambulance services and possible harm. Eur J Vasc Endovasc Surg. 2010;40(1):54–9.
6. McPhee J, Eslami MH, Arous EJ, Messina LM, Schanzer A. Endovascular treatment of ruptured abdominal aortic aneurysms in the United States (2001–2006): a significant survival benefit over open repair is independently associated with increased institutional volume. J Vasc Surg. 2009;49(4):817–26.
7. Dueck AD, Kucey DS, Johnston KW, Alter D, Laupacis A. Survival after ruptured abdominal aortic aneurysm: effect of patient, surgeon, and hospital factors. J Vasc Surg. 2004;39(6):1253–60.
8. Holt PJ, Poloniecki JD, Gerrard D, Loftus IM, Thompson MM. Meta-analysis and systematic review of the relationship between volume and outcome in abdominal aortic aneurysm surgery. Br J Surg. 2007;94(4):395–403.
9. Hafez H, Owen LW, Lorimer CF, Bajwa A. Advantage of a one-stop referral and management service for ruptured abdominal aortic aneurysms. Br J Surg. 2009;96(12):1416–21.
10. Mehta M, Taggert J, Darling 3rd RC, Chang BB, Kreienberg PB, Paty PS, et al. Establishing a protocol for endovascular treatment of ruptured abdominal aortic aneurysms: outcomes of a prospective analysis. J Vasc Surg. 2006;44(1):1–8. discussion 8.
11. Starnes BW, Quiroga E, Hutter C, Tran NT, Hatsukami T, Meissner M, et al. Management of ruptured abdominal aortic aneurysm in the endovascular era. J Vasc Surg. 2010;51(1):9–17. discussion 17–8.
12. Hinchliffe RJ, Powell JT, Cheshire NJ, Thompson MM. Endovascular repair of ruptured abdominal aortic aneurysm: a strategy in need of definitive evidence. J Vasc Surg. 2009;49(4):1077–80.
13. Mastracci TM, Garrido-Olivares L, Cina CS, Clase CM. Endovascular repair of ruptured abdominal aortic aneurysms: a systematic review and meta-analysis. J Vasc Surg. 2008;47(1):214–21.
14. Hinchliffe RJ, Powell JT. Improving the outcomes from ruptured abdominal aortic aneurysm: interdisciplinary best practice guidelines. Ann R Coll Surg Engl. 2013;95(2):96–7.
15. Hoornweg LL, Storm-Versloot MN, Ubbink DT, Koelemay MJ, Legemate DA, Balm R. Meta analysis on mortality of ruptured abdominal aortic aneurysms. Eur J Vasc Endovasc Surg. 2008;35(5):558–70.
16. Veith FJ, Lachat M, Mayer D, Malina M, Holst J, Mehta M, et al. Collected world and single center experience with endovascular treatment of ruptured abdominal aortic aneurysms. Ann Surg. 2009;250(5):818–24.
17. Hinchliffe RJ, Bruijstens L, MacSweeney ST, Braithwaite BD. A randomised trial of endovascular and open surgery for ruptured abdominal aortic aneurysm - results of a pilot study and lessons learned for future studies. Eur J Vasc Endovasc Surg. 2006;32(5):506–13; discussion 514–5.
18. Desgranges P, Kobeiter H, Castier Y, Senechal M, Majewski M, Krimi A. The endovasculaire vs chirurgie dans les anevrysmes rompus PROTOCOL trial update. J Vasc Surg. 2010;51(1):267–70.

19. Reimerink JJ, Hoornweg LL, Vahl AC, Wisselink W, van den Broek TA, Legemate DA, et al. Endovascular repair versus open repair of ruptured abdominal aortic aneurysms: a multicenter randomized controlled trial. Ann Surg. 2013;258(2):248–56.
20. Investigators IT, Powell JT, Sweeting MJ, Thompson MM, Ashleigh R, Bell R, et al. Endovascular or open repair strategy for ruptured abdominal aortic aneurysm: 30 day outcomes from IMPROVE randomised trial. BMJ. 2014;348:f7661.
21. Mayer D, Rancic Z, Veith FJ, Lachat M. Part two: against the motion. EVAR offers no survival benefit over open repair for the treatment of ruptured abdominal aortic aneurysms. Eur J Vasc Endovasc Surg. 2015;49(2):119–27.
22. Veith FJ, Rockman CB. The recent randomized trials of EVAR versus open repair for ruptured abdominal aortic aneurysms are misleading. Vascular. 2015;23(2):217–9.
23. Dubois L, Mayer D, Rancic Z, Veith FJ, Lachat M. Debate: whether endovascular repair offers a survival advantage over open repair for ruptured abdominal aortic aneurysms. J Vasc Surg. 2015;61(2):546–55.
24. Prytherch DR, Sutton GL, Boyle JR. Portsmouth POSSUM models for abdominal aortic aneurysm surgery. Br J Surg. 2001;88(7):958–63.
25. Knaus WA, Wagner DP, Draper EA, Zimmerman JE, Bergner M, Bastos PG, et al. The APACHE III prognostic system. Risk prediction of hospital mortality for critically ill hospitalized adults. Chest. 1991;100(6):1619–36.
26. Samy AK, Murray G, MacBain G. Glasgow aneurysm score. Cardiovasc Surg. 1994;2(1):41–4.
27. Visser JJ, Williams M, Kievit J, Bosch JL, Group AS. Prediction of 30-day mortality after endovascular repair or open surgery in patients with ruptured abdominal aortic aneurysms. J Vasc Surg. 2009;49(5):1093–9.
28. Hardman DT, Fisher CM, Patel MI, Neale M, Chambers J, Lane R, et al. Ruptured abdominal aortic aneurysms: who should be offered surgery? J Vasc Surg. 1996;23(1):123–9.
29. Tambyraja A, Murie J, Chalmers R. Predictors of outcome after abdominal aortic aneurysm rupture: Edinburgh ruptured aneurysm score. World J Surg. 2007;31(11):2243–7.
30. Robinson WP, Schanzer A, Li Y, Goodney PP, Nolan BW, Eslami MH, et al. Derivation and validation of a practical risk score for prediction of mortality after open repair of ruptured abdominal aortic aneurysms in a US regional cohort and comparison to existing scoring systems. J Vasc Surg. 2013;57(2):354–61.

Chapter 18
Quality of Life After RAAA

April Rodriguez and Elina Quiroga

Over the last 20 years, the treatment and management of ruptured abdominal aortic aneurysms (rAAA) has been studied extensively [1–6]. Perioperative outcomes such as mortality, major complications, and re-intervention rates have been the major focus of many of these studies. However, the success of an operation lies in more than just these factors, and the patients' quality of life after surgery is an area that has been neglected. This is especially evident when looking at the quality of life after endovascular versus open repair of rAAA. Nonetheless, this is an area that should be focused on, not only for the benefit of patients and their families when making medical decisions but also for the surgical community, enhancing the ability to better treat patients and improve long-term quality of life.

Discharge disposition can be seen as a surrogate of quality of life after the procedure, assuming that the patients' quality of life and medical condition are better if they can be discharged home. The IMPROVE trial [7, 8], discussed below, interviewed some of its participants asking what were the key outcome measures they were interested in. Return to home was identified as one of the positive outcomes by patients or their families. Wallace et al. [9] compared discharge disposition for patients that had an open versus and endovascular repair for a rAAA. The authors found that patients undergoing endovascular repair were ten times more likely to be discharged home than patients having an open repair (OR, 9.96, $p = .002$). Similarly, the recently released 1-year outcomes of the IMPROVE [8] trial showed that patients undergoing endovascular repair were significantly more likely to be discharged home than patients having an open repair ($p = 0.001$)

Multiple small case series have looked at the quality of life after treatment of open rAAA (Table 18.1) [10]. Although the overall number of patients analyzed was

A. Rodriguez, MD • E. Quiroga, MD, FACS (✉)
Division of Vascular Surgery, Department of Surgery, University of Washington, Seattle, WA, USA
e-mail: elinaq@uw.edu

B.W. Starnes et al. (eds.), *Ruptured Abdominal Aortic Aneurysm*,
DOI 10.1007/978-3-319-23844-9_18

Table 18.1 Summary of studies evaluating quality of life after rAAA

Author	Year	Number of patients[a]			Mean follow-up time (months)	Questionnaire used	Results
		Total	Open	EVAR			
Hennessy	1998	14	14		33	Rosser QoL	No difference between rupture and elective surgery
Bohmer	1999	28	28	0	48	SF-36	No difference with general population
Korhonen	2003	82	82	0	33	RAND-36	No difference in seven domains, only decreased scores in:
Hinterseher	2004	24	24	0		WHO-QoL BREF-test	Same QoL as general population
Hill	2007	71	71	0	33	SF-36	Similar QoL than elective AAA repair and general population
IMPROVE trial	2015	229	102	127	12	EQ-5D	Better scores for EVAR than open

[a]Patients that completed the QoL questionnaire tool

small (ranging between 14 and 82 patients), these studies consistently demonstrated a good quality of life after open rAAA repair, equivalent to that of patients undergoing elective repair of abdominal aortic aneurysms.

The Rosser index evaluates eight levels of disability (physical mobility) and four levels of distress (freedom from pain). Answers are weighted and scored. "Perfect health" equals a score of 1, and equal to and less than 1 are the only two possible results. Hennessy et al. [11] in 1998 analyzed a group of 14 rAAA survivors who had a Rosser index of 1.000 (range, 0.680–1.000), and this was similar to the scores of patients having an elective AAA repair.

The Medical Outcomes Study Short Form-36 (SF-36) health survey is a 36-item, patient-reported questionnaire of current (last four weeks) health. The SF-36 and its derivative form, the RAND-36, have been widely used to compare the quality of life in different patient populations. The SF-36 has eight rated score areas: vitality, physical functioning, bodily pain, general health perceptions, physical role functioning, emotional role functioning, social role functioning, and mental health. The SF-36 has been used in several studies to evaluate the quality of life after ruptured AAA. Bohmer et al. [12], in 1999, using the SF-36, reported that at a mean of 48 months after repair, the quality of life of survivors of a rAAA was similar to the quality of life of the age-adjusted general population. In 2007, Hill et al. [13] compared patients undergoing elective open AAA repair to patients that survived an rAAA and the general population and found that they all reported a similar quality of life. Korhonen et al. [14], in 2003, evaluated patients using the RAND-36 and found no difference in seven of the eight domains at a mean of 33 months after the procedure when compared to the general population. However, they did note that the rAAA survivors scored lower in the physical functioning domain. Interestingly, these authors commented that a "stormy" (complicated) postoperative course did not correlate with poor quality of life when evaluated years after the procedure.

Hinterseher and colleagues [15] used the WHO-QoL-BREF-test to evaluate the quality of life after rAAA. The WHO-QoL-BREF-test is a self-administered questionnaire that contains 26 items to be answered on a scale of 1–5. The categories evaluated are global life quality; physical, psychological, and social relations; and environment. They compared the results of 24 patients that had an open repair for a rAAA to the results of age- and sex-matched subjects in the German population. At 6 months the quality of life between both groups was not different.

A Cochrane database [16] review published in July 2014 aimed to evaluate the advantages of endovascular treatment for rAAA in comparison to open surgical repair. One of the outcomes that the review aimed to evaluate was quality of life, measured via standardized questionnaires. However, no studies were identified that met inclusion criteria for evaluating quality of life.

More recently the question of quality of life after endovascular versus open rAAA has come to attention, and the IMPROVE trial [8] is probably the first study reporting this data. This multicenter trial randomized patients who presented with rAAA to either open or endovascular repair provided data on many factors, including health-related quality of life at 1 year and quality-adjusted life years (QALYs). The EQ-5D (previously known as the EuroQoL) was used in the IMPROVE trial to measure quality of life. The EQ-5D is a standardized, non-disease-specific tool used to describe health-related quality of life. The EQ-5D analyzes five dimensions of "health": mobility, self-care, usual activities, pain/discomfort, and anxiety/depression [17]. The IMPROVE trial found that patients who underwent endovascular repair had a shorter overall hospital stay, were more likely to be discharged to home, and, as evaluated using the EQ-5D questionnaire, had superior early QoL, compared to those who underwent open repair.

While treatment of rAAA has evolved over time with the development of endovascular techniques, the disease process continues to carry a significant operative mortality. Patients who are able to survive the initial insult of an open surgery have been shown to have a quality of life comparable to patients who have undergone elective AAA repair. Furthermore, endovascular repair of rAAA has been shown to have an early quality of life superior to that of patients undergoing open repair. These patients are also discharged faster, are more likely to be discharged to home, and possibly have a higher quality of life. Aggressive treatment should be considered in all patients who present with a rAAA, and endovascular repair should be favored in those who demonstrate suitable anatomy.

References

1. Yusef SW, Whitaker SC, Chuter T, Wenham PW, Hopkinson BR. Emergency endovascular repair of leaking aortic aneurysm. Lancet. 1994;344:1645.
2. Albuquerque FC, Tonnessen BH, Noll RE, Cires G, Kim JK, Sternbergh WC. Paradigm shifts in the treatment of abdominal aortic aneurysm: trends in 721 patients between 1996 and 2008. J Vasc Surg. 2010;51:1348–53.
3. Marin ML, Veith FJ, Cynamon J, Sanchez LA, Lyon RT, Levine BA, et al. Initial experience with transluminally placed endovascular grafts for the treatment of complex vascular lesions. Ann Surg. 1995;222:449–65.
4. Chagpar RB, Harris JR, Lawlor DK, DeRose G, Forbes TL. Early mortality following endovascular versus open repair of ruptured abdominal aortic aneurysms. Vasc Endovascular Surg. 2010;44:645–9.
5. Ten Bosch JA, Teijink JA, Willigendael EM, Prins MH. Endovascular aneurysm repair is superior to open surgery for ruptured abdominal aortic aneurysms in EVAR-suitable patients. J Vasc Surg. 2010;52:13–8.
6. Starnes BW, Quiroga E, Hutter C, Tran NT, Hatsukami T, Meissner M, Tang G, Kohler T. Management of ruptured abdominal aortic aneurysm in the endovascular era. J Vasc Surg. 2010;51(1):9–17.
7. IMPROVE Trial Investigators, Powell JT, Sweeting ML, Thompson MM, Ashleigh R, Bell R, Gomes M, Greenhalgh RM, Grieve R, Heatly F, Hinchlifee RJ, Thompson SG, Ulug P. Endovascular or open repair strategy for ruptured abdominal aortic aneurysm: 30 day outcomes from IMPROVE randomized trial. BMJ. 2014;348:f7661.
8. Greive R, Gomes M, Sweeting MJ, Ulug P, Hinchliffe RJ, Thompson MM, Thompson SG, Ashleigh R, Greenhalgh RM, Powell JT. Endovascular strategy or open repair for ruptured abdominal aortic aneurysm: one year outcomes from the IMPROVE randomized trial. Eur Heart J. 2015. Pii:ehv125 [Epub ahead of print].
9. Wallace GA, Starnes BW, Hatsukami TS, Quiroga E, Tang GL, Kohler TR, Tran NT. Favorable discharge disposition and survival after successful endovascular repair of ruptured abdominal aortic aneurysm. J Vasc Surg. 2013;57(6):1495–502.

10. Tambyraja AL, Fraser SCA, Murie JA, Chalmers RTA. Quality of life after repair of ruptured abdominal aortic aneurysm. Eur J Vasc Endovasc Surg. 2004;28(3):229–33.
11. Hennessy A, Barry MC, McGee H, O'Boyle C, Hayes DB, Grace PA. Quality of life following repair of ruptured and elective abdominal aortic aneurysms. Eur J Surg. 1998;164:673–7.
12. Bohmer RD, Freischl J, Knight D. Quality of life after emergency abdominal aortic aneurysm repair. Aust N Z J Surg. 1999;69:447–9.
13. Hill AB, Palerme LP, Brandys T, Lewis R, Steinmetz OK. Health-related quality of life in survivors of open ruptured abdominal aortic aneurysm repair: a matched, controlled cohort study. J Vasc Surg. 2007;46(2):223–9.
14. Korhonen SJ, Kantonen I, Pettila V, Keranen J, Salo JS, Lepantalo M. Long-term survival and health-related quality of life of patients with ruptured abdominal aortic aneurysm. Eur J Vasc Surg. 2003;25:350–3.
15. Hinterseher I, Saeger HD, Koch R, Bloomenthal A, Ockert D, Berger H. Quality of life and long-term results after ruptured abdominal aortic aneurysm. Eur J Vasc Endovasc Surg. 2004;28:262–9.
16. Badger S, Bedenis R, Blair PH Ellis P, Kee F, Harkin DW. Endovascular treatment for ruptured abdominal aortic aneurysm. Cochrane Database Syst Rev. 2014;(7):CD005261.
17. Rabin R, de Charro F. EQ-5D: a measure of health status from the EuroQoL group. Ann Med. 2001;33:337–43.

Chapter 19
Ethical Issues Regarding rAAA

Deepika Nehra and Samuel P. Mandell

Key Points

- The fundamental ethical principles that should govern all medical care are beneficence, nonmaleficence, autonomy, and justice.
- In modern medicine, especially in the Western world, we have embraced the concept of shared decision-making, or a collaborative process by which patients and their providers make healthcare decisions together.
- Timely, clear, compassionate, and ongoing communication between clinicians, nurses, and family members of critically ill patients is of utmost importance.
- One of the most important aspects of an effective family conference is taking the time to listen to the family.
- Palliative care services may be offered to patients and families dealing with critical illness at any time and is not limited to end-of-life care.
- It is our duty as physicians to learn to recognize patients who are going to die despite aggressive medical care and guide patients and their families through the myriad medical options that exist in an attempt to balance prolongation of life with quality of life.

D. Nehra, MD
Department of Surgery, Harborview Medical Center, 325 9th Ave, Seattle, WA 98104, USA

S.P. Mandell, MD, MPH (✉)
Department of Surgery, University of Washington, Harborview Medical Center, 325 9th Ave, Seattle, WA 98104, USA
e-mail: mandells@uw.edu

B.W. Starnes et al. (eds.), *Ruptured Abdominal Aortic Aneurysm*,
DOI 10.1007/978-3-319-23844-9_19

Introduction

Medical advances and technological progress have affected the management of ruptured abdominal aortic aneurysms (rAAAs) as much as almost any other pathology. With modern skills we now rescue, resuscitate, and perform surgical procedures on patients who in the past were unsalvageable, often with excellent results. Such progress makes it even more difficult to recognize those times when our best is not good enough. It is imperative that we work with patients to identify when we are faced with a problem that medicine cannot fix. Recognizing these situations is not easy nor is it easy to translate the same tremendous energy and effort that we put into saving lives toward quality end-of-life care. This is a reality that must be confronted in the care of the critically ill patient. Regardless of whether the goal is to pursue aggressive life-sustaining care or quality end-of-life care, the basic ethical principles remain the same, as does the need for constant, effective, and clear communication between the interdisciplinary medical team and the patient and his or her family.

In this chapter, we will explore ethical issues that will likely arise in the care of a critically ill patient with a ruptured AAA. We will discuss some of the most basic ethical principles that should be at the core of all medical care. In the intensive care unit, the patient in question is oftentimes unable to make decisions, meaning a family member or surrogate must make critical life-and-death decisions. With this come a host of ethical issues and challenges that we will also discuss. We will then provide some evidence-based strategies for most effectively communicating with critically ill patients and their families followed by a discussion of the role of palliative care and issues specific to end-of-life care.

Body

Basic Ethical Principles

Despite the tremendous changes that have and will continue to occur in the field of medicine, the basic ethical principles that are at the heart of medicine have not changed since they were first described in the Hippocratic oath in the late fifth century BCE. These fundamental ethical principles that should govern all medical care are (1) beneficence, or the physician's obligation to do good for patients; (2) nonmaleficence, or the duty to avoid harm; (3) autonomy, or respect for a patient's right to self-determination; and (4) justice, or the fair allocation of healthcare resources. These very principles form the basis of the physician-patient relationship, and it is the duty of the physician to keep these basic principles at the center of all medical decisions that are made to ensure that they are always acting in the best interest of the patient.

Decision-Making

In modern medicine, especially in the Western world, we have embraced the concept of shared decision-making, or a collaborative process by which patients and their providers make healthcare decisions together. Ideally this is done by taking into account the best scientific evidence available in context with the patient's values and beliefs. This concept can quickly become problematic in the intensive care unit where patients are often unable to participate in discussions about their care. In some instances, a patient's wishes regarding care in the case of his or her incapacity may be known in advance; however, in many instances they are not.

The process by which patients can, with or without the help of their families and healthcare providers, plan for future medical care is known as *advance care planning* [1]. The results of these deliberations are known as *advance* directives, a very broad term that refers to any verbal or written, formal or informal, instructions to healthcare providers, family members, or others involved in a patient's care regarding treatment that may be required while the patient is unable to participate in medical decision-making [2]. Unfortunately, these advance directives are rarely specific enough to provide meaningful guidance regarding day-to-day care in the ICU [3], and as such, physicians most often rely on surrogate decision-makers for patients who are unable to make decisions for themselves.

The determination of the most appropriate surrogate decision-maker can be complex. A patient can complete a legal document that gives statutory authority to an individual to make medical decisions for a patient in case of incapacity, a document referred to as a *durable power of attorney for health care.* If the patient has assigned a *durable power of attorney for health care*, the decision with regard to who the legal surrogate decision-maker should be becomes easy. However, it does not mean that the identified individual is prepared for or desires the role. Not surprisingly, most patients have not completed a form legally making someone their surrogate decision-maker in the event of incapacity. In many cultures, in these instances, we turn to a designated hierarchy of surrogates determined by law. A typical sequence might be: (1) spouse, (2) eldest child, (3) next eldest child, (4) parent, and (5) sibling. In addition to such legal standing however, it is important to consider the person's moral standing to act as a surrogate decision-maker. Additionally, regardless of documentation that exists or family members that are present, it is prudent, if the opportunity exists, to ask any patient who may become incapable of making medical decisions for themselves who they would like to appoint as their surrogate decision-maker.

Code status is a more limited form of an advance directive that should be sought on admission to the hospital and certainly on admission to the intensive care unit. This is an advance directive that specifically addresses a patient's (or surrogate's) preferences regarding cardiopulmonary resuscitation and other measures in the event of a cardiopulmonary arrest. Patients and family members often link limitation in code status to less aggressive care overall. It is imperative when having these discussions that code status be completely disentangled from the aggressiveness of disease-oriented care.

In order to respect a patient's autonomy, all decision-making, even that which occurs via a surrogate, must involve an *informed consent*. The basic tenants of informed decision-making are (1) the patient or surrogate must be competent, meaning they must be capable of understanding and manipulating the relevant information in order to formulate and communicate a choice; (2) the patient or surrogate must have enough information in order to be able to make an informed decision about their medical care; and (3) the decision by the patient or surrogate must be voluntary and free of coercion.

Making critical and often life-or-death decisions in the intensive care unit on behalf of a loved one is never easy and can easily be overwhelming for a surrogate decision-maker. It is important to remember, and to remind family members, that the surrogate is not necessarily being asked to independently make medical decisions for the patient but rather that this is a shared responsibility by the patient's surrogate and other people close to the patient with input from the care team as to the best course of therapy. Most surrogate decision-makers really prefer such a shared decision-making approach, and there is consensus among multiple critical care societies in Europe and North America that the shared decision-making model should be the default in the intensive care unit setting [4, 5]. However, there is considerable heterogeneity among patients and families regarding their desired role in decision-making, and one must be able to individualize one's approach in order to best meet the needs of the individual patient and family.

Effective Communication with Families of Critically Ill Patients

There is no substitute for timely, clear, compassionate, and ongoing communication between clinicians, nurses, and family members of critically ill patients. A focus on communication with the families of *all* critically ill patients is important, not just those expected to die. Not surprisingly, surrogate decision-makers report improved satisfaction when physicians are accessible and when they are comprehensive in their communication [6], and there is a higher risk of posttraumatic stress disorder among family members who feel that communication in the intensive care unit is inadequate [7].

Family conferences play a key role in the care of the critically ill patient. These are seminal events for family members and surrogate decision-makers who sometimes feel ill equipped to make decisions on behalf of their loved one. This type of meeting, when done well, with skilled communication by an interdisciplinary ICU team, has the potential to improve outcomes for both patients and family members [8]. There are some core, teachable, evidence-based communication skills that are vital in leading an effective family conference. In this section, we will highlight some of these skills while providing a basic framework for leading an effective family meeting.

Timing of family conferences should be determined on an individual basis taking into consideration the clinical situation and the specific needs of the family. It should, however, be noted that studies suggest that family conferences early in the intensive care unit stay are beneficial, with both decreased use of critical care resources among patients who die and higher quality of death and dying reported by family members when family conferences are held within 72 h of ICU admission [9, 10]. One of the very important tenants of a good family meeting is consistent communication among different members of the medical team, and as such, having a "preconference" immediately prior to a scheduled family meeting can be invaluable [11]. Having a dedicated room for a family conference has also been associated with decreased anxiety among family members and whenever possible should be arranged [12].

The crux of leading an effective family conference, however, is really taking the time to listen to the family while communicating with them in an empathic fashion. Most physicians spend the majority of time when meeting with patients and families talking rather than listening. Families have been shown to have a higher level of satisfaction with lower levels of perceived conflict with clinicians who speak less and listen more [8, 13]. When having a family meeting, it is imperative for the clinician to really focus on listening to the patient and family. Expressions of empathy while relating medical information are important but should not predominate or interrupt family members.

There is an approach called the "Ask-Tell-Ask" approach that can be a helpful tool to assess baseline understanding and evaluate understanding of the information provided [14]. This consists of first "asking" the patient or surrogate to describe his/her understanding of their medical disease and prognosis followed by "telling" the patient or surrogate what you understand about their medical disease and prognosis and then "asking" the patient or surrogate to explain things in their own words in order to allow for an assessment of their understanding.

Once you have gained an appreciation for the family's level of understanding and have had a chance to provide a medical update, a useful tool in enhancing clinician-family communication that has been shown to improve mental health outcomes of family members is the VALUE tool [15]. This is a mnemonic that features five key components to an effective family meeting that stands for: value family statements, acknowledge family emotions, listen to the family, understand the patient as a person, and elicit family questions.

One of the hardest things for physicians to discuss at family meetings is prognosis, which is at least in part a result of the uncertainty often involved in trying to accurately prognosticate. It is worth noting that this uncertainty is not lost on family members and surrogates who report that they understand and appreciate explanations of the uncertainty involved in prognostication [16]. When it comes to prognosis, physicians in the ICU are more likely to discuss functional prognosis rather than the likelihood of survival in general, and it is important to recognize that both types of prognostication are of critical importance to the surrogate decision-maker. When discussing prognosis, experts recommend framing prognosis numerically rather than in nonspecific terms (i.e., "1 in every 100 patients" rather than "rare"), framing prognosis both positively and negatively, and using consistent denominators when presenting rates of risk [17]. Avoiding mixed messages that exacerbate this feeling of uncertainty is also critical. The ICU team should ensure that surgical and consultant services are involved with the planning and, if possible, the conduct of meetings. If multiple teams are present, a huddle should be held prior to meeting with the family so that care providers have a common plan.

Whether or not a specific tool is used, the goal during every family meeting should really be to take a step back to try to listen to the family in order to appreciate their understanding of the situation while also taking the time to listen to them talk about their loved one as a person in order to better guide them through the difficult decisions that often need to be made for critically ill patients.

The Role of Palliative Care

Palliative care is an interdisciplinary medical specialty that focuses on preventing and relieving suffering as well as supporting the best possible quality of life for patients and families facing serious illness. Patients and medical providers alike often equate palliative care with hospice, and while all care that is delivered by hospice can be considered palliative care, not all palliative care delivered is hospice. Palliative care services may be offered to patients and families dealing with critical illness at any time, and palliative care is actually often optimally provided together with life-prolonging care. This coordinated approach that has been supported by major societies representing critical care professions [4, 18] is a practice that is embraced by patients and families [19]. Therefore, palliative care should not be seen as a sequel to failed attempts at life-prolonging care, but rather as an integral component of the care provided to patients with critical or life-threatening illness.

The primary tenets of palliative care are several-fold and include: (1) symptom management; (2) elucidation of the patient's goals of care that are in keeping with their personal values and preferences; (3) consistent and sustained communication between the patient and those involved in his or her care; (4) psychosocial, spiritual, and practical support for patients and their families; and (5) coordination across sites of care.

Despite data that access to palliative care services enhances quality of care in the intensive care unit [20], palliative care services continue to be underutilized in the intensive care unit setting. Potential barriers or explanations include: a lack of awareness by clinicians regarding the availability and benefits of this service, a misconception that palliative care is only for patients who are actively dying, and a limited availability of palliative care services. Although these and other barriers can prevent the effective incorporation of palliative care into the care of critically ill patients in general, the surgical patient can pose a unique set of challenges. Surgeons often feel a strong sense of personal responsibility for patient outcomes [21–23], and the surgeon can feel at odds with the intensivists and nurses with respect to appropriate goals of postoperative care [24]. Given these challenges, it becomes even more important that in these situations all healthcare providers communicate effectively among one another and openly discuss the potential benefits of palliative care interventions prior to engaging this service.

Published guidelines attempt to identify patients and families that may benefit from a palliative care consultation. According to these guidelines, a palliative care consultation may be considered for any patient who has a chronic critical illness, an indication for specific medical procedures, is >80 years old, has significant medical comorbidities or poor baseline functional status, has a chronic or life-limiting illness, and has specific acute illnesses with a poor prognosis or an overall poor prognosis as determined by an attending physician [25–27].

There are many different ways of incorporating palliative care services in the care of the surgical patient and in the intensive care unit, and the optimal method of doing this has not yet been established. It is thus each clinician's responsibility to determine the best way of incorporating this service into the care of their patients within their practice setting.

End-of-Life Issues

The remarkable changes in medicine and technology over the last century brought notable change in the process of dying. We are now able to keep patients alive despite multi-system organ failure and with this ability come a whole host of complex medical and ethical issues. More than 75 % of Americans now die in healthcare facilities, although one might find that the vast majority say that they would prefer to die in their homes [28, 29]. Perhaps even more notable is the fact that about 20 % of Americans will die in an intensive care unit [30]. A tremendous amount of healthcare dollars are being spent on delivering medical care to dying patients [31].

A seminal study published in 1995 looked for the first time at how seriously ill people in the United States die. The investigators looked at multiple aspects of end-of-life care and found that only 47 % of the time did the physician even know when a patient wanted to avoid cardiopulmonary resuscitation and that 50 % of patients were dying with moderate to severe pain [32]. Subsequent studies focusing on the dying experience in intensive care units found that the vast majority of deaths in the intensive care unit occur only after a decision to limit life support has been made [33, 34].

Intensive care units today have, in some ways, expanded into facilities that care for chronically, seriously, ill people and often become repositories for patients who have little or no chance for survival. Healthcare providers can get caught up in the day-to-day care of these patients and may forget to take a step back to make well-considered decisions regarding the end of human life. When asked, most patients want to die at home, but logistical and medical issues in critically ill patients may preclude this from happening. More often, we fail to ask the question when it matters most. It is critical that when caring for patients in the intensive care unit who are dying, we focus on, acknowledge, and address important end-of-life issues.

Evidence strongly suggests that patients and families are unhappy with the care they receive once a decision has been made to limit or withdraw life support [32] and furthermore that we do a poor job of providing comfort care during the dying process [35].

Since many of the deaths in the ICU and hospital are preceded by a decision to withhold or withdraw life support, high-quality decision-making and end-of-life care are essential and can improve patient and family outcomes. The elements required to make such decisions include adequate training, good communication between the clinician and the patient or family, and the collaboration of a well-functioning interdisciplinary team. In this new era, it is our duty as physicians to learn to recognize patients who are dying despite aggressive medical care and guide patients and their families through the myriad of medical options that exist in an effort to balance duration of life with quality of life.

Conclusion

The ethical care of a patient with a ruptured AAA, or any other critical illness, should be founded on the very same four basic principles common to all disciplines of medicine, namely, beneficence, nonmaleficence, autonomy, and justice. The provision of ethical and high-quality critical care for patients with a ruptured AAA requires training and emphasis on ethical decision-making and communication, collaboration among an interdisciplinary team, effective communication with patients and their families, and identification and resolution of conflict within the team and with patients and their families.

References

1. Emanuel LL, von Gunten CF, Ferris FD. Advance care planning. Arch Fam Med. 2000;9(10): 1181–7.
2. Teno JM, Lynn J. Putting advance-care planning into action. J Clin Ethics. 1996;7(3):205–13.
3. Tonelli MR. Pulling the plug on living wills. A critical analysis of advance directives. Chest. 1996;110(3):816–22.
4. Carlet J, Thijs LG, Antonelli M, et al. Challenges in end-of-life care in the ICU. Statement of the 5th International Consensus Conference in Critical Care: Brussels, Belgium, April 2003. Intensive Care Med. 2004;30(5):770–84.
5. Davidson JE, Powers K, Hedayat KM, et al. Clinical practice guidelines for support of the family in the patient-centered intensive care unit: American College of Critical Care Medicine Task Force 2004–2005. Crit Care Med. 2007;35(2):605–22.
6. Fumis RR, Nishimoto IN, Deheinzelin D. Families' interactions with physicians in the intensive care unit: the impact on family's satisfaction. J Crit Care. 2008;23(3):281–6.
7. Azoulay E, Pochard F, Kentish-Barnes N, et al. Risk of post-traumatic stress symptoms in family members of intensive care unit patients. Am J Respir Crit Care Med. 2005;171(9):987–94.
8. Lautrette A, Darmon M, Megarbane B, et al. A communication strategy and brochure for relatives of patients dying in the ICU. N Engl J Med. 2007;356(5):469–78.

9. Glavan BJ, Engelberg RA, Downey L, Curtis JR. Using the medical record to evaluate the quality of end-of-life care in the intensive care unit. Crit Care Med. 2008;36(4):1138–46.
10. Lilly CM, De Meo DL, Sonna LA, et al. An intensive communication intervention for the critically ill. Am J Med. 2000;109(6):469–75.
11. Curtis JR, Rubenfeld GD. Improving palliative care for patients in the intensive care unit. J Palliat Med. 2005;8(4):840–54.
12. Pochard F, Azoulay E, Chevret S, et al. Symptoms of anxiety and depression in family members of intensive care unit patients: ethical hypothesis regarding decision-making capacity. Crit Care Med. 2001;29(10):1893–7.
13. McDonagh JR, Elliott TB, Engelberg RA, et al. Family satisfaction with family conferences about end-of-life care in the intensive care unit: increased proportion of family speech is associated with increased satisfaction. Crit Care Med. 2004;32(7):1484–8.
14. Back AL, Arnold RM, Baile WF, Tulsky JA, Fryer-Edwards K. Approaching difficult communication tasks in oncology. CA Cancer J Clin. 2005;55(3):164–77.
15. Cook DJ, Guyatt GH, Jaeschke R, et al. Determinants in Canadian health care workers of the decision to withdraw life support from the critically ill. Canadian Critical Care Trials Group. JAMA. 1995;273(9):703–8.
16. Evans LR, Boyd EA, Malvar G, et al. Surrogate decision-makers' perspectives on discussing prognosis in the face of uncertainty. Am J Respir Crit Care Med. 2009;179(1):48–53.
17. Paling J. Strategies to help patients understand risks. BMJ. 2003;327(7417):745–8.
18. Truog RD, Campbell ML, Curtis JR, et al. Recommendations for end-of-life care in the intensive care unit: a consensus statement by the American College [corrected] of Critical Care Medicine. Crit Care Med. 2008;36(3):953–63.
19. Nelson JE, Puntillo KA, Pronovost PJ, et al. In their own words: patients and families define high-quality palliative care in the intensive care unit. Crit Care Med. 2010;38(3):808–18.
20. Scheunemann LP, McDevitt M, Carson SS, Hanson LC. Randomized, controlled trials of interventions to improve communication in intensive care: a systematic review. Chest. 2011;139(3):543–54.
21. Cassell J, Buchman TG, Streat S, Stewart RM. Surgeons, intensivists, and the covenant of care: administrative models and values affecting care at the end of life--Updated. Crit Care Med. 2003;31(5):1551–7; discussion 1557–1559.
22. Buchman TG, Cassell J, Ray SE, Wax ML. Who should manage the dying patient?: rescue, shame, and the surgical ICU dilemma. J Am Coll Surg. 2002;194(5):665–73.
23. Schwarze ML, Bradley CT, Brasel KJ. Surgical "buy-in": the contractual relationship between surgeons and patients that influences decisions regarding life-supporting therapy. Crit Care Med. 2010;38(3):843–8.
24. Paul Olson TJ, Brasel KJ, Redmann AJ, Alexander GC, Schwarze ML. Surgeon-reported conflict with intensivists about postoperative goals of care. JAMA Surg. 2013;148(1):29–35.
25. Norton SA, Hogan LA, Holloway RG, Temkin-Greener H, Buckley MJ, Quill TE. Proactive palliative care in the medical intensive care unit: effects on length of stay for selected high-risk patients. Crit Care Med. 2007;35(6):1530–5.
26. Mosenthal AC, Weissman DE, Curtis JR, et al. Integrating palliative care in the surgical and trauma intensive care unit: a report from the Improving Palliative Care in the Intensive Care Unit (IPAL-ICU) Project Advisory Board and the Center to Advance Palliative Care. Crit Care Med. 2012;40(4):1199–206.
27. Nelson JE, Curtis JR, Mulkerin C, et al. Choosing and using screening criteria for palliative care consultation in the ICU: a report from the Improving Palliative Care in the ICU (IPAL-ICU) Advisory Board. Crit Care Med. 2013;41(10):2318–27.
28. Higginson IJ, Sen-Gupta GJ. Place of care in advanced cancer: a qualitative systematic literature review of patient preferences. J Palliat Med. 2000;3(3):287–300.
29. Wilson DM, Cohen J, Deliens L, Hewitt JA, Houttekier D. The preferred place of last days: results of a representative population-based public survey. J Palliat Med. 2013;16(5):502–8.
30. Angus DC, Barnato AE, Linde-Zwirble WT, et al. Use of intensive care at the end of life in the United States: an epidemiologic study. Crit Care Med. 2004;32(3):638–43.

31. Cher DJ, Lenert LA. Method of medicare reimbursement and the rate of potentially ineffective care of critically ill patients. JAMA. 1997;278(12):1001–7.
32. A controlled trial to improve care for seriously ill hospitalized patients. The study to understand prognoses and preferences for outcomes and risks of treatments (SUPPORT). The SUPPORT Principal Investigators. JAMA. 1995;274(20):1591–1598.
33. Prendergast TJ, Claessens MT, Luce JM. A national survey of end-of-life care for critically ill patients. Am J Respir Crit Care Med. 1998;158(4):1163–7.
34. Faber-Langendoen K. A multi-institutional study of care given to patients dying in hospitals. Ethical and practice implications. Arch Intern Med. 1996;156(18):2130–6.
35. Hall RI, Rocker GM, Murray D. Simple changes can improve conduct of end-of-life care in the intensive care unit. Can J Anaesth. 2004;51(6):631–6.

Chapter 20
US Coding and Reimbursement

Sean P. Roddy

Introduction

Vascular surgical practices focus, in the treatment of ruptured abdominal aortic aneurysms (AAAs), on patient presentation, operative care, post-procedure management, and quality outcomes. Despite the importance of these issues, continuous assessment of the process by which care is rendered in order to optimize billing, coding, and ultimately reimbursement remains essential as well. The billing department in each medical practice produces an insurance claim for each medical provider by linking a diagnosis code with a procedure code and adding modifiers as needed. Typically, claims are submitted to the insurance carrier electronically. The appropriateness of this coding translates into timely reimbursement for the practice. Each time a submission is rejected for any reason, the chance of that service ever being paid to the physician decreases significantly. Therefore, the ultimate goal is to generate a claim that is without error, medically appropriate, and correctly describes the intervention. This chapter should be used only as a guideline for the physician and coder since each insurance payer has their own rules and regulations.

The resource-based relative value scale (RBRVS) was implemented by the Centers for Medicare and Medicaid Services (CMS) in 1992. This methodology relies on a basic element termed the relative value unit (RVU). The Medicare Physician Fee Schedule (MPFS) assigns a set amount of RVUs to the majority of procedure codes within the Current Procedural Terminology (CPT) manual. Each code is apportioned a specific amount of physician work, practice expense, and malpractice risk. These RVU sets are then summed and multiplied by a variable termed the "conversion factor" which is determined every year by statute (or recently

S.P. Roddy, MD
Albany Medical College/Albany Medical Center Hospital,
43 New Scotland Avenue (MC157), Albany, NY, USA
e-mail: roddys@albanyvascular.com

B.W. Starnes et al. (eds.), *Ruptured Abdominal Aortic Aneurysm*,
DOI 10.1007/978-3-319-23844-9_20

by congressional override). In 2015, the Medicare conversion factor is $35.7547 from 1 January 2015 to 31 May 2015 and $35.9335 from 1 June 2015 to 31 December 2015. Reimbursement is also tied to the cost of living in each region. The United States is broken down into districts that each has a geographic practice cost index (GPCI) which can alter payment based on the economy in the location that a medical practice serves.

Since 2004, Congress has overridden a sustainable growth rate (SGR) decrease in the conversion factor over a dozen times. In April 2015, the Medicare Access and CHIP Reauthorization Act of 2015 (MACRA, Public Law No. 114–10) legislation was passed without a "pay for" in Congress abolishing the SGR mandated changed to the conversion factor for a 10-year period. In each of the first 5 years, providers will receive a 0.5 % payment increase and 0 % update in the latter five. This must also be weighed against the cost of living which typically is estimated as a 3 % rate of inflation annually. The negative effect on each medical practice over the next 10 years is staggering.

Open Surgical Repair

The CPT manual describes open surgical repair of aneurysmal disease as "direct repair of aneurysms or excision (partial or total) and graft insertion for aneurysm, pseudoaneurysm, ruptured aneurysm, and occlusive disease." Therefore, reporting open aneurysmorrhaphy is not altered based on conduit required for the reconstruction (i.e., autogenous or prosthetic) or the presence/absence of arterial occlusive disease. The route of aortic exposure (transabdominal or retroperitoneal) also does not matter. All codes have an associated 90-day global period. Separate CPT codes exist for treatment in the setting of a ruptured abdominal aortic aneurysm (AAA). Asymptomatic or symptomatic non-ruptured aneurysms are considered identical from a billing standpoint. If the patient expires during repair of a ruptured AAA, modifier −53 (discontinued procedure) is appended to the appropriate CPT code. The insurance carrier will usually require a medical record submission to determine what fraction of the global fee should be reimbursed in such a situation.

Infrarenal AAA repair with a tube graft is reported by CPT code 35081 electively and 35082 in the setting of a ruptured AAA. Juxta- or pararenal AAA repair is describe by CPT code 35091 electively and 35092 when the aneurysm is ruptured. The official wording for these two code descriptions is "abdominal aorta involving visceral vessels (mesenteric, celiac, renal)." Combined aorta and iliac artery aneurysm repair using a bifurcated graft is illustrated in CPT code 35102 when elective and 35103 when the aneurysm has ruptured. Common or internal iliac artery aneurysm repair through an open approach as an isolated entity is reported by CPT code 35131, while treatment of the same vessels in the ruptured setting is described by CPT code 35132. If reimplantation of a visceral vessel such as the inferior mesenteric artery is required onto the aortic graft during open aortic surgery, the add-on CPT code 35697 is also reported for the additional work involved. Table 20.1 summarizes these services and their associated RVU content in 2015.

Table 20.1 CPT codes used in open infrarenal AAA repair and their total RVU content in the 2015 Medicare Physician Fee Schedule

CPT code	Total RVUs	Description
35081	51.45	Open infrarenal AAA repair with tube graft, non-ruptured
35082	64.60	Open infrarenal AAA repair with tube graft, ruptured
35091	52.84	Open juxtarenal AAA repair with tube graft, non-ruptured
35092	76.91	Open juxtarenal AAA repair with tube graft, ruptured
35102	55.70	Open infrarenal AAA repair with bifurcated graft, non-ruptured
35103	66.36	Open infrarenal AAA repair with bifurcated graft, ruptured
35131	40.92	Open iliac aneurysm repair, non-ruptured
35132	48.21	Open iliac aneurysm repair, ruptured
+35697	4.36	Reimplantation of visceral artery to infrarenal graft during open aortic surgery

Note: + listed before a CPT code denotes an add-on code

Infrarenal Endovascular Repair

Endovascular aneurysm repair (EVAR) of an infrarenal abdominal aortic aneurysm is governed by component coding which generally consists of separate CPT codes for catheter, imaging, and intervention. There are five steps to consider when reporting such a repair. These include the appropriate main body description with extensions, arterial catheter placements, open arterial exposure, radiological supervision and interpretation (S&I), and finally any separately reportable service including its associated S&I coding, if appropriate. Unlike open surgery CPT coding, ruptured and elective EVARs are reported similarly.

Endovascular therapies typically allow the provider to bill multiple CPT codes in one claim. The CPT code with the highest RVU content is paid in full. All subsequent non-radiologic codes are paid at 50 % of their independent value. This decrease is termed the "multiple procedure discount" taking into account the overlap in work before, during, and after multiple procedures done on the same date of service. Imaging codes (i.e., the radiology codes that begin with the number 7) are not subject to this discount and are paid in full. Additionally, add-on codes are exempt from this fee reduction since they are created solely for use with other codes.

Occlusive disease may limit endovascular access such that angioplasty is employed to facilitate sheath insertion in the common or external iliac arteries. Any angioplasty performed within the "treatment zone" of the graft to allow for appropriate cannulation, advancement of a sheath, and stent graft deployment is bundled. "Treatment zone" is defined simply as any area of the aorta or iliac arteries where the endoprosthesis is touching the arterial wall after deployment. However, angioplasty or endovascular stent placement in the native artery distal to the "treatment zone" may be billed to the insurance carrier.

EVAR is reported based on the main body graft configuration. The first description is an aorta-to-aorta tube stent graft (CPT code 34800). This type of graft is no longer available for implantation in the United States, and therefore, this code is rarely appropriate in current practice. The next configuration is a modular bifurcated endoprosthesis with one docking limb (CPT code 34802). Reporting this CPT code includes deployment of the ipsilateral graft, cannulation of the contralateral gate, and insertion of the contralateral stent graft docking limb. The third option is a modular bifurcated device with two docking limbs (CPT code 34803). CPT code 34803 contains the work of deploying an initial main body stent graft, cannulation of the contralateral gate, insertion of the contralateral docking limb, and insertion of the ipsilateral stent graft docking limb. In total, three pieces of prosthetic stent graft are contained within this main body description. The fourth in this series comprises the use of a bifurcated unibody graft (CPT code 34804). All manipulation to appropriately seat this single-piece device into both iliac arteries is bundled. The last description is the aorto-uni-iliac endoprosthesis (CPT code 34805). When a bifurcated graft (modular or unibody) is transformed into an aorto-uni-iliac configuration with either a formal graft converter, an aortic cuff placed proximally, or even the deployment of a second main body stent graft, the two devices are collectively reported with this single CPT code. Angioplasty to iron out folds or kinks after deployment is considered inherent to all five of these main body code descriptions.

Additional stent graft extensions both proximally in the aorta and distally after docking limb insertion in the iliac vasculature may be reported separately. Similar to bare metal stent insertion in the superficial femoral artery, they are coded per vessel treated and not per number of devices implanted. This implies a maximum of five extensions (one in the aorta proximally, one in each common iliac artery, and one in each external iliac artery). A single endoprosthesis extension that traverses two vessels is only reported once. Remember that deployment of the docking limb(s) is part of the main body coding. The first endoprosthesis is described by CPT code 34825. Each additional vessel treated by endograft extension is represented by CPT code 34826. If three or more stent graft extensions are necessary, keep in mind that subsequent submissions would require the use of a −59 modifier on the CPT code 34826 to identify that the replication of an identical code is not an accidental duplicate bill.

Next, the arterial catheter placements are considered. Most patients will have two nonselective aortic catheters (CPT code 36200 billed twice): one in each femoral artery that extends into the aorta. If selective catheterization is performed, appropriate component coding rules apply for first-, second-, or third-order selection. Percutaneous access with or without the use of a closure device is bundled and does not allow for additional reporting. However, open arterial access has separate CPT code descriptions. Usually, femoral artery exposure and simple repair are coded with 34812, but complex primary repair (35226), prosthetic patch angioplasty (35286), and common femoral endarterectomy (35371) may supersede an exposure code. CPT code 34820 denotes iliac artery exposure as necessary and 34833 conveys iliac artery exposure with the additional creation of a prosthetic graft conduit to assist in sheath insertion when small or heavily diseased external iliac arteries are encountered.

Table 20.2 CPT codes used in endovascular infrarenal AAA repair and their total RVU content in the 2015 Medicare Physician Fee Schedule

CPT code	Total RVUs	Description
34800	33.16	EVAR main body – aorto-aortic tube endoprosthesis
34802	36.67	EVAR main body – modular bifurcated endoprosthesis w/1 docking limb
34803	37.85	EVAR main body – modular bifurcated endoprosthesis w/2 docking limbs
34804	36.61	EVAR main body – bifurcated unibody endoprosthesis
34805	35.29	EVAR main body – aorto-uni-iliac endoprosthesis
34825	20.44	EVAR stent graft extension, first vessel
+34826	6.03	EVAR stent graft extension, each additional vessel
34812	9.91	Femoral artery exposure for EVAR
+34813	6.97	Cross femoral bypass at the time of EVAR
34820	14.41	Iliac artery exposure for EVAR
36200	4.46	Nonselective aortic catheterization
36245	7.36	First-order selective arterial catheterization (below diaphragm)
36246	7.83	Second-order selective arterial catheterization (below diaphragm)
75952–26	6.51	EVAR main body – radiology supervision and interpretation
75953–26	1.97	EVAR stent graft extension, radiology supervision and interpretation, each vessel

Note: + listed before a CPT code denotes an add-on code

All radiological supervision and interpretation is then summarized. CPT code 75952 is reported with main body stent graft placement, and 75953 is reported for each vessel treated with a stent graft extension (after all docking limbs are deployed). Any separately reportable services are then added such as stenting or angioplasty outside of the endograft landing zone (e.g., left renal stent placement) or embolization of arteries that do not contain an endograft (e.g., internal iliac artery or inferior mesenteric artery). Cross femoral bypass with prosthetic conduit at the time of EVAR is described by the add-on code 34813. Table 20.2 contains a listing of these CPT codes and their assigned total RVU content for 2015 by CMS.

Fenestrated Endovascular Repair

The fenestrated endovascular aortic aneurysm repair (FEVAR) category I CPT codes first published in 2014 are based on the number of fenestrations in the visceral segment and whether or not the aortic device extends into the common iliac arteries or terminates in the aorta above the aortic bifurcation. The fenestrations allow for selective catheterization of the visceral and/or renal arteries and subsequent placement of an endoprosthesis. The codes were constructed on the presence of one, two, three, or "four or more" fenestrations. Unlike EVAR, these code descriptions bundle all nonselective aortic catheterizations as well as all selective arterial catheterization that extend into the visceral and/or renal arteries that receive a stent graft, as well as all radiology supervision and interpretation for the FEVAR procedure.

CPT codes 34841–34844 report deployment of a fenestrated endoprosthesis that extends from the visceral aorta through the infrarenal aorta but does not extend into the common iliac arteries (i.e., a tube graft and not a bifurcated device). Alternatively, CPT codes 34845–34848 report deployment of a fenestrated endoprosthesis that spans from the visceral aorta through the infrarenal aorta into the common iliac arteries (i.e., a bifurcated graft). CPT codes 34845–34848 include placement of unilateral or bilateral docking limbs (depending on the device) into the iliac system similar to infrarenal EVAR. Proximal abdominal aortic stent graft extension prostheses are never separately reported with FEVAR. Any additional distal stent graft extensions that are deployed in the infrarenal aorta (when codes 34841–34844 are performed) or in the common iliac arteries (when codes 34845–34848 are performed) are bundled. However, distal stent graft extension endoprostheses that terminate in the internal iliac, external iliac, or common femoral artery may be billed by codes 34825 and 34826.

Catheterization of the hypogastric artery(ies) and/or arterial families outside the treatment zone of the graft may be reported separately as well as interventional procedures performed at the time of FEVAR outside the treatment zone (e.g., embolization of the hypogastric artery, stent placement in the distal native artery for dissection, etc.). Lastly, exposure of the access vessels (e.g., CPT code 34812), extensive repair of an artery (e.g., CPT codes 35226 and 35286), or endarterectomy (e.g., CPT code 35371) is not bundled.

After any CPT code is created, that service is then measured for appropriate relative value across the entire physician fee schedule. Care is taken to identify the work done before the procedure (preservice), during the procedure (intraservice), and after the procedure (post-service) within the assigned global period. When the eight new FEVAR codes were assessed by survey, a large quantity of preservice time was identified. This included several hours of physician time on a workstation reviewing high-resolution cross-sectional imaging, utilizing three-dimensional software for center line of flow analysis, and ordering a patient-specific endoprosthesis which was markedly longer than standard preservice values in the fee schedule. It became readily apparent during discussions of these FEVAR codes at the American Medical Association/Specialty Society Relative Value Scale Update Committee (or RUC) that the preservice work could not be adequately valued for the 2014 MPFS.

As a result, a new category I CPT code (34839) was created for 2015 which states, "Physician planning of a patient-specific fenestrated visceral aortic endograft requiring a minimum of 90 min of physician time." Similar to the radiation oncology planning codes, direct patient contact is not needed to report this service. Also, physician planning time does not need to be continuous but must be clearly documented in the patient record. CPT code 34839 is reported on the date that the planning work concludes. However, it may not be reported on the day before or the day

Table 20.3 CPT codes used in FEVAR and their total RVU content in the 2015 Medicare Physician Fee Schedule

CPT code	Total RVUs	Description
34839	N/A	FEVAR planning, 90 min minimum of physician time
34841	N/A	FEVAR (does NOT extend distally into the iliac arteries), 1 visceral artery endoprosthesis
34842	N/A	FEVAR (does NOT extend distally into the iliac arteries), 2 visceral artery endoprostheses
34843	N/A	FEVAR (does NOT extend distally into the iliac arteries), 3 visceral artery endoprostheses
34844	N/A	FEVAR (does NOT extend distally into the iliac arteries), 4+ visceral artery endoprostheses
34845	N/A	FEVAR (extends distally into the iliac arteries), 1 visceral artery endoprosthesis
34846	N/A	FEVAR (extends distally into the iliac arteries), 2 visceral artery endoprostheses
34847	N/A	FEVAR (extends distally into the iliac arteries), 3 visceral artery endoprostheses
34848	N/A	FEVAR (extends distally into the iliac arteries), 4+ visceral artery endoprostheses

Note: These 9 codes are "carrier priced" in the 2015 MPFS, so there are no specific RVU values listed

of the fenestrated endovascular repair procedure (i.e., 34841–34848). If the formal planning of a patient-specific fenestrated visceral aortic endograft concludes on the day of or on the day before the actual FEVAR deployment, no code is reported and that work is considered inherent to CPT codes 34841–34848. The code description mandates that at least 90 min of physician time be spent on the planning. If less than 90 min of physician time is documented, no code is reported and that work is also considered inherent to the FEVAR deployment. Lastly, non-physician planning time (e.g., radiologic technologists, sales representatives, etc.) may not be used in these time calculations.

Because of the above issues, CPT codes 34841–34848 were "carrier-priced" and not given standard values in the MPFS. That means each vascular surgeon must call their regional Medicare carrier medical director and/or the private carriers in his/her area and negotiate a reimbursement for each of the codes before doing the surgery. If one simply does the procedure and then submits a claim with these codes without a prior discussion with the insurance carrier (and a response in writing), the claim will most likely be denied. Formal work values for these CPT codes are expected in the MPFS by 2018. The SVS website (http://www.vascularweb.org) has downloadable template forms to assist members when contacting their insurance carriers in the meantime. Table 20.3 provides a summary of the FEVAR CPT codes and their total RVU values for 2015.

Upcoming Changes

The RUC established the "Relativity Assessment Workgroup" with the purpose of identifying potentially "misvalued" services using objective mechanisms. They screen the fee schedule focused on new technology use, changes in site of service, excessive growth, services originally surveyed/valued by one specialty that are now performed by a different specialty, "Harvard-valued" (codes never reviewed by the RUC and given a value in 1992 through the original resource-based relative value study) codes, and CPT services that may require bundling (i.e., two services reported together to CMS 75 % or more of the time). The RUC identified codes with allocated "pre-time" (i.e., time allotted to the value of the CPT code in the time before the actual skin incision) that was high. This screen identified three codes (34802, 34812, 34825) used to report endovascular repair of abdominal aortic aneurysms. The RUC referred the codes to the CPT Editorial Panel for revision. The Society for Vascular Surgery is currently working on a bundling proposal for infrarenal AAA coding with tentative implementation in 2018.

References

1. 2015 Physicians' Professional ICD-9-CM International. Classification of diseases, Vols 1 and 2. Salt Lake City: The Medical Management Institute; 2014.
2. Current procedural terminology cpt 2015. Professional ed. Chicago: American Medical Association; 2014.
3. 2015 medicare physician fee schedule final rule. Federal Register Vol. 79, No. 219. 2014. p. 67547–68092.
4. Medicare Access and CHIP Reauthorization Act of 2015 (MACRA, Public Law No. 114–10).

Chapter 21
Technique of Supraceliac Balloon Control of the Aorta During Endovascular Repair of Ruptured Abdominal Aortic Aneurysms

Todd L. Berland, Frank J. Veith, Neal S. Cayne, Manish Mehta, Dieter Mayer, and Mario Lachat

Since 1994, endovascular aneurysm repair (EVAR) has been used with increasing frequency to treat ruptured abdominal aortic aneurysms (RAAAs) [1–3]. Even though the results of prospective randomized trials comparing open vs. endovascular repair for RAAAs failed to show decreased mortality with EVAR [4, 5], these trials have flaws (see Chapter 14B) and retrospective pooled data from several centers around the world indicate that there is decreased morbidity and mortality for endovascular repair of RAAAs [6]. The technical success of the endovascular approach hinges on several key strategies, techniques, and adjuncts [2, 6]. Approximately 25 %

Based on a video presentation at the 2010 Vascular Annual Meeting of the Society for Vascular Surgery, Boston, Mass, June 10–13, 2010.
Reprint requests: Dr Frank J. Veith, New York University Medical Center, 530 First Ave, Suite 6 F, New York, NY 10016 (e-mail: fjvmd@msn.com).
The editors and reviewers of this article have no relevant financial relationships to disclose per the JVS policy that requires reviewers to decline review of any manuscript for which they may have a conflict of interest.

T.L. Berland, MD • N.S. Cayne, MD
Division of Vascular Surgery, New York University Langone Medical Center, New York, NY, USA

F.J. Veith, MD (✉)
Division of Vascular Surgery, New York University Langone Medical Center, New York, NY, USA

The Division of Vascular Surgery, The Cleveland Clinic, Cleveland, OH, USA
e-mail: fjvmd@msn.com

M. Mehta, MD
The Division of Vascular Surgery, Albany Medical Center, Albany, NY, USA

D. Mayer, MD
Hospital of Zurich, Zurich, Switzerland

M. Lachat, MD
The Division of Vascular Surgery, University Hospital of Zurich, Zurich, Switzerland

B.W. Starnes et al. (eds.), *Ruptured Abdominal Aortic Aneurysm*,
DOI 10.1007/978-3-319-23844-9_21

of patients with RAAAs experience complete circulatory collapse [6]. The survival of such patients depends on obtaining and maintaining aortic balloon control continuously until the endograft is fully deployed and the RAAA is excluded [7]. The technique for doing so is one of many important steps for achieving good results with EVAR for RAAA. This article details the steps necessary for effectively accomplishing supraceliac balloon control in this setting.

Technique

The procedure must be performed in a facility equipped for digital cine fluoroscopy and open operative procedures. Appropriately size endografts and other catheters, guidewires, and sheaths must be available. With the patient under local anesthesia, a percutaneous puncture is made in one common femoral artery, preferably the left. If the patient has no palpable pulse, ultrasound may be used to gain access. Alternatively, a small cutdown can be made to expose the anterior surface of the common femoral artery. Through this puncture, a floppy wire, such as a Bentson wire (Cook Medical, Bloomington, Ind), and a 7 F sheath are placed. An angled catheter is used to navigate the iliac arteries, and a pigtail catheter is placed above the renal arteries. A cine angiogram may be obtained if information concerning the aortic neck and iliac arteries is not available from a preoperative computed tomographic scan. A Superstiff Lunderquist (Cook Medical) wire or Meier wire (Boston Scientific, Natick, Mass) is inserted into the thoracic aorta, and both the catheter and the 7 F sheath are removed while maintaining digital control in the groin. Although controversial, to prevent thrombotic complications, we administer heparin at the time of large sheath insertion to maintain an activated clotting time >250 s. A 14 F×40-cm length sheath is then placed over the stiff guidewire to a location well above the renal arteries, and its dilator is removed. A compliant balloon, such as the Coda balloon (Cook Medical), is placed under fluoroscopic guidance through the large sheath to an appropriate level in the suprarenal aorta (usually above the celiac axis) and inflated under fluoroscopic control until the aorta is occluded. It is important to fix the sheath in position securely and to use the distal end of the sheath to support and maintain the position of the compliant balloon as the blood pressure rises (Fig. 21.1a). The sheath should be sutured to the drapes or skin of the patient, or it should be held manually because loss of sheath position will make successful balloon control and removal impossible. This is important because the balloon would otherwise migrate distally as a hypotensive patient's arterial pressure returns to normal levels. Femoral access is obtained on the contralateral side using either open or percutaneous technique. A Bentson wire, 7 F sheath, and angled catheter are used to gain catheter-guided wire access above the previously placed aortic control balloon. Slight balloon deflation may be required but usually is unnecessary with proper catheter support. A Superstiff Lunderquist wire is placed through this catheter and an angiogram performed through the large sheath supporting the balloon. After the 7 F sheath and catheter are removed, a properly sized endograft device (main body) is inserted over the Lunderquist wire. The tip of the device and its

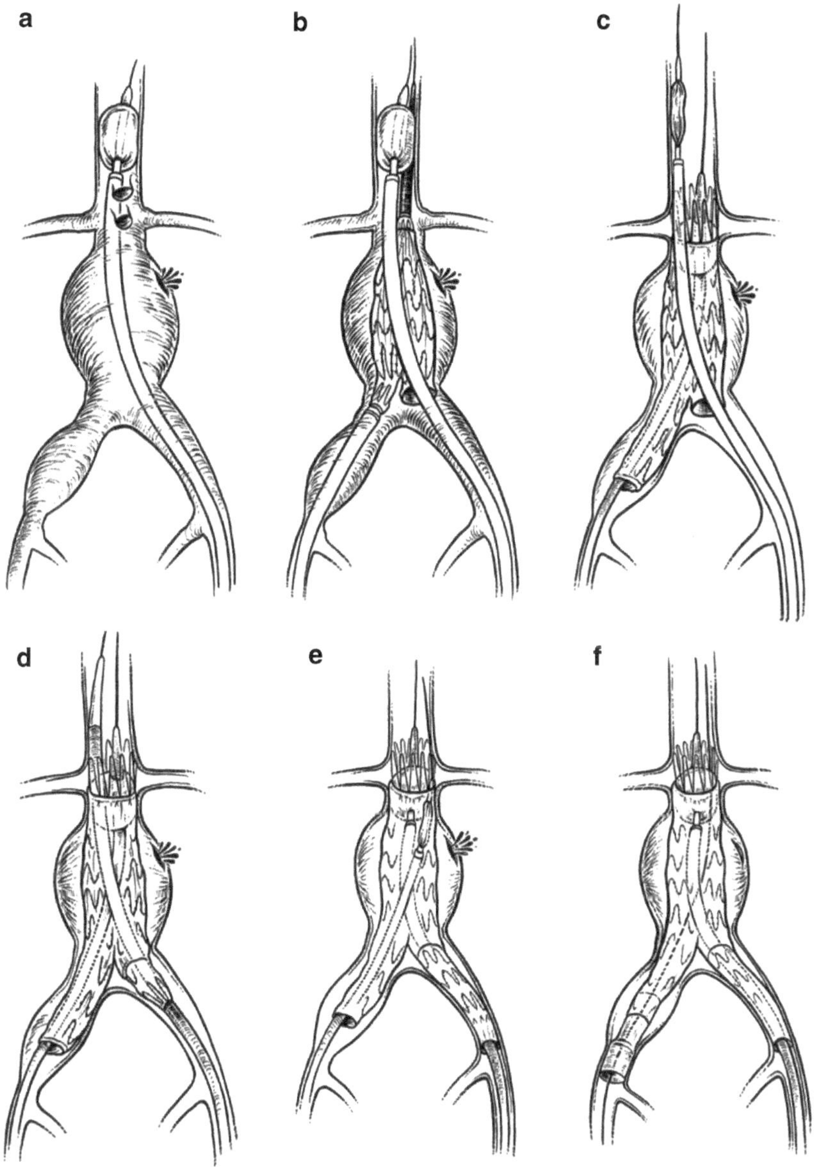

Fig. 21.1 (**a**) Supraceliac balloon control via a large contralateral sheath. (**b**) Main body of endograft is deployed via ipsilateral access. Slight temporary deflation of the balloon may be required to allow for passage of the tip of the device. (**c**) After the endograft body and ipsilateral limb are deployed, a second balloon is placed via the ipsilateral groin and inflated within the main body of the graft, maintaining continuous aortic control. (**d**) The contralateral gate is cannulated and the contralateral limb is deployed while maintaining balloon control from the ipsilateral side. (**e**) To allow for extension of the ipsilateral limb without losing aortic control, a third balloon is placed through the contralateral groin, maintaining wire access on the ipsilateral side. (**f**) With the third balloon still inflated via the contralateral groin, the ipsilateral limb is extended to allow for a distal seal. The balloon is then deflated and angiography is performed (see text for details)

sheath must pass beyond the balloon (Fig. 21.1b). This requires careful manipulation under fluoroscopic control and occasionally slight balloon deflation.

By injecting into the contralateral (side with first balloon) sheath, below the balloon, the renal arteries can be visualized and the most proximal covered portion of the endograft positioned precisely below their orifices. The ipsilateral sheath is retracted, deploying the covered portion of the main body of the endograft along with the remaining ipsilateral limb. Its delivery system is removed, leaving the wire and a large sheath in place on that (ipsilateral) side.

A second large, compliant balloon is passed over that (ipsilateral) wire into the main body of the endograft and infrarenal aneurysm neck and inflated under fluoroscopic control to occlude aortic flow. The first (supraceliac) balloon is fully deflated and removed through its large contralateral sheath (Fig. 21.1c), which had been fixed in place. At this point, the visceral and renal vessels are perfused.

The contralateral wire and sheath (which are outside the deployed endograft) are withdrawn into the aneurysm sac. The contralateral gate is cannulated, and the contralateral limb is placed as in a standard EVAR procedure for an unruptured AAA. The only difference is that the wire and tip of the deployment system for the contralateral limb must be carefully guided above the inflated second balloon in the body of the main graft using the precautions already described. Using similar techniques, any extensions needed to obtain a distal seal in the contralateral iliac system are placed (Fig. 21.1d).

If the ipsilateral iliac system has not been sealed, a third large compliant balloon must be placed in the body of the graft via the contralateral side and inflated within the graft as the second (ipsilateral) balloon is deflated and removed (Fig. 21.1e). With this third balloon maintaining aortic control, any extensions are placed on the ipsilateral side to obtain a distal seal, again taking care to pass the tip of any extension device carefully alongside the balloon without losing this control. Only when the aneurysm is fully excluded with appropriate proximal and distal seals should aortic balloon control be given up and all balloons removed (Fig. 21.1f).

Discussion

EVAR has been used increasingly to treat patients with RAAAs and offers many theoretical advantages over open repair. In addition to being less invasive, it eliminates the complications that can occur during laparotomy, minimizes hypothermia, and can be performed with the patient under local anesthesia [6, 8]. Because of these advantages, many investigators have deemed EVAR to be superior to open repair for the treatment of RAAAs [2]. Combined results from centers committed to EVAR treatment of RAAAs indicate that the 30-day mortality for EVAR is 19.7 % vs. 36.3 % for open repair [6]. With increasing enthusiasm and procedural experience, the more modern series in the literature attribute lower mortality to several key strategies, adjuncts, and technical factors [6]. These include a standardized approach, hypotensive hemostasis [6], local anesthesia [8], recognition and treatment of abdominal compartment syndrome [2], and supraceliac balloon control of the aorta [7–10]. Variations in these techniques may account for the variable results reported in the literature [6].

This article focuses on supraceliac control of the aorta and describes the transfemoral approach for balloon placement. Others performing this technique have used a transbrachial or axillary route for balloon placement. This is simpler, facilitates balloon fixation, and decreases manipulation within the aortic sac. However, it has the disadvantages of risking injury to the smaller upper extremity arteries, interfering with C-arm manipulation, and increasing stroke risk by manipulations near the aortic arch. One of the advantages of the transfemoral technique described herein is that it minimizes renal and visceral ischemia. It is generally well accepted that patients with longer ischemic times become increasingly acidotic, have a higher incidence of renal failure, and may have poorer outcomes. In addition, when done correctly, this technique provides continuous aortic control until the rupture site in the aneurysm is sealed. Many patients requiring balloon control are sufficiently ill that they cannot tolerate loss of this control with further blood loss. Use of an aorto-uni-iliac endograft may be required if bilateral groin access is impaired; it also provides rapid exclusion of the rupture site. However, we favor bifurcated endograft systems if possible because they provide more dependable pelvic and extremity revascularization, avoid use of extra-vascular prosthetic material, and prevent possible-related complications such as infection. Our technique also allows rapid balloon control until the rupture site is excluded. In RAAA cases where the anatomy may be unsuitable for endovascular repair, this technique of achieving rapid supraceliac balloon control may also be used to facilitate open repair.

We have used this technique successfully to maintain aortic control in 32 patients with RAAAs and circulatory collapse, and we believe mastery of its technical steps is crucial for obtaining good outcomes in these patients.

References

1. Marin ML, Veith FJ, Cynamon J, Sanchez LA, Lyon RT, Levine BA, et al. Initial experience with transluminally placed endovascular grafts for the treatment of complex vascular lesions. Ann Surg. 1995;222:449–65; discussion 465–9.
2. Mayer D, Pfammatter T, Rancic Z, Hechelhammer L, Wilhelm M, Veith FJ, et al. 10 years of emergency endovascular aneurysm repair for ruptured abdominal aortoiliac aneurysms: lessons learned. Ann Surg. 2009;249:510–5.
3. Yusuf SW, Whitaker SC, Chuter TA, Wenham PW, Hopkinson BR. Emergency endovascular repair of leaking aortic aneurysm. Lancet. 1994;344:1645.
4. Ruptured Aorta-Iliac Aneurysms: Endo vs. Surgery (ECAR). ClinicalTrials.gov Identifier: NCT00577616.
5. The AJAX Trial. Acute endovascular treatment to improve outcome of ruptured aorto-iliac aneurysms. Available at: http://controlled-trials.com/ISRCTN66212637/isrctn66212637.

6. Veith FJ, Lachat M, Mayer D, et al. Collected world and single center experience with endovascular treatment of ruptured abdominal aortic aneurysms. Ann Surg. 2009;250:818–24.
7. Malina M, Veith F, Ivancev K, Sonesson B. Balloon occlusion of the aorta during endovascular repair of ruptured abdominal aortic aneurysm. J Endovasc Ther. 2005;12:556–9.
8. Lachat ML, Pfammatter T, Witzke HJ, Bettex D, Künzli A, Wolfensberger U, et al. Endovascular repair with bifurcated stent-grafts under local anaesthesia to improve outcome of ruptured aortoiliac aneurysms. Eur J Vasc Endovasc Surg. 2002;23:528–36.
9. Larzon T, Lindgren R, Norgren L. Endovascular treatment of ruptured abdominal aortic aneurysms: a shift of the paradigm? J Endovasc Ther. 2005;12:548–55.
10. Veith FJ, Ohki T. Endovascular approaches to ruptured infrarenal aorto-iliac aneurysms. J Cardiovasc Surg (Torino). 2002;43:369–78.

Index

B.W. Starnes et al. (eds.), *Ruptured Abdominal Aortic Aneurysm*,
DOI 10.1007/978-3-319-23844-9

Kolibri 360 GmbH
Ferdinand-Jühlke-Straße 7
99095 Erfurt, Deutschland
produktsicherheit@kolibri360.de